Musculoskeletal MRI

PHOEBE A. KAPLAN, M.D.
Musculoskeletal Radiologist
Massachusetts General Hospital
Harvard Medical School
Boston, Massachusetts
Formerly:
University of Virginia
Charlottesville, Virginia

CLYDE A. HELMS, M.D.
Professor of Radiology
Duke University Medical Center
Durham, North Carolina

ROBERT DUSSAULT, M.D.
Musculoskeletal Radiologist
Massachusetts General Hospital
Harvard Medical School
Boston, Massachusetts
Formerly:
University of Virginia
Charlottesville, Virginia

MARK W. ANDERSON, M.D.
Associate Professor of Radiology
University of Virginia Health System
Charlottesville, Virginia

NANCY M. MAJOR, M.D.
Assistant Professor of Radiology
Division of Musculoskeletal Imaging
Duke University Medical Center
Durham, North Carolina

SAUNDERS
An Imprint of Elsevier

SAUNDERS
An Imprint of Elsevier
The Curtis Center
Independence Square West
Philadelphia, PA 19106

Library of Congress Cataloging-in-Publication Data

Musculoskeletal MRI / Phoebe A. Kaplan . . . [et al.].—1st ed.

p.   cm.

Includes bibliographical references and index.

ISBN 0–7216–9027–0

1. Musculoskeletal system—Magnetic resonance imaging.   2. Musculoskeletal
system—Diseases—Diagnosis.   I. Kaplan, Phoebe.
[DNLM: 1. Musculoskeletal Diseases—diagnosis.   2. Magnetic Resonance
Imaging.   3. Musculoskeletal system—anatomy & histology.
WE 141 M9388 2001]

RC925.7.M342 2001   616.7′07548—dc21

DNLM/DLC   00-058854

Acquisitions Editor: Lisette Bralow
Project Manager: Tina Rebane
Production Manager: Natalie Ware
Illustration Specialist: Robert Quinn
Book Designer: Matt Andrews

MUSCULOSKELETAL MRI   ISBN 0–7216–9027–0

Some illustrations from Chapter 15 are reproduced from Helms CA: Fundamentals of Skeletal
Radiology, 2nd edition. Philadelphia, W.B. Saunders, 1995.

Printed in the United States of America.

Last digit is the print number: 9   8   7   6

To each other; we make one hell of a team.

PAK and RD

To Austin Michael. Teaching you is the greatest joy in our lives.

NMM and CAH

To the residents and fellows who have made me a
better radiologist and my job worth doing.

MWA

PREFACE

Why did we write this book anyway? There are several excellent reference books already available on musculoskeletal MRI. It was our collective opinion, however, that residents in training and physicians in practice are overwhelmed at the prospects of using these in-depth textbooks when they are initially trying to figure out how to approach an MRI or even recognize that an abnormality exists. Our premise is that "less is more." We have included practical material that we believe is necessary to know in order to perform quality musculoskeletal MRI, but we have tried to keep the details down to a low roar.

Chapters include basic technical information on how to obtain a quality examination. We then discuss the normal appearance and immediately follow it by a discussion of the abnormal for each small unit that composes a joint. We have short attention spans, and this method works best for us. For example, the normal triangular fibrocartilage of the wrist is described, and this is followed by a section on abnormalities of the triangular fibrocartilage. This approach differs from many books where normal anatomy of the entire wrist is described (ligaments, bones, tendons, muscles, and so forth) and then a long section on abnormalities follows. We hope this method is helpful for others.

We have also included some basic information as to the clinical relevance of many of the MRI findings because, regardless of how much we know about the MR image, we may look like idiots to our referring physicians without this knowledge.

There are "boxes of information" throughout the chapters that summarize things that we think are important or difficult to understand or remember. These boxes are similar to information we put on slides when we give lectures, and they will hopefully allow for a quick review of pertinent material.

We hope that this book helps people to learn musculoskeletal MRI to the point that they can then enjoy using the in-depth masterpieces that already exist. . . . One must be able to walk before one can run.

CONTENTS

1 BASIC PRINCIPLES OF
    MUSCULOSKELETAL MRI 1

2 MARROW 23

3 TENDONS AND MUSCLES 55

4 PERIPHERAL NERVES 89

5 MUSCULOSKELETAL INFECTIONS 101

6 ARTHRITIS 117

7 TUMORS 125

8 OSSEOUS TRAUMA 151

9 TEMPOROMANDIBULAR JOINT 169

10 SHOULDER 175

11 ELBOW 225

12 WRIST AND HAND 247

13 SPINE 279

14 HIPS AND PELVIS 333

15 KNEE 363

16 FOOT AND ANKLE 393

    INDEX 439

1 BASIC PRINCIPLES OF MUSCULOSKELETAL MRI

WHAT MAKES A GOOD IMAGE?
Lack of Motion
Signal and Resolution
  Voxel Principle
  Slice Thickness
  Field of View
  Matrix
  Signal Acquisitions
  Gap
  Coil Selection
Tissue Contrast
  Pulse Sequences

Spin Echo
  T1
  T2
  Proton Density
Fast Spin Echo
Inversion Recovery
Gradient Echo
Fat Saturation
  Frequency Selective
  Inversion Recovery
Gadolinium
  Cystic versus Solid

Tumor
Infection
Spine
MR ARTHROGRAPHY
MUSCULOSKELETAL TISSUES
Bone
Articular Cartilage
Fibrocartilage
Tendons and Ligaments
Muscle
Synovium
APPLICATIONS

Although a detailed understanding of nuclear physics is not necessary to interpret magnetic resonance imaging (MRI) studies, it also is not acceptable to passively read whatever images you are given without concern for how the images are acquired or how they might be improved. Radiologists should have a solid understanding of the basic principles involved in acquiring excellent images. This chapter describes the various components that go into producing high-quality images, stressing the fundamental principles shared by all MRI scanners.

Unfortunately, every machine is different. Each vendor has its own language for describing its hardware, software, and scanning parameters, and an entire chapter could be devoted to deciphering the terms used by different manufacturers. Time spent learning the details of your machine with your technologists or physicists will be time well spent. And, if you are interested, by all means feel free to read one of the excellent discussions of MRI physics in other textbooks,[1–3] because, for the most part, we will leave the physics to the physicists.

WHAT MAKES A GOOD IMAGE?

Lack of Motion

Motion is one of the greatest enemies of MRI (Fig. 1–1). It can arise from a variety of sources, such as cardiac motion, bowel peristalsis, respiratory movement, and so forth. For most musculoskeletal applications, motion usually stems from body movement related to patient discomfort. Patient comfort is, therefore, of paramount importance, because even if all the other imaging parameters are optimized, any movement will ruin the entire image.

Patient comfort begins with positioning. Every effort should be made to make the patient comfortable, such as placing a pillow beneath the knees when the patient is supine to reduce the stress on the back, or providing padding at pressure points. Once the patient is in a comfortable position, passive restraints, such as tape, foam rubber, or sandbags can be used for maximal immobilization. Music via headphones can help alleviate anxiety, and oral sedation may be required for claustrophobic patients.

Another cause of patient motion is a prolonged examination, which is one reason why set imaging protocols are useful. By designing streamlined imaging sequences, the necessary scans are obtained in as short a time as possible, resulting in better patient compliance, improved technologist efficiency, and maximal scanner throughput. Standardized protocols also reduce the need for direct physician oversight during the scan and allow for improved image interpretation, because the radiologist views the same anatomy in the same imaging planes and using the same sequences each time.

Signal and Resolution (Box 1–1)

Signal is the amount of information on an image. Other factors are important, but if the image is signal-poor (ie, "noisy"), even the best radiologist will not be able to interpret it (Fig. 1–2).

Each image is composed of *voxels* (volume elements) that correspond to small portions of tissue within the patient. One dimension of the voxel is defined by the *slice thickness*. The other dimensions are determined by the *field of view* and *imaging matrix* (number of squares in the imaging grid) (Fig.

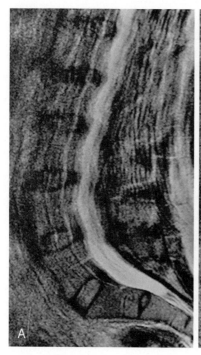
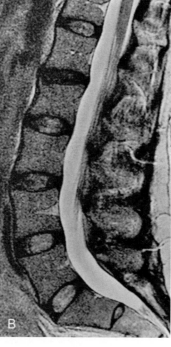

Figure 1–1. MOTION ARTIFACT.
A, Fast spin echo-T2 sagittal image, lumbar spine. The image is not diagnostic due to patient motion artifact. **B**, Fast spin echo-T2 sagittal image, lumbar spine (same patient as in *A*). Note the improved image quality in this scan, obtained after the patient was made more comfortable.

1–3). Because the signal is proportional to the number of protons resonating within each voxel, anything that increases the size of the voxel will increase the signal (Fig. 1–4). Therefore, increasing slice thickness or field of view or, alternatively, decreasing the matrix (spreading the imaging volume over fewer but larger boxes), will increase the signal.

Another factor that affects the signal is the number of *signal acquisitions* (also known as the number of *signal averages*). A signal average of 2 means that the signal arising from the protons in each voxel is collected twice, resulting in a doubling of the overall signal, but this also doubles the imaging time.

Finally, signal may be adversely affected if the slices are obtained too close together due to the phenomenon of "cross talk." When adjacent slices are acquired, some interference from one slice may spill over into the adjacent slice, resulting in increased noise. This is especially true for T2-weighted sequences. This effect is lessened by interposing a "gap" between the slices (a small portion of tissue that is not imaged), resulting in decreased noise and increased signal. Typical gaps

range from 10% to 25% of the slice thickness. Be aware that the larger the gap, the greater the amount of unimaged tissue and the greater the possibility of missing a small lesion.

Now that we have discussed several ways to improve the signal of the image (also known as increasing the signal-to-noise ratio), we need to look at the second major factor that makes for a good image: *resolution*.

Resolution is the ability to distinguish small objects. It is absolutely critical in most musculoskele-

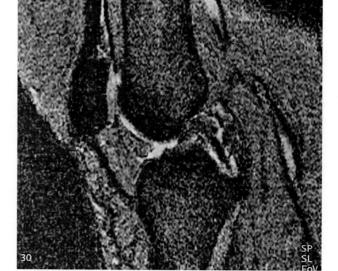

Figure 1–2. IMAGE NOISE.
T2* sagittal image, knee. The scan is of extremely poor quality due to pronounced image noise related to the use of the body coil. Because of the patient's body habitus, her knee would not fit in the standard extremity surface coil.

BOX 1–1: SIGNAL AND RESOLUTION:
Life's Trade Offs

↑ **SIGNAL/** ↓ **RESOLUTION:**	↑ **RESOLUTION/** ↓ **SIGNAL:**
↑ Slice thickness	↓ Slice thickness
↑ Field of view	↓ Field of view
↓ Imaging matrix	↑ Imaging matrix

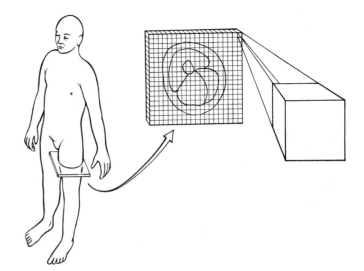

Figure 1–3. IMAGING VOXEL.
Schematic diagram illustrating the imaging matrix and an individual voxel from an axial MR image of the proximal thigh.

tal applications. As in life, there is no such thing as a free lunch in MR imaging, and any changes designed to improve resolution will negatively affect the signal. Decreasing the size of the voxel (by decreasing slice thickness, decreasing the field or view, or increasing the imaging matrix) will improve resolution but also will decrease the number of protons in each voxel and thereby decrease the signal. Consequently, when designing imaging protocols, there is always a compromise between maximizing signal and optimizing resolution. A third factor, *coil selection*, can help to minimize this trade off.

The MR image is created using the signal that returns from resonating protons within tissue. Just as it is easier to hear a speaker's voice the closer he is to you, the closer the receiver coil is to the tissues of interest, the better the signal and the lower the noise (Fig. 1–5).

In MR imaging, every attempt should be made to use the smallest coil possible to produce the maximum signal. Coils that can be placed on or close to the body part of interest are called *surface coils* and result in markedly improved signal compared to the *body coil*. One factor that must be considered when selecting a coil relates to its size. It must be able to detect signal from the entire length and depth of the tissues of interest; for a flat surface coil, the depth of penetration equals roughly half of the coil's diameter or width. Beyond this distance, the signal begins to drop off, as evidenced by decreasing signal in that region of the image (Fig. 1–6). To avoid this problem, "volume" coils often are used in the extremities. These encircle the arm or leg, thereby providing uniform signal throughout the tissues of interest. Most newer coils also are constructed with a phased array design. A phased array coil is composed of several smaller coils placed in a series, resulting in maximal signal from each small coil and from each segment of tissue covered by the coils.

The use of a surface coil usually provides more than adequate signal and allows for the use of high-resolution imaging parameters.

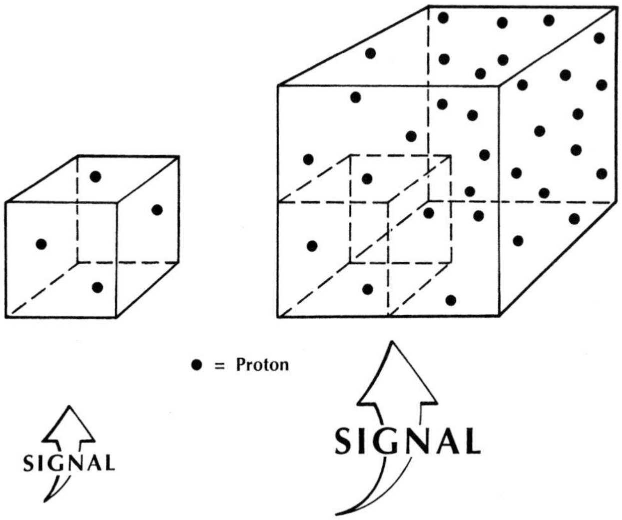

● = Proton

SIGNAL

SIGNAL

Figure 1–4. VOXEL SIZE VERSUS SIGNAL.
Signal is directly proportional to the number of protons within the voxel. Note the larger number of protons and the resulting increased signal in the larger imaging voxel.

Tissue Contrast

Both computed tomography (CT) and MRI are capable of producing high-resolution scans, but the superior soft tissue contrast of MRI (the ability to differentiate different types of tissue based on their signal intensities) sets it apart. Whereas a CT image is based on the x-ray attenuation properties of tissues, soft tissue contrast in MRI is related to differences in proton resonance within the tissues. The protons within fat resonate differently than those in fluid, and by changing the imaging parameters at the MRI console, differences in these tissue-specific properties can be emphasized. This is known as *weighting* the image. Tissues can then be differentiated based on their signal intensities on various sequences. The signal intensity of a tissue on MRI

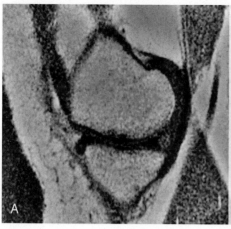 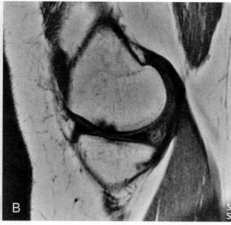

Figure 1–5. EFFECT OF SURFACE COIL.
A, T1 sagittal image, knee. Note the image noise in this scan, which was obtained with the large body coil. *B*, T1 sagittal image, knee (same patient as in *A*). A dedicated extremity coil, in closer proximity to the knee, results in better signal, less noise, and improved overall image quality.

should be described in relative terms (eg, hyperintense relative to muscle), because the gray scale values of the image are not assigned in a quantitative fashion as with CT, but are scaled relative to the brightest voxel on the image.

Pulse Sequences (Boxes 1–2 and 1–3)

The specific imaging parameters selected for a single scan are called a pulse sequence. A typical musculoskeletal examination will include three to six sequences obtained in various anatomic planes. There are many different kinds of sequences, each with its strengths and weaknesses. We do not want to get bogged down in technical details at this point but, in the following discussion, typical imaging

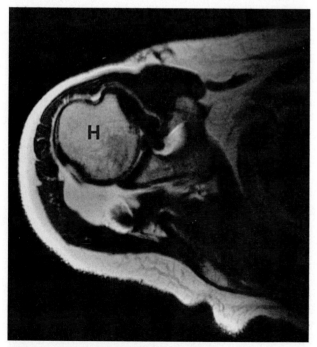

Figure 1–6. COIL SIZE AND SIGNAL DROP-OFF.
T1 axial image, shoulder after the intraarticular injection of a dilute gadolinium solution. The use of a dedicated shoulder surface coil results in excellent signal in the region of interest; however, note the relatively rapid drop-off in signal intensity in the deeper tissues of the axilla and chest wall. H—humerus.

parameters for each pulse sequence are provided in parentheses after each title. These are summarized in Box 1–3, and there is a glossary at the end of the chapter to help with understanding any unfamiliar terms.

Spin Echo. Conventional spin echo pulse sequences include T1, T2, and proton density-weighted sequences (Box 1–4).

T1 (TR <800 msec; TE <30 msec). This is considered a "short TR, short TE" sequence. Fat and subacute hemorrhage are bright on these images (Fig. 1–7). Proteinaceous fluid (as in an abscess or ganglion cyst) may be of intermediate or even high signal intensity due to the protein content. Most other soft tissues are of intermediate to low signal intensity on T1-weighted (T1W) images and fluid is especially low (hypointense relative to muscle) (Fig. 1–8). T1W images are useful for delineating anatomic planes, marrow architecture, fat content within masses, and subacute hemorrhage. T1W sequences also are used to evaluate tissue enhancement after the intravenous administration of gadolinium-DTPA (see later in this chapter).

T2 (TR >2000 msec; TE >60 msec). This is considered a "long TR, long TE" sequence. Fluid is bright on T2-weighted (T2W) images (Fig. 1–8). An easy way to remember this is that fluid (H_2O) is bright on T2W images. Likewise, most pathologic processes (eg, tumor, infection, injury) often are highlighted on T2W images due to their increased fluid content. Fat is less bright than on T1W images, and muscles remain of intermediate signal intensity. Conventional T2W spin echo sequences have been a part of most imaging protocols in the past, but now are used much less frequently because of their relatively long imaging times.

Proton Density (TR >1000 msec; TE <30 msec). This is considered an "intermediate TR, short TE" sequence. Also known as "spin density," these images represent a mixture of T1 and T2 weighting, with contrast being primarily a function of the number of protons within each tissue. This sequence also provides good anatomic detail but relatively little overall tissue contrast due to its intermediate weighting. Proton density images most often are ac-

BOX 1–2: PULSE SEQUENCES: Strengths and Weaknesses

SEQUENCE	STRENGTH	WEAKNESS
Spin Echo		
T1	- Anatomic detail - Fat, subacute hemorrhage - Meniscal pathology - Gadolinium enhancement (with fat saturation) - Marrow pathology	- Poor detection of soft tissue edema and other T2-sensitive pathology - Not as sensitive as STIR or fast spin echo-T2 with fat sat for marrow pathology
Proton Density	- Anatomic detail - Meniscal pathology	- Poor detection of fluid and marrow pathology
T2	- Detection of fluid and many pathologic processes	- Long imaging times
Fast Spin Echo		
Proton Density	- Anatomic detail	- Potential blurring artifact can lead to missing meniscal tears
T2	- T2 contrast obtained with shorter imaging times - Excellent detection of marrow pathology when combined with fat saturation - Good in patients with metal hardware ($\downarrow$ susceptibility effects)	- Poor detection of marrow pathology when not combined with fat sat
Gradient Echo		
T2*	- Ligaments - Tendons - Loose bodies and subtle hemorrhage ($\uparrow$ susceptibility effects) - 3D imaging	- Poor detection of marrow pathology at high field strengths - Metallic hardware ($\uparrow \uparrow$ artifacts due to susceptibility effects)
STIR	- Marrow and soft tissue pathology	- Should not be used with Gadolinium

BOX 1–3: PULSE SEQUENCES: Imaging Parameters (or "How to Recognize a Sequence by the Numbers")

SEQUENCE	TR (Msec)	TE (Msec)	TI (Msec)	FLIP ANGLE	ETL
T1	≤ 1000	≤ 30	N/A	90°	N/A
Proton Density	≥ 1000	≤ 30	N/A	90°	N/A
T2	≥ 2000	≥ 60	N/A	90°	N/A
FSE T2	≥ 2000	≥ 60	N/A	90°	2–16
GRE T1	variable	≤ 30	N/A	70–110°	N/A
T2*	variable	≤ 30	N/A	5–20°	N/A
FSE STIR	≥ 2000	≥ 60	120–150	180→90°	2–16

TR = Repetition Time; TE = Echo Time; TI = Inversion Time; ETL = Echo Train Length; FSE = Fast Spin Echo; GRE = Gradient Echo.

quired simultaneously with T2W images as part of a double echo sequence (Fig. 1–8).

Fast Spin Echo (FSE; also known as turbo spin echo). This technique allows for much more rapid acquisition of images than does the conventional spin echo method. This is accomplished by acquiring several samples in the time one sample is obtained with a conventional spin echo technique (Fig. 1–9). The time saved is directly proportional to the number of samples (also designated as the *echo train length*). For example, a fast spin echo sequence with an echo train length of 4 will acquire the same amount of information as a conventional spin echo sequence in one fourth the time. This provides for decreased overall imaging time, thereby

lessening the potential for patient motion. Alternatively, the time saved can be used for obtaining additional signal averages to improve signal. Therefore, fast spin echo sequences commonly are used in musculoskeletal imaging.

However, this technique has some drawbacks. First, the signal intensity of fat remains quite bright on fast spin echo-T2W images. Consequently, pathology in subcutaneous fat or marrow may be obscured on these images because of the similar signal intensity of fat and fluid (Fig. 1–10). This problem can be overcome by combining this technique with fat saturation (see later in this chapter).

Second, the fast spin echo technique can result in blurring along tissue margins, especially when proton density-weighted images are acquired using long echo train lengths (>4). Although it is tempting to use a longer echo train length to decrease imaging time, the associated increase in blurring may result in missing some types of pathology, such as meniscal tears in the knee (Fig. 1–11).

Inversion Recovery (STIR) (TR >2000 msec; TE >30 msec; TI = 120 to 150 msec). Historically known as STIR imaging, this is a fat saturation technique that results in markedly decreased signal intensity from fat and strikingly increased signal from fluid and edema (Figs. 1–11 and 1–12). As a result, it is an extremely sensitive tool for detecting most types of soft tissue and marrow pathology. We use a fast spin echo-STIR sequence with most of our musculoskeletal protocols. The fast spin echo-STIR sequence does not suffer from the long imaging times, limited number of slices, and poor signal that plagued older, conventional STIR sequences. For

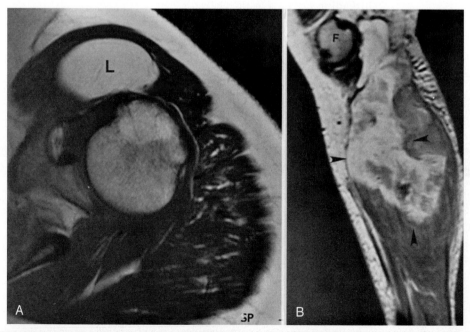

Figure 1–7. T1-WEIGHTED IMAGES: High Signal Intensity Tissues.
A, T1 axial image, left shoulder. Note the high signal–intensity subcutaneous fat and intramuscular lipoma (L) within the anterior portion of the intermediate signal deltoid muscle. *B,* T1 sagittal image, calf. There is extensive, somewhat heterogeneous, high signal intensity infiltrating the soft tissues of the proximal calf related to a subacute hematoma *(arrowheads).* F—medial femoral condyle.

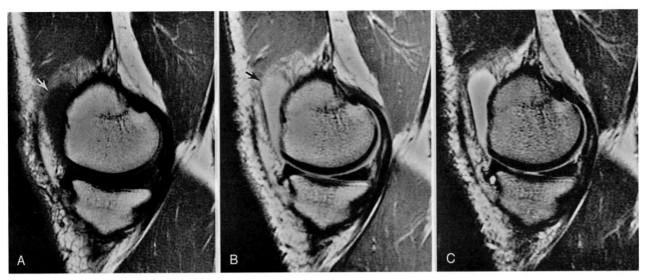

Figure 1–8. FLUID SIGNAL INTENSITY.
A, T1 sagittal image, knee. There is a small amount of fluid in the medial recess of the patellofemoral compartment *(arrow)*, displaying signal intensity lower than that of adjacent intermediate signal intensity muscle. **B**, Proton density sagittal image, knee. The fluid *(arrow)* is hyperintense to muscle. **C**, Spin echo-T2 sagittal image, knee. The signal intensity of the fluid is strikingly hyperintense to muscle and even slightly brighter than adjacent fat.

Figure 1–9. CONVENTIONAL VERSUS FAST SPIN ECHO PULSE SEQUENCES.
Diagram demonstrating the efficiency of a fast spin echo (FSE) sequence in which four echoes are obtained within a single repetition time, compared with one echo using a conventional spin echo (CSE) technique.

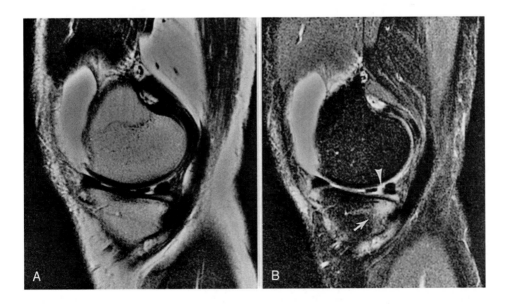

Figure 1–10. PITFALL OF FAST SPIN ECHO IMAGING.
A, Fast spin echo-T2 sagittal image, knee. There is a bone contusion of the posterior, medial tibial plateau. The contusion is difficult to detect because it does not contrast with the relatively bright marrow fat. **B**, STIR sagittal image, knee (same patient as in *A*). The contusion *(arrow)* is much more conspicuous against the dark, saturated fat. Note also the vertical tear in the posterior horn of the medial meniscus *(arrowhead)*.

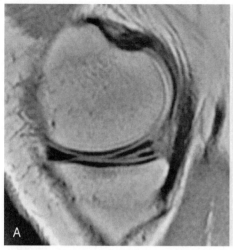
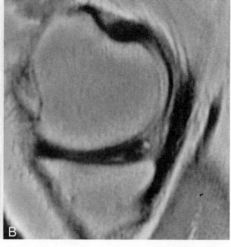

Figure 1–11. BLURRING ARTI-FACT, FAST SPIN ECHO SE-QUENCE.
A, Conventional spin echo-proton density sagittal image, knee. An oblique tear in the posterior horn of the medial meniscus is well demonstrated. B, Fast spin echo-proton density sagittal image, knee (echo train length = 16). Note the decreased conspicuity of the meniscal tear and blurring of all tissue margins.

the remainder of this book, when the term STIR is used, it refers to the fast spin echo-STIR technique, unless otherwise indicated. On a practical note, fast spin echo-STIR imaging is, in many respects, equivalent to a fast spin echo-T2W sequence with fat saturation, and many people use these sequences interchangeably.

Gradient Echo (TR variable; TE <30 msec; flip angle = 10 to 80 degrees). This family of pulse sequences was originally developed to produce T2W images in less time than was possible with a conventional spin echo technique. As their names imply, gradient echo and spin echo pulse sequences acquire images in different ways. Consequently, although fluid appears bright on both gradient echo-T2W images (designated T2*W) and spin echo-T2W images, the appearance of other tissues differs between the two. Ligaments and articular cartilage are particularly well demonstrated with gradient echo sequences, as are fibrocartilagenous structures such as the knee menisci and glenoid labrum. Contrast

between other soft tissues, however, is relatively poor on gradient echo images.

Gradient echo imaging can be performed using a two-dimensional technique (in which slices are obtained individually) or with a three-dimensional (3D) "volume" technique. In 3D imaging, the signal from an entire volume of tissue is obtained at one time, and these data can then be partitioned into extremely thin (less than 1 mm) slices such that the voxel dimensions are nearly isotropic (equal in all dimensions) (Fig. 1–13). This allows for high-resolution imaging and is especially useful when evaluating extremely small structures, such as ligaments in the wrist. These 3D sequences also provide the ability to create reformatted images in virtually any plane without a significant loss of resolution (Fig. 1–14). Although most 3D sequences require relatively lengthy imaging times, if the reformatted images are of adequate quality, other sequences may be omitted from the protocol, thereby minimizing this effect.

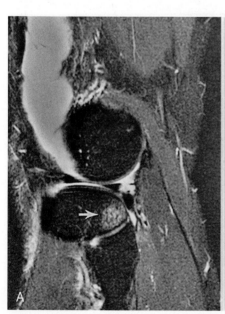
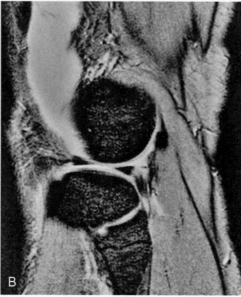

Figure 1–12. STIR VERSUS GRADIENT ECHO SEQUENCES FOR MARROW PATHOLOGY.
A, STIR sagittal image, knee. There is a focal contusion in the posterior lateral tibial plateau (arrow). Note the conspicuity of the contusion relative to the dark, suppressed marrow fat. B, Gradient echo-T2* sagittal image, knee. The contusion is not visible due to susceptibility effects of the trabecular bone in the tibial plateau.

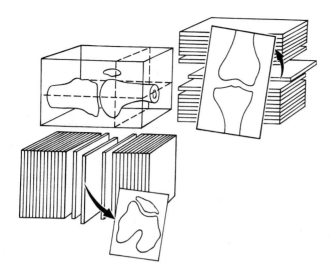

Figure 1–13. THREE-DIMENSIONAL IMAGING.
Diagram demonstrating axial and coronal reconstructions from a single acquisition 3D volume sequence.

One feature of gradient echo sequences is a heightened sensitivity to *susceptibility effects*. This refers to artifactual signal loss at the interface between tissues of widely different magnetic properties, such as metal and soft tissue. This can be advantageous when searching for subtle areas of hemorrhage, because these will be highlighted on gradient echo images due to susceptibility effects of the hemoglobin breakdown products within the tissue (Fig. 1–15). Similarly, these sequences are useful for detecting loose bodies and soft tissue gas, again because of susceptibility effects.

Conversely, drawbacks of these susceptibility effects include overestimating the size of osteophytes in spine imaging and missing marrow pathology, when trabecular bone is not destroyed, because of susceptibility artifact at the interfaces between trabecular bone and marrow fat (see Fig. 1–12). They also can be problematic when imaging patients with metallic hardware due to the obscuring of adjacent normal tissue by the susceptibility artifacts. Fast spin echo sequences tend to minimize susceptibility artifacts and therefore are useful when imaging patients with a history of prior surgery, especially if it is known that metallic hardware is present (Fig. 1–16).

Fat Saturation

There are certain clinical situations in which it is advantageous to suppress the high signal intensity of fat. Two main techniques are used to accomplish this: frequency-selective (chemical) fat saturation and STIR imaging.

Frequency-selective. This technique exploits the differences in resonant frequencies between fat and water by applying a "spoiler" pulse at the frequency of fat. This wipes out the signal from fat without affecting the signal from water. Likewise, the signal from gadolinium (either intravenous or intraarticular) is preserved.

This technique can be used with T1W imaging to confirm the fatty nature of a mass (Fig. 1–17), to distinguish between fat and hemorrhage (both of which will be bright on non–fat-saturated T1W images), and to make tissue enhancement more conspicuous after the intravenous administration of gadolinium contrast material (Fig. 1–18). Fat-saturated T1W images also are used with gadolinium arthrography.

Fast spin echo-T2W imaging often is combined with frequency-selective fat saturation to highlight areas of soft tissue and marrow pathology, because the high signal intensity of fluid and edema is extremely conspicuous against the dark background of suppressed fat.

A major problem with frequency-selective fat saturation is the potential for inhomogeneous suppression of fat signal. Because the technique is sensitive to magnetic field inhomogeneities and susceptibility

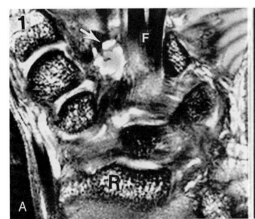
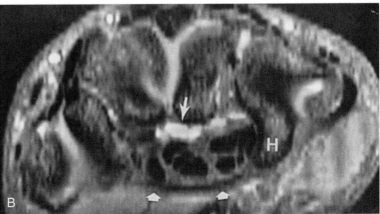

Figure 1–14. THREE-DIMENSIONAL VOLUME IMAGING.
A, T2*-gradient echo coronal image, wrist. This 1.5-mm-thick section through the volar extrinsic ligaments of the wrist demonstrates a small multilocular ganglion cyst *(arrow)* adjacent to the flexor tendons (F) within the carpal tunnel. R—distal radius; 1—first metacarpal. *B*, Axial reformatted image from data set acquired in *A* demonstrates the ganglion cyst *(arrow)*, flexor tendons, and overlying flexor retinaculum *(small arrows)* attaching to the hook of the hamate (H).

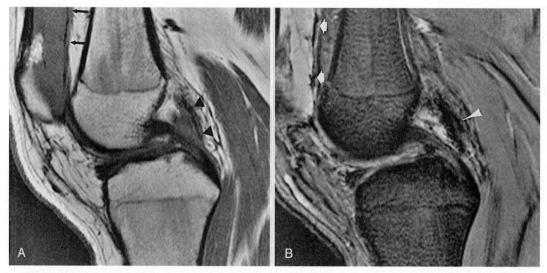

Figure 1–15. GRADIENT ECHO IMAGING: Improved detection of hemorrhage.
A, T1 sagittal image, knee. There is a large joint effusion in the suprapatellar bursa *(arrows)*, as well as a small focus of low signal–intensity hemorrhage in the posterior joint *(arrowheads)*. *B*, T2*-gradient echo sagittal image, knee. Note the increased conspicuity of the hemorrhage in the posterior joint *(arrowhead)* caused by the "blooming" artifact, which is related to susceptibility effects of the hemoglobin breakdown products. Other areas of hemorrhage are also evident in the suprapatellar bursa *(small arrows)*.

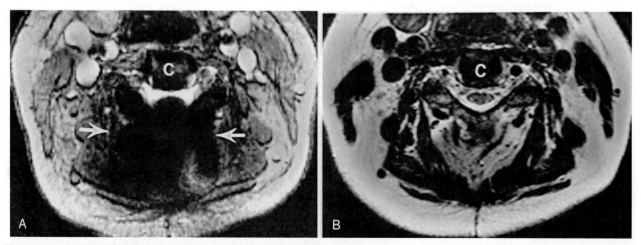

Figure 1–16. FAST SPIN ECHO IMAGING: Decreased susceptibility artifacts.
A, T2*-gradient echo axial image, cervical spine. There is a large area of susceptibility artifact in the posterior cervical spine *(arrows)* related to fixation hardware. This obscures adjacent structures, including portions of the spinal canal and cord. *B*, Fast spin echo-T2 axial image, cervical spine (same level as in *A*). Note the decreased artifact related to the metal hardware and improved depiction of the spinal canal and contents. C—cervical vertebral body.

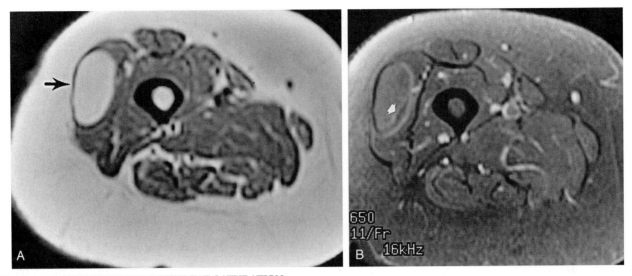

Figure 1–17. FREQUENCY-SELECTIVE FAT SATURATION.
A, T1 axial image, thigh. There is an ovoid intramuscular lipoma *(arrow)* in the vastus lateralis muscle. *B,* Fast spin echo-T2W axial image, thigh with fat suppression. There is complete suppression of the signal arising from this mass, with the exception of a thin intralesional septum *(small arrow),* confirming its lipomatous nature.

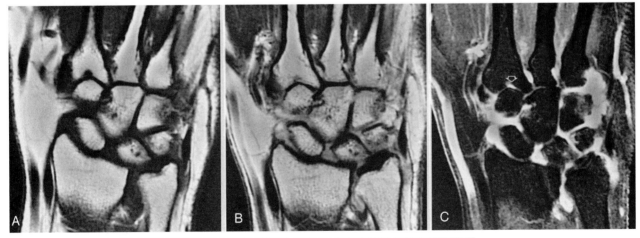

Figure 1–18. FREQUENCY-SELECTIVE FAT SATURATION AND GADOLINIUM ENHANCEMENT.
A, T1 coronal image, wrist. It is impossible to differentiate hypertrophied synovium from joint fluid in this patient with rheumatoid arthritis. *B,* T1 coronal image, wrist, with intravenous contrast. Note the diffuse enhancement of the hypertrophied synovium between the carpal bones. No joint fluid is evident. *C,* T1 coronal image, wrist, with intravenous contrast and fat suppression. There is strikingly increased conspicuity of the enhancing synovial pannus when the fat is suppressed. Note also the multiple erosions in the carpal bones and at the base of the second metacarpal *(open arrow).*

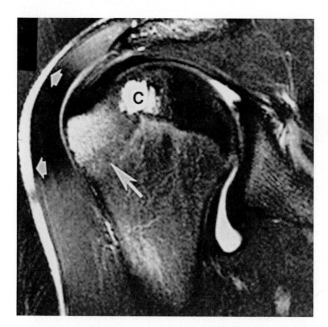

Figure 1–19. PITFALL: Heterogeneous fat saturation.
Fast spin echo-T2 coronal image, right shoulder (MR arthrogram). High signal intensity within the greater tuberosity of the humerus *(arrow)* mimics a focal contusion. However, note the lack of adequate suppression of the overlying subcutaneous fat *(short arrows)*, a clue that the humeral signal intensity is related to nonsuppressed fat. Note the true cyst (C) in the central humeral head is surrounded by a rim of better suppressed, low signal fat.

effects, the fat saturation may be incomplete across an imaging volume. This may even result in inadvertent suppression of water signal in these areas. This is especially common along curved surfaces, such as the shoulder and ankle, and may result in spurious signal intensity that mimics pathology (Fig. 1–19). This often can be identified by noticing the lack of suppression of the overlying subcutaneous fat signal in these regions, but it can be difficult to recognize and may result in diagnostic errors.

Frequency-selective fat saturation relies on adequate separation of the fat and water peaks, which occurs only at high field strengths (greater than or equal to 1.0 Tesla). Consequently, another drawback of this technique is that it is not available on mid- and low field strength machines.

STIR. The STIR technique also results in fat saturation, but it is based on the relaxation properties of fat protons rather than their resonant frequency, as is the case with frequency-selective fat saturation. Many people use a fast spin echo-T2W sequence with fat saturation rather than STIR imaging, and although these appear very similar in terms of image contrast, there are some differences, because the two techniques are based on different mechanisms. The STIR technique tends to produce more homogeneous fat suppression, because it is not as sensitive to field inhomogeneity as the frequency-selective technique. Secondly, a STIR sequence should not be used with intravenous or intraarticular gadolinium because the contrast agent has similar relaxation properties to fat protons and therefore its signal intensity will be saturated along with fat on the STIR images.

Gadolinium (Box 1–5)

This brings us to the question of when gadolinium is useful in musculoskeletal MR imaging. Gadolin-

ium-DTPA (Gd-DTPA) is a paramagnetic compound that demonstrates increased signal intensity on T1W images. It has two major routes of administration: intravenous and intraarticular. Its intraarticular use in MR arthrography is discussed in the next section.

When administered intravenously, Gd-DTPA is analogous to iodinated radiographic contrast agents and results in enhancement proportional to soft tissue vascularity. Contrast enhancement is best evaluated on T1W-fat saturated images. However, by administering gadolinium *and* applying fat saturation, two variables affecting tissue contrast have been changed, and care must be taken to avoid diagnostic errors. For example, when pre-gadolinium T1W images are obtained *without* fat saturation, a hematoma may demonstrate apparent "enhancement" on T1W-fat saturated, post-contrast images, not because of true tissue enhancement, but because the subacute blood products within the hematoma may *appear* brighter because of the suppression of adjacent fat.

Intravenous Gd-DTPA is not administered for most musculoskeletal MR examinations but is indicated in certain situations:

Cystic Versus Solid. Gadolinium is useful for distinguishing cystic lesions from cystic-appearing solid masses. A true cyst will demonstrate thin peripheral enhancement without enhancement of the

---

BOX 1–5: GADOLINIUM:
When to Use It

- Mass: cyst vs. solid
- Mass: viable tumor vs. necrosis (biopsy guidance)
- Infection: abscess vs. phlegmon
- Spine: disc herniation vs. scar

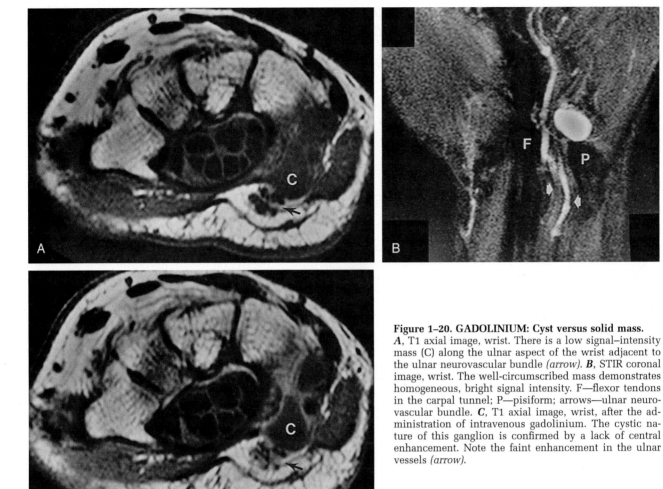

Figure 1–20. GADOLINIUM: Cyst versus solid mass.
A, T1 axial image, wrist. There is a low signal–intensity mass (C) along the ulnar aspect of the wrist adjacent to the ulnar neurovascular bundle *(arrow)*. *B*, STIR coronal image, wrist. The well-circumscribed mass demonstrates homogeneous, bright signal intensity. F—flexor tendons in the carpal tunnel; P—pisiform; arrows—ulnar neurovascular bundle. *C*, T1 axial image, wrist, after the administration of intravenous gadolinium. The cystic nature of this ganglion is confirmed by a lack of central enhancement. Note the faint enhancement in the ulnar vessels *(arrow)*.

cyst fluid centrally (Fig. 1–20). A solid mass will show diffuse enhancement, or at least large areas of enhancement.

Tumor. We do not use gadolinium routinely in the evaluation of soft tissue or osseous tumors, with the exception of differentiating cystic from solid lesions. It can be helpful in directing a biopsy by differentiating enhancing, viable tumor tissue from areas of nonenhancing necrosis.

Infection. In cases of soft tissue infection, gadolinium enhancement can assist in differentiating soft tissue edema or phlegmon from a focal abscess, which can be difficult on T2W or STIR images alone. An abscess will show a thick enhancing wall and lack of central enhancement. Similarly, small sinus tracts are more easily detected on enhanced images. Marrow enhancement is a nonspecific finding, because it can result from both osteomyelitis and areas of noninfected, reactive marrow edema with hyperemia.

Spine. Gd-DTPA is useful in the postoperative patient for differentiating enhancing scar tissue from nonenhancing disk material. It also is helpful for evaluating cord lesions (tumor, demyelinating dis-

ease) and intradural/extramedullary lesions (metastases, nerve sheath tumors).

MR ARTHROGRAPHY

Distension of a joint with a solution containing dilute gadolinium is extremely useful for detecting certain types of pathology, such as labral tears in the shoulder and hip. MR arthrography of the knee also is useful in patients with a history of prior surgery, because it allows for differentiating between a meniscal tear (contrast extends into the tear) and scar within a healed meniscal tear.

We mix 10 mL of sterile saline with 3 mL of iodinated radiographic contrast in order to confirm the intraarticular needle position under fluoroscopy; to this mixture, we add 0.1 mL of gadolinium-DTPA immediately prior to joint puncture. Only this small amount of the gadolinium is administered because if the gadolinium is too concentrated, it actually will result in a loss of signal from the fluid.

T1W images are sufficient for arthrographic imaging, and fat saturation often is employed to distin-

BOX 1–6: MUSCULOSKELETAL TISSUES: Best Sequences		
Bone	• STIR	• Fast T2 with fat saturation	• T1
Cartilage	• STIR	• Fast T2 with fat saturation	• GRE (especially with fat saturation)
Meniscus	• GRE T2*	• T1	• Spin echo proton density
Labrum	• T1 after intraarticular gad. injection	• GRE T2*	
Tendons/ ligaments	• GRE T2*	• STIR	• Fast T2 +/− fat saturation
Muscle	• STIR	• T1	• T1

guish gadolinium from fat (eg, in the subacromial/ subdeltoid bursa in the shoulder). A T2W sequence in at least one plane is also necessary to detect edema, cysts, or other T2-sensitive abnormalities in the soft tissues or marrow.

MUSCULOSKELETAL TISSUES

This is a summary of the appearance of various musculoskeletal tissues on MRI and the sequences we have found most helpful in their evaluation (Box 1–6).

Bone

Normal Appearance

Cortical bone is black on all imaging sequences because protons within the mineralized matrix are unable to resonate and produce signal. Within the medullary cavity, fat and hematopoietic marrow are identified. Hematopoietic marrow is slightly hypo-intense to fat on T1W images and mildly hyperintense to muscle on all sequences (Fig. 1–21).

Most Useful Sequences

1. STIR—Extremely sensitive for detecting even subtle marrow pathology.
2. Fast spin echo-T2 with fat saturation—Similar sensitivity as STIR, but may demonstrate heterogeneous fat suppression.
3. T1—Good for detecting tumors and prominent marrow edema. It is not as sensitive as the STIR technique for more subtle pathology.
4. Gradient echo (T2*)—On mid- and low field strength machines, some gradient echo sequences are useful for detecting marrow pathology. Also, once trabecular or cortical bone has

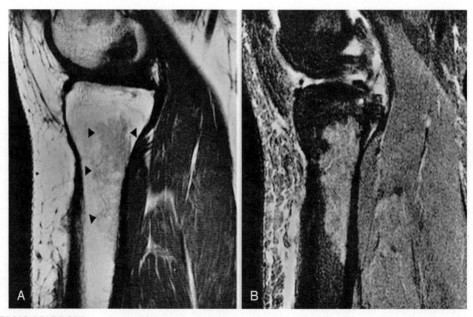

Figure 1–21. NORMAL MARROW.
A, T1 sagittal image, proximal tibia. There is patchy intermediate signal intensity within the proximal tibial shaft and metaphysis *(arrowheads)*, which is slightly brighter than skeletal muscle. *B*, STIR sagittal, proximal tibia. The hematopoietic marrow is even more conspicuous due to suppression of the adjacent marrow fat. Note once again that the marrow remains brighter than skeletal muscle.

been destroyed, this is a sensitive sequence for detecting lesions.

Pitfalls

1. Marrow pathology may be obscured on fast spin echo-T2W images without fat suppression because of the similar high signal intensity of both fat and pathologic lesions on these images.
2. Marrow pathology is easily missed on gradient echo images (on high field strength machines) due to the susceptibility effects of trabecular bone, as described previously.

Articular Cartilage

Normal Appearance

Variable, depending on sequence.

Most Useful Sequences

1. STIR or fat-saturated fast spin echo-T2—Cartilage is dark gray and easily distinguished from joint fluid, making focal defects quite conspicuous (Fig. 1–22). The cartilage is difficult to separate from underlying subchondral bone, but this distinction is less important than identifying abnormalities of the articular surface.
2. 3D-T1W gradient echo with fat saturation—Cartilage is very bright and easily distinguished from subchondral bone and fluid. But because this sequence is quite time consuming and must be added to the standard imaging sequences (unlike a STIR sequence), it is impractical for most uses.

Fibrocartilage

Normal Appearance

Dark on all sequences.

Useful Sequences: Meniscus

Meniscal tears are best demonstrated with short TE sequences. These include

1. T1.
2. Spin echo proton density.
3. Gradient echo-T2*.

Pitfalls

1. Most tears are less well seen with long TE, T2W images (spin echo or fast spin echo).
2. The inherent blurring artifact of fast spin echo-proton density sequences obscures some meniscal tears.

Useful Sequences: Glenoid or Acetabular Labrum (Fig. 1–23)

1. T1W images after intraarticular gadolinium injection (with or without fat suppression).
2. Gradient echo T2*.

Tendons and Ligaments

Normal Appearance

These structures are generally dark on all sequences, with the exception of the anterior cruciate ligament, which demonstrates a somewhat striated appearance due to the thickness and orientation of its collagen bundles. The quadriceps and triceps tendons normally have longitudinal striations as

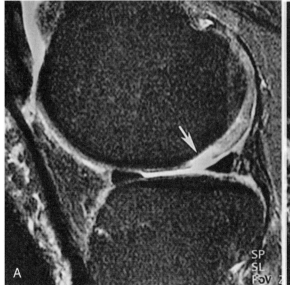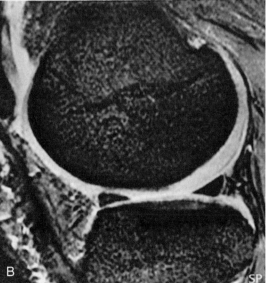

Figure 1–22. FOCAL CARTILAGE DEFECT.
A, STIR sagittal image, knee. There is a small focal defect within the articular cartilage of the medial femoral condyle *(arrow)*. Note the excellent contrast between the intermediate signal intensity of the articular cartilage and the high-signal joint fluid. **B,** T2*-gradient echo sagittal image, knee. The cartilage defect is much more difficult to identify due to the relative isointensity of joint fluid and articular cartilage.

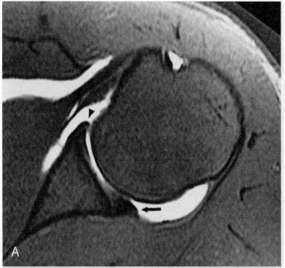
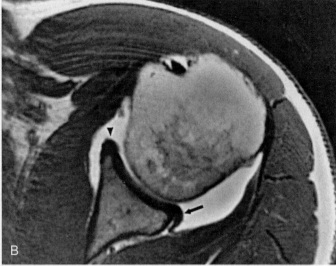
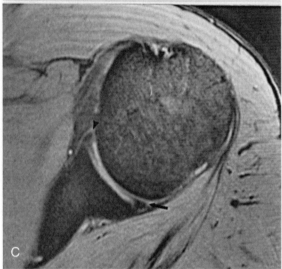

Figure 1–23. FIBROCARTILAGE: Glenoid labrum.
A, T1 axial image, with fat suppression, left shoulder after the intraarticular administration of dilute gadolinium solution. The anterior labrum *(arrowhead)* and posterior labrum *(arrow)* are well demonstrated, primarily due to the excellent joint distention and contrast between the gadolinium solution and low signal–intensity labral tissue. Fibrocartilage is normally low signal on all pulse sequences. *B*, T1 axial image, left shoulder after the intraarticular administration of dilute gadolinium solution. There is better contrast between the low-signal labrum and underlying bone when fat suppression is not performed. *C*, T2*-gradient echo axial image, left shoulder. The low-signal anterior labrum *(arrowhead)* and posterior labrum *(arrow)* are again well demonstrated, but the lack of joint distention limits labral/capsular evaluation overall.

well. Some tendons, such as the posterior tibial, demonstrate increased signal near their insertions due to multiple osseous attachments.

Most Useful Sequences (Fig. 1–24)

1. Gradient echo T2*.
2. T1.
3. STIR/fast spin echo-T2 with or without fat saturation.

Pitfalls

Magic angle: Spuriously increased signal intensity may occur within any tissue containing highly structured collagen fibers (tendon, ligament, meniscus, labrum), depending on its position within the magnetic field. This magic angle effect is due to the orientation of the collagen bundles and occurs when the structure lies at an angle near 55 degrees to the main magnetic field. The resulting increased signal is seen on images obtained with a short TE (T1, proton density, and most gradient echo sequences) but disappears on long TE (T2W) images (Fig. 1–25). This latter feature allows for differentiation from

true tendon pathology. Other supportive signs include a lack of tendon enlargement or peritendinous edema.

Muscle

Normal Appearance

Intermediate signal intensity on all sequences.

Useful Sequences (Fig. 1–26)

1. T1—Good depiction of overall muscle architecture and of fatty atrophy of the muscle.
2. STIR—Extremely sensitive for detecting most types of muscle pathology other than atrophy.

Synovium

Normal Appearance

Not usually evident unless it is pathologically thickened.

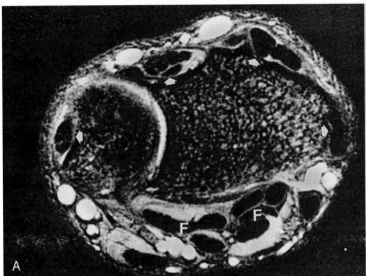

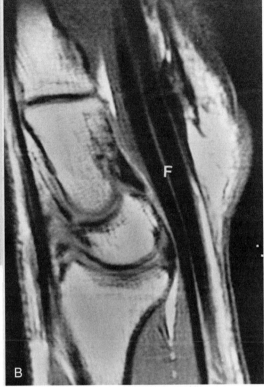

Figure 1–24. NORMAL TENDONS.
A, T2*-gradient echo axial image, wrist. The low-signal flexor tendons (F) within the carpal tunnel and the extensor tendons *(arrows)*, along the dorsum of the wrist, are well demonstrated. *B*, T1 sagittal image, wrist. The low signal flexor tendons (F) are well demonstrated within the carpal tunnel.

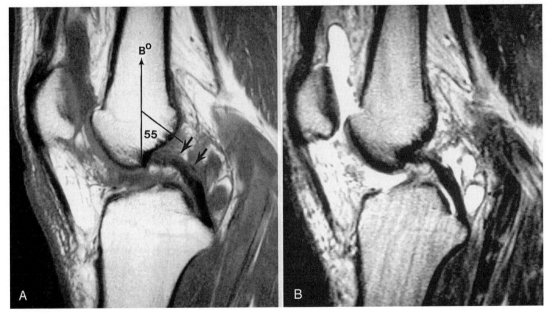

Figure 1–25. MAGIC ANGLE ARTIFACT.
A, Spin echo-T1 sagittal image, knee. There is intermediate signal intensity within the proximal to mid posterior cruciate ligament *(arrows)* where it arches near 55 degrees to the main magnetic field (B°). *B*, Spin echo-T2 sagittal image, knee. The intermediate signal intensity disappears, and the ligament displays normal size and low signal intensity.

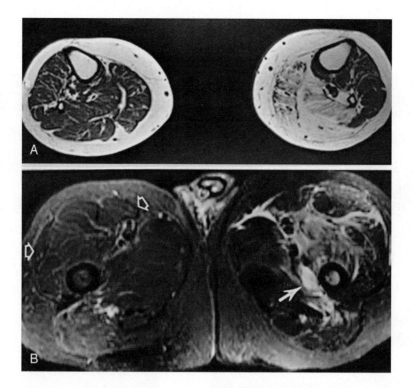

Figure 1–26. MUSCLE.
A, T1 axial image, proximal lower legs. There is extensive muscular atrophy in the left calf, as evidenced by high signal–intensity fatty infiltration of the gastrocnemius and soleus muscles. Note the normal fatty septa distributed within the muscles of the right calf. *B*, STIR axial image, proximal thighs. Note the normal low signal muscles in the anterior compartment of the right thigh *(small arrows)*. There is extensive intramuscular and perifascial fluid within the proximal left thigh of this patient with necrotizing fasciitis. There is also a small abscess *(arrow)* along the medial aspect of the femoral shaft.

Useful Sequences (Fig. 1–27)

1. T1 fat-saturated images after the administration of intravenous gadolinium.
2. T1W images without gadolinium enhancement will demonstrate synovial pannus as intermediate signal intensity tissue that is slightly higher in signal intensity than adjacent joint fluid or muscle. This can be detected with careful scrutiny of the images, but is much less conspicuous than after gadolinium enhancement.

Pitfalls

It usually is not possible to distinguish hypertrophied synovium from joint fluid on T2W and STIR images.

APPLICATIONS

Because each anatomic site contains multiple different structures within the volume being imaged (tendons, cartilage, bone, muscle, spinal cord, and so forth), it is necessary to use protocols that adequately demonstrate all of these varied structures. Pulse sequences and imaging planes must be carefully selected to optimally demonstrate these structures in a relatively short period of time. The clinical indications for obtaining an MR examination further help to determine which pulse sequences and imaging planes should be selected. There is no added value in obtaining every pulse sequence or imaging plane known to man; it will not improve your ability to make a diagnosis when compared to using tailored protocols. Clinicians also appreciate the use of standardized protocols, because this consistency allows them to become familiar with the anatomy and pathology demonstrated on the studies.

It is hoped that the basic information presented in this chapter regarding MR imaging as it relates to the musculoskeletal system will allow you to be street smart about MRI without being plagued by details of the physics (unless you want to be). It is our impression that name dropping various MR terms in front of clinicians serves little to no useful purpose. Our orthopedists are not impressed if they hear us discussing flip angles, TRs, TEs, and signal intensity. They are much more pleased if we point to a white line traversing the black triangle of a meniscus and assure them that they will find a meniscal tear at arthroscopy.

The protocols presented in each chapter are based on our approach to musculoskeletal MR imaging. These work well for us, but we certainly recognize that there is more than one way to properly perform any given MR examination. Our protocols are meant to serve as a useful guide. Because of the different types of equipment available, we cannot specify all of the parameters, such as repetition times (TR), echo times (TE), and so forth, but have concentrated on the field of view, section thickness, imaging planes, and pulse sequences used for different indications. The precise TR, TE, number of signal aver-

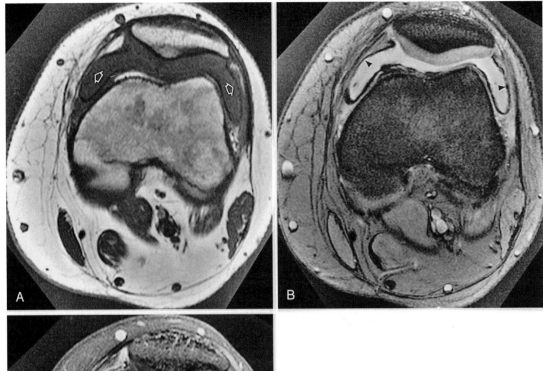

Figure 1–27. SYNOVIUM.
A, T1 axial image, knee. The synovium is not distinguishable from joint fluid because both are of intermediate signal intensity *(open arrows)*. *B*, T2*-gradient echo axial image, knee (same patient as in *A*). The synovium is not distinguishable from joint fluid because both display increased signal intensity. Note the low signal–intensity hemosiderin lining the joint *(arrowheads)* related to the patient's known hemophilia. *C*, T1 axial image, knee, with fat saturation, after the intravenous administration of gadolinium (same patient as in *A*.). A thin rim of enhancing synovium *(open arrows)* is easily distinguishable from the low signal–intensity joint fluid.

ages, matrix size, and so on, will need to be optimized for the particular machine you work with.

Remember, all scanners are *not* created equal. If you try to duplicate the results from an article written by investigators using one type of MR scanner by using their protocol on a different brand of scanner, it probably will not work because each machine uses different methods to acquire and display the data. The point is that you need to first work at understanding the fundamentals that go into producing a high-quality MR image, and then work just

as hard at understanding how this can be achieved with your particular machine.

References

1. Westbrook C, Kaut C. *MRI in Practice.* Oxford: Blackwell Scientific; 1993.
2. Elster AD. *Questions and Answers in Magnetic Resonance Imaging.* St. Louis: Mosby; 1994.
3. NessAvier M. *All You Really Need to Know About MRI Physics.* Baltimore: Simply Physics; 1997.

GLOSSARY: COMMON TERMS IN MUSCULOSKELETAL MRI

Coil: A piece of hardware that can transmit or receive radiofrequency pulses during MR imaging. All scanners are equipped with a large body coil within the scanner itself. For most musculoskeletal applications, a surface coil is used. This is a smaller coil that can be placed on or around the body part of interest for improved imaging.

Cross talk: This phenomenon occurs due to some "spill over" of radiofrequency excitation between adjacent tissue slices during MR imaging and results in increased image noise. This effect can be minimized by inserting small "gaps" of non-imaged tissue between adjacent slices.

Echo: This refers to the radiofrequency returning from tissues, which is then used to create the final image. Various types of echoes (eg, spin echo, gradient echo, etc.) will be produced, depending on which pulse sequence is used.

Echo train: (see also *fast spin echo*) Specialized rapid pulse sequences can produce a series of echoes, known as an echo train, in the same amount of time that conventional sequences produce a single echo. The reduction in imaging time is directly proportional to the length of the echo train (typically 2 to 16).

Fast spin echo: A family of pulse sequences that include RARE, fast spin echo (General Electric term) and turbo spin echo (Siemens/Phillips term). These pulse sequences produce images with contrast similar to conventional spin echo sequences but in less time.

Fat saturation: Certain scanning techniques result in the suppression (reduction) of the signal intensity arising from fat. The two main techniques are inversion recovery imaging and frequency-selective fat suppression.

Field of view: The amount of tissue included on each cross sectional image. Typically expressed in mm^2 or cm^2.

Gadolinium: A paramagnetic compound that forms the basis for most MR contrast agents. Its primary effect is to cause increased signal intensity on T1-weighted images within tissues (if administered intravenously) or within a joint (if administered intraarticularly after being diluted in saline).

Gap: A small slice of non-imaged tissue inserted between two adjacent imaging slices to reduce cross talk.

Gradient echo: A family of pulse sequences originally developed to produce T2-weighted images in less time than with the spin echo technique. Because of differences between these two types of sequences, gradient echo-T2W images are designated T2*W and are especially useful for imaging ligaments, fibrocartilage, and hyaline articular cartilage. They are also useful for identifying areas of hemorrhage, metal, bone, or air due to heightened susceptibility effects.

Inversion recovery: Commonly known as STIR (short tau inversion recovery). This technique results in excellent fat suppression and high signal intensity from areas of fluid or edema; thus, it is extremely sensitive for detecting many types of acute pathology.

Matrix: The grid of voxels which compose each MR image. Typical matrix values range from 128 x 128 to 512 x 512 (width x height).

Noise: The quality of an MR image is determined largely by two competing factors, signal and noise. Image noise refers to the background graininess that results from several factors, including the background electrical noise of the imaging system, the presence of the patient in the magnet, the imaging coil used, and other factors. For a given patient, the noise is constant, and maneuvers employed to improve the signal of the image will result in an improved signal-to-noise ratio (SNR) and a better image.

Proton density sequence:	A pulse sequence that is relatively balanced in terms of T1 and T2 weighting (TR <1000, TE >30). Tissue contrast on these images is based on the number of protons within each tissue, rather than their T1 or T2 relaxation properties. (Fat is relatively bright, whereas fluid is gray due to the higher number of protons per unit volume in the fat.)
Pulse sequence:	A combination of imaging parameters that are selected at the MRI console to produce images of predictable tissue contrast. The most common families of pulse sequences include spin echo, fast spin echo, gradient echo, and inversion recovery (STIR).
Resolution:	The ability to distinguish between two objects. The better the resolution of an image, the easier it is to distinguish objects of increasingly smaller size. In general, the smaller the voxels in an image, the better the resolution, but this also will result in decreased image signal.
Signal average:	The number of times each portion of tissue (voxel) is sampled to generate an MR image. Increasing the number of signal averages improves the signal-to-noise ratio of an image, but also prolongs imaging time proportionately.
Slice thickness:	The thickness of the MR image. Although each image is projected two-dimensionally on a monitor or film, it actually represents a three-dimensional slice of tissue, typically ranging from 1 to 10 mm in depth. The smaller the slice thickness, the better the resolution.
Spin echo sequence:	A family of pulse sequences that includes T1-, proton density-, and T2-weighted sequences.
STIR:	See *inversion recovery.*
Susceptibility:	The degree to which a tissue distorts the magnetic field around it. Certain materials, such as surgical hardware, metal fragments, or the iron-containing hemoglobin found within areas of hemorrhage, have large susceptibilities and tend to create artifactual signal loss on MR images. Gradient echo pulse sequences accentuate these artifacts. Fast spin echo sequences tend to minimize them.
T1, T2:	These are inherent properties of tissue that define how a proton will react during MR imaging. Each tissue has unique T1 and T2 values. As a result, contrast between tissues on an MR image is based primarily on differences in T1 or T2 properties, depending on the imaging parameters selected. (T1 or T2 "weighted")
TE:	Also known as echo time. This is a parameter selected at the imaging console that controls the T2 weighting of an image. A short TE minimizes T2 differences, whereas a long TE maximizes T2 weighting.
TR:	Repetition time. This is an imaging parameter selected at the console that controls the amount of T1 weighting in an image. A short TR maximizes T1 differences, whereas a long TR minimizes T1 weighting.
Turbo spin echo:	See *fast spin echo.*
Voxel:	The basic unit of the MR image, this represents a small portion of tissue within the patient that is sampled during the MR examination. Also known as volume elements, the size of each voxel is determined by the field of view, imaging matrix, and the slice thickness.
Weighting:	This refers to the contrast properties of a particular imaging sequence. This is determined by selecting specific scanning parameters at the console that will emphasize contrast differences between tissues based on tissue-specific properties (eg, T1- or T2-weighted images).

HOW TO IMAGE BONE MARROW
**Normal Marrow Anatomy and
Function**
 Trabecular Bone
 Red Marrow
 Yellow Marrow
 Marrow Conversion
 Variations in Normal Red Marrow
MRI of Normal Marrow
 Yellow Marrow
 Red Marrow
 Marrow Heterogeneity
Marrow Pathology
 Marrow Proliferative Disorders
  Benign
   *Reconversion of Yellow to Red
   Marrow*

   Leukemias
   Monoclonal Gammopathies
  Malignant
   *Aggressive Gammopathies
   (Plasma Cell Dyscrasias)*
 Marrow Replacement Disorders
  Skeletal Metastases
  Osteoporotic Versus Pathologic
   Vertebral Compression Fracture
  Lymphoma
  Benign and Malignant Primary
   Bone Tumors
 Marrow Depletion
  Aplastic Anemia
  Chemotherapy
  Radiation

 Vascular Abnormalities (Hyperemia
  and Ischemia)
   *Transient Osteoporosis of the
   Hip*
   Regional Migratory Osteoporosis
  Ischemia
 Miscellaneous Marrow Diseases
  Gaucher Disease
  Paget's Disease
  Osteopetrosis
  Hemosiderin Deposition
  Serous Atrophy (Gelatinous
   Transformation)

HOW TO IMAGE BONE MARROW

Magnetic resonance imaging (MRI) of suspected bone marrow abnormalities should be directed to the site of clinical symptoms, or where abnormalities or confusing findings are present on bone scintigraphy or other imaging studies. Thus, the coil used, patient position, planes of imaging, and field of view will vary for each site. The parameters generally should be the same as those used for imaging the nearest joint.

When diffuse marrow disease is suspected, a marrow survey of the entire body or, more commonly, of the entire spine, pelvis, and proximal femora is performed. These areas are surveyed because they are where the bulk of hematopoietic marrow (and marrow pathology) exists. The imaging parameters given below are for a marrow survey of the spine, pelvis, and proximal femora.

Coils/Patient Position. For a marrow survey, the patient is supine in the magnet. Spine phased array coils are used for the spine, and the body coil is used for the pelvis and proximal femora.

Image Orientation. Sagittal images of the spine and coronal images of the pelvis and proximal femora are obtained.

Pulse Sequences/Regions of Interest. Large field-of-view sagittal T1W images of the cervical and upper thoracic spine and of the lower thoracic and entire lumbar spine are routine. We also use coronal T1W and STIR images of the pelvis and proximal femora. Section thickness in the spine is 4 mm and in the pelvis is 7 mm.

Contrast. Intravenous gadolinium generally serves no useful purpose for routine diagnosis of marrow disorders. In fact, it may camouflage the lesions by giving them signal characteristics similar to fatty marrow on T1W images, unless fat suppression is used.

Normal Marrow Anatomy and Function (Box 2–1)

It is important to understand the function and distribution of normal marrow in order to be able to

---

**BOX 2–1: BONE MARROW: Functions of the
Three Components**

Trabecular bone
 Architectural support for red and yellow
 marrow
 Mineral depot
Red marrow
 Produces red cells, white cells, platelets
Yellow marrow
 ? Surface/nutritional support for red
 marrow

---

diagnose abnormalities and understand how to best image for marrow disease. In simplest terms, bone marrow consists of three components: (1) trabecular bone, (2) red marrow, and (3) yellow marrow. Red marrow is the hematopoietically active fraction of marrow that produces blood cells. Yellow marrow is hematopoietically inactive and composed mainly of fat cells, the purpose of which is uncertain. Red and yellow marrow elements are supported by a system composed of reticulum cells, nerves, and vascular sinusoids. The trabecular bone serves as a framework to support the red and yellow marrow elements.[1-3]

Trabecular Bone

Synonyms for trabecular bone include cancellous, spongy, and medullary bone. It is composed of primary and bridging secondary trabeculae that serve for architectural support and as a mineral depot. The number of trabeculae decreases with age.

Red Marrow (Box 2-2)

Synonyms for red marrow are cellular, active, myeloid, or hematopoietic marrow. Red marrow is composed of cellular elements that include erythrocytes (red cells), granulocytes (white cells), and thrombocytes (platelets), which are responsible for satisfying an individual's needs for oxygenation, immunity, and coagulation, respectively. Within islands of red marrow, there is a supporting stroma, the reticulin (or reticulum), which includes two major groups of cells: phagocytes (or macrophages) and the undifferentiated nonphagocytic cells. There is a rich sinusoidal vascular supply in red marrow.

Yellow Marrow

Synonyms for yellow marrow include fatty or inactive marrow. The theory for the purpose of fat cells in yellow marrow is that they provide surface or nutritional support for red marrow elements. The vascular supply to yellow marrow is sparse.

For convenience, red and yellow marrow generally are discussed as if they are completely separate entities that exist in precise anatomic locations; however, this is not the case. Red marrow is not composed entirely of hematopoietic cells, but always has a significant amount of fat cells scattered throughout the active cellular elements. Conversely, normal yellow marrow is never composed entirely of fat cells, but always has some small amount of active cellular elements present. Thus, red marrow is the portion of marrow where the largest concentrations of active cellular elements exist, and yellow marrow is the portion of marrow where fat cells predominate. This composition of marrow elements accounts for the MRI appearance discussed later in this chapter. The fraction of yellow marrow increases with age as trabecular bone resorbs from osteoporosis and fat fills in the spaces created.

Marrow Conversion (Box 2-3)

The amount and distribution of red and yellow marrow change with age.[4-10] This normal conversion from red to yellow marrow occurs in a predictable and progressive manner and is completed by an individual's middle 20s (Fig. 2-1). At birth, nearly the entire osseous skeleton is composed of red marrow. When epiphyses and apophyses ossify, they have red marrow within them only transiently, for a matter of a few weeks, before conversion to yellow marrow occurs. Conversion of the remainder of the skeleton occurs over the following 2 decades.

Conversion from red to yellow marrow proceeds from the extremities to the axial skeleton, occurring in the distal bones of the extremities (feet and hands) first, and progressing finally to the proximal bones (humeri and femora). This process occurs in a roughly symmetric manner on each side in a given individual.

Progression of conversion from red to yellow marrow within an individual long bone occurs in the following sequence: epiphyses and apophyses first, then the diaphysis, followed by the distal metaphysis, and finally the proximal metaphysis. Conversion also occurs in a centripetal fashion within a bone,

---

BOX 2-3: PROGRESSION OF CONVERSION FROM RED TO YELLOW MARROW

ENTIRE SKELETON (Extremities to axial skeleton)	INDIVIDUAL LONG BONES:
Hands/feet ↓	Epiphyses/apophyses ↓
Forearms/lower legs ↓	Diaphysis ↓
Humeri/femora ↓	Distal metaphysis ↓
Pelvis/spine	Proximal metaphysis

BOX 2-2: CHARACTERISTICS OF RED AND YELLOW MARROW

RED MARROW	YELLOW MARROW
• Rich vascular supply	• Poor vascular supply
• Reticulin stroma	• Paucity of reticulin
• Small fraction of fat cells	• Small fraction of red marrow elements
• Increases if demand for hematopoiesis increases (reconversion)	• Increases with age

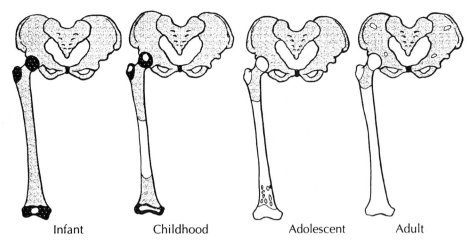

Figure 2–1. MARROW CONVERSION.
Diagram of axial and appendicular marrow distribution as a function of age, as red marrow progressively converts to yellow marrow.

Infant   Childhood   Adolescent   Adult

▨ Red Marrow
▨ Cartilage
☐ Yellow Marrow

with fat predominating centrally, whereas red marrow predominates at the outer margins or periphery (subcortical region) of the medullary space of flat bones, long bones, and vertebral bodies.

The rate of conversion may vary from one individual to another, but generalities have been established that are important to know (Box 2–4). The reverse process of conversion can occur, called reconversion. This is a process of yellow marrow being reconverted to red marrow when there is an increased demand for hematopoiesis. Reconversion affects marrow in the entire skeleton and in individual long bones in exactly the reverse sequence as conversion.

BOX 2–4: RATE OF CONVERSION FROM RED TO YELLOW MARROW

AGE GROUP	MARROW FINDINGS
Infants (<1 year)	→ Diffuse red marrow, except for ossified epiphyses and apophyses
Children (1–10 years)	→ Yellow marrow below knees and elbows, and in diaphyses of femora and humeri
Adolescents (10–20 years)	→ Progressive yellow marrow in distal and proximal metaphyses of proximal long bones
Adults (>25 years)	→ Yellow marrow except in axial skeleton and proximal metaphyses of proximal long bones

Variations in Normal Red Marrow
(Box 2–5)

There are several normal variations in appearance of red marrow that are important to know in order not to misinterpret them as pathology.

Variations in red marrow distribution may be confusing. Some individuals have virtually no red marrow in the femora or humeri, whereas others have large amounts; most fall somewhere between these two extremes (Fig. 2–2). Small differences in the amount and distribution of red marrow from side to side are normal, but marked asymmetry is suspicious for a disease process.

An important and common exception to early and complete conversion in the epiphyses occurs in the proximal humeral and femoral epiphyses, where a small amount of red marrow may persist normally throughout life. This normal epiphyseal red marrow is curvilinear in configuration and located in the subchondral regions of these bones (Fig. 2–3).[11]

Variations in the red marrow pattern commonly are encountered and could be a source of error if not recognized as normal. Heterogeneous patterns of red and yellow marrow distribution occur with

BOX 2–5: NORMAL VARIATIONS IN RED MARROW

- Amount/distribution varies from person to person, but not from side to side in the same person
- Persistent curvilinear, subchondral red marrow in proximal epiphyses of humeri and femora
- Heterogeneous, focal islands of red marrow

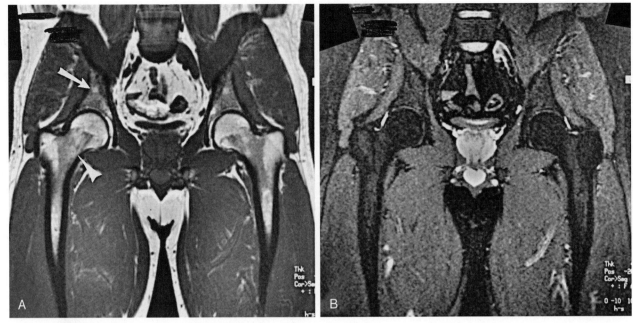

Figure 2–2. NORMAL RED AND YELLOW MARROW.
A, T1 coronal image, pelvis/femora. Yellow marrow has signal identical to that of the high-signal subcutaneous fat. It is present in apophyses, epiphyses, the femoral diaphyses, and focal regions in the pelvis *(arrow)*. Red marrow is intermediate signal (higher signal than muscle) and located in the pelvis and proximal femoral metaphyses *(arrrowhead)*. Note the striking symmetry of the distribution of red and yellow marrow bilaterally. *B*, STIR coronal image, pelvis/femora. Fatty marrow becomes black from fat suppression in this sequence. Red marrow is intermediate signal, somewhat similar in appearance to muscle; this is best seen in the pelvis.

isolated islands of red marrow in predominately yellow marrow, or foci of yellow marrow in regions of predominately red marrow.[12] Foci of red marrow are often juxtacortical and located around the periphery of the marrow space (Fig. 2–4). Central foci of yellow marrow within islands of red marrow

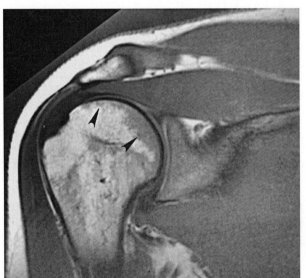

Figure 2–3. NORMAL RED MARROW: variation in distribution. T1 coronal oblique image, shoulder. Intermediate signal normal red marrow is seen in the scapula and proximal humeral metaphysis, as expected. Curvilinear red marrow in the subchondral bone of the humeral head *(arrowheads)* is present. This can be seen as a normal variation in the humeral and femoral heads without disease being present.

indicate a benign appearance. Focal islands of conversion to fatty marrow may be the result of chronic stress and biomechanical stimuli causing decreased vascularity at involved sites, which stimulates conversion.[13, 14]

MRI of Normal Marrow

The most important pulse sequence used to evaluate marrow is the T1W spin echo sequence. T2W and STIR sequences commonly are used also.[1–3, 15–17] Gadolinium has no apparent effect on normal adult yellow or red marrow; children's abundant red marrow may show mild enhancement. Red and yellow marrow should be distributed in predictable locations, based on age, as discussed previously in the section on normal marrow anatomy.

Yellow Marrow

On T1W MR images, yellow marrow has signal characteristics similar to subcutaneous fat, with relatively high signal intensity. On T2W or STIR images, the signal intensity again follows that of subcutaneous fat, being relatively intermediate signal intensity on T2W images and completely suppressed and demonstrating low signal intensity on STIR images (see Fig. 2–2).

Fat signal in marrow is interrupted by groups of low signal intensity stress trabeculae. A thin, low signal intensity line where a physeal plate closed (the "physeal scar") often is evident (Fig. 2–5). Bone islands are oval, low signal intensity regions on all pulse sequences.

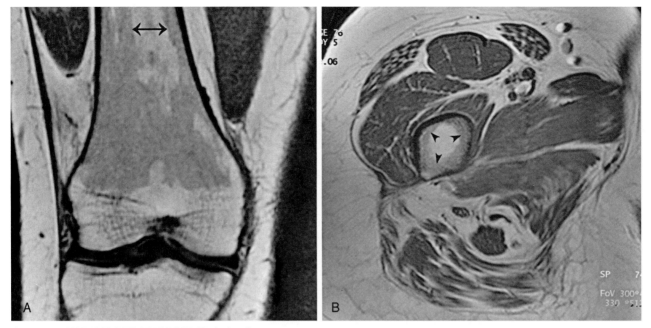

Figure 2–4. NORMAL RED MARROW: Variation in pattern.
A, T1 coronal image, knee. Patchy foci of intermediate-signal red marrow are located in the peripheral juxtacortical region of bone *(arrow)*. *B,* T1 axial image, thigh. Arrowheads point to the red marrow located around the periphery of the marrow space, just deep to the low-signal cortical bone of the femur.

Red Marrow

When red marrow exists in enough concentration, it is evident on both T1W and T2W images as intermediate signal intensity (see Fig. 2–2). Thus, on T1W images, it will be lower in signal intensity than yellow marrow and relatively easy to identify.

Because both yellow and red marrow show intermediate signal intensity on T2W images, they can be difficult to distinguish from each other on this sequence. On STIR or fat-suppressed T2W images, red marrow demonstrates intermediate signal intensity that is more hyperintense than yellow marrow and very similar in appearance to muscle (see Fig. 2–2).

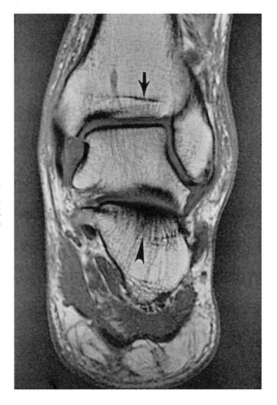

Figure 2–5. NORMAL YELLOW MARROW.
T1 coronal image, ankle. In the distal extremities, high-signal fatty marrow predominates. The yellow marrow is interrupted by low-signal normal structures, including the physeal scar *(arrow)* where the growth plate closed, and stress trabeculae in the calcaneus *(arrowhead)*. There is also a low-signal bone island evident just above the distal tibial epiphyseal scar.

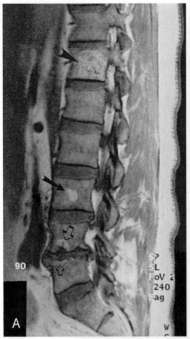
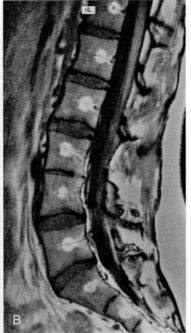
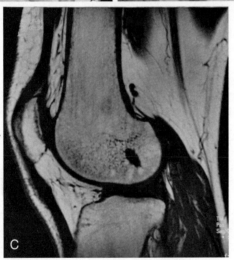

Figure 2–6. NORMAL MARROW HETEROGENE-ITY: Foci of fatty marrow.
A, T1 sagittal image, lumbar spine. Overall, the marrow has intermediate signal (higher signal than intervertebral disks) from normal red marrow. In addition, several foci of high-signal fat that are of no real clinical significance are evident. There is a large hemangioma in T12 *(arrowhead)* and a central focus of fat in L3 *(solid arrow)* from either focal marrow conversion or a small hemangioma; curvilinear fat surrounds a Schmorl's node in the inferior endplate of L4 *(large open arrow)*, and linear fat along the superior endplate of L5 *(small open arrow)* is the result of adjacent degenerative disk disease. *B*, T1 sagittal image, lumbar spine. Focal conversion to high-signal fatty marrow in the center of each vertebral body at the level of the basivertebral vessels is present. *C*, T1 image, sagittal knee. Numerous foci of high-signal fatty marrow are scattered throughout the distal femoral metaphysis and epiphysis from disuse ("aggressive") osteoporosis. The oval, low-signal structure in the epiphysis is a benign bone island (enostosis).

A very important feature of normal red marrow is that it is always slightly higher in signal intensity than normal muscle or normal intervertebral disks on T1W images (Figs. 2–2 and 2–6). It is never normal for marrow to have lower signal intensity than normal muscle or disk on the same T1W image. The reason red marrow is always slightly higher in signal intensity than muscle or disk on T1W images is because of the normal red marrow composition, where a significant number of fat cells are scattered throughout the red marrow elements, contributing to the higher signal intensity. When red marrow becomes equal or lower in signal intensity than normal disk or muscle on T1W images, pathology is almost certainly present.

Marrow Heterogeneity (Boxes 2–5 and 2–6)

Red and yellow marrow may be either homogenous or focal in appearance. The focal marrow patterns sometimes are difficult to distinguish from pathology without careful analysis of the location and signal intensity involved. Focal islands of red marrow may have high signal intensity fat centers of a benign nature on T1W images from focal conversion, called the "bull's-eye" appearance.[18] Focal islands of yellow marrow are common in the spine, especially in the posterior elements, around the central venous channels in the vertebral bodies, or adjacent to the endplates of vertebral bodies (see Fig. 2–6).[12]

In general, identification of focal areas of fat within the marrow on MRI should never be a cause for concern. Focal regions of fat in marrow are common in normal marrow or may result from extremely common disease-related alterations, but never from anything of a serious nature (see Fig. 2–6). Chronic stresses and biomechanical stimuli cause a decrease in the vascularity to specific sites in marrow and stimulate conversion of red to yellow marrow, which probably accounts for many focal areas of conversion to fat. A classic example of this phenomenon occurs in the marrow adjacent to vertebral endplates that border on a degenerated disk. A band-like focal alteration in marrow signal occurs as a result of the ischemia associated with the disk disease.

Focal areas of red marrow can be particularly difficult to distinguish from pathologic lesions, such as metastases. There have been publications regarding the use of certain "designer" pulse sequences to try to determine if such lesions are red marrow or not (in- and out-of-phase gradient echo imaging and diffusion imaging).[19, 20] The theory behind these sequences is that foci of red marrow have some fat intermixed, whereas neoplasm completely replaces normal marrow, including the fatty elements. On in-phase and out-of-phase gradient echo imaging, the signal contribution of fat and water cycle in and out of phase with respect to each other as the echo time increases. The signal generated from tissue that has fat in it is different from the signal generated from tissue without fat in it. Benign foci of red marrow (which has some fat cells in it) are low signal intensity on the out-of-phase images, whereas neoplasm should be high signal intensity as compared to the in-phase images because of the lack of fat in the lesion (Fig. 2–7). Large studies to prove the value of these sequences have not yet been performed.

Marrow Pathology

Abnormalities of bone marrow sometimes have a diagnostic appearance, but they often are nonspecific in their MRI features.[1-3, 21] It is best to have an approach to the lesions and offer a reasonable differential diagnosis in the many instances where a specific diagnosis is not possible.

Five broad categories of marrow disease can be used to facilitate an approach to evaluating the images and forming an appropriate differential diagnosis: (1) marrow proliferative disorders, (2) marrow replacement disorders, (3) marrow depletion, (4) vascular abnormalities, and (5) miscellaneous marrow diseases.

Marrow Proliferative Disorders
(Box 2–7)

Marrow proliferative disorders will be considered as both benign and malignant diseases that arise from proliferation of cells that normally exist in the marrow. These diseases should be distinguished from the closely related category of marrow replacement disorders, which consists of replacement of normal marrow by implantation of cells that do not arise from normally existing marrow elements.

BENIGN

The benign marrow proliferative abnormalities include myelodysplastic syndrome, polycythemia vera, myelofibrosis, mastocytosis, and reconversion from yellow to red marrow. Malignant conditions that arise from existing marrow elements are leukemias, multiple myeloma, primary amyloidosis, and Waldenstrom's macroglobulinemia. The general MRI appearance of these entities will be discussed first,

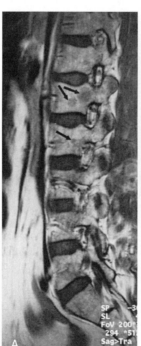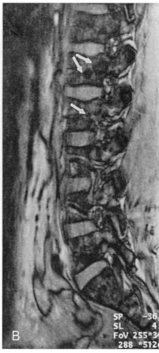

Figure 2–7. NORMAL MARROW HETEROGENEITY: Foci of red marrow.
A, T1 sagittal image, lumbar spine. Foci of low signal in the vertebral bodies of L1 and L2 *(arrows)* were suspicious for metastases in this elderly woman with a history of breast and colon cancer. The suspicious areas are slightly higher signal than the disks; therefore, islands of red marrow should be strongly considered for the diagnosis. *B*, Out-of-phase gradient echo sagittal image, lumbar spine. This special sequence determines if fat is present in the marrow lesions. Any lesion with fat cells remaining should be benign and low signal on this sequence *(arrows)*. The larger lesion at L1 was biopsied and was normal red marrow.

BOX 2–7: PROLIFERATIVE MARROW DISORDERS

- Arise from existing marrow elements
- Diffuse disease, usually. Major exception: focal multiple myeloma.

Benign	*Malignant*
Myelofibrosis	Leukemia
Reconversion	Multiple
Polycythemia vera	myeloma
Mastocytosis	Amyloidosis
Myelodysplastic	Waldenström's
syndrome	macroglobulinemia

- MRI
  - Normal signal and distribution (low tumor burden, higher signal than muscle or disk on T1)
  - Abnormal signal: equal or lower than muscle on T1; variable on T2, usually some increased signal.
  - Abnormal distribution: replacement of yellow marrow
  - Both abnormal signal and distribution

and specifics of some of the diseases will be delineated later. In general, marrow proliferative disorders involve the marrow in a diffuse manner rather than with focal lesions, except for the focal form of multiple myeloma.

MRI of marrow proliferative disorders can have several appearances. First, it must be emphasized that the normal appearance of marrow on MRI does not eliminate the possibility of a significant marrow disease being present. Proliferation of abnormal cells may be indistinguishable from normal red marrow early in the disease when the tumor burden is low, because of the fact that not all fat cells have yet been replaced. This is the situation in about 10% to 20% of patients with multiple myeloma and leukemia, and it is important to understand this weakness of the imaging technique.

The major abnormalities we look for on MRI to indicate a marrow proliferative disease are (1) abnormal signal intensity, (2) abnormal distribution of what appears to be normal signal intensity red marrow, or (3) both abnormal marrow distribution and signal intensity (Figs. 2–8 and 2–9). Only if there is an abnormal distribution of what appears to be red marrow can the disease be diagnosed on MRI prior to the signal intensity becoming abnormal. Conversely, only if the signal intensity is abnormal as compared to normal red marrow can the disease be diagnosed if there is a normal red marrow distribution. Thus, as abnormal numbers of cells continue to proliferate, fat cells in the marrow will be replaced, and the signal intensity will become equal to or lower than muscle or disk on T1W images.

The cells will appear in areas where red marrow should not exist for the age of the patient (distal femora or humeri, diaphyses of long bones, below the knee or elbow, in epiphyses or apophyses along the central venous channels in the vertebral body). Increased cellular elements generally lead to STIR or T2W images showing increased signal intensity relative to muscle.

Several of these diseases alter the appearance of the marrow for reasons other than proliferation of the abnormal cellular elements, and the MRI appearance may vary. When the cells proliferate, they replace normal marrow elements and cause induction of reconversion from yellow to red marrow in order to increase hematopoiesis; reconversion affects the appearance of marrow in ways indistinguishable from proliferation of cells from other benign or malignant causes. Also, some of the marrow proliferative disorders, such as mastocytosis and myelofibrosis, stimulate fibrosis of the reticulin of the marrow, and sclerosis of adjacent trabecular bone occurs, which results in extremely low signal intensity on all pulse sequences. Finally, some patients will have hemolysis (eg, sickle cell anemia and thalassemia) and develop hemosiderosis, which causes diffuse, very low signal intensity (black) in marrow from deposition of hemosiderin.

Reconversion of Yellow to Red Marrow (Box 2–8). If existing red marrow cannot meet an individual's needs for hematopoiesis, hyperplasia of red marrow elements will occur in exactly the reverse sequence that conversion from red to yellow mar-

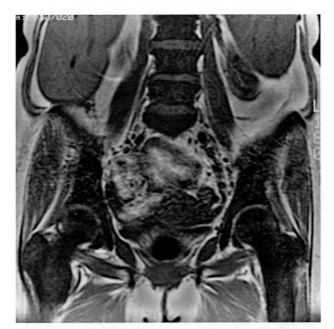

Figure 2–8. MARROW PROLIFERATIVE DISORDERS: Mastocytosis.
T1 coronal image, pelvis. The marrow, including the epiphyses and apophyses, is diffusely lower signal than disks and muscle. The spleen is enlarged. Thus, the marrow is abnormal in signal and distribution, which is typical of a marrow proliferative disorder. This patient has mastocytosis.

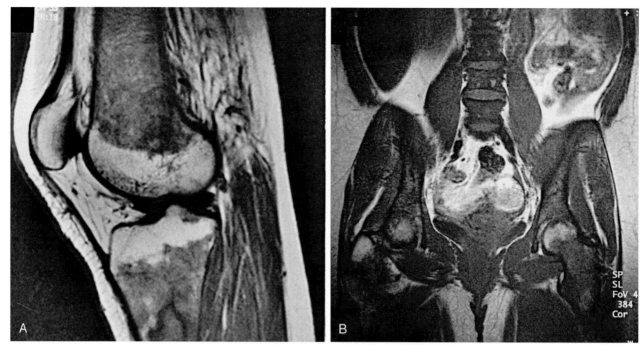

Figure 2–9. MARROW PROLIFERATIVE DISORDERS: Reconversion from sickle cell anemia.
A, T1 sagittal image, knee. The red marrow in the distal femur and proximal tibia of this 27-year-old woman has normal signal that is higher than muscle, but the distribution is abnormal for her age. There is also a low-signal serpiginous line in the tibial diametaphysis from osteonecrosis. *B*, T1 coronal image, pelvis. The signal of the marrow in the spine is lower than disk, and in the femora and pelvis it is equal to or lower than muscle. These findings are from reconversion from yellow to red marrow in response to sickle cell anemia. The linear signal in the left femoral head is from osteonecrosis.

row occurred during normal maturation (Fig. 2–10). Marrow reconversion starts in areas that are predominately red marrow and progresses to areas that are predominately yellow marrow. Regarding the progression of changes in the entire skeleton, the axial skeleton undergoes red marrow hyperplasia ⋆ earliest, followed by the peripheral (appendicular) skeleton. The humeri and femora are affected before the bones of the forearm and lower leg. In an individual long bone, marrow reconversion first affects the proximal metaphysis, followed by the distal metaphysis, then the diaphysis. If there is an extreme

need to recruit red marrow in response to an increased demand for hematopoiesis, the epiphyses and apophyses of long bones will convert to cellular red marrow. ⋆

MRI of marrow reconversion shows an abnormal distribution of marrow signal, with replacement of areas expected to be composed of yellow marrow by focal or diffuse areas of red marrow that have signal characteristics identical to normal red marrow (see Fig. 2–9). If red marrow hyperplasia is massive, the signal intensity is abnormal and isointense or even lower signal than muscle and disk on T1W images because of near-complete replacement of all fatty elements in the marrow.

An increased demand for hematopoiesis may exist in circumstances of replacement or destruction of normal red marrow by diffuse marrow proliferative disorders or marrow replacement disorders. It also may be seen in severe anemias such as sickle cell anemia and thalassemia from hemolysis, in high-level athletes with increased oxygen requirements (marathon runners), in high altitudes, or as an incidental finding, usually in obese women smokers. Hematopoiesis also is stimulated by administration of human hematopoietic growth factors in patients being treated with high-dose chemotherapy.

Mild marrow reconversion as an incidental finding in adult women who are obese (and who are often smokers) is probably the most common cause of marrow reconversion seen on MRI. The proposed theory for this incidental marrow expansion is that

---

BOX 2–8: RECONVERSION OF YELLOW TO RED MARROW

Increased demand for hematopoiesis
- Incidental finding, obese women
- Hemolytic anemias (sickle cell, thalassemia, sports)
- Increased oxygen requirements
  - High altitudes
  - High-level athletes
- Replacement/destruction of normal red marrow from marrow proliferative or replacement disorders
- Granulocyte colony-stimulating factor given as part of chemotherapy

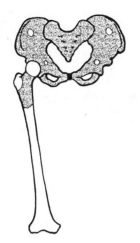
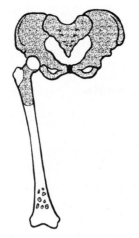
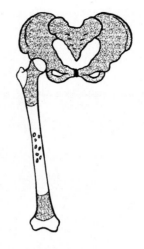

Figure 2–10. MARROW PRO-LIFERATIVE DISORDERS: Reconversion.
Diagram of the axial and appendicular skeleton's response to an increased demand for hematopoeisis, which leads to marrow reconversion from yellow to red marrow. This occurs in exactly the reverse order as does normal conversion from red to yellow marrow. If severe enough, even the epiphyses will undergo reconversion.

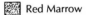 Red Marrow

 Cartilage

☐ Yellow Marrow

these patients have a leukocytosis, possibly on the basis of chronic bronchitis, which may cause recruitment of myeloid elements in marrow. These women are of menstruating age, and this may contribute to the increased requirement for red marrow hyperplasia.

Sickle cell anemia results in an altered configuration of the red blood cells, preventing them from flowing through small vessels, which causes vascular obstruction and tissue infarction. Thus, the two MRI features of sickle cell anemia in the marrow are those of reconversion with red marrow hyperplasia and bone infarction (see Fig. 2–9) (Box 2–9). Other severe anemias, such as thalassemia, cause identical changes as sickle cell anemia regarding marrow reconversion, but bone infarctions are not typical.

Leukemias. The proliferation of leukemic cells in bone marrow replaces normal red marrow elements, ultimately leading to anemia, neutropenia, and thrombocytopenia. Marrow aspiration or biopsy is required for definitive diagnosis.

MRIs of marrow in patients with leukemia show focal or, much more commonly, diffuse abnormalities, usually in the metaphyses and diaphyses of bones. Infiltration of marrow by leukemic cells also may extend into the epiphyses and apophyses of patients with leukemia, which is an indication of a large tumor load. Abnormal signal intensity in

---

BOX 2–9: OSTEONECROSIS SUPERIMPOSED ON DIFFUSE MARROW ABNORMALITIES

- Sickle cell anemia
- Waldenström's macroglobulinemia
- Gaucher disease
- Marrow proliferative or replacement disorders treated with steroids

---

epiphyses and apophyses also may represent red marrow hyperplasia occurring because of replacement of red marrow elsewhere by leukemic infiltrate. On T1W images, there is abnormal marrow signal intensity that is lower than muscle and disk; the signal intensity increases so it is somewhat higher than fat on T2W images (or higher signal than muscle on STIR images) because of the high water content of leukemic cells (Fig. 2–11). The T2W findings, however, are variable; often leukemic infiltrate will have little increased signal intensity and may resemble an excessive amount of red marrow (Fig. 2–11). Serial MRI has been shown to allow accurate monitoring of the disease for remission and relapse in children with acute lymphocytic leukemia.

Monoclonal Gammopathies. Monoclonal gammopathies consist of a spectrum of diseases, categorized by severity. The *aggressive monoclonal gammopathies* are multiple myeloma, primary amyloidosis, Waldenström's macroglobulinemia, and lymphoproliferative disorder.

The *nonmyelomatous monoclonal gammopathies* (further divided into monoclonal gammopathy of undetermined significance and monoclonal gammopathy of borderline significance) are less aggressive marrow disorders. These two types of gammopathy constitute a large subgroup of asymptomatic patients who are discovered, usually incidentally, to have small amounts of monoclonal protein in their blood; they require no therapy. However, 19% of these patients will progress within 10 years to an aggressive monoclonal gammopathy that requires treatment. The current method of determining which patients progress to aggressive disease is by routine measurements of monoclonal protein in the urine and blood, and often by bone marrow aspirates as well. MRI has been shown to be a valuable adjunct in predicting which patients are likely to have disease progression, allowing for more appropriate management of patients. Those patients who

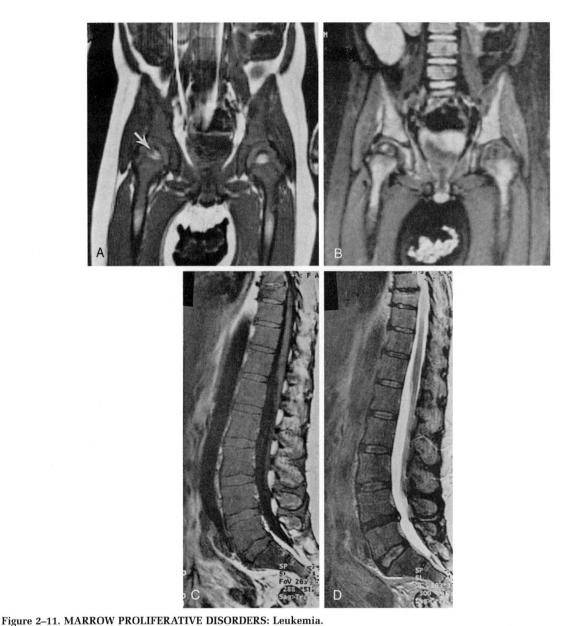

Figure 2–11. MARROW PROLIFERATIVE DISORDERS: Leukemia.
A, T1 coronal image, pelvis. This is a 2-year-old child who presented with a limp and had normal radiographs and an abnormal radionuclide bone scan at the right iliac wing above the acetabulum. The MRI shows diffuse marrow signal that is equal to muscle, which is abnormal. In addition, there is an abnormal distribution with a focal round area of abnormal signal in the right femoral head *(arrow)*, which should be entirely fat at this age. **B**, STIR coronal image, pelvis. The marrow becomes significantly higher signal than muscle, which is abnormal. Abnormal signal in the soft tissues adjacent to the right iliac wing corresponds to the only abnormal focus on bone scan. The high signal between the legs is the dirty diaper (like almost everything else, a dirty diaper is low signal on T1 and high signal on T2). Biopsy of the iliac crest demonstrated leukemia. **C**, T1 sagittal image, lumbar spine (different patient than in *A* and *B*). There is diffuse abnormal signal throughout the vertebral bodies that is slightly lower signal than adjacent intervertebral disks. There is a fracture at T9, which is why the patient presented with back pain. Marrow aspirate showed leukemia. **D**, Fast T2 sagittal image, lumbar spine (same patient as in *C*). There is no increased signal except in the fractured T9 vertebral body. This is the typical appearance of most leukemias on T2 types of sequence.

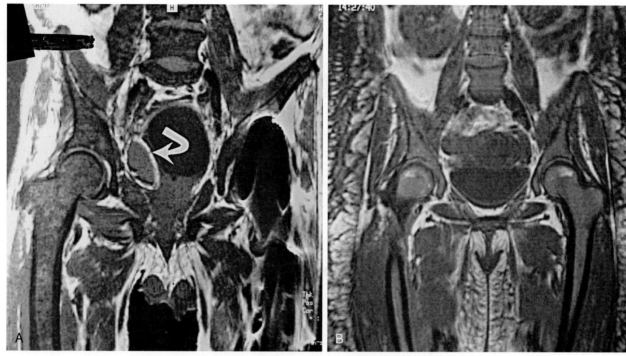

Figure 2–12. MARROW PROLIFERATIVE DISORDERS: Aggressive gammopathies.
A, T1 coronal image, pelvis. There is diffuse marrow signal and distribution abnormalities from Waldenström's macroglobulinemia. The marrow is equal to or lower in signal to muscle and disks and involves the diaphysis of the femur as well as the epiphysis. There is a hematoma *(curved arrow)* adjacent to a fracture in the pubic ramus. *B,* T1 coronal image, pelvis (different patient than in *A*). This woman has primary amyloidosis. The marrow distribution is abnormal, with replacement of fatty marrow in the diaphyses of the femora, of the greater trochanters, and patchy replacement in the femoral heads. The signal of the marrow is normal, being slightly higher than muscle. There is diffuse subcutaneous edema.

are likely to progress to an aggressive gammopathy will have MRI abnormalities that consist of diffuse or focal marrow lesions in the spine or pelvis, similar to those seen in multiple myeloma.[22, 23]

Malignant

Aggressive Gammopathies (Plasma Cell Dyscrasias). Multiple myeloma, amyloidosis, and Waldenström's macroglobulinemia are very closely related to one another and have essentially identical MRI appearances (Fig. 2–12). One difference that may be evident with Waldenström's disease is bone infarctions, which occur as a result of the hyperviscosity of the blood.

Multiple myeloma is a common disease of uncontrolled, malignant proliferation of plasma cells in the absence of an antigenic stimulus. Proliferation of plasma cells causes production of an osteoclastic stimulating factor and inhibition of osteoblastic activity, which in turn leads to trabecular destruction and diffuse osteopenia. Radionuclide bone scans are often normal because of the lack of osteoblastic response in this disease. Laboratory findings are extremely important for making the diagnosis of myeloma, but they are not always present or conclusive, either initially or later in the disease. Bone biopsy or marrow aspiration is an important method of documenting the diagnosis. MRI is probably the most valuable imaging technique to establish

the presence and precise location of abnormalities in order to guide a marrow biopsy, because the process may be focal or diffuse and blind marrow aspirates in the pelvis may not accurately reflect the nature of the problem. MRI may be useful in patients with a presumed solitary plasmacytoma; more than one marrow lesion is seen on MRI in 25% of these patients, which may alter therapy.[22]

The marrow patterns of multiple myeloma on MRI, in increasing order of severity of disease, are (1) normal marrow pattern, (2) focal lesions, (3) variegated pattern, and (4) diffuse homogeneous pattern (Figs. 2–13 through 2–15) (Box 2–10).[3, 24]

Focal lesions on MRI from myeloma may be equal to or lower in signal intensity than muscle or disk on T1W images; hemorrhage into a lesion occasionally results in high signal intensity in a focal lesion on T1W images. On T2W images, lesions may either be low or high signal intensity in approximately equal numbers in untreated patients. The findings are identical to those of metastatic disease, unless a pattern known as the "mini-brain" is present (Fig. 2–13). The mini-brain appearance occurs in some focal myeloma lesions as thick bone struts radiating inward from the outer margins of a focal lesion, resembling the sulci and gyri pattern of the brain.

The variegated pattern of myeloma has the appearance of many small, low signal intensity foci on T1W images, as if cracked black pepper were sprinkled on the marrow. There may be some mild,

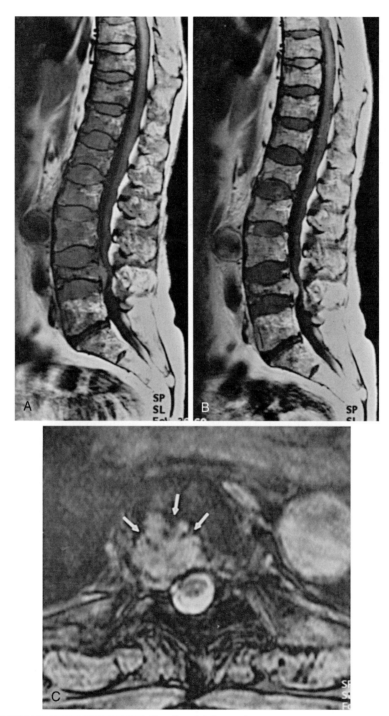

Figure 2–13. MARROW PROLIFERATIVE DISORDERS: Focal multiple myeloma.
A, T1 sagittal image, lumbar spine. There are multiple focal marrow lesions, indistinguishable from metastases. Many vertebral bodies are compressed as a result of the myeloma. There is an epidural mass posterior to the L4 vertebral body. *B*, T1 contrast-enhanced sagittal image, lumbar spine. Many of the lesions show contrast enhancement, obscuring the lesions. If the patient has received therapy for the myeloma, this indicates a poor response. The epidural mass is easier to see because of the enhancement. *C*, T2* axial image, spine (different patient than in *A* and *B*). A focal lesion of multiple myeloma demonstrates the "mini-brain" appearance that, when present, helps to distinguish myeloma from metastatic disease. Thick bone struts *(arrows)* are radiating into the lesion from its outer margin, creating the sulci and gyri pattern.

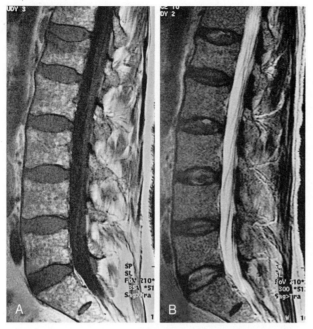

Figure 2–14. MARROW PROLIFERATIVE DISORDERS: Variegated pattern of myeloma.
A, T1 sagittal image, lumbar spine. There is a diffuse, stippled appearance to the marrow that looks like pepper has been sprinkled on fatty marrow. This is a more aggressive pattern of myeloma than focal lesions. There is a fracture of L1. *B*, Fast T2 sagittal image, lumbar spine. The marrow appears normal on this sequence.

increased signal intensity on T2W images. This pattern is relatively specific for myeloma (Fig. 2–14).

The diffuse pattern of myeloma is a homogeneous pattern of marrow replacement without features to distinguish it from many other marrow proliferative entities (Fig. 2–15). There may be a mix of more than one of the four marrow patterns in a single patient with myeloma, as a result of the disease progressing or regressing.

A successful response to therapy can be inferred in patients with myeloma who initially have high signal intensity lesions on T2W images that become

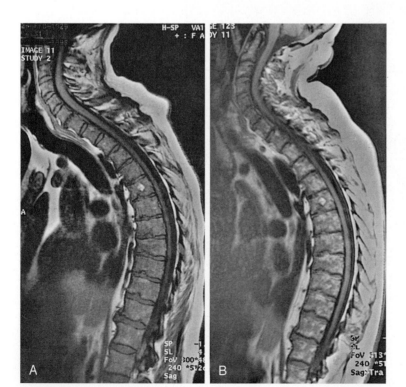

Figure 2–15. MARROW PROLIFERATIVE DISORDERS: Diffuse pattern of myeloma.
A, T1 sagittal image, cervical and upper thoracic spine. The marrow is diffusely and homogeneously intermediate signal, similar to the intervertebral disks. This is a 70-year-old man who should have much more fatty marrow present. *B*, T1 postcontrast sagittal image, spine. There is heterogenous marrow with many areas of contrast enhancement. Normal red marrow in adults does not show contrast enhancement. This patient has received therapy for his myeloma and the enhancement indicates a poor response.

low signal intensity after treatment. Because 50% of myeloma lesions are low signal intensity on T2W images before treatment, this finding is of no significance unless patients have had both pre- and post-treatment scans. Because of this confusing picture, gadolinium has been used after therapy to try to determine if there has been a successful response.

The preliminary work with gadolinium after therapy for myeloma suggests it is useful for predicting therapeutic response and prognosis. Complete response to chemotherapy includes the following post-contrast enhancement patterns: (1) complete resolution of abnormality, (2) persistent abnormality with no enhancement, and (3) peripheral rim enhancement only.[24] A partial response to chemotherapy showed conversion of a diffuse to a focal or variegated pattern with persistent contrast enhancement.

The Bottom Line. The benign and malignant proliferative disorders arising from existing marrow elements may have a variable appearance, either focal or diffuse, or both. All of the disorders have a very similar appearance to one another, and cellular red marrow hyperplasia may look like benign or malignant cellular deposition. So, why do MRI?

MRI establishes that a disease is present, which is not always easy on a clinical or laboratory basis. Even if laboratory findings are abnormal, a marrow biopsy or aspirate often is required to establish the diagnosis. Blind marrow aspirates usually are performed for this purpose. Sampling error can be great, considering the variability in extent and location of disease as demonstrated on MRI. A biopsy can be properly directed toward an abnormal site in the marrow based on MRI. Response of a disease to therapy can be monitored with serial MRI examinations.

Marrow Replacement Disorders
(Box 2–11)

Unlike marrow proliferative diseases, which usually are diffuse and arise from cells that originate in

---

BOX 2–11: MARROW REPLACEMENT DISORDERS

- Implantation of cells in marrow that do not normally exist there
- Focal lesions, usually

Benign	Malignant
Primary bone tumors	Metastases
Osteomyelitis	Lymphoma
	Primary bone tumors

- MRI
  - T1: low signal (equal or lower than muscle, disk)
  - T2: variable, but usually high signal

BOX 2–12: HALO SIGNS

T1 halo ("the angel")
  Resolving lesion; high-signal fat on T1 images surrounding periphery of shrinking marrow lesion
T2 halo ("the devil")
  Active lesion; high-signal edema on T2 images surrounding a focal marrow lesion

---

the bone marrow, the most common marrow replacement diseases usually are focal abnormalities that arise from cells other than those inherent in the bone marrow. The major marrow replacement disorders include metastatic disease, lymphoma, primary bone tumors, and osteomyelitis.

Skeletal Metastases. The typical MRI appearance of metastatic disease in the bone marrow is that of focal, often multiple lesions characterized by low signal intensity on T1W images that become higher signal intensity than surrounding marrow on T2W sequences (Fig. 2–16). Sclerotic metastases usually, but not always, show low signal intensity on all pulse sequences. Marrow and soft tissue edema surrounding a metastatic lesion may be extensive or nonexistent. Benign lesions such as bone islands, Paget's disease, and hemangiomas can have appearances similar to metastases, and evaluation of MRI studies should always be done by correlating with other imaging examinations to avoid errors. Although most metastatic lesions are focal, metastases also may show a diffuse pattern in the marrow that is either homogeneous or heterogeneous in appearance (Fig. 2–17).

MRI is exquisitely sensitive to detecting metastatic disease and surpasses all other imaging techniques in this regard. Screening MRI studies of the entire skeleton for metastases (Fig. 2–18) may become the standard of practice in the future, but currently MRI generally is used as a problem-solving tool to clarify abnormalities of uncertain significance detected by other imaging.[25] Patients with bone pain or abnormal laboratory values may have metastases not evident on other studies, whereas MRI will show lesions (Figs. 2–16 and 2–18).[25–27]

MRI can show that lesions change in size with time. Monitoring the response of metastases to therapy may allow appropriate and early alteration of therapy (Box 2–12). A focal lesion surrounded by a halo of high signal intensity edema on T2W images (the T2 halo sign) indicates an active lesion (Fig. 2–19). A rim of high signal intensity yellow marrow surrounding a focal marrow lesion on T1W images (the T1 halo sign) is observed in treated lesions that have responded (Fig. 2–19).[18] Complete fatty replacement of marrow where lesions once existed can occur after treatment for metastases (Fig. 2–20).[28]

MRI also is useful in demonstrating the extent of a lesion in the bone as well as relative to other

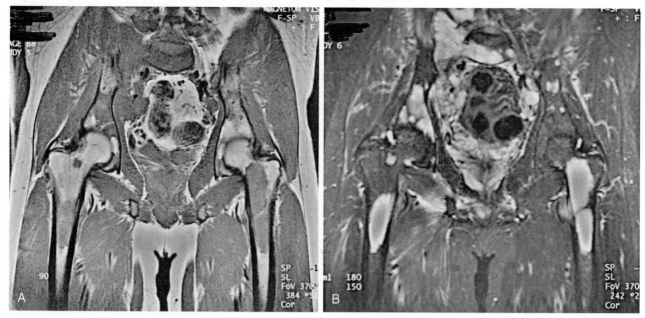

Figure 2–16. MARROW REPLACEMENT DISORDERS: Focal metastases.
A, T1 coronal image, pelvis. This 32-year-old patient with adenocarcinoma of the urachis had posterior pelvis pain but a normal bone scan and radiographs. MRI shows multiple intermediate signal focal bone metastases involving the proximal femora and scattered throughout the pelvic bones and the sacrum. *B,* STIR coronal image, pelvis. The metastatic lesions become very high signal on this sequence, which is typical of most metastases.

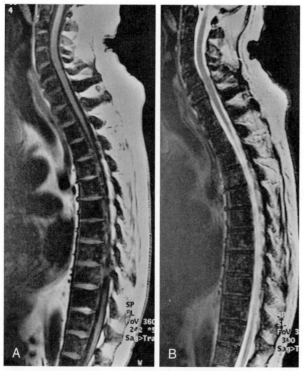

Figure 2–17. MARROW REPLACEMENT DISORDERS: Diffuse metastases.
A, T1 sagittal image, cervical and upper thoracic spine. Patient with prostate cancer and diffuse skeletal metastases. The image gives an appearance identical to many of the marrow proliferative disorders. The metastases are sclerotic, which gives the very low signal on the MRI. *B,* Fast T2 sagittal image, spine. The diffuse metastases remain low signal on the T2 sequence, which is typical of most sclerotic metastases.

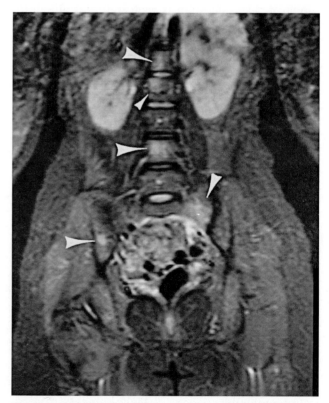

Figure 2–18. MARROW REPLACEMENT DISORDERS: Screening for metastases.
STIR coronal image, spine/pelvis. This is part of an MR marrow survey that covers the entire body from head to toe. Multiple high-signal bone metastases *(arrowheads)* were discovered in this 41-year-old with breast cancer, whereas bone scintigraphy was negative.

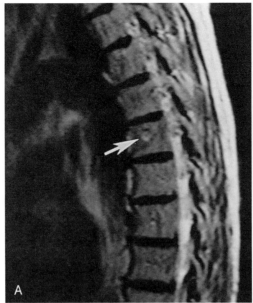
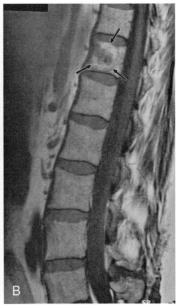

Figure 2–19. MARROW REPLACEMENT DISORDERS: The halo signs.
A, Fast T2 sagittal image, thoracic spine. There is a small lesion with surrounding edema (the T2 halo sign; *arrow*). This indicates active disease, and this proved to be metastatic lung cancer. *B*, T1 sagittal image, lumbar spine (different patient than in *A*). There is a low-signal lesion in the T12 vertebral body surrounded by fat *(arrows)*. This is the T1 halo sign, which indicates a positive response of a metastasis to therapy. The fatty rim is where tumor previously existed. This patient was undergoing treatment for metastatic carcinoid.

adjacent structures, such as the spinal cord (Fig. 2–21).

Areas of increased activity on a radionuclide bone scan in patients with a known primary carcinoma have been shown to be from benign causes in many instances.[29] The superior anatomic resolution of MRI compared to radionuclide studies allows more specific diagnoses to be made. Many patients with cancer are older and osteoporotic. Chemotherapy (especially steroids) and radiation therapy contribute to osteoporosis. Thus, insufficiency fractures, often multiple, are common in this group. Osteonecrosis from steroid therapy is also a common finding. Bursitis, fasciitis, tendinitis, and other soft tissue inflammatory changes can incite a hyperemic response in adjacent marrow that may be suspicious for metastases on a bone scan but is clearly from a benign process on MRI. The nonspecificity of bone scans has led us to require an MRI prior to biopsy of bone lesions in patients who have normal conventional radiographs, in order to establish that there is indeed a lesion present that should be biopsied.

Osteoporotic Versus Pathologic Vertebral Compression Fracture (Box 2–13). Determining if an

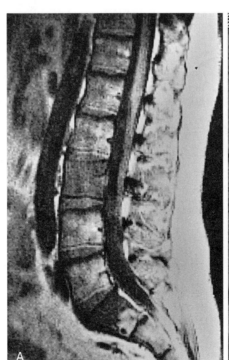
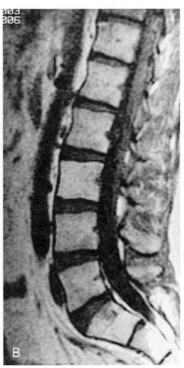

Figure 2–20. MARROW REPLACEMENT DISORDERS: Treated lesions replaced by fat.
A, T1 sagittal image, lumbar spine. Several focal marrow replacement lesions are seen, most pronounced at L3 and S1, from Hodgkin's lymphoma. This MRI was done prior to treatment. *B*, T1 sagittal image, lumbar spine. Following therapy, all of the focal marrow lymphoma lesions have disappeared (as has the red marrow). Complete fatty replacement where the lesions previously existed indicates a positive response.

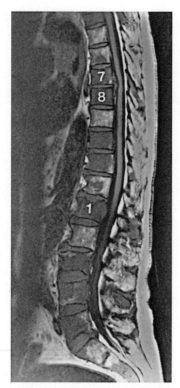

Figure 2–21. MARROW REPLACEMENT DISORDERS.
T1 sagittal image, thoracic and lumbar spine. MRI demonstrates the presence of metastatic lesions in the spine of this woman with breast cancer. In addition, it shows the relationship of the lesions to adjacent structures. There are epidural masses extending into the anterior epidural space posterior to T7 and T8 with compression of the spinal cord, and also posterior to L1.

acute fracture of a vertebral body occurred on the basis of tumor from metastasis or from osteoporosis is a commonly encountered dilemma, especially in patients with a known primary tumor. Both entities will show a fractured vertebral body with replacement of normal marrow by low signal intensity on T1W MRI. The low signal in the marrow either

represents tumor or hemorrhage and edema from a nonpathologic fracture (Figs. 2–22 and 2–23). T2W features vary and are not helpful in making a distinction between benign and malignant. Features that suggest tumor are abnormal low signal intensity extending into the pedicles and other posterior spinal elements, involvement of the entire vertebral body by abnormal signal intensity, associated soft tissue mass, and multiple bone lesions. Features suggestive of an osteoporotic fracture are absence of the above features; abnormal signal does not involve the entire vertebral body, but has a horizontal straight line or band separating the abnormal signal intensity from the normal fatty marrow signal.[3, 30, 31] A linear horizontal fracture line from compressed trabeculae also has been proposed as a sign of benignancy, whereas a vertebral body that collapses from tumor will not have a fracture line evident because the trabeculae are destroyed by tumor. The posterior vertebral body wall often has an angled appearance from a benign fracture, whereas fractures related to metastases more often result in a bowed or convex posterior wall.

The signs that help differentiate tumor from osteoporotic compression fractures are interesting and it is valuable to be aware of them. However, for an individual patient, the difference between having metastatic disease or not is of such importance that it is usually not adequate to depend on these signs to declare a patient tumor-free or not (Figs. 2–22 and 2–23). In patients who are at risk for having metastatic disease, we recommend following the lesion with a limited MRI examination in about 8 weeks or else performing a biopsy to establish a definitive diagnosis. Osteoporotic fractures will show partial or complete resolution of the marrow abnormalities on follow-up MRI, whereas tumor will be unchanged or will progress during the same interval.

Lymphoma. About 95% of lymphomas in bone are deposited in the marrow from circulating blood, which carried the cells from an extraskeletal primary site. MRI characteristics are indistinguishable from those of metastatic carcinoma. In general, lymphoma affecting bone has low signal intensity on both T1 and T2W images. Osseous dissemination of lymphoma is seen in 20% to 50% of patients with a primary extraskeletal lymphoma at postmortem examination. Blind marrow aspirates in patients with lymphoma show marrow involvement much less frequently. The focal nature of lymphoma accounts for this discrepancy, and biopsies directed to a specific lesion seen on MRI would allow more accurate staging and treatment of the disease to occur.

Benign and Malignant Primary Bone Tumors. These are focal lesions of bone marrow. The precise nature of the lesions is best diagnosed by conventional radiographs. The extent of the tumor in the marrow and the relationship to adjacent structures can be determined best with MRI. Monitoring the response to therapy is valuable with MRI. This is a varied and large group of diseases, and this topic as well as osteomyelitis are marrow replacement diseases that are covered elsewhere.

BOX 2–13: OSTEOPOROTIC VERSUS PATHOLOGIC VERTEBRAL FRACTURES

OSTEOPOROTIC	PATHOLOGIC
• Abnormal signal limited to vertebral body	• Abnormal signal in pedicles, other posterior elements
• Usually no soft tissue hematoma/mass	• Associated soft tissue mass
• Some fatty marrow persists in vertebral body	• Entire vertebral body involved
• Usually solitary	• Convex posterior wall
• Angled posterior wall	• No fracture line
• Fracture line	

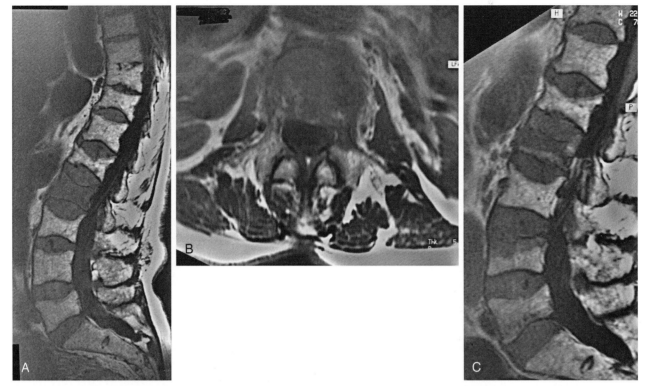

Figure 2–22. OSTEOPOROTIC VERSUS PATHOLOGIC COMPRESSION FRACTURE.
A, T1 sagittal image, lumbar spine. Several compression fractures are present in this woman with a history of primary malignancy. The L2 vertebral body is fractured and completely replaced by low signal, a feature suspicious for tumor. *B*, T1 axial image through L2. There is extension of abnormal signal from the vertebral body into the left pedicle, another sign suspicious for tumor as the basis for the fracture. *C*, T1 sagittal image, lumbar spine. This follow-up MRI was obtained 8 weeks after the study in *A* and *B* above. The L2 vertebral body has collapsed a bit more in the interval, but there is partial regression of the low signal so that the inferior vertebral body shows linear high signal, paralleling the endplate. This could only occur with a benign fracture, because untreated tumor would not regress spontaneously in this short interval. The L4 vertebral body has collapsed partially since the first study, and it also has a straight line separation between fat marrow (below) and low-signal marrow (above). This is a typical acute benign fracture.

Marrow Depletion (Box 2–14)

Diffuse or regional absence of normal red marrow may occur as a consequence of aplastic anemia, chemotherapy, and radiation therapy. We do not image in order to diagnose these entities. Rather, we often image patients who have had radiation or chemotherapy to look for evidence of tumor. The typical reason to image patients with aplastic anemia is that they have pain from osteonecrosis secondary to the steroids they took as part of the treatment for their disease. We must recognize the findings of marrow depletion and subsequent marrow regeneration in order not to misinterpret the findings.

Aplastic Anemia. There are two marrow MRI patterns that may be seen in patients with aplastic anemia.[32, 33] One pattern is that of diffuse yellow marrow throughout the skeleton in areas where red marrow is expected to exist (Fig. 2–24). This pattern may be difficult to recognize as abnormal in older individuals, who normally have large proportions of fatty marrow. The second pattern is seen in patients who have been treated for aplastic anemia and develop focal islands of red marrow regeneration scattered throughout the yellow marrow (Fig. 2–24). These islands of red marrow can be very focal in appearance and may simulate other diseases.

Chemotherapy. There may be no changes in the MRI of patients receiving chemotherapy. Others have diffuse ablation of the red marrow elements and an appearance identical to that of untreated aplastic anemia, with diffuse fatty marrow that has

---

BOX 2–14: MARROW DEPLETION

- Ablation of red marrow elements
- Diffuse or regional distribution
- Causes
  - Chemotherapy
  - Radiation therapy
  - Aplastic anemia
- MRI
  - T1: diffuse or regional high signal, typical of fat
  - T2: marrow signal follows fat (low signal on STIR or fat saturation, intermediate on T2, high on turbo T2 without fat saturation)

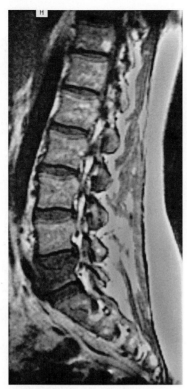

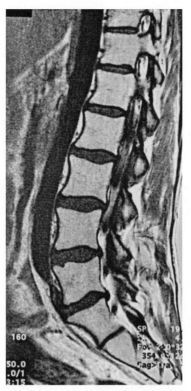

Figure 2–23. OSTEOPOROTIC VERSUS PATHOLOGIC COMPRESSION FRACTURE.
T1 sagittal image, lumbar spine. There is a straight line cutoff between low signal in the upper portion of the fractured L5 vertebral body and high-signal fat in the lower portion, paralleling the endplate. This suggests a benign osteoporotic fracture. The angled posterior vertebral body wall fragments also suggest this is benign. The vertebra was biopsied because of a history of breast cancer. This was metastatic disease. The point is to follow or biopsy these lesions in people at risk, because the rules for differentiating these lesions are not very good.

Figure 2–25. MARROW DEPLETION: Chemotherapy.
T1 sagittal lumbar spine. The marrow is diffusely high-signal intensity from fat as the result of ablation of the red marrow elements from systemic chemotherapy.

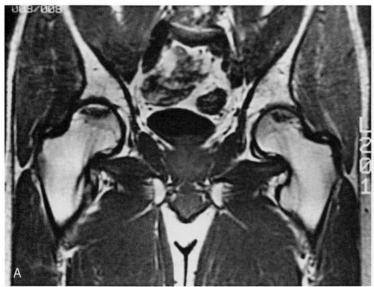

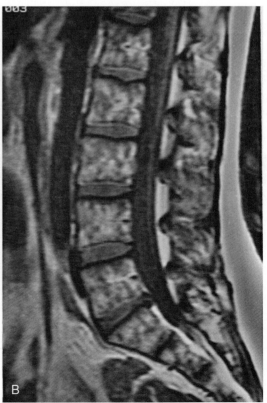

Figure 2–24. MARROW DEPLETION: Aplastic anemia.
A, T1 coronal image, pelvis. There is high-signal fatty marrow throughout the pelvis and hips (with the exception of avascular necrosis in both femoral heads). The marrow normally should be more intermediate in signal. This is from aplastic anemia. *B*, T1 sagittal image, lumbar spine (same patient as in *A*). There is diffuse heterogeneous marrow signal. This was biopsied and showed islands of regenerating red marrow in this patient, who was treated for aplastic anemia.

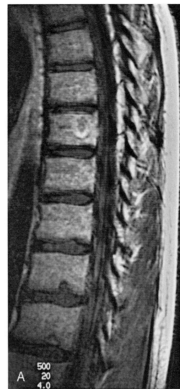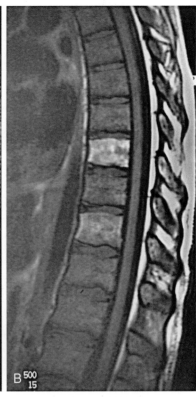

Figure 2–26. INCREASED RED MARROW FROM HEMATOPOIETIC GROWTH FACTOR CHEMO-THERAPY.
A, T1 sagittal image, thoracic spine. The marrow is generally a patchy intermediate signal intensity that is higher than adjacent disks. There are no definite signs of metastases in this 16-year-old patient with a primitive neuroectodermal tumor. *B*, T1 sagittal image, thoracic spine. The marrow has become diffusely intermediate signal, and much lower signal than on the original MRI done 9 months earlier *(A)*. The diffuse intermediate signal is from red marrow stimulation that occurred from receiving granulocyte colony-stimulating factor. The high-signal fatty marrow in the two vertebral bodies indicate there was tumor present at the time of the original MRI that has been destroyed by the therapy.

MRI signal characteristics that follow those of subcutaneous fat on all pulse sequences (Fig. 2–25).

An important caveat regarding chemotherapy is that some patients being treated for musculoskeletal malignancies (usually primary bone tumors) receive human hematopoietic growth factors (granulocyte or granulocyte–macrophage colony-stimulating factor) with their neoadjuvant chemotherapy regimen.[34] This is given in order to boost the patient's red marrow production and prevent the negative sequelae of chemotherapy-induced myelosuppression, allowing earlier and more intense therapy to be administered. This iatrogenic red marrow stimulation appears as diffuse or patchy areas of low signal intensity on T1W images similar to muscle, and unchanged or slightly high signal intensity on T2W images, similar to normal red marrow in its signal intensity (Fig. 2–26). The changes in the marrow can be striking and rapid from this therapy (Box 2–15).

Radiation. Metastases and multiple myeloma often are treated with local radiation. Red marrow elements are preferentially destroyed as compared to fatty marrow cells, because of the greater sensitivity of the immature red marrow cells to radiation.

The extent of ablation of red marrow and its ability to recover is dose dependent. Changes in marrow signal intensity on MRI relate to the dose of radiation received as well as to the amount of time elapsed since treatment.[35]

Patients who receive radiation to the spine usually show no marrow changes by MRI during the first 2 weeks after treatment. Between 3 and 6 weeks post-treatment, most of the red marrow disappears and there is diffuse fatty marrow centrally in the vertebral body. A second pattern that may be seen is that of an increased heterogeneity of the marrow because of partial red marrow ablation. After 6 weeks, all patients have homogeneous high signal intensity fatty marrow on T1W images because of ablation of the red marrow elements. Within 1 year of cessation of radiation therapy that was less than 30 Gy (relatively low dose), red marrow regeneration occurs diffusely in the radiated marrow so that it looks normal, or there may be a peripheral distribution of red marrow in the margins of the vertebral body only (Fig. 2–27). This pattern must not be confused with tumor. Marrow that receives doses greater than 50 Gy will never show regeneration of red marrow. MRI will show diffuse fatty marrow in

---

BOX 2–15: MARROW REGENERATION

- Occurs after
  - Chemotherapy
  - Treatment of aplastic anemia
  - Low-dose radiation
- MRI
  - T1: intermediate/low signal (higher or equal to muscle, disk)
  - T2: usually mild increased signal
  - Patterns: Focal islands
    Periphery of bone only
    Diffusely in bone

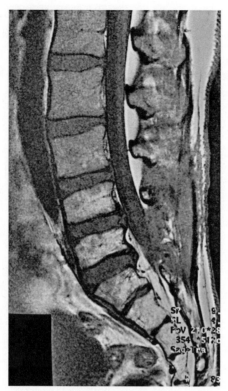

Figure 2–27. MARROW DEPLETION: Radiation.
T1 sagittal image, lumbar spine. This patient received pelvic radiation as a child for a sarcoma. The lower two lumbar vertebrae, as well as the sacrum, are hypoplastic as the result of radiation given during growth. The sacrum and lower lumbar spine also have more fatty marrow than the normal lumbar spine, seen from L1 through L3. A small amount of red marrow exists in the periphery of the radiated vertebral bodies, but most of the red marrow has been ablated and will never regenerate.

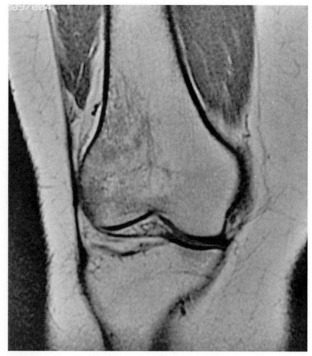

Figure 2–28. HYPEREMIA: Trauma.
T1 coronal image, knee, showing intermediate signal with no discrete pattern in the marrow of the lateral and distal aspects of the femur. This is typical of marrow edema, in this case from a lateral patellar dislocation that traumatized the femur.

the region of the treatment portal with a straight line cut-off between normal cellular red marrow and abnormal fatty marrow at the margin of the radiation port.

Vascular Abnormalities (Hyperemia and Ischemia)

The underlying cause of extracellular bone marrow edema is probably hyperemia. Different clinical abnormalities may lead to localized bone marrow edema, including trauma (bone contusions, stress and insufficiency fractures), transient osteoporosis of the hip, regional migratory osteoporosis, reflex sympathetic dystrophy syndrome, osteonecrosis (early), infection, tumors, and joint abnormalities (cartilage abrasion in degenerative joint disease).

The MRI appearance of marrow edema is that of intermediate signal intensity on T1W images and very high signal intensity on T2W images. The T1 signal intensity is almost always higher than muscle or disk on T1W images. The signal characteristics are the result of fatty marrow cells intermixed with the edema fluid (Fig. 2–28). It has a somewhat heterogeneous appearance without a discrete pattern. Tumor and infection generally have edema at the periphery of the underlying lesion (Fig. 2–29). Marrow edema from the other causes is not associated with an underlying mass (Box 2–16).

Transient Osteoporosis of the Hip. Mainly young and middle-aged men are affected in either hip by

---

BOX 2–16: VASCULAR ABNORMALITIES (HYPEREMIA)

- Hyperemia causes marrow edema
- Focal lesions, often involving epiphyses
- Causes
  - Trauma
  - Transient osteoporosis, hip
  - Regional migratory osteoporosis
  - Reflex sympathetic dystrophy syndrome
  - Infection
  - Tumors
  - Joint abnormalities (degenerative joint disease, cartilage abrasion)
  - Early osteonecrosis
- MRI
  - T1: intermediate signal (higher than muscle, disk)
  - T2: high signal
  - Heterogeneous, no discrete pattern

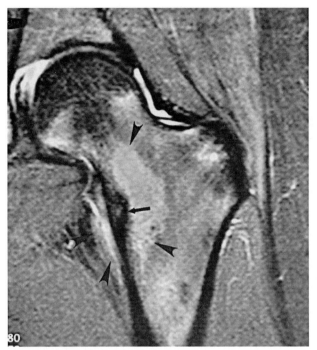

Figure 2–29. HYPEREMIA: Tumor.
STIR coronal image, left hip. There is a large area of high-signal marrow edema from hyperemia involving the medial aspect of the femoral neck and the soft tissues adjacent to the neck *(arrowheads)*. This edema surrounds an underlying osteoid osteoma *(arrow)*.

this painful process. Women with transient osteoporosis of the hip often are affected in the last trimester of pregnancy, with a predilection for the left hip. Osteoporosis may be so severe that fractures occur. The joint space remains normal, but joint effusions are common. Bone marrow edema usually affects

the femoral head and neck down to the intertrochanteric region (Fig. 2–30). Follow-up studies show resolution of edema and osteoporosis as the clinical symptoms subside in 3 to 12 months.[36, 37]

Regional Migratory Osteoporosis. This has the same MRI and clinical features as transient osteoporosis of the hip. The major difference is that abnormalities are not confined to the hip and are migratory in nature. The subchondral regions of the knee, ankle, and hip each may be affected in turn, and both extremities may be involved over several years (Fig. 2–31). Spontaneous recovery also occurs in this entity.

The pathogenesis of transient osteoporosis of the hip and regional migratory osteoporosis is not known, but clinical similarities to reflex sympathetic dystrophy syndrome are striking. The MRI findings for all of these entities are compatible with ischemic changes of the small vessels that supply proximal nerve roots, with loss of control of the normal vascular supply more distally, leading to localized hyperemia. If any abnormalities are seen in marrow from reflex sympathetic dystrophy, they are similar to the other two diseases, with patchy areas of intermediate signal intensity (higher than muscle or disk) on T1W images that become bright on T2W images.

The relationship between transient osteoporosis of the hip and regional migratory osteoporosis to osteonecrosis is not clear. Biopsy of these lesions shows areas of bone necrosis. There have been reports of typical changes of transient osteoporosis of the hip that, rather than undergoing spontaneous resolution, went on to develop typical MRI and biopsy changes of osteonecrosis in the femoral heads. Why this should occur in some patients, and in which patients, is not clear.

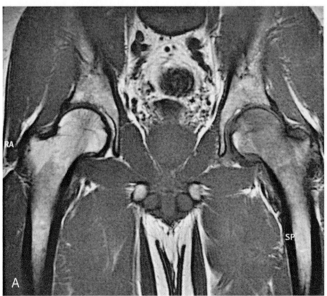
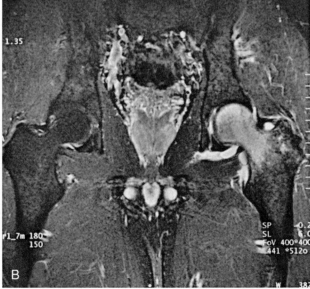

Figure 2–30. HYPEREMIA: Transient osteoporosis of the hip.
A, T1 coronal image, pelvis. There is abnormal intermediate signal in the left femoral head and neck, down to the intertrochanteric region. *B*, STIR coronal image, pelvis. The abnormality in the left hip becomes very high signal so that it looks like a light bulb, and there is a left hip joint effusion. The distribution of marrow edema is typical of transient osteoporosis of the hip.

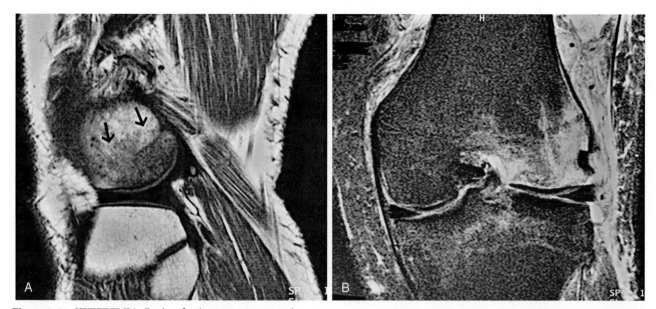

Figure 2–31. HYPEREMIA: Regional migratory osteoporosis.
A, T1 sagittal image, knee. There is intermediate signal in the lateral femoral condyle with fat mixed in *(arrows),* an appearance typical of marrow edema. *B,* STIR coronal image, knee. The marrow edema becomes very high signal, and there is edema in the adjacent soft tissues as well. This patient previously had transient osteoporosis of the hip, and later had it in the ankle.

Ischemia (Box 2–17). The causes of bone marrow infarction are numerous and include traumatic disruption of the blood supply, steroids, sickle cell anemia, Gaucher disease, alcoholism, pancreatitis, dysbaric causes, systemic lupus erythematosus, idiopathic causes, and other causes. Many people refer to ischemic changes in the epiphyses as avascular necrosis and to those in the shafts of bone as bone infarction. The MRI findings are the same regardless of the location of the lesions, and here we use the term osteonecrosis to mean ischemic

changes to bone and do not further differentiate by name as to the location of the lesions.

Osteonecrosis most commonly affects areas where yellow marrow (with its poor vascular supply) predominates: the epiphyses and diaphyses of long bones. In fact, patients with osteonecrosis of the femoral head have been shown by MRI to have more fatty than red marrow elements at an earlier age in the femoral neck and intertrochanteric region than did a control group, and this indicates a decreased blood supply to the region, which may predispose to developing osteonecrosis.[38]

The sensitivity of MRI for osteonecrosis exceeds that of all other imaging techniques. In addition to a high sensitivity, MRI also usually allows a specific diagnosis to be made. Early diagnosis is difficult by other imaging techniques and can resemble subtle metastases or infection.[39] An accurate and early diagnosis by MRI can avoid inappropriate therapy and allow early core decompression or other treatment, which will give the patient the best chance of recovery without the debilitating sequelae of bone collapse and secondary degenerative joint disease.

The MRI appearance of osteonecrosis varies somewhat, based on the age and stage of the lesion. The earliest manifestation seen with MRI is a nonspecific focal area of what looks like marrow edema, intermediate signal intensity on T1W and high signal intensity on T2W images, in the typical anatomic locations for infarction, that is, in the epiphyses and diametaphyses (Fig. 2–32).[40, 41] This appearance rapidly progresses to a distinctive, well-defined pattern that allows a specific diagnosis to be made.

A characteristic, low signal intensity serpentine rim develops in well over 90% of cases on both T1W and T2W images (Fig. 2–33).[42–49] This forms

---

BOX 2–17: VASCULAR ABNORMALITIES (ISCHEMIA)

- Ischemia causes osteonecrosis in poorly vascularized fatty marrow
- Focal lesions in epiphyses or diaphyses
- Usual causes
  - Trauma
  - Steroids
  - Sickle cell anemia
  - Dysbaric causes
  - Systemic lupus erythematosus
  - Gaucher disease
  - Alcoholism
  - Pancreatitis
  - Idiopathic
- MRI
  - Marrow edema early (intermediate signal, T1; high signal, T2)
  - Serpiginous, geographic patterns later
    T1: low-signal margin; center usually isointense to fat or may be low signal
    T2: low-signal margin (± double-line sign); center isointense to fat or may be low or high signal

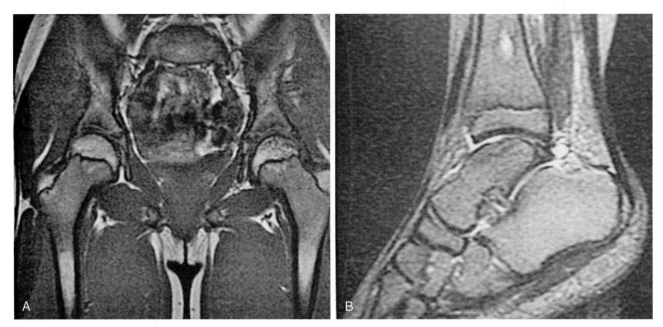

Figure 2–32. ISCHEMIA: Early changes.
A, T1 coronal image, pelvis. Vague, patchy abnormal signal is present in the left femoral head of this child, with early MR evidence of osteonecrosis. *B*, Spin echo-T2 sagittal image, ankle. There is an oblong high-signal abnormality in the distal tibial diametaphysis from early changes of osteonecrosis in this 5-year-old patient, who had a bone marrow transplant and was on steroids.

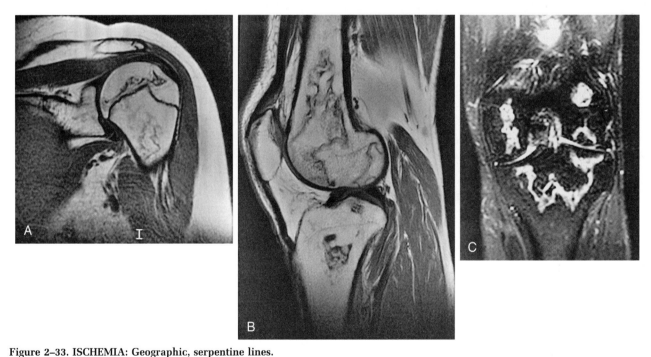

Figure 2–33. ISCHEMIA: Geographic, serpentine lines.
A, T1 coronal image, shoulder. This is a 16-year-old girl with Hodgkin's disease who had a bone marrow transplant. She had bone pain and a positive bone scan at multiple sites, with negative radiographs. MRI shows several areas of serpentine low-signal lines involving the proximal humeral epiphysis and diametaphysis from osteonecrosis. The thickest of the low-signal lines is the growth plate. Note that there is high-signal fatty marrow in the scapula and proximal humerus, which is abnormal at any age, as a result of the therapy that ablated her red marrow. *B*, T1 sagittal image, knee (different patient than in *A*). Serpiginous lines from osteonecrosis due to steroid therapy are evident in the distal femur and proximal tibia. This forms the geographic pattern typical of osteonecrosis (look closely and you can see Canada in the distal femur, with Hudson Bay dipping down to the articular surface). *C*, STIR coronal image, knee (same patient as in *B*). The serpiginous lines can become high signal on heavily T2W sequences, as seen here in both femoral condyles and the proximal tibia.

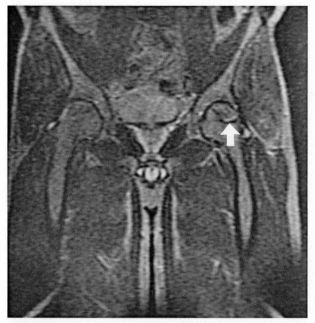

Figure 2–34. ISCHEMIA: The double-line sign.
Spin echo-T2 coronal image, pelvis. There is osteonecrosis of the left femoral head *(arrow)*, with a high-signal line just proximal to a low-signal line. This is the double-line sign of osteonecrosis. This is not necessary to make the diagnosis and is not always present. It is, however, frequently discussed.

what has been called a geographic pattern, because the areas of osteonecrosis resemble the shapes of different countries and states on a map. This serpentine line represents the interface at the junction between living and dead bone. This is the site of active bone repair, where new bone and an advancing front of granulation tissue is seen histologically. In approximately 80% of cases of osteonecrosis, a high signal intensity line will be present on T2W images just inside the low signal intensity serpentine line, called the "double-line sign" (Fig. 2–34). This probably occurs as a result of chemical shift misregistration or perhaps reflects the pathologic changes at the reactive bone interface.[50] A double-line sign is certainly not required to make the diagnosis of osteonecrosis. The area of bone within the infarcted segment usually has signal intensity identical to fat. Occasionally, the infarcted bone has signal that is low intensity on T1W and high signal on T2W images (edema), or low signal intensity on both T1W and T2W images (fibrosis, sclerosis, trabecular collapse). Symptoms tend to be least severe in lesions that are isointense with fat and most severe in those with low signal intensity on all pulse sequences. Joint effusions usually are present in cases of painful osteonecrosis that involve the epiphysis of a bone that makes up the joint.

MRI can be used to determine the volume and location of bone involved with osteonecrosis, and if there is collapse of bone or if degenerative changes are present.

Miscellaneous Marrow Diseases

There is an important group of abnormalities that affects bone marrow, but these abnormalities do not fit neatly into the other categories of marrow disease. These abnormalities are Gaucher disease, Paget's disease, osteopetrosis, hemosiderosis, and serous atrophy (gelatinous transformation) of marrow.

Gaucher Disease. This is a rare disease of cerebroside metabolism, where the enzyme glucocerebroside hydrolase is absent. This leads to accumulation of lipid material (glucocerebroside) in histiocytes throughout the reticuloendothelial system. Infiltration of marrow in the axial and proximal appendicular skeleton is common.

MRI findings of the marrow infiltration are nonspecific; however, there often are areas of osteonecrosis that significantly limit the differential diagnostic possibilities (Fig. 2–35). The marrow infiltration may be patchy or diffuse, and the signal intensity will be low on both T1W and T2W images. Erlenmeyer flask deformities of the distal femora are obvious on MRI. Occasionally, the Gaucher cells can be seen breaking out of the cortex and into the soft tissues surrounding the bone.

Treatment of Gaucher disease may consist of administration of an enzyme to break down the glucocerebroside. MRI often is used for monitoring the changes in the liver, spleen, and marrow in these patients. Decreased amounts of marrow infiltration are evident on serial images in patients who respond to the therapy (Fig. 2–36).

Paget's Disease. The MRI appearance of this disease varies, depending on the balance between osseous matrix and normal marrow. Common MRI findings in pagetic bone include areas of normal high signal intensity from fat and areas of intermediate or low signal intensity on T1W images (Fig. 2–37). The low signal intensity reflects fibrovascular connective tissue, dilated vascular channels, or uncalcified osteoid. Thick bone trabeculae and cortical bone can be seen, but not as easily as on conventional radiographs or computed tomography. This diagnosis often either is overlooked or misinterpreted as a hemangioma in the spine because of the large areas of fatty marrow that result in a nearly normal appearance. The diagnosis is so easy to make by correlating the MRI with conventional radiographs that there is no excuse to misdiagnose it unless there are no existing radiographs. Sarcomatous degeneration of pagetic bone, giant cell tumors within it, or metastases to areas of Paget's disease can be easily demonstrated on T1W MRI as low signal intensity marrow lesions or soft tissue masses replacing the bone; these lesions are high signal intensity on T2W images (Fig. 2–37). There is a higher incidence of metastases to pagetic bone because of its hypervascularity.

Osteopetrosis. This is a hereditary bone dysplasia with different manifestations, depending on the severity of disease. There is a decreased level of osteoclastic activity, so that there is not the normal differentiation between cortical and medullary bone. Cortical bone predominates, with mild or near complete obliteration of the marrow space, depending on which type of disease is present (there are four types, of varying severity). The recessive or lethal

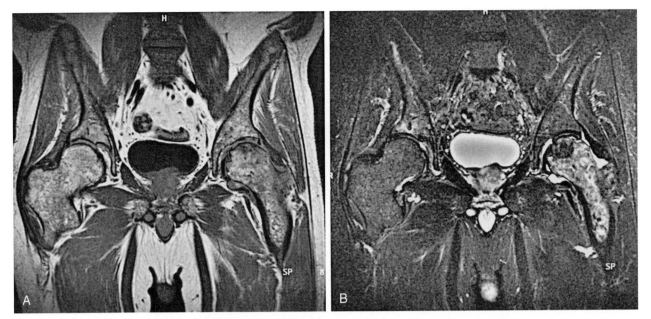

Figure 2–35. MISCELLANEOUS: Gaucher disease.
A, T1 coronal image, pelvis. There is diffuse, patchy abnormal intermediate signal throughout the visualized marrow, including the femoral epiphyses and apophyses. There is also osteonecrosis of the left femoral head and low-signal serpiginous lines in the right supraacetabular region from osteonecrosis. *B*, STIR coronal image, pelvis. The Gaucher cells in the marrow remain low signal. There is high signal in the left femoral neck and the right supraacetabular regions from the osteonecrosis.

form recently has been successfully treated with bone marrow transplants. MRI of the most severe cases shows low-signal cortical bone on all pulse sequences with little to no high signal intensity fatty bone marrow on T1W images (Fig. 2–38). After marrow transplant, the modeling abnormalities disappear and a marrow space with normal-appearing marrow develops. Milder forms of

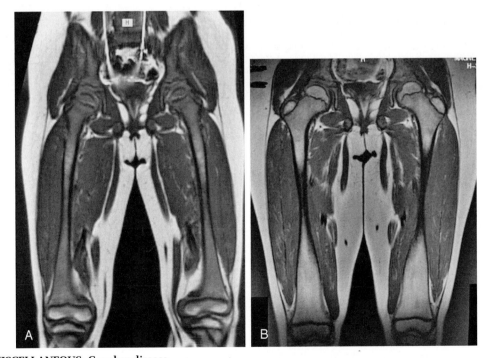

Figure 2–36. MISCELLANEOUS: Gaucher disease.
A, T1 coronal image, pelvis/femora. This is a 5-year-old child with Gaucher disease prior to treatment with enzyme therapy. There is abnormal marrow distribution with intermediate signal in the proximal and distal femoral epiphyses, the apophyses, and in the diaphyses. *B*, T1 coronal image, femora. Just over a year after initiating enzyme therapy for treatment of Gaucher disease, the marrow distribution has returned to normal, with fatty epiphyses and apophyses in the proximal and distal femora, and the marrow is not as low signal as it was pretreatment. Erlenmeyer flask deformities of the femora remain.

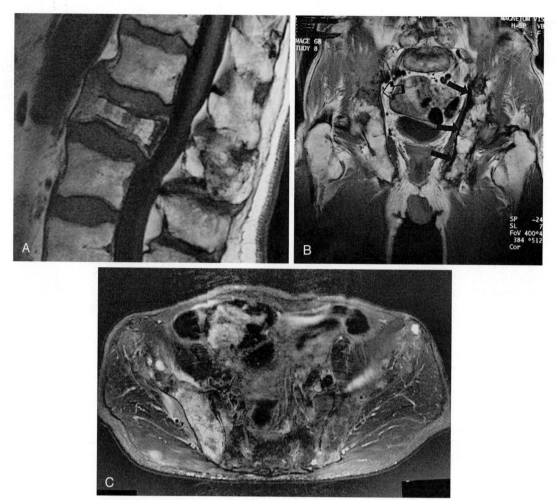

Figure 2–37. MISCELLANEOUS: Paget's disease.
A, T1 sagittal image, spine. There is a fracture of L1, and mixed regions of intermediate signal and high signal, with a peripheral rim of intermediate signal (the "picture frame" seen on radiography). Taking the fracture into account, the vertebra is still enlarged. There are thickened trabeculae. *B*, T1 coronal image, pelvis (different patient than in *A*). The bones of the pelvis are enlarged with thickened cortex *(solid arrows)* and thickened trabeculae. The signal of the marrow is high on the left side from fat in the pagetic bone, but on the right side there are focal areas of intermediate signal *(open arrow)*. *C*, STIR axial image, pelvis (same patient as in *B*). The fatty marrow is suppressed on this sequence, but large focal areas of high signal on the right side are evident with surrounding soft tissue edema. Biopsy of the right iliac showed metastatic disease to Pagetic bone.

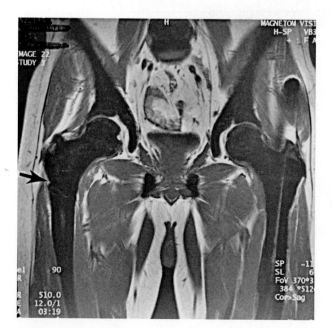

Figure 2–38. MISCELLANEOUS: Osteopetrosis.
T1 coronal image, pelvis. The bone is diffusely very low signal intensity. This is the result of osteopetrosis with lack of medullary bone and the presence of cortical bone diffusely. There is a pathologic fracture *(arrow)* in the right subtrochanteric region, which was much better seen on the STIR sequence. The left femur previously had an intramedullary rod placed for a pathologic fracture.

BOX 2–18: DIFFUSE VERY LOW SIGNAL (BLACK) MARROW

- Focal
  - Bone islands
  - Sclerotic metastases
  - Vacuum phenomenon (intraosseous)
- Diffuse
  - Mastocytosis
  - Hemosiderosis
  - Myelofibrosis
  - Osteopetrosis

osteopetrosis have greater amounts of marrow (although still decreased), and the characteristic bone-in-bone appearance seen on conventional radiographs can be seen on MRI as low signal intensity within higher signal intensity marrow on T1W images. Stress fractures are common in bones weakened by osteopetrosis, and these can be shown easily on MRI, if the diagnosis is not clear from radiographs.

Hemosiderin Deposition (Box 2–18). Hemosiderin (iron) deposition in macrophages located in bone marrow and other organs occurs from either chronic breakdown of red blood cells (sickle cell anemia, thalassemia), chronic blood transfusions, or metabolic abnormalities in chronic inflammatory disorders and acquired immunodeficiency syndrome (AIDS). The marrow appears extremely low signal intensity (signal void, black marrow) on all pulse sequences, and there is the blooming effect on gradient echo imaging (Fig. 2–39). The liver and spleen have the same low signal intensity as bone marrow, which helps to distinguish this process from similar-appearing diseases on MRI.

Serous Atrophy (Gelatinous Transformation). Severely cachectic patients, people with anorexia nervosa, and AIDS patients may all develop this entity, which consists of bone marrow essentially turning to mush. The process occurs in exactly the same progression and sequence as does conversion of red to yellow marrow. Thus, the hands and feet, followed by the bones of the forearms and lower legs, are affected first. Ultimately, the proximal long bones and axial skeleton become abnormal. The MRI signal characteristics are identical to those of water, with low signal intensity (equal to or lower than muscle) on T1W images that becomes high

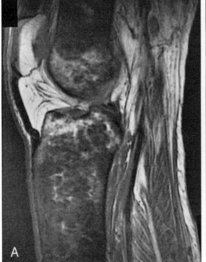

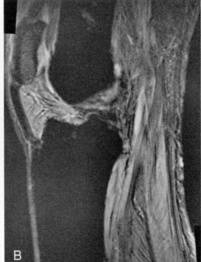

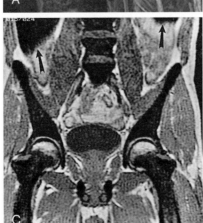

Figure 2–39. MISCELLANEOUS: Hemosiderin deposition.
A, T1 sagittal image, knee. There is diffuse abnormal low signal in the femur and tibia, involving the epiphyses as well as the shafts of the bones in this patient with sickle cell anemia. *B*, T2* sagittal image, knee. The bones become diffusely very low signal from blooming that occurs from the hemosiderin deposited in the marrow. *C*, T1 coronal image, pelvis (different patient than in *A* and *B*). The bones are diffusely black, except for the femoral heads. The liver and spleen are also black *(arrows)*. This patient has hemosiderosis.

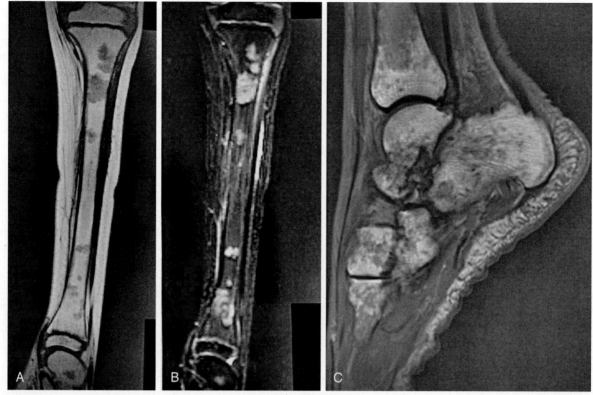

Figure 2–40. MISCELLANEOUS: Serous atrophy (gelatinous transformation).
A, T1 coronal image, lower leg. This patient was previously treated for Ewing's sarcoma and was cachectic (note the lack of muscle in the calf). The focal areas of intermediate signal intensity were of concern for metastatic disease. **B**, STIR coronal image, lower leg. The focal marrow abnormalities are high signal. Biopsy of the proximal large lesion showed fluid in the marrow, and this was diagnosed as serous atrophy. **C**, T1 sagittal image, foot (different patient than in A and B). This patient had acquired immunodeficiency syndrome (AIDS). There are multiple foci of intermediate signal in the marrow of the foot and tibia, as well as in the subcutaneous fat, compatible with serous atrophy.

signal on T2W images (Fig. 2–40). This process may start out as focal lesions, but it rapidly progresses to large, confluent regions of abnormality on MRI. Histologically, the marrow is necrotic and composed of serous fluid.[51]

References

1. Vogler JB, Murphy WA. Bone marrow imaging. *Radiology* 1988; 168:679–693.
2. Steiner RM, Mitchell DG, Rao VM, Schweitzer ME. Magnetic resonance imaging of diffuse bone marrow disease. *Radiol Clin North Am* 1992; 31:383–409.
3. Kaplan PA, Dussault RG. Magnetic resonance imaging of the bone marrow. In Higgins CB, Hricak H, Helms CA (eds). *Magnetic Resonance Imaging of the Body*, edn 3. New York: Lippincott-Raven; 1997:101–126.
4. Dooms GC, Fisher MR, Hricak H, et al. Bone marrow imaging: magnetic resonance studies related to age and sex. *Radiology* 1985; 155:429–432.
5. Jaramillo D, Laor T, Hoffer FA, et al. Epiphyseal marrow in infancy: MR imaging. *Radiology* 1991; 180:809–812.
6. Ricci C, Cova M, Kang YS, et al. Normal age-related patterns of cellular and fatty bone marrow distribution in the axial skeleton: MR imaging study. *Radiology* 1990; 177:83–88.
7. Dawson KL, Moore SG, Rowland JM. Age-related marrow changes in the pelvis: MR and anatomic findings. *Radiology* 1992; 183:47–51.
8. Kricun ME. Red-yellow marrow conversion: its effect on the location of some solitary bone lesions. *Skeletal Radiol* 1985; 14:10–19.
9. Moore SG, Dawson KL. Red and yellow marrow in the femur: age-related changes in appearance at MR imaging. *Radiology* 1990; 175:219–223.
10. Moore SG, Bisset GS, Siegel MJ, Donaldson JS. Pediatric musculoskeletal MR imaging. *Radiology* 1991; 179:345–360.
11. Mirowitz SA. Hematopoietic bone marrow within the proximal humeral epiphysis in normal adults: investigation with MR imaging. *Radiology* 1993; 188:689–693.
12. Hajek PC, Baker LL, Goobar JE, et al. Focal fat deposition in axial bone marrow: MR characteristics. *Radiology* 1987; 162:245–249.
13. Roos AD, Kressel H, Spritzer C, Dalinka M. MR imaging of marrow changes adjacent to end plates in degenerative lumbar disk disease. *AJR* 1987; 149:531–534.
14. Modic MT, Steinberg PM, Ross JS, et al. Degenerative disk disease: assessment of changes in vertebral body marrow with MR imaging. *Radiology* 1988; 166:193–199.
15. Jones KM, Unger EC, Granstrom P, Seeger JF, et al. Bone marrow imaging using STIR at 0.5 and 1.5 T. *Magn Reson Imaging* 1992; 10:169–176.
16. Sebag GH, Moore SG. Effect of trabecular bone on the appearance of marrow in gradient-echo imaging of the appendicular skeleton. *Radiology* 1990; 174:855–859.
17. Vande Berg BC, Malghem J, Lecouvet FE, Maldague B. Magnetic resonance imaging of the normal bone marrow. *Skeletal Radiol* 1998; 27:471–483.
18. Schweitzer ME, Levine C, Mitchell DG, et al. Bull's-eyes and halos: useful MR discriminators of osseous metastases. *Radiology* 1993; 188:249–252.
19. Disler DG, McCauley TR, Ratner LM, et al. In-phase and out-of-phase MR imaging of bone marrow: prediction of neopla-

sia based on the detection of coexistent fat and water. *AJR* 1997;169:1439–1447.

20. Baur A, Stäbler, Brüning R, et al. Diffusion-weighted MR imaging of bone marrow: differentiation of benign versus pathologic compression fractures. *Radiology* 1998; 207:349–356.

21. Vande Berg BC, Mallghem J, Lecouvet FE, Maldague B. Classification and detection of bone marrow lesions with magnetic resonance imaging. *Skeletal Radiol* 1998; 27:529–545.

22. Vande Berg BC, Lecouvet FE, Michaux L, et al. Stage I multiple myeloma: value of MR imaging of the bone marrow in the determination of prognosis. *Radiology* 1996; 201:243–246.

23. Vande Berg BC, Michaux L, Lecouvet FE, et al. Nonmyelomatous monoclonal gammopathy: correlation of bone marrow MR images with laboratory findings and spontaneous clinical outcome. *Radiology* 1997; 202:247–251.

24. Moulopoulos LA, Dimopoulos MA, Alexanian R, et al. Multiple myeloma: MR patterns of response to treatment. *Radiology* 1994; 192:441–446.

25. Eustace S, Tello R, DeCarvalho V, et al. A comparison of whole-body TurboSTIR MR imaging and planar ^{99m}Tc-methylene diphosphonate scintigraphy in the examination of patients with suspected skeletal metastases. *AJR* 1997; 169:1655–1661.

26. Frank JA, Ling A, Patronas NJ, et al. Detection of malignant bone tumors: MR imaging vs scintigraphy. *AJR* 1990; 155:1043–1048.

27. Algra PR, Bloem JL, Tissing H, et al. Detection of vertebral metastases: comparison between MR imaging and bone scintigraphy. *Radiographics* 1991; 11:219–232.

28. Lien HH, Holte H. Fat replacement of Hodgkin disease of bone marrow after chemotherapy: report of three cases. *Skeletal Radiol* 1996;25:671–674.

29. Mink J. Percutaneous bone biopsy in the patient with known or suspected osseous metastases. *Radiology* 1986; 161: 191–194.

30. Yuh WTC, Zachar CK, Barloon TJ, et al. Vertebral compression fractures: distinction between benign and malignant causes with MR imaging. *Radiology* 1989; 172:215–218.

31. Baker LL, Goodman SB, Inder P, et al. Benign versus pathologic compression fractures of vertebral bodies: assessment with conventional spin-echo, chemical shift, and STIR MR imaging. *Radiology* 1990; 174:495–502.

32. Kaplan PA, Asleson RJ, Klassen LW, Duggan MJ. Bone marrow patterns in aplastic anemia: observations with 1.5-T MR imaging. *Radiology* 1987; 164:441–444.

33. McKinstry CS, Steiner RE, Young AT, et al. Bone marrow in leukemia and aplastic anemia: MR imaging before, during, and after treatment. *Radiology* 1987; 162:701–707.

34. Fletcher BD, Wall JE, Hanna SL. Effect of hematopoietic growth factors on MR images of bone marrow in children undergoing chemotherapy. *Radiology* 1993; 189:745–751.

35. Stevens SK, Moore SG, Kaplan ID. Early and late bone-marrow changes after irradiation: MR evaluation. *AJR* 1990; 154:745–750.

36. Wilson AJ, Murphy WA, Hardy DC, Totty WG. Transient osteoporosis: transient bone marrow edema? *Radiology* 1988; 167:757–760.

37. Bloem J. Transient osteoporosis of the hip: MR imaging. *Radiology* 1988; 167:753–755.

38. Mitchell DG, Rao VM, Dalinka M, et al. Hematopoietic and fatty bone marrow distribution in the normal and ischemic hip: new observations with 1.5-T MR imaging. *Radiology* 1986; 161:199–202.

39. Munk PL, Helms CA, Holt RG. Immature bone infarcts: findings on plain radiographs and MR scans. *AJR* 1989; 152:547–549.

40. Turner DA, Templeton AC, Selzer PM, et al. Femoral capital osteonecrosis: MR finding of diffuse marrow abnormalities without focal lesions. *Radiology* 1989; 171:135–140.

41. Guerra JJ, Steinberg ME. Distinguishing transient osteoporosis from avascular necrosis of the hip. *J Bone Joint Surg [Am]* 1995; 77:616–624.

42. Totty WG, Murphy WA, Ganz WI, et al. Magnetic resonance imaging of the normal and ischemic femoral head. *AJR* 1984; 143:1273–1280.

43. Mitchell MD, Kundel HL, Steinberg ME, et al. Avascular necrosis of the hip: comparison of MR, CT, and scintigraphy. *AJR* 1986; 147:67–71.

44. Mitchell DG, Rao VM, Dalinka MK, et al. Femoral head avascular necrosis: correlation of MR imaging, radiographic staging, radionuclide imaging, and clinical findings. *Radiology* 1987; 162:709–715.

45. Bettran J, Herman LJ, Burk JM, et al. Femoral head avascular necrosis: MR imaging with clinical-pathologic and radionuclide correlation. *Radiology* 1988; 166:215–220.

46. Genez BM, Wilson MR, Houk RW, et al. Early osteonecrosis of the femoral head: detection in high risk patients with MR imaging. *Radiology* 1988; 168:521–524.

47. Coleman BG, Kressel HY, Dalinka MK, et al. Radiographically negative avascular necrosis: detection with MR imaging. *Radiology* 1988; 168:525–528.

48. Tervonen O, Mueller DM, Matteson EL, et al. Clinically occult avascular necrosis of the hip: prevalence in an asymptomatic population at risk. *Radiology* 1992; 182:845–847.

49. Glickstein MF, Burk DL, Schiebler ML, et al. Avascular necrosis versus other diseases of the hip: sensitivity of MR imaging. *Radiology* 1988; 169:213–215.

50. Sugimoto H, Okubo RS, Ohsawa T. Chemical shift and the double-line sign in MRI of early femoral avascular necrosis. *J Comput Assist Tomogr* 1992; 16:727–730.

51. Vande Berg BC, Malghem J, Devuyst O, et al. Anorexia nervosa: correlation between MR appearance of bone marrow and severity of disease. *Radiology* 1994; 193:859–864.

3 TENDONS AND MUSCLES

HOW TO IMAGE TENDONS
Normal Tendons
  Anatomy
  MRI of Normal Tendons
Tendon Abnormalities
  Degeneration
  Tenosynovitis
  Tendon Tears
  Tendon Subluxation/Dislocation
  Miscellaneous Tendon Lesions
HOW TO IMAGE MUSCLES
Normal Muscle
  MRI Appearance
Muscle Abnormalities

Muscle Trauma
  Indirect Muscle Injuries
    Delayed-Onset Muscle Soreness
    Muscle Strains
  Direct Muscle Injuries
    Intramuscular Hemorrhage
    Hematoma
    Hemorrhage into Tumor
    Myositis Ossificans
  Miscellaneous Traumatic Injuries
    Compartment Syndromes
    Exertional Compartment
      Syndrome
    Fascial Herniation of Muscle

Inflammatory Myopathies
  Pyomyositis
  Necrotizing Fasciitis
  Idiopathic Inflammatory
    Polymyopathies
Primary Muscle Diseases
  Dystrophies and Myopathies
Denervation
Tumors
Miscellaneous Muscle
  Abnormalities
  Rhabdomyolysis
  Muscle Infarction
  Accessory Muscles
  Radiation/Surgery/Chemotherapy

HOW TO IMAGE TENDONS

Coils/Patient Position. Whether or not a coil should be used is based entirely on the anatomy to be imaged. In general, surface coils improve images and should be used. Obviously, for large areas such as the thighs or pelvis, this approach is not practical, and coils are not used. Patients should be positioned as if the nearest joint were being imaged. For example, ankle tendons are imaged by positioning the patient and using a coil for an ankle examination.

Image Orientation. In general, tendons are best imaged transversely (perpendicular to their long axis). Occasionally, other planes are helpful to image tendons in their entire length. For example, the triceps, quadriceps, and Achilles tendons are depicted very well on both axial and sagittal images. The hamstring tendons in the pelvis and the supraspinatus tendon in the shoulder are demonstrated well on coronal as well as axial images. Given only one option for an imaging plane through a tendon, however, axial images generally are the most useful.

Pulse Sequences/Regions of Interest. T1W as well as some type of T2W images are required for complete evaluation of tendons. The T2W sequences are useful for demonstrating abnormal fluid surrounding the tendon (tenosynovitis). We prefer gradient echo and STIR sequences for the T2W images of tendons. Slice thickness and fields of view are determined by the size of the body part being imaged. A good rule of thumb is that the same field of view and slice thickness that is used to image the adjacent joint will suffice to image a tendon in that same region.

Contrast. There is no need to do contrast-enhanced studies for tendon evaluation.

Normal Tendons

Anatomy

Tendons are relatively avascular structures that attach muscles to bones. They are made of dense fascicles of collagen fibers. The fascicles of collagen are composed of smaller units, called microfibrils. Microfibrils interdigitate with one another in a regular and structured fashion to form extremely tight bonds, giving tendons their strength. The microfibrils are made of a protein called tropocollagen, which consists of three polypeptide chains arranged in a triple-helix configuration. The helical configuration of the protein tightly binds molecules of water, so that tendons have low signal intensity because the hydrogen ions in water are not mobile.

Most tendons are invested with a tendon sheath, which either partially or completely covers the tendon. Tendon sheaths are present where tendons pass through fascial slings, beneath ligamentous bands, or through fibro-osseous tunnels. In other words, they exist where closely apposed structures move relative to one another, in order to decrease friction. The microscopic structure of a tendon sheath is similar to the synovial membrane that lines joints. During fetal development, the tendon invaginates the tendon sheath so that there are inner (visceral)

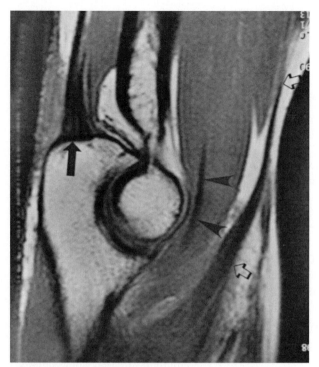

Figure 3–1. NORMAL TENDONS.
T1 sagittal image, elbow. The anteriorly located biceps tendon *(open arrows)* is low signal and has a long segment that is not surrounded by muscle. The brachialis tendon *(arrowheads)* is also a typical low-signal tendon, but it is surrounded by muscle with little exposed tendon. The triceps *(solid arrow)*, unlike most tendons, normally has vertical striations of low and intermediate signal.

and outer (parietal) layers of the sheath that are closely apposed to each other. A mesotendon is formed where the tendon invaginated the sheath. The mesotendon carries blood vessels and is located on the nonfrictional surface of the tendon. A thin layer of synovial fluid exists between the visceral and parietal layers of the tendon sheath and allows for smooth gliding of the tendon.

Some tendons are located mainly outside of the muscle, such as the distal biceps tendon at the elbow. Other tendons have long segments that are surrounded by muscle and have very little exposed tendon, such as the brachialis at the elbow (Fig. 3–1).

MRI of Normal Tendons

Normal tendons have so few mobile protons that they are usually low signal intensity on all pulse sequences. The major exceptions to this rule include the quadriceps tendon at the knee and distal triceps tendon at the elbow, which have a striated appearance with alternating areas of linear low and intermediate signal intensity (similar to the distal anterior cruciate ligament in the knee) (see Fig. 3–1). This striated appearance is caused by the longitudinal arrangement of coarse fasciculi and also by the fact that several tendons are fusing to form a single, conjoined tendon.[1] The longitudinal striations in

the triceps and quadriceps tendons must not be mistaken for pathology. Similarly, there is a solitary vertical line of high signal intensity in the midsubstance of many normal Achilles tendons, which probably represents the site where the soleus and gastrocnemius tendons (which make up the Achilles tendon) are apposed to one another, or else a vascular channel in the tendon.

There are certain other exceptions to the rule that normal tendons are low signal intensity on all pulse sequences (Box 3–1). Many tendons may show slightly increased signal intensity near their osseous insertions. This occurs because tendons may fan out as they come to attach to a bone and nontendinous fatty material is interposed between tendon fibers (Fig. 3–2).

A second major reason for a normal tendon having

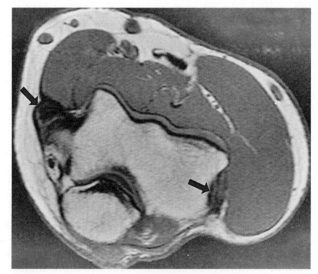

Figure 3–2. NORMAL TENDON HIGH SIGNAL.
T1 axial image, elbow. The attachment sites of some tendons to bone *(arrows)* result in areas of high signal within the tendon, which is normal and is caused by diverging collagen fascicles, rather than from partial tendon tears.

BOX 3–2: TENDON ABNORMALITIES

Degeneration
Tenosynovitis
Partial or complete tears
} Most common by far

Subluxation or dislocation
Xanthoma formation
Gout, hydroxyapatite, or other crystals
Giant cell tumor of tendon sheath
Clear cell sarcoma

Tendon Abnormalities (Box 3–2)

The major abnormalities that may affect tendons include tendon degeneration, tenosynovitis, partial tears, complete tears, subluxation or dislocation, xanthoma formation, deposits of calcium hydroxyapatite or calcium pyrophosphate crystals, gouty tophi, and clear cell sarcoma. Giant cell tumor of the tendon sheath is a relatively common mass that arises from the tendon sheath. By far the most common abnormalities seen on MRI are tendon degeneration, tenosynovitis, and tendon tears (Fig. 3–3).

Degeneration

Myxoid degeneration of tendons occurs with aging or from chronic overuse (Fig. 3–4). This is a painless process, but it weakens the tendon so that it is predisposed to partial or complete tears with minimal trauma. The quadriceps tendon is a good example of a tendon that may rupture in an elderly population with no or minimal trauma because of preexisting underlying tendon degeneration. Rupture results in weakness of the extensor mechanism and patients are often initially worked up for a neurologic abnormality rather than a tendon problem.

On MRI examination, a degenerated tendon has high signal intensity within the substance of the tendon on both T1W and any type of T2W sequences. The tendon is generally normal or enlarged in caliber. This cannot be distinguished from partial tears of a tendon. Many people use terms such as tendinitis, tendinopathy, or tendinosis to indicate that such abnormal signal intensity of a tendon exists, but that it is impossible to give the precise cause for the findings. The term tendinitis should probably not be used, because an inflammatory response in the tendon does not occur. Another way to describe the nonspecific findings of intrasub-

increased signal intensity is the result of the magic angle phenomenon.[2] The magic angle phenomenon results from the fact that tendons are anisotropic structures. When tendons are oriented at an angle of about 55 degrees to the bore of the magnet, there will be high signal intensity within the tendon on short TE sequences (such as T1W, proton density, and gradient echo sequences). Determining if high signal on short TE sequences is from the magic angle phenomenon or from pathology generally can be done by (1) using a pulse sequence with a long TE that will show the high signal intensity disappears, (2) observing that the tendon is of normal caliber, or (3) repositioning the body part being imaged so that the tendon is imaged at a different angle relative to the bore of the magnet.

Most tendons are round, oval, or flat when imaged transversely. Tendon sheaths are not normally seen on MRI, unless fluid is present in the sheath. Small amounts of fluid may be seen in certain tendon sheaths, particularly in the ankle and wrist. Our general rule is that the fluid should not be considered abnormal unless it completely surrounds the circumference of the tendon.

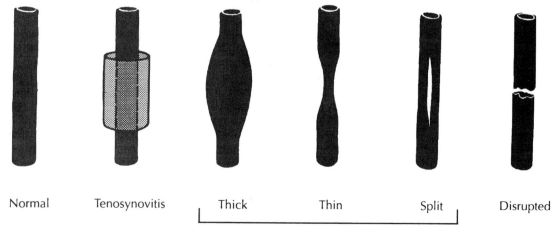

| Normal | Tenosynovitis | Thick | Thin | Split | Disrupted |

PARTIAL TEARS

Figure 3–3. TENDON INFLAMMATION/TEARS.
Diagram demonstrating the changes that occur in tendons from inflammatory tenosynovitis through different types of partial tears and complete tendon disruption.

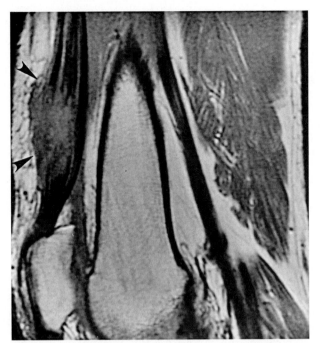

Figure 3–4. TENDON DEGENERATION/PARTIAL TEARS. T1 sagittal image, knee. The quadriceps tendon normally has vertical striations within it. The normal architecture of the tendon is disrupted by intermediate signal *(arrowheads)* representing myxoid degeneration and partial tears. This person had no injury or pain, but presented with a palpable mass.

BOX 3–3: TENOSYNOVITIS

Causes
  • Overuse, increased stresses
  • Inflammatory arthritis
  • Infection
Stenosing tenosynovitis
  • Focal, loculated fluid collections in tendon sheath, often with septations in fluid
MRI
  • Underlying tendon may be normal or abnormal
  • Fluid (low signal, T1; high signal, T2) must surround the entire circumference of a tendon—meaningless if tendon sheath communicates with adjacent joint.
  • Septations in loculated fluid of stenosing tenosynovitis are thin, linear, low-signal structures. Do not confuse with mesotendon.
  • Pannus may be present in tendon sheaths in rheumatoid arthritis.

stance high signal in a tendon is simply to state that it is compatible with degeneration or partial tears, because they generally coexist anyway.

Tenosynovitis (Box 3–3)

Fluid that completely surrounds the circumference of a tendon indicates an inflammatory process of the tendon sheath, called tenosynovitis. The underlying tendon may be normal or abnormal. The abnormal presence and amount of fluid is required to make this diagnosis regardless of the status of the tendon fibers. This may occur from chronic repetitive motion or stress on the tendon from overuse, from an inflammatory arthritis, or from a purulent infection.

Stenosing tenosynovitis can occur when there are focal, loculated collections of fluid in the tendon sheath. This is a common finding in the flexor hallucis longus tendon about the ankle in patients with the os trigonum syndrome, and also in the wrist from De Quervain's stenosing tenosynovitis.

MRI of tenosynovitis demonstrates a rounded collection of fluid that is low signal intensity on T1W and high signal intensity on T2W images, completely surrounding a tendon on images obtained transversely through it. The mesotendon may be identified as a thin, low signal intensity line extending from the tendon to the outer layer of the tendon sheath (Fig. 3–5). The underlying tendon may be normal or abnormal in signal intensity and caliber.

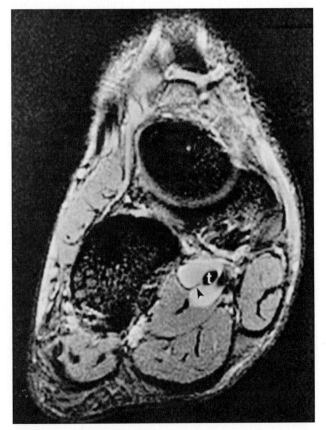

Figure 3–5. TENOSYNOVITIS. T2* axial image, hindfoot. The flexor hallucis longus tendon (t) is normal in size and signal. It is surrounded by high-signal fluid, representing tenosynovitis. The thin line within the fluid *(arrowhead)* is the mesotendon, where the tendon invaginated the tendon sheath during fetal development.

Stenosing tenosynovitis can be diagnosed on MRI by the presence of focal distension of a tendon sheath with fluid, as well as thin, linear low signal intensity septations that course through the fluid in the sheath (Fig. 3–6).

Tendon sheaths that communicate directly with an adjacent joint (such as the long head of the biceps tendon in the shoulder and the flexor hallucis longus tendon at the ankle) should not be considered to have tenosynovitis simply because of the finding of fluid surrounding the circumference of the tendon. If there is an effusion of the joint, fluid can surround the tendon without the tendon or its sheath being abnormal. Only if there is no adjacent joint effusion do we consider fluid around these specific tendons to have possible clinical significance.

Tendons that do not have a sheath may have inflammatory changes surrounding the tendon, which is called paratendinitis (Fig. 3–7). MRI will show abnormal signal intensity typical of edema (low signal intensity on T1 and hyperintense on T2W images) in the soft tissues surrounding the tendon. The Achilles tendon is a classic location for these findings, because it has no tendon sheath.

Tendon Tears (Box 3–4)

There are several conditions that cause weakened tendons and predispose to tears: chronic repetitive

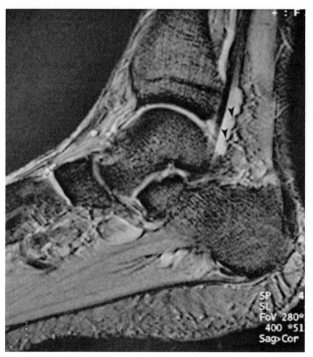

Figure 3–6. STENOSING TENOSYNOVITIS.
T2* sagittal image, hindfoot. High signal fluid from tenosynovitis surrounds the flexor hallucis tendon at the level of the ankle joint. There are small, linear septations in the margin of the tendon sheath *(arrowheads)* and lobulated margins of the tendon sheath, indicating this is stenosing tenosynovitis with scarring and inflammatory changes of the sheath.

BOX 3–4: FACTORS PREDISPOSING TO TENDON RUPTURE

- Tendon degeneration—occurs with age and from chronic stresses
- Chronic, repetitive stresses (overuse)
- Acute major trauma
- Diabetes
- Systemic steroids and other medications
- Rheumatoid arthritis and other inflammatory arthritides
- Chronic renal failure/hyperparathyroidism
- Infection of tendon sheath
- Gout

---

stresses, tendon degeneration, inflammatory processes of tendons (such as from rheumatoid arthritis, the seronegative spondyloarthropathies, systemic lupus erythematosus, or infection of the tendon sheath), chronic renal disease, use of chronic systemic steroids and certain other medications, diabetes, and gout.[3]

Partial tendon tears represent incomplete disruption of the fibers. Complete tendon tears indicate total disruption of the fibers of the tendon so that there are two separate fragments. Partial tears often are difficult to diagnose on clinical grounds, whereas complete tears are more obvious.

Partial tendon tears can have a variable appearance on MRI (Fig. 3–8). The tendon may be thickened (hypertrophic partial tear), thinned (atrophic partial tear), or remain of normal caliber with abnormal signal being the only evidence of the partial tear. An attenuated tendon is closer to complete rupture than a thickened tendon. A classification system has been proposed to describe tears based on the caliber of the tendon; we prefer to simply describe the findings (partial tear with a normal-caliber, thickened, or attenuated tendon) rather than assign a number from a classification system, because we cannot remember the system ourselves and especially because the referring physicians are unaware of the classification system. Tendons sometimes become partially torn in a longitudinal or vertical manner, rather than transversely (Fig. 3–9). This results in a split tendon that may be functionally incompetent and acts as if it is completely torn, even though it is still in continuity with the muscle and the bone. Usually there is high signal intensity in the tendon on all pulse sequences with partial tendon tears, but with chronic partial tears, there may be low signal intensity because of scarring and fibrosis; an abnormal tendon size or tenosynovitis are the only ways to recognize the tendon as abnormal in this situation. Tenosynovitis often coexists with partial tendon tears.

Complete tendon rupture on MRI appears as a focal disruption with absence of the tendon fibers for variable distances (Fig. 3–10). MRI is valuable

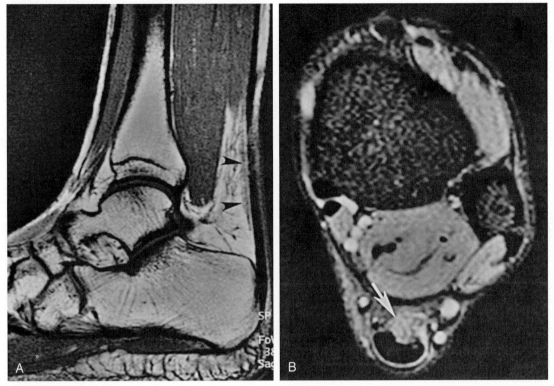

Figure 3–7. PARATENDINITIS.
A, T1 sagittal image, ankle. The Achilles tendon does not have a tendon sheath, so inflammatory changes appear as edema in the fat adjacent to the tendon *(arrowheads)*. *B*, T2* axial image, ankle. Edema anterior to the Achilles tendon is manifest as high signal in Kager's fat *(arrow)*, indicating paratendinitis.

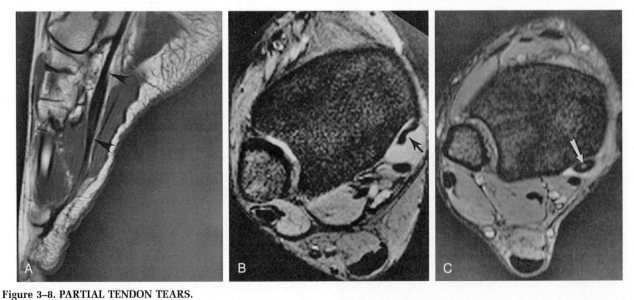

Figure 3–8. PARTIAL TENDON TEARS.
A, T1 sagittal image, foot (different patient than in *B* or *C*). There is focal thickening of the flexor hallucis longus tendon evident between the arrowheads from hypertrophic partial tendon tears. *B*, T2* axial image, ankle (different patient than in *A* or *C*). Thinning of the posterior tibial tendon *(arrow)* indicates atrophic partial tendon tears. *C*, T2*axial image, ankle (different patient than in *A* or *B*). The posterior tibial tendon is of normal caliber, but partial tendon tears can be diagnosed by the presence of intrasubstance high signal *(arrow)*.

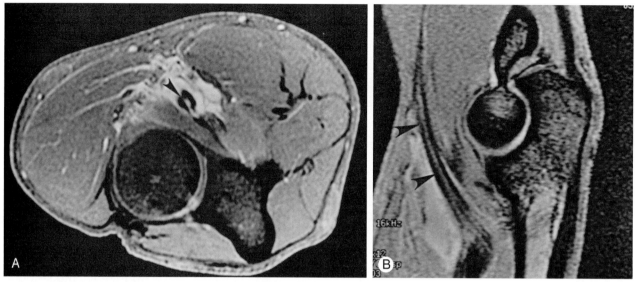

Figure 3–9. PARTIAL TENDON TEAR: Longitudinal split.
A, Fast-T2 with fat suppression axial image, elbow. The distal biceps tendon is split *(arrowhead)* into anterior and posterior halves. The fluid surrounding the tendon is in the inflamed bicipito-radial bursa (there is no tendon sheath around this tendon, so tenosynovitis cannot be the diagnosis). **B,** T2* sagittal image, elbow. The distal biceps tendon is identified longitudinally *(arrowheads)*, with a longitudinal split tear seen as a high-signal line down the center of the tendon.

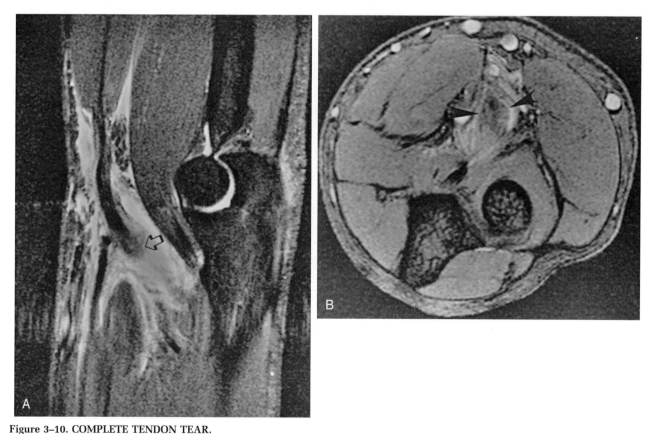

Figure 3–10. COMPLETE TENDON TEAR.
A, STIR sagittal image, elbow. The distal end of the distal biceps tendon is completely torn. The end of the fragment is seen *(open arrow)* retracted proximally, along with a large amount of surrounding high-signal edema/hemorrhage. The tendon is thickened and has high signal in it distally. **B,** T2* axial image, elbow. The distal end of the ruptured biceps tendon is markedly enlarged and has internal high signal *(arrowheads)*. Distal to this point, only high-signal fluid was seen in the gap where the tendon previously existed.

BOX 3–5: TENDONS THAT SUBLUX OR DISLOCATE

Wrist
    Extensor carpi ulnaris (medial)
Shoulder
    Long head of biceps (medial)
Ankle
    Peroneal tendons (lateral or medial)
    Posterior tibial (medial and anterior)

---

in documenting the presence of a complete tear, demonstrating the quality of the remnants of tendon, and showing how far retracted the remnants are; all of these features may contribute to determining how to manage the patient. Careful search for tendons on every image is essential in order not to overlook tears, because abnormalities may be present on only one image.

Tendon Subluxation/Dislocation
(Box 3–5)

Most tendons maintain a normal relationship to adjacent osseous structures by way of retinacula that hold them in place. If the retinacula become disrupted, the tendons may sublux or dislocate from their normal positions (Fig. 3–11). The tendons may have no intrinsic, underlying abnormalities, but partial tears, complete tears, and tenosynovitis are common from irritation with chronic subluxation and wear and tear on adjacent bones.

The tendons that may sublux or dislocate include the extensor carpi ulnaris in the wrist, the long head of the biceps in the shoulder, the peroneal tendons over the lateral malleolus at the ankle, and the posterior tibial tendon on the medial side of the ankle.[4]

Miscellaneous Tendon Lesions

Abnormalities other than tears, tenosynovitis, and dislocations are relatively uncommon. Xanthomas occur in patients with familial hyperlipidemia syndrome and most commonly affect the Achilles tendon and the extensor tendons of the hand (Fig. 3–12).

Deposits of gout crystals also may affect tendons (Fig. 3–13). It is usually impossible to distinguish gouty tophi or xanthomas from partial tendon tears by MRI, and they should simply be kept in mind in the appropriate setting. Calcific tendinitis from deposition of calcium hydroxyapatite crystals is common and easy to diagnose on radiographs, which is a good thing, because MRI does not usually demonstrate the abnormality well. The hydroxyapatite crystals have low signal intensity on all pulse sequences that are usually difficult or impossible to distinguish from the low signal intensity tendon. If the crystal deposit is large enough, it may show lower signal than the tendon on all pulse sequences, making it visible on MRI (Fig. 3–14).

Tumors of tendons are exceedingly rare, but clear cell sarcoma (malignant melanoma of soft parts) should be considered if one is considering a tumor at all. Tumors arising from the tendon sheath are much more common than a tumor of the tendon itself. Giant cell tumor of the tendon sheath is a relatively common cause of a mass in the hands and feet. It is a localized and extraarticular form of pigmented villonodular synovitis. It presents as a nonpainful, soft tissue mass. On MRI it usually is lobulated with intermediate signal on both T1 and T2W images, closely apposed to a low signal tendon (Fig. 3–15).

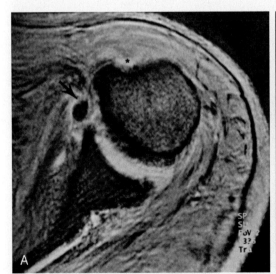 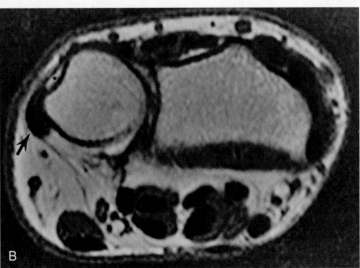

Figure 3–11. DISLOCATED TENDONS.
A, T2* axial image, shoulder. The long head of the biceps tendon *(arrow)* has dislocated medially from the bicipital groove (*) and lies over the anterior glenohumeral joint. The subscapularis tendon is avulsed from its attachment to the lesser tuberosity of the humerus. *B*, T1 axial image, wrist. The extensor carpi ulnaris tendon *(arrow)* has dislocated medially from the notch in the ulna (*) where it normally exists.

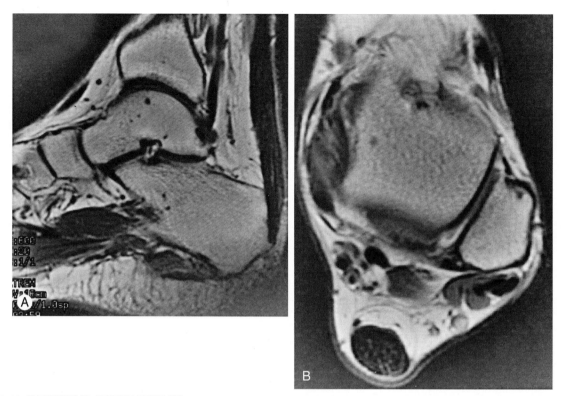

Figure 3–12. XANTHOMA OF THE TENDON.
A, T1 sagittal image, ankle. The Achilles tendon is thickened and has abnormal high-signal striations within it. *B*, T1 axial image, ankle. The Achilles tendon has a stippled appearance of low and high signal and is thickened with a convex anterior margin. These findings are from familial hyperlipidemia with xanthoma formation but cannot be distinguished from partial tendon tears by MRI.

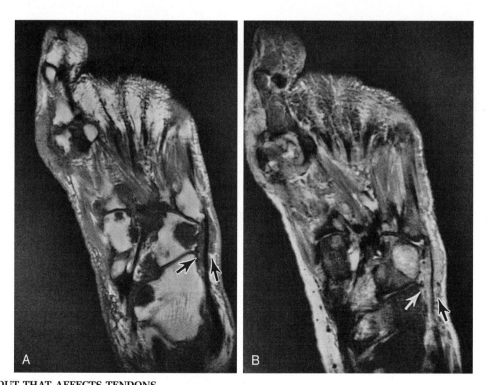

Figure 3–13. GOUT THAT AFFECTS TENDONS.
A, T1 coronal image, foot. An intermediate signal lobulated mass *(arrows)* representing a gouty tophus surrounds a tendon. Intraosseous gout deposits can be seen in several bones as well. *B*, STIR coronal image, foot. Same findings as in *A* above, but the gouty tophi change signal slightly. They are intermediate signal on this STIR image but may be even lower signal on other types of T2W sequences.

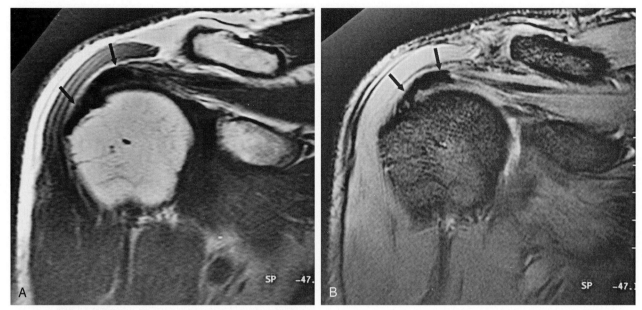

Figure 3–14. CALCIUM HYDROXYAPATITE IN TENDONS.
A, T1 coronal oblique image, shoulder. The supraspinatus tendon *(arrows)* is lower signal than a normal tendon and slightly thickened from calcium hydroxyapatite crystal deposition (calcific tendinitis). *B*, T2* coronal oblique image, shoulder. Same findings as in *A*, but the features are more conspicuous with this sequence.

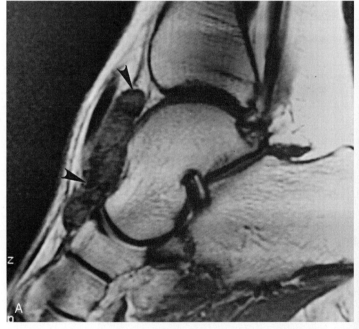

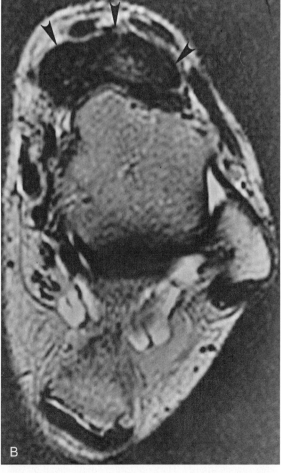

Figure 3–15. GIANT CELL TUMOR OF THE TENDON SHEATH.
A, T1 sagittal image, ankle. There is an intermediate signal mass *(arrowheads)* anterior to the ankle. *B*, Spin echo-T2 axial image, ankle. The mass remains intermediate to low signal intensity on this sequence *(arrowheads)* and is seen running along the extensor tendons.

HOW TO IMAGE MUSCLES

Coils/Patient Position. Injured or abnormal muscle often affects large muscles in large body parts where surface coils are not used. The use of coils is dependent on the size of the region being imaged. In general, the patient should be imaged in the same position as if the adjacent joint were being imaged.

Image Orientation. In general, most muscles and muscle groups are best evaluated in the axial plane. Longitudinal (coronal or sagittal) planes are used for orientation of abnormalities relative to osseous landmarks and to demonstrate the extent of the disease.

Pulse Sequences/Regions of Interest. Both T1W and some types of T2W images are required. For the T2 sequence, we prefer using STIR, because this sequence is exquisitely sensitive to most muscle pathology. T1 sequences are also necessary in order to show anatomic detail and configuration of the muscle, subacute hemorrhage, and fatty atrophy of muscle. Fields of view and slice thickness are entirely dependant on the body part being imaged and the extent of the suspected abnormality. We often do a large field-of-view coronal, fast STIR sequence as a scout view. The edema that is present will indicate the region that needs to be covered with a smaller field of view and other pulse sequences, as well as whether or not a surface coil can be used.

Contrast. Contrast-enhanced sequences are unnecessary, unless one is attempting to identify abscesses or areas of muscle necrosis.

Normal Muscle

MRI Appearance

Normal skeletal muscle has intermediate signal intensity on all pulse sequences (Fig. 3–16). T1W images demonstrate a feathery or marbled appearance because of fat that is interposed between adjacent muscles and between muscle fibers within a muscle. In some locations, individual muscle groups can be distinguished because of interposed fat. Where intermuscular fat is sparse, such as in the calf, individual muscle groups blend together and are difficult to identify. Low signal intensity tendons may course through a muscle for long distances or may arise near the periphery of a muscle; this myotendinous junction is usually the weakest link in the chain from a perspective of strength of the entire unit. On T2W sequences, normal muscle remains intermediate signal intensity and no high signal is evident between muscles, with the exception of normal vascular structures.

Muscle Abnormalities

Several abnormalities of muscle occur that can be evaluated well by MRI. These include abnormalities from trauma, inflammatory disorders, tumors, denervation, muscular dystrophies, neuromuscular disorders, and ischemia. MRI is exquisitely sensitive to muscle abnormalities but is usually nonspecific. Because of this, it is important to have a list of differential diagnoses available when a muscle abnormality is encountered on MRI (like the abnormalities listed in the outline for this chapter). Clinical findings and biopsy of abnormal tissue play important roles in making a specific diagnosis when abnormalities are proved by MRI, and MRI is useful in directing where a biopsy should be done.

Abnormal muscle may have a normal, increased, or decreased size. There may be fatty replacement, manifested as high signal intensity in the muscle on T1W images, or there may be areas of high signal

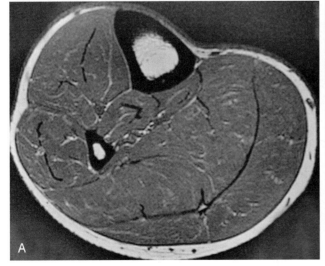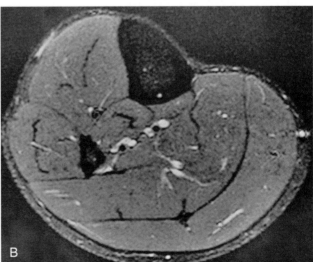

Figure 3–16. NORMAL SKELETAL MUSCLE.
A, T1 axial image, calf. Muscle has intermediate signal intensity with a feathery appearance created by small amounts of interspersed fat. Little to no intermuscular fat is present in this person, making identification of individual muscles somewhat difficult. *B*, STIR axial image, calf. Muscle remains intermediate signal on this sequence, but the feathery pattern disappears because of suppression of the fat.

intensity on T2W images. A focal mass within muscle is another manifestation of disease.

Muscle Trauma

Traumatic muscle injuries can be divided into indirect injuries, direct muscle injuries, and miscellaneous other muscle injuries. Usually, traumatic injuries are imaged in order to assess the exact cause of pain and the extent of the injured area.

Indirect Muscle Injuries (Box 3–6)

This category of muscle injuries includes (1) delayed-onset muscle soreness (DOMS) and (2) strains (muscle tears). When the force of a contracting muscle exceeds the load placed upon it, the muscle shortens, and this is called concentric action (like the action of the biceps when lifting a weight). Conversely, eccentric action is when a muscle lengthens or stretches as it contracts; for example, the action of the biceps when lowering a weight. Concentric contractions produce fatigue, whereas eccentric contractions are responsible for indirect muscle injuries with muscle strains (partial or complete muscle tears).

Injuries often occur along the myotendinous junction. These are generally sports-related injuries.[6–9] Muscles at highest risk for indirect injuries are those that span two joints and are eccentrically activated, like the biceps femoris, gastrocnemius, and rectus femoris muscles in the lower extremity.

Delayed-Onset Muscle Soreness (DOMS). This is a fancy name for stiff muscles. We have all experienced this problem, which begins hours or days after participating in unaccustomed physical exertion. Symptoms peak 2 to 3 days after the activity. There is ultrastructural damage to the contractile elements of muscle, but no irreversible damage is done. Training prevents or reduces DOMS. Serum creatine kinase levels are elevated because of the myonecrosis that is present.

MRI is never done to diagnose DOMS, because we are all familiar with what it is and there is no diagnostic dilemma. We might inadvertently image someone who happens to have DOMS for unrelated reasons. It is in the differential diagnosis for a certain constellation of MR findings, and that is the main reason to be aware of it.

T1W images show no abnormality with DOMS. On T2W images, increased signal intensity may be seen about the periphery of muscles or in the perifascial and intermuscular spaces closely apposed to the injured muscle (Fig. 3–17). This abnormal rim develops 3 to 5 days after the inciting event. A feathery interstitial pattern of increased signal intensity also may be evident throughout the entire muscle from the extracellular fluid that causes increased intramuscular pressure.

MR abnormalities persist long after clinical symptoms abate and after the creatine kinase levels return to normal; however, the abnormalities on MR persist for the same period that biopsy-proved ultrastructural damage is identified. Findings may take weeks to resolve on MRI.

Muscle Strains. Strains are muscle tears, either partial or complete, that occur as a sudden event during eccentric muscle contraction. DOMS and certain types of muscle strains can have identical appearances on MRI, but the history serves to distinguish the two entities. Muscle strains occur with an acute onset during activity, versus delayed onset of symptoms and no acute injury for DOMS. Muscles can absorb more energy and be protected from muscle strains by warming up and stretching; these activities have no protective effect for DOMS.

Muscle strains are the most frequent injury in sports. Powerful, eccentric muscle contractions

---

BOX 3–6: INDIRECT MUSCLE INJURIES

Delayed-onset muscle soreness (DOMS; muscle stiffness)
- Pain peaks 2 days after unaccustomed activity
- No acute injury or painful event
- Damage is at ultrastructural level and reversible

Muscle strains (partial or complete tears)
- Pain is sudden onset during activity
- Occurs during eccentric muscle contraction (ie, muscle lengthens as it contracts, such as the biceps while lowering a weight)
- Often affects muscles crossing two joints (rectus femoris, biceps femoris, gastrocnemius) and affects myotendinous junction
- *Grade I:* few muscle fibers torn, no functional loss, interstitial blood
  Grade II: more fibers torn, some loss of strength, focal defect and interstitial blood in muscle, blood surrounding tendon from myotendinous junction injury
  Grade III: muscle completely torn, loss of strength, focal and interstitial blood

MRI of muscle strains
- *DOMS and grade I (T2)*
  - Feathery, interstitial signal in muscle
  - ± ↑ signal between muscles
- *Grade II (T2)*
  - Feathery, interstitial ↑ signal in muscle
  - ↑ signal between muscles
  - ± focal muscle defect
  - Tendon thinned, irregular, lax
  - ↑ signal surrounding tendon
- *Grade III (T2)*
  - Feathery, interstitial ↑ signal in muscle
  - Complete muscle disruption with ↑ signal in gap between retracted segments
  - ↑ signal between muscle fragments—discontinuity of tendon within muscle

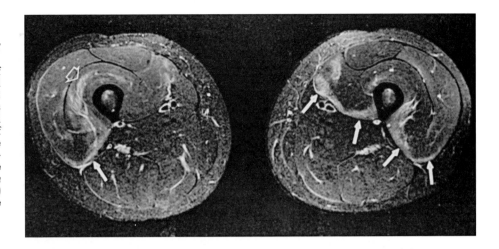

Figure 3–17. DELAYED-ONSET MUSCLE SORENESS (DOMS). STIR axial image, thighs. One of our fellows ran a marathon, and these are her thighs less than 2 days later (she said they felt as bad as they look). High-signal edema is seen in the periphery of some of the vastus musculature *(solid arrows)*. More diffuse interstitial muscle edema is seen in the right vastus intermedius *(open arrow)*. Intermuscular (perfascial) edema was not present at the time of this MRI.

while a muscle is being stretched tear the muscle fibers at and just proximal to the myotendinous junction. With healing, the muscle can regain most of its strength. Until full recovery, the muscle is at increased risk for a second injury because of the decreased strength and stiffness of the injured muscle. The myotendinous junction is the weakest point because it has less ability to absorb energy than either the muscle or the tendon. At the myotendinous junction, the muscle cells have multiple projections that form intervening recesses, into which collagen fibrils from the tendon insert. This ultrastructural arrangement allows for increased contact area between the muscle and tendon that helps to dissipate forces and lessen the risk of injury; however, the myotendinous junction remains the area most susceptible to injury.

One exception to muscle strains presenting as an acute painful event relates to the rectus femoris muscle in the anterior thigh. Chronic repetitive stresses, usually in runners, may result in a nonpainful muscle strain that presents as a palpable mass. Many of these patients come to medical attention for work-up of a tumor mass (Fig. 3–18).

Strains are divided into three grades. Grade I and grade II strains can be difficult to distinguish from

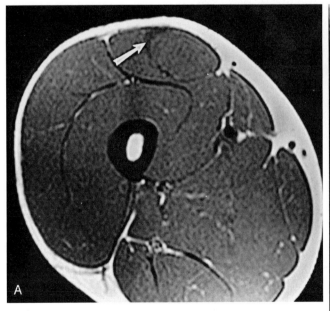
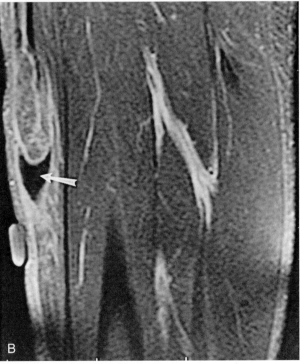

Figure 3–18. MUSCLE TEAR MASQUERADING AS A TUMOR.
A, T1 axial image, thigh. This patient was referred for work-up of a tumor (painless mass) in the anterior thigh. The rectus femoris muscle is enlarged focally and there is a defect within it *(arrow)*, indicating a grade II muscle strain (tear) rather than a tumor mass.
B, T1 sagittal image, thigh, with fat suppression after gadolinium enhancement. The gap in the muscle *(arrow)* from the tear is seen again. Hyperemia surrounds the torn muscle. No mass is evident. This patient was a runner, which is typically the inciting event for (often painless) tears of this muscle.

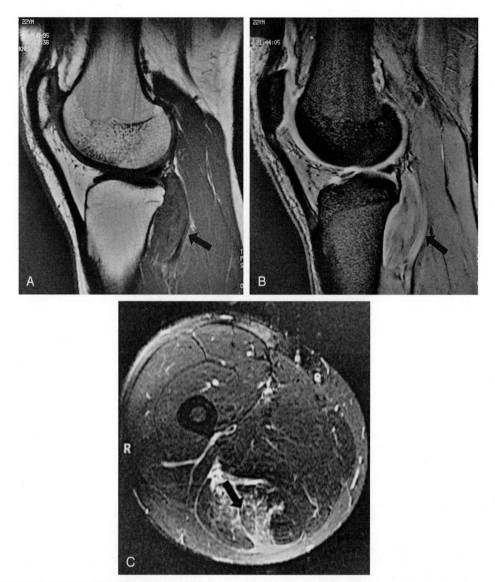

Figure 3–19. GRADE I MUSCLE STRAINS.
A, T1 sagittal image, knee. The popliteus muscle *(arrow)* is enlarged and the feathery fat pattern is absent when compared to adjacent muscles. *B*, T2* sagittal image, knee. High signal within the enlarged popliteus muscle *(arrow)* has a feathery pattern from interstitial edema/hemorrhage, and there is perifascial edema anterior and posterior to the muscle. *C*, STIR axial image, thigh (different patient than in *A* and *B*). The interstitial feathery pattern from edema/hemorrhage is seen well with STIR in grade I strain of the hamstrings *(arrow)*. There is also intermuscular (perifascial) edema.

each other, or from DOMS or a direct blow to muscle on MRI. A grade I strain consists of tearing of only a few muscle fibers, with no loss of function or permanent defect in the muscle (essentially, the muscle was stretched). There is edema, which causes enlargement of the muscle, a feathery interstitial increased signal intensity on T2W images, and perifascial edema (Fig. 3–19). We rarely seem to do MRI for grade I strains, probably because the symptoms are not severe enough to warrant the imaging examination. A grade II strain is a larger partial tear of the muscle with some loss of muscle strength. On MRI, there is the same feathery increased signal intensity from edema and hemorrhage in muscle as in grade I strains; additionally, a focal, mass-like lesion or stellate defect in the mus-

cle may be found as the result of a focal disruption of muscle fibers, and perifascial edema/hemorrhage is evident between muscles (Fig. 3–20). A grade II strain has a myotendinous junction that is partially torn, so that mild thinning, irregularity, or laxity of the tendon may be evident (Figs. 3–21 and 3–22). Hematoma surrounding the myotendinous junction is diagnostic of a grade II partial tear, indicating a true defect in the muscle tissue (Fig. 3–22). A grade III strain is a complete rupture of the muscle with near complete loss of function (strength). MRI demonstrates discontinuity of muscle and of the tendon traversing the muscle, retraction of fragments with wavy margins, and a hematoma that forms between the fragments (Fig. 3–23).[10, 11]

Muscle strains take a long time to heal because it

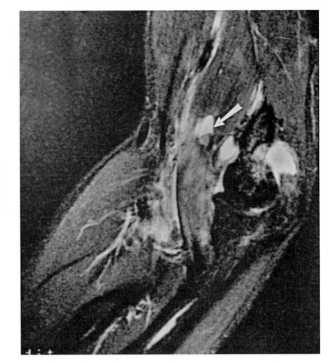

Figure 3–20. GRADE II MUSCLE STRAIN.
STIR sagittal image, elbow. Persistent pain and weakness following a posterior elbow dislocation led to this MRI, which demonstrates interstitial high-signal muscle edema in the brachialis, as well as a focal defect in the brachialis muscle *(arrow)*, clearly making this a grade II tear.

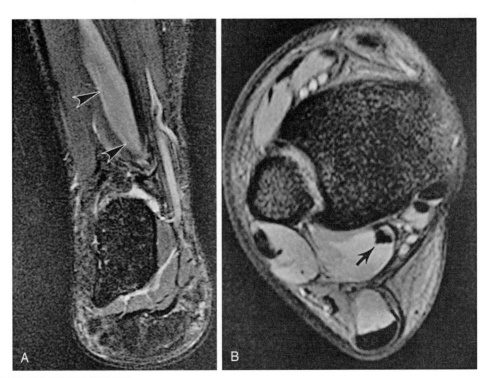

Figure 3–21. GRADE II MUSCLE STRAIN.
A, STIR coronal image, ankle. High signal is seen in the flexor hallucis longus muscle *(arrowheads)* adjacent to the tendon. *B,* T2* axial image, ankle. The flexor hallucis longus tendon in cross section *(arrow)* is irregular with high signal around it, indicating a grade II myotendinous junction muscle strain.

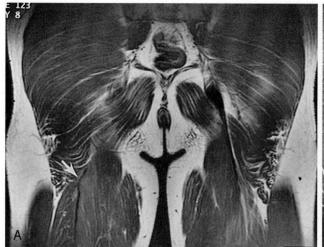
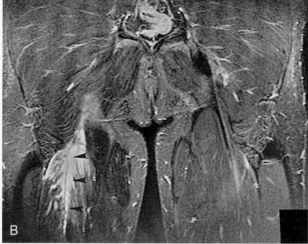

Figure 3–22. GRADE II MUSCLE STRAIN.
A, T1 coronal image, pelvis. The hamstring tendon is undulating *(arrow)*, and the feathery pattern in the adjacent muscle is obliterated. *B*, STIR coronal image, pelvis. There is high-signal hematoma surrounding the myotendinous junction *(arrowheads)* from a defect in the muscle tissue, a diagnostic finding of a grade II partial muscle tear.

is so difficult to put a muscle at rest for purposes of healing. Persistent contractions of the injured muscle can result in repeated microtears and hemorrhage months after the initial injury. For this reason, it is not unusual to see fatty infiltration from muscle atrophy secondary to disuse or injury, with superimposed blood products of varying age at the site of the muscle strain.

Direct Muscle Injuries (Box 3–7)

Direct trauma to muscles can be blunt or penetrating. Blunt trauma results in muscle contusions with intraparenchymal (interstitial) bleeds, hematoma formation, or myositis ossificans as a late sequela. Direct muscle lacerations can occur from penetrating injuries. Both blunt trauma and lacerations produce hemorrhage within the muscle belly at the point of insult. Lacerations also may cause denervation with muscle abnormalities distal to the injury.

Acutely, T2W images show increased signal intensity within the muscle due to the blood, edema, and inflammation that accompany bleeding from a contusion. This may have a feathery pattern within the muscle. Hematomas less than 48 hours old are usually isointense to muscle on T1W images, whereas subacute hemorrhage characteristically has high signal intensity on T1W images.

Intramuscular (Intraparenchymal or Interstitial) Hemorrhage. When blood dissects freely between muscle fibers, it is referred to as intraparenchymal, interstitial, or intramuscular hemorrhage. The integrity of the muscle is not violated. Interstitial hemorrhage is caused by direct injury to the muscle with

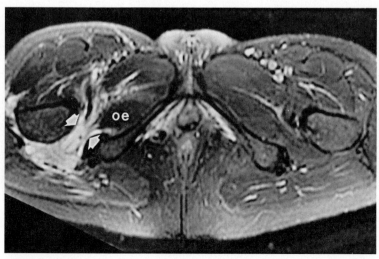

Figure 3–23. GRADE III MUSCLE STRAIN.
Fast T2 with fat suppression axial image, pelvis. There is complete disruption of the obturator externus (oe) muscle at the point indicated by the arrows. High-signal hematoma fills the gap. Compare with the normal obturator externus on the left side.

BOX 3–7: DIRECT MUSCLE INJURIES

Muscle Contusions
  Interstitial hemorrhage
    - Intraparenchymal bleeding
    - High signal on T2 with muscle fibers coursing through the abnormal area
    - No focal defect; muscle may be enlarged
Hematoma
    - Confined, mass-like collection of blood
    - No muscle fibers coursing through mass
    - Focal, heterogeneous mass with muscle enlargement
    - Signal of blood on T1 and T2 are age dependent
Myositis Ossificans
    - Intramuscular granulation tissue that may ossify or calcify
    - Acute (<8 weeks)
    Heterogeneous mass
        T1: isotense to muscle
        T2: mixed high- and low-signal lesion; surrounding high-signal edema
    - Chronic (>8 weeks)
    Variable appearance:
    Fatty marrow—T1 and T2: low-signal rim, center isotense with fat
        T1: diffuse, intermediate-signal center
        T2: slight increased signal in center
            Low-signal rim, all sequences

a contusion, usually by a blunt object, rather than from exertional physical activity (indirect muscle injury).

MRI demonstrates focal muscle enlargement, which may be subtle, and separation of fibers by blood, creating a feathery pattern on T2W images (Fig. 3–24). T1W images may appear normal or may show the enlarged muscle. No focal collections of blood or edema are evident. Muscle fibers are always evident coursing through the abnormal area in the muscle. This obviously can have an appearance similar to grade I muscle strains, and the history

is necessary for reliable differentiation of the two entities.

Hematoma (Box 3–8). Injury to soft tissues can cause subcutaneous or intramuscular hematomas. Hematomas are confined collections of blood that are well defined with a mass-like character and no interspersed muscle parenchyma or stroma.

The appearance of hematomas on MRI is highly variable, is age dependent, and follows the same changes as blood in the brain and spinal cord, but the time course tends to be longer and less predictable because of the lower oxygen tension outside of the brain (Figs. 3–25 through 3–27). What is considered isointense signal relative to the brain or cord can be considered as intermediate signal intensity in the extremities, similar to muscle. Hyperacute blood is rarely imaged but is intermediate signal intensity on T1W (similar to muscle) and high signal intensity on T2W images. Acute blood has intermediate signal intensity on T1W and T2W images. Subacute hematomas show hyperintensity on T1W images, similar to that of fat. Early subacute hematomas have low signal intensity on T2W images, whereas older subacute hematomas and chronic hematomas have high signal intensity on T2W images. Chronic hematomas may have low signal intensity, especially around their rims, because of hemosiderin deposition and fibrosis (Fig. 3–27).

The easiest way we know to remember the progression of signal intensity changes in hematomas that occurs over time is by using a sophisticated mnemonic imported by one of our fellows from Canada, who clearly had nothing better to do on those long, cold northern nights: "**It Be IdDy BiDdy BaBy DooDoo**." This is a phrase that helps to organize the sequence of events. If I = Intermediate signal, B = Bright signal, and D = Dark (low) signal, then the bold letters in the phrase refer to the signal intensity on T1W and T2W images, respectively, in each of the five stages of hematoma progression (hyperacute, acute, early subacute, late subacute, and chronic).

There often is heterogeneity of the hematoma, probably from repeated bleeding from recurrent injury, because placing muscles at rest is difficult (Figs. 3–25 and 3–26). Both fat and subacute blood can cause high signal intensity on T1W images in the musculoskeletal system and could have a similar appearance; fat-suppressed images allow differentiation of fat (which suppresses) from blood (which does not).

BOX 3–8: PROGRESSION OF HEMATOMA SIGNAL ON MRI

	BLOOD PRODUCTS	T1 SIGNAL	T2 SIGNAL	MNEMONIC	
Hyperacute	Oxyhemoglobin/serum	*I*ntermediate	*B*right	It Be	(IB)
Acute	Deoxyhemoglobin	*I*ntermediate	*D*ark	IdDy	(ID)
Subacute, early	Intracellular methemoglobin	*B*right	*D*ark	BiDdy	(BD)
Subacute, late	Extracellular methemoglobin	*B*right	*B*right	BaBy	(BB)
Chronic	Hemosiderin	*D*ark	*D*ark	Doo Doo	(DD)

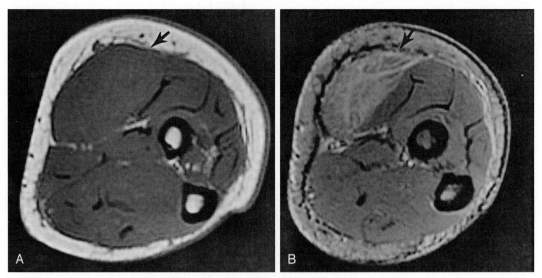

Figure 3–24. INTRAMUSCULAR (INTERSTITIAL) MUSCLE HEMORRHAGE (DIRECT BLOW).
A, T1 axial image, forearm. The brachioradialis muscle is enlarged *(arrow)*. *B*, T2* axial image, forearm. The brachioradialis muscle *(arrow)* has a feathery interstitial increased signal pattern from blood dissecting between muscle fibers, without disrupting the muscle.

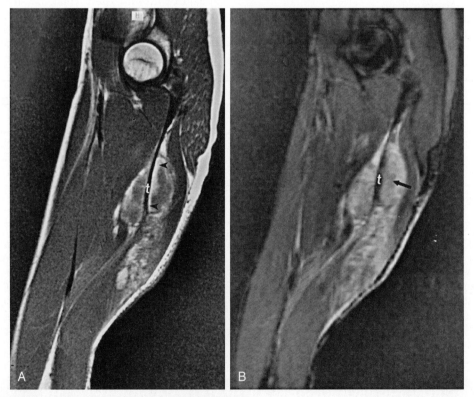

Figure 3–25. HEMATOMA WITH BLOOD AT DIFFERENT STAGES.
A, T1 sagittal image, thigh. There is a hematoma surrounding the biceps femoris tendon (t) from a large grade II muscle strain. The outer rim of the hematoma *(arrowheads)* has high signal from late subacute blood products. The inner portion of the hematoma is intermediate signal. *B*, STIR sagittal image, thigh. The hematoma around the biceps femoris tendon (t) has a heterogeneous pattern. The areas that were high signal on T1 remain high signal on STIR (late subacute blood). Some of the area that was intermediate signal on T1 became high signal on STIR (hyperacute blood), and still other areas were intermediate on T1 and remained low signal on STIR *(arrow)* (acute blood).

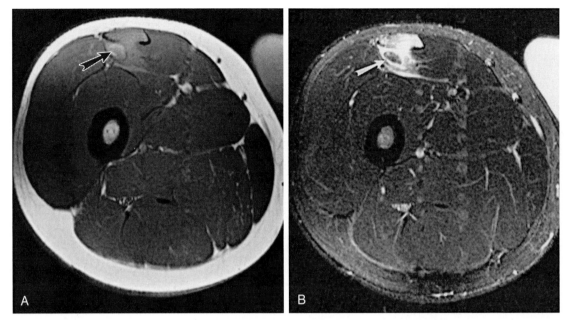

Figure 3–26. HEMATOMA WITH BLOOD AT VARYING STAGES.
A, T1 axial image, thigh. High signal in the rectus femoris muscle is evident adjacent to the tendon. A more focal area of higher signal is present laterally *(arrow)*. *B*, STIR axial image, thigh. The lateral half of the muscle generally remains high signal (late subacute blood), whereas the focal area *(arrow)* becomes low signal (early subacute blood).

With healing, scarring with fibrosis is produced along with muscle regeneration. The amount of fibrosis produced can be monitored with MR examinations and predicts whether full tensile strength and functional recovery will occur. Chronic scar tissue and fibrosis have low signal intensity on all

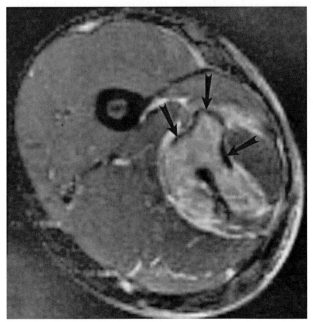

Figure 3–27. CHRONIC HEMATOMA.
STIR axial image, thigh. Heterogeneous high and low signal are evident in the hematoma surrounding one of the hamstring tendons. In addition, there is a rim of low signal forming *(arrows)* around the margin of the hematoma, typical of a chronic hematoma with fibrosis and hemosiderin deposition.

MR pulse sequences. A defect in muscle from a tear may eventually fill in with fat rather than fibrosis (Fig. 3–28).

Hemorrhage into Tumor. The presence of a hematoma in or between muscle may be the manifestation of bleeding into a necrotic soft tissue tumor, rather than simply being a benign post-traumatic hematoma (Fig. 3–29). It can sometimes be difficult to determine if a hematoma exists within or between muscles, because intermuscular masses may significantly displace and thin overlying muscle so that the appearance in both circumstances is very similar. If the history is inconsistent so that the patient reports minimal trauma but a large hematoma is present, or if there is any solid-appearing component in the hematoma, one must suspect a soft tissue sarcoma and evaluate it by other means, such as angiography or biopsy. Other helpful signs to differentiate a hematoma from a hemorrhagic neoplasm are that neoplasms will not have complete or partial tears of the tendon, and the mass effect of the neoplasm will cause displacement of the tendon rather than abnormal signal surrounding it, the latter finding being more typical of a traumatic hematoma at the myotendinous junction.

Myositis Ossificans. Blunt trauma to muscle can cause myositis ossificans, which is a circumscribed mass of granulation tissue that may calcify or ossify with time. If the trauma is not recalled and no calcification is seen on radiographs, this entity is generally not thought of and patients are worked up for a soft tissue mass.

The MR appearance depends on the histology and the stage of evolution of the lesion (Fig. 3–30).[12] In general, the appearance is variable and nonspecific,

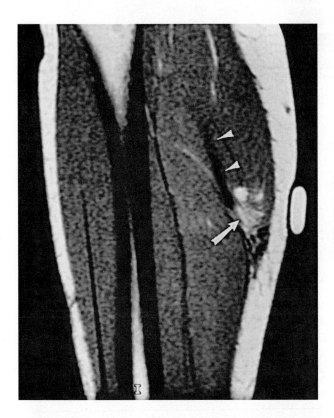

Figure 3–28. CHRONIC MUSCLE TEAR.
T1 sagittal image, calf. A defect in the muscle from a strain may heal with low-signal fibrosis, scarring, and muscle regeneration, or it may simply fill in with fat *(arrow)* as in this case of a remote gastrocnemius grade II strain. The linear low-signal structure proximal to the muscle defect *(arrowheads)* is an abnormally thickened plantaris tendon that previously ruptured.

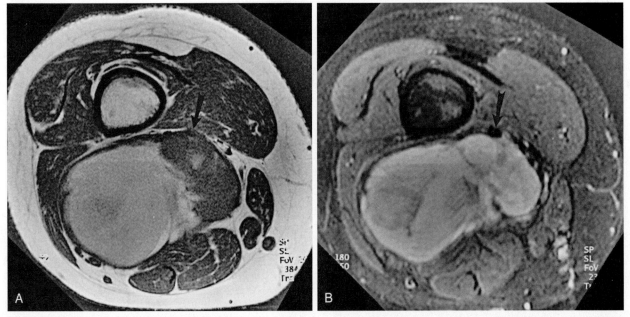

Figure 3–29. HEMORRHAGE INTO A TUMOR.
A, T1 axial image, distal thigh. There is a large mass posteriorly with high signal throughout most of it, indicating blood. There is a tendon displaced by the hemorrhagic mass *(arrow)*. *B*, STIR axial image, distal thigh. The posterior mass is heterogeneous, but mainly high signal, and again consistent with blood. The displaced tendon is seen *(arrow)*. This initially was diagnosed elsewhere as a hematoma and left alone for a year. The patient came to see our orthopedists because the mass did not decrease in size. The fact that the blood does not surround the tendon is a good clue that this is not a traumatic hematoma. The medial portion of this mass (on the side where the tendon is displaced) is actually solid, and showed a synovial sarcoma at biopsy.

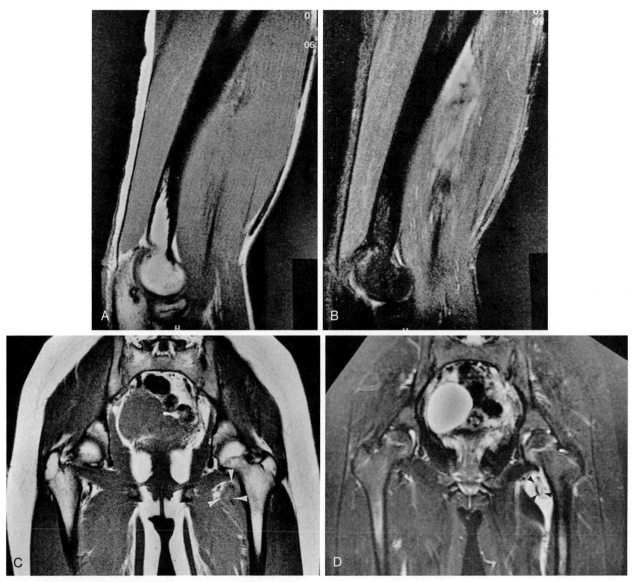

Figure 3–30. MYOSITIS OSSIFICANS.
A, T1 sagittal image, arm. There was a palpable mass in this patient's anterior arm. There is vague heterogeneity in the brachialis muscle anterior to the humerus, but overall the signal is isointense to muscle. *B*, STIR sagittal image, arm (same patient as in *A*). There is mixed signal, but mainly high signal in the muscle and adjacent to the humerus, compatible with acute changes of myositis ossificans. *C*, T1 coronal image, pelvis (different patient than in *A* and *B*). A palpable mass with negative radiographs led to this MR, which demonstrates a mass in the adductors of the left thigh medial to the intertrochanteric region of the hip *(arrowheads)*. There is a low-signal rim and intermediate-signal center. *D*, STIR coronal image, pelvis (same patient as in *C*). The center of the mass is slightly high signal, the rim around it remains low signal *(arrowheads)*, and there is a large area of surrounding high-signal edema. This is compatible with a diagnosis of myositis ossificans greater than 8 weeks old with fibrosis in the center of the lesion.

and it can be confused with a soft tissue tumor, especially early.

Acute lesions under 2 months old are isointense to muscle on T1W images and mixed signal (mainly high signal) intensity on T2W images, especially centrally, because of proliferating cellular fibroblasts and myofibroblasts. There may be a large area of surrounding edema.

Lesions of myositis ossificans more than 8 weeks old may have two different patterns on MRI: (1) central signal intensity that is isointense with fat on T1W and T2W images, representing bone marrow surrounded by a low signal intensity rim of lamellar bone, or (2) diffuse intermediate signal intensity on T1W images from fibrosis that is slightly high signal intensity on T2W images. Edema generally is not present surrounding the mass after the first few weeks postinjury. Radiographs and computed tomography (CT) can be very helpful in making the specific diagnosis of myositis ossificans if it is unclear from the MRI.

Miscellaneous Traumatic Injuries

Compartment syndromes and fascial herniation of muscle are considered here. Denervation of muscle

BOX 3–9: COMPARTMENT SYNDROMES

Traumatic
  Acute:
  - Fracture, hemorrhage, edema, usually in calf
  - ↑ pressure, ↓ circulation
  - Muscle necrosis: T2: increased signal diffusely in and between muscle of affected compartment
  Chronic:
  - Muscles atrophied, fibrotic, or necrotic with calcified rim (calcific myonecrosis)
Exertional
  - Exercise normally causes extracellular, intramuscular fluid that disappears 10 minutes after cessation of exercise.
  - If the intramuscular edema persists more than 15–25 minutes after exercise, acute or chronic exertional compartment syndromes may occur from the increased pressure.
  - T2: increased signal in and between muscles, 25 minutes after provocative exercise.

and rhabdomyolysis may occur from trauma but are discussed elsewhere.

Compartment Syndromes (Box 3–9). *Acute traumatic compartment syndrome* can affect the calf following trauma with a fracture. Compartment syndrome occurs when hemorrhage or edema within closed fascial boundaries leads to increased pressure with compromise of the circulation. MRI can show the extent of edema and rhabdomyolysis, because necrotic muscle is much higher signal intensity than normal muscle on T2W images. This is a surgical emergency and MRI generally does not play a role in the work-up of this entity.

In *chronic compartment syndrome*, muscles are atrophied and may be densely fibrotic. Calcification of the involved muscle compartment may exist, and this is especially common in the peroneal compartment. A chronic compartment syndrome may rarely lead to *calcific myonecrosis*. There is typically a remote history of trauma, usually several decades prior to the development of calcific myonecrosis. Patients have a painless mass, usually in the calf. The mass consists of liquefied necrotic muscle surrounded by a thin shell of calcification (Fig. 3–31). Peripheral peroneal nerve damage commonly is associated with this condition.

MRI is useful for showing the anatomic extent of the abnormalities and the extent of muscle loss that exists.

Exertional Compartment Syndrome. During intense activity, extracellular free water increases in the affected muscles, particularly in concentrically exercised muscles. This increased intramuscular fluid leads to increased pressure in the anatomic compartment that contains the muscles. MRI can show this normal, exercise-induced phenomenon, which will cause no changes on T1W images, but will show increased signal intensity on T2W images immediately after exercise. The signal intensity returns to baseline by 10 minutes after cessation of exercise. The increased signal intensity is seen diffusely throughout the affected muscles.[13]

Intramuscular pressure increases more than normal in some patients after exercise and does not quickly return to baseline. Such changes may lead to an acute or chronic exertional compartment syndrome, requiring fasciotomy for cure. Chronic exertional compartment syndromes are difficult to diagnose because symptoms abate between episodes of exertion. Intramuscular wick pressure measurements before and after exercise may be useful for diagnostic purposes, but it is an invasive test and pressure criteria for the diagnosis are not universally accepted.

On MR images, exertional compartment syndromes are characterized by swelling within a compartment, which manifests as intramuscular diffuse high signal intensity on T2W images (Fig. 3–32). Performing the MR examination immediately after a provocative exercise may be necessary. Failure of the edematous muscles to return to a baseline normal appearance by 15 to 25 minutes after the completion of exercise is diagnostic.

Fascial Herniation of Muscle. Muscle can herniate through a traumatic fascial defect and present

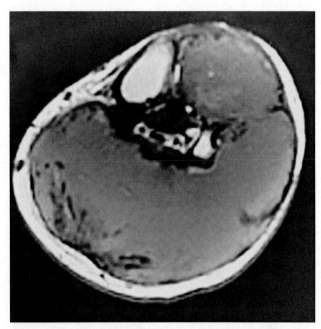

Figure 3–31. CALCIFIC MYONECROSIS FROM CHRONIC COMPARTMENT SYNDROME.
T1 axial image, calf. There is intermediate to high signal in the muscles of the calf, with a low-signal rim. There is absence of the feathery pattern of normal musculature. The conventional radiographs showed diffuse calcification in the calf musculature. There was a history of trauma 15 years earlier.

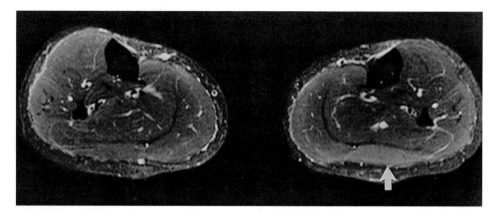

Figure 3–32. EXERTIONAL COMPARTMENT SYNDROME. STIR axial image, calves. There is diffuse intramuscular high signal in the lateral head of the left gastrochemius muscle 30 minutes after provocative exercise *(arrow)*. The T1 images were normal, as were the preexercise STIR images (not shown). Postexercise muscle edema normally disappears within about 10 minutes of the activity.

clinically as a soft tissue mass (Fig. 3–33). The lesions are usually asymptomatic, although pain or cramping may occur with activity. It sometimes is difficult to demonstrate the mass during the MR examination without contracting the muscle by placing the foot in dorsal and plantar flexion, but this may lead to motion and degraded images. Very short pulse sequences during muscle contraction may allow demonstration of muscle tissue protruding in the region of the patient's palpable mass. The mass may disappear on images obtained without muscle contraction. MRI can confirm the diagnosis by showing normal muscles with no mass, even though the herniated muscle is not demonstrated on the study. In other cases, the muscle remains herniated at all times and is not significantly affected by muscle contraction; the diagnosis is easier to make in this circumstance. Occasionally, a defect in the low signal intensity fascia through which the muscle herniates can be seen by MRI. This is a traumatic injury and most commonly is seen in the anterior lower leg or thigh in athletes, may be multiple, and usually is asymptomatic.

Inflammatory Myopathies

Bacterial or viral pyomyositis, necrotizing fasciitis, sarcoidosis, and the autoimmune idiopathic inflammatory polymyopathies are all relatively unusual diseases that may affect muscle.

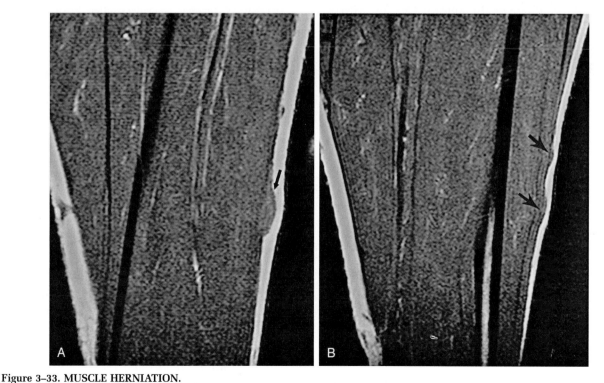

Figure 3–33. MUSCLE HERNIATION.
A, T1 coronal image, calf. There is a soft tissue mass *(arrow)* protruding into the subcutaneous fat at the site of a painless, palpable abnormality. The signal intensity followed that of muscle on all pulse sequences, and this represents herniation of the peroneus longus muscle through fascia. **B**, T1 coronal image, calf. Two separate fascial muscle herniations are evident on this cut *(arrows)* from the same patient as in *A*.

BOX 3–10: INFECTION

Pyomyositis
- Penetrating injury or hematogenous
- Rare; usually in immune-compromised host
- Nonspecific MRI with high signal on T2 images in and around muscle

Necrotizing Fasciitis
- Infection of intermuscular fascia, pyomyositis rarely associated
- Severe systemic toxicity, high mortality
- Difficult clinical distinction from cellulitis, which affects only subcutaneous fat
- MRI:
  T2: Increased signal between muscles
      Possible increased signal in muscles (from hyperemia)
  Easy distinction from cellulitis that shows strand-like abnormal signal (low on T1, high on T2) limited to the subcutaneous fat

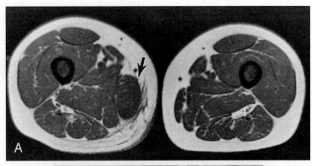

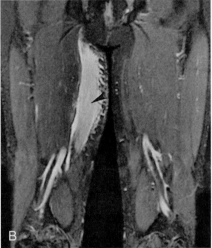

Figure 3–34. PYOMYOSITIS.
A, T1 axial image, thighs. The gracilis muscle is enlarged on the right side *(arrow)*. The muscle also has lower signal than adjacent muscles and there is edema in the subcutaneous fat overlying the gracilis. The marrow of both femora is intermediate signal (the same signal as muscle), indicating a diffuse marrow infiltrative process, which was from leukemia. *B*, STIR coronal image, thighs. The gracilis has diffuse abnormal high signal within it and in the adjacent subcutaneous fat. The center of the muscle shows a focal area of slightly higher signal *(arrowhead)* that proved to be an abscess when aspirated.

Pyomyositis (Box 3–10)

Infection of muscle may be introduced either during a penetrating injury or by hematogenous spread and must be considered as a cause for abnormal size and signal intensity in musculature by MRI. Bacterial myositis is unusual except in immune-compromised hosts, such as transplant patients and those with acquired immunodeficiency syndrome (AIDS). Pyomyositis generally occurs where there was blunt trauma, with a coexisting source in the body for bacteremia, usually in someone who is immune compromised.[14] There is diffuse muscle involvement, sometimes with a focal abscess (Fig. 3–34). Nothing specific is seen on MRI in pyomyositis. There will be increased signal intensity throughout the affected muscle on T2W images. The muscle often is enlarged, and there may be high signal intensity fluid in fascial planes surrounding the abnormal muscle.

Muscle abscesses are fluid-filled cavities that are bright on T2W images, with a thick rim (Box 3–11). The center does not enhance with intravenous contrast material, whereas the rim typically does. Such a pattern is typical of an abscess, but it may be seen in other entities, including ischemic foci in muscle and necrotic soft tissue tumors.

Necrotizing Fasciitis (Box 3–10)

This is a relatively rare, rapidly progressive infection characterized by extensive necrosis of subcutaneous tissue and the fascia between muscles, and usually accompanied by severe systemic toxicity.

The mortality rate is over 70% if not recognized and appropriately treated.

Early clinical recognition of necrotizing fasciitis may be difficult and the differentiation between this entity and cellulitis may be impossible on clinical grounds. Cellulitis involves infection of only subcutaneous fatty tissue and can be treated adequately with antibiotics in most cases. Necrotizing fasciitis requires early surgical intervention in addition to

BOX 3–11: RIM ENHANCEMENT OF FOCAL MUSCLE LESION

MRI shows: Low signal on T1
           High signal on T2
           Rim enhancement post-contrast
Differential diagnosis: Abscess
                        Necrotic tumor
                        Ischemic foci (diabetics)

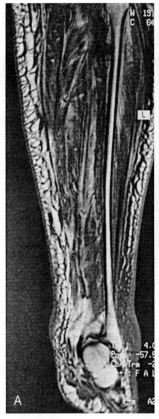
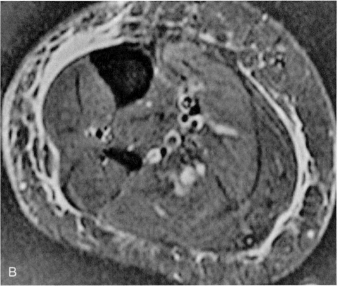

Figure 3–35. CELLULITIS.
A. T1 coronal image, calf. There is a low-signal reticular pattern throughout the subcutaneous fat from edema as the result of cellulitis. *B,* STIR axial image, calf. The reticular edema pattern in the subcutaneous fat becomes high signal on this sequence. Of key importance is that there is no high signal in or between muscles.

antibiotics. Early fasciotomy and debridement in necrotizing fasciitis have been associated with improved survival, compared with delayed surgical exploration.

Prior to MRI, the only way to diagnose necrotizing fasciitis was at the time of surgery, when no resistance to probing was discovered in the fascial planes between muscles. MRI has the ability to make the differentiation between cellulitis and necrotizing fasciitis in a noninvasive manner and constitutes a legitimate reason for an emergency MRI examination (Figs. 3–35 and 3–36).[15, 16]

The MRI appearance in necrotizing fasciitis is that of high signal intensity and thickening between muscles along deep fascial sheaths on T2W images. The adjacent muscles also may have high signal intensity secondary to hyperemia and edema from the adjacent inflammatory process. Contrast-enhanced images show high signal intensity on T1W images in fascial planes because of the hyperemia associated with the infection; occasionally, muscle abscesses or focal necrotic tissue with ring enhancement also can be seen. In general, there is no need to do contrast-enhanced imaging for this diagnosis, especially because muscle pyomyositis is rarely associated with this disease.

MRI has a high sensitivity for detecting necrotizing fasciitis and showing its extent, but the findings are nonspecific. This is not a real problem, however, because the clinical setting in conjunction with the typical MRI appearance allows the diagnosis to be made, even though the MRI findings are seen in other entities.

Idiopathic Inflammatory Polymyopathies

The common diseases in this category are polymyositis and dermatomyositis. Active myositis

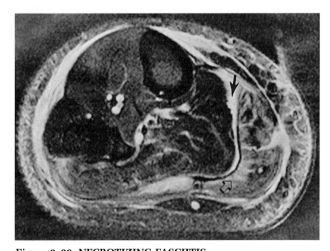

Figure 3–36. NECROTIZING FASCIITIS.
STIR axial image, calf. There is edema in the subcutaneous fat. There is also high signal between muscles *(solid arrow)* in deep fascial planes, and diffuse interstitial edema in the gastrocnemius muscle *(open arrow)* from hyperemia and edema as the result of the adjacent fascial infection.

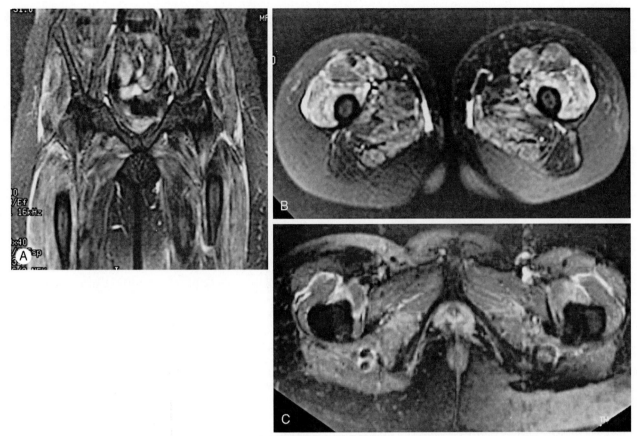

Figure 3–37. IDIOPATHIC INFLAMMATORY POLYMYOPATHIES.
A, Fast T2 with fat suppression coronal image, pelvis. There is high signal within multiple muscles as well as surrounding them. This was an 11-year-old child with diffuse pain. This is juvenile dermatomyositis. *B*, Fast T2 with fat suppression axial image, thighs (same patient as in *A*). Most of the muscles demonstrate diffuse abnormal high signal, but posteriorly muscles are spared bilaterally. Muscle involvement is typically non-uniform in these diseases. *C*, STIR axial image, pelvis (different patient than in *A* and *B*). This patient presented with bilateral hip pain. The MR shows abnormal signal between muscles of the hips bilaterally, as well as some intramuscular abnormal high signal. This ultimately proved to be from polymyalgia rheumatica.

demonstrates increased signal intensity on T2W images, which is more conspicuous with fat-suppression techniques (Fig. 3–37). Burned-out disease shows fatty replacement of muscles that is high signal intensity on T1W images. Muscle involvement is typically non-uniform in these diseases, and MRI is useful to direct a biopsy to an abnormal muscle early in the disease process in order to make a diagnosis. Non–image-guided biopsies have up to a 25% false-negative rate, because the needle is in abnormal muscle only by chance.[17, 18]

Once disease is established, increased weakness in these patients can be from several sources, such as an inflammatory flare involving the muscles (which will respond to steroid therapy), a steroid-induced myopathy, or progressive muscle atrophy. MR imaging is useful to distinguish among these possibilities.

Primary Muscle Diseases

Dystrophies and Myopathies

Muscular dystrophies and congenital myopathies can sometimes be differentiated on the pattern of muscle involvement. For example, Duchenne's muscular dystrophy tends to have symmetric involvement progressing from proximal to distal, whereas myotonic dystrophy tends to progress from distal to proximal.[19, 20]

MRI can show the pattern of muscle involvement, which may help to confirm a diagnosis, or MRI also can be valuable in guiding a biopsy to an involved muscle. Similarly, MRI can identify muscles that are selectively spared by the disease process and can be used for muscle transfer operations. MRI more accurately depicts progression of disease than serum enzyme levels.

Early in the disease, MRI generally demonstrates increased signal intensity on T2W images as the result of edema and inflammation in the abnormal muscle. Atrophy of the muscle is the predominant finding late in the disease, and high signal intensity from fatty infiltration of the atrophied muscle will be seen on T1W images.

Denervation (Boxes 3–12 and 3–13)

Muscles and the nerves that supply them can be considered as a single motor or neuromuscular unit.

BOX 3–12: FATTY ATROPHY OF MUSCLE

• High signal intensity on T1 images
• Differential diagnoses
  - Denervation
  - Burned-out dermatomyositis or polymyositis
  - Disuse
  - Muscular dystrophies
  - Congenital myopathies

BOX 3–13: MRI APPEARANCE OF DENERVATION

Acute (<2 weeks)
  - Normal signal in muscle
1–12 months
  - High signal in affected muscles on T2 from extracellular, intramuscular edema
>12 months
  - High signal on T1 from fatty infiltration of atrophied muscle

Damage to a nerve causes changes in the muscle supplied by that nerve. Several traumatic, vascular, congenital, metabolic, and infiltrative processes can disrupt the nerve supply to muscle.

The MRI changes after denervation follow a predictable course. Acutely, MRI may be normal. After about 2 weeks, extracellular water increases within muscle, resulting in increased signal intensity on T2W images, especially fat-suppressed images such as STIR (Fig. 3–38). This appearance tends to persist for about 1 year after the insult. If reinnervation does not occur, fatty atrophy develops in the muscle, which is easily detected on T1W images as high signal intensity replacing muscle fibers (Fig. 3–39). These early and late changes in muscle are not specific unless the pattern of muscle involvement correlates with a known nerve distribution, which would suggest the diagnosis.[21, 22]

MRI can predict that a muscle will not be salvageable from reinnervation or nerve grafting by showing that the muscle has undergone fatty atrophy, which is irreversible at that point. MRI can be useful to map out muscles that are spared and could be used in muscle-tendon transfer operations. Occasionally, the cause of the neuropathy can be shown with MRI. MRI has several advantages over electromyographic (EMG) evaluation: it is noninvasive, has excellent resolution, and can demonstrate pathology in muscles with aberrant or dual nerve supplies.

Tumors (Box 3–14)

MRI frequently is used in the work-up of soft tissue masses, many of which arise in muscle. The MR appearance of some masses, such as intramus-

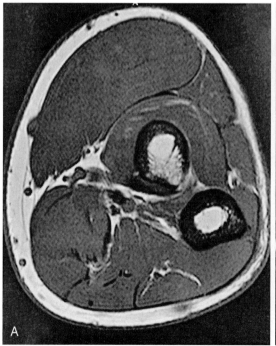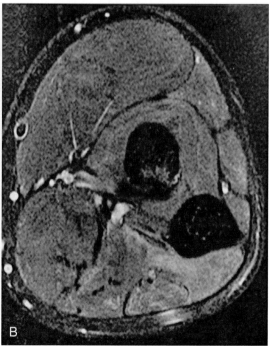

Figure 3–38. ACUTE DENERVATION.
A, T1 axial image, forearm. No abnormalities are evident. *B*, STIR axial image, forearm. There is diffuse intramuscular high signal in the flexor digitorum profundus and flexor carpi ulnaris muscles from early denervation (prior to muscle atrophy).

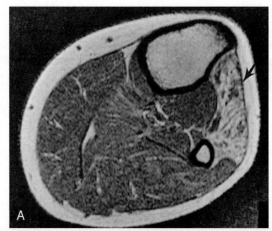

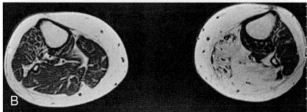

Figure 3–39. LATE DENERVATION.
A, T1 axial image, calf. The tibialis anterior muscle shows fatty atrophy *(arrow)* compared to the normal adjacent muscles. *B*, T1 axial image, calves (different patient than in *A*). Profound fatty replacement of the posterior calf musculature of the left thigh is evident from long-standing denervation in this diabetic patient.

cular lipomas, hematomas, and hemangiomas, is sufficiently specific so that no further tests are necessary. Most disorders, however, have a nonspecific appearance with increased signal on T2W images and variable enhancement. Although biopsy is often

BOX 3–14: INTRAMUSCULAR TUMORS

LESION	DISCRIMINATORS
Hemangioma	Contains fat
Lipoma	Is fat
Myxoma	Many cyst characteristics
Sarcoma	No surrounding edema
Metastases	Often surrounding edema
Lymphoma	Infiltrates entire muscle
Neurofibroma	Target sign possible; resembles myxoma, but diffuse enhancement

necessary, MRI is still useful to localize the most viable and therefore diagnostic tissues for biopsy.

Among the most common intramuscular tumors are hemangioma, lipoma, myxoma, neurofibroma, sarcoma, metastases, and lymphoma. Hemangiomas usually have serpiginous channels surrounded by fat that are diagnostic by MRI (Fig. 3–40). Lipomas also are easily diagnosed as masses with fat signal intensity on all pulse sequences (Fig. 3–41). Lymphoma often infiltrates an entire muscle, rather than appearing as a rounded mass (Fig. 3–42); metastases to muscle are rounded masses that often have large areas of edema surrounding them (Fig. 3–43).[23] Metastases from malignant melanoma may have a classic MRI appearance, consisting of focal lesions in muscle that are high signal intensity on T1W images and very low signal on STIR or T2W images, as a consequence of melanin (Fig. 3–43). Soft tissue sarcomas are rounded masses, but they do not generally have edema surrounding them; they may be-

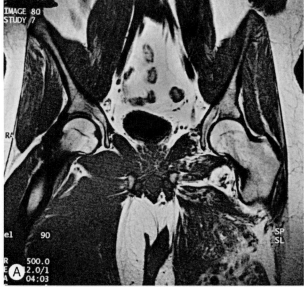

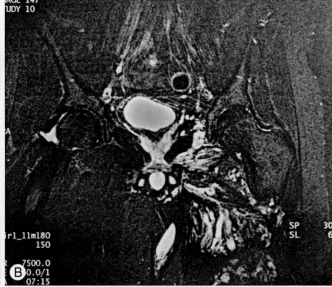

Figure 3–40. INTRAMUSCULAR TUMOR: Hemangioma.
A, T1 coronal image, pelvis. There is fatty infiltration of several muscles of the left proximal thigh (compare to the normal right side). *B*, STIR coronal image, pelvis. Numerous tubular, serpiginous vessels are seen as high-signal structures in and between muscles of the proximal left thigh and extending into the left pelvis from a hemangioma.

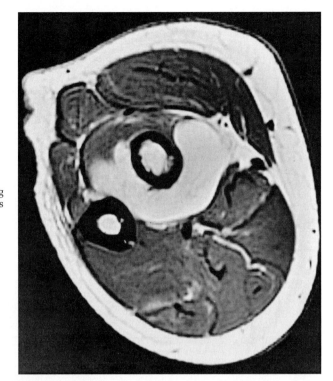

Figure 3–41. INTRAMUSCULAR TUMOR: Lipoma.
T1 axial image, forearm. There is a high-signal fatty mass replacing most of the supinator muscle and extending between the radius and ulna.

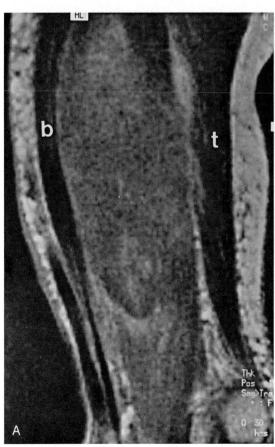

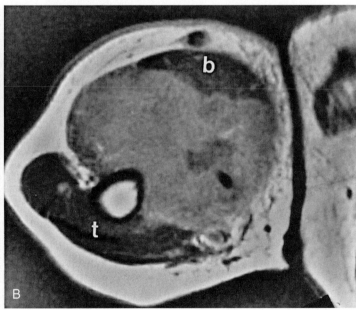

Figure 3–42. INTRAMUSCULAR TUMOR: Lymphoma.
A, Spin echo-T2 sagittal image, arm. There is mild increased signal throughout the enlarged brachialis muscle. The biceps muscle (b) is draped anterior to the brachialis and the triceps (t) is seen posterior to it. *B,* T1 with contrast enhancement axial image, arm. There is heterogeneous high signal throughout the markedly enlarged brachialis muscle from lymphoma. Again, the normal biceps (b) is seen anterior and the triceps (t) posterior to the mass.

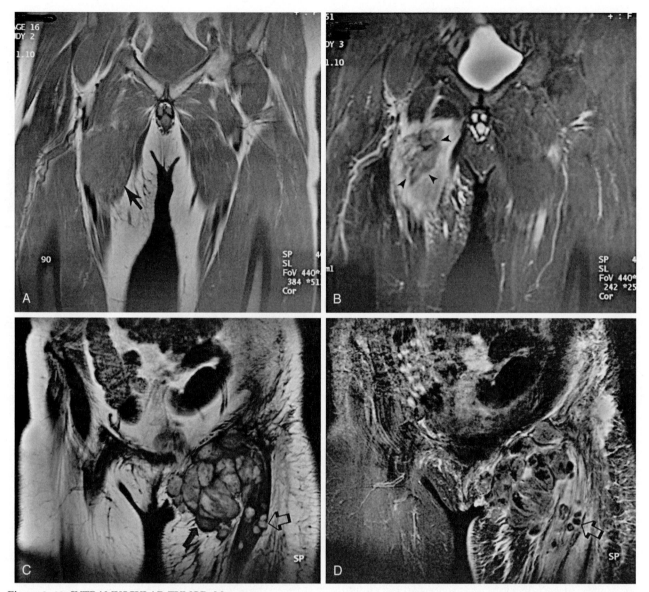

Figure 3–43. INTRAMUSCULAR TUMOR: Metastases.
A, T1 coronal image, pelvis. Mass in the right adductor muscles *(arrow).* *B,* STIR coronal image, pelvis (same patient as in *A*). The mass is heterogeneous and intermediate to high signal *(arrowheads).* The mass is surrounded by a large amount of high-signal edema. This was metastatic transitional cell cancer from the bladder. *C,* T1 coronal image, pelvis (different patient than in *A* and *B*). A mass of enlarged lymph nodes is present in the left groin. Several rounded high-signal masses are evident in the left sartorius muscle *(open arrow).* *D,* STIR coronal image, pelvis (same patient as in *C*). The intramuscular masses in the sartorius *(open arrow),* as well as several focal areas in the enlarged lymph nodes, have become profoundly low-signal intensity. In addition, there is edema in the sartorius muscle surrounding the focal lesions. These masses are from metastatic malignant melanoma. The signal intensity changes are typical for melanoma as compared to other metastases.

come necrotic, and hemorrhage into the necrotic tumor could be mistaken for a traumatic hematoma. Myxomas have signal characteristics that resemble fluid (very low signal on T1W, and very bright signal on T2W images) with heterogeneous or only peripheral enhancement when contrast is administered (Fig. 3–44). Intramuscular neurofibromas generally have a nonspecific appearance, being a mass that is low signal on T1 that is difficult to distinguish from normal surrounding muscle, and diffuse increased signal on T2W images. It has an MR appearance very similar to a myxoma, but there should be diffuse enhancement of a neurofibroma after intravenous

gadolinium is given. A target sign may be evident on T2W or contrast-enhanced images (low signal in the center of the mass).

Miscellaneous Muscle Abnormalities

Rhabdomyolysis

Many entities may cause massive destruction of muscle with increased serum levels of creatine kinase enzyme. This may result from massive trauma, prolonged immobilization, vascular ischemia, ex-

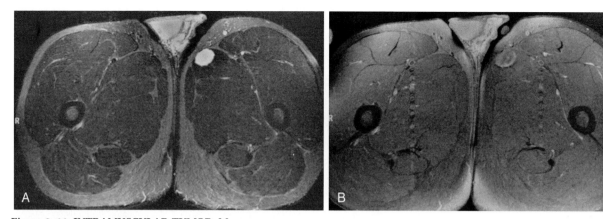

Figure 3–44. INTRAMUSCULAR TUMOR: Myxoma.
A, STIR axial image, thighs. There is a very high-signal mass in the left adductor musculature. *B*, T1 contrast-enhanced with fat suppression axial image, thighs. This myxoma shows peripheral enhancement.

cessive exercise, drug or alcohol overdose, and metabolic disorders such as hypokalemia, among others. The involved muscles show diffuse increased signal intensity on T2W images due to edema, necrosis, and hemorrhage. T1W images are not helpful, and the muscles usually are not enlarged.

Muscle Infarction (Box 3–15)

Ischemia to muscles is particularly common in diabetics and those with sickle cell anemia. Ischemic changes are very painful and result in edema with focal and diffuse areas of increased signal intensity in and surrounding muscle on T2W images.[24, 25]

Diabetic muscle infarction occurs from thrombosis of medium and small arterioles in patients with atherosclerosis and poorly controlled diabetes. Clinical symptoms consist of severe pain with or without swelling or a mass. The white count is normal. Over half of the patients have coexistent diabetic nephropathy, neuropathy, and retinopathy.

BOX 3–15: MUSCLE ISCHEMIA

- Common in diabetics and sickle cell anemia
- Diabetic muscle infarction
  - Severe pain with or without swelling/ mass
  - Normal white blood cell count
  - Thigh involved in 80%
    Calf involved in 20%
  - Bilateral in one third of patients
- MRI appearance
  - T1: Muscle swelling, obliteration of fat planes
  - T2: Diffuse intramuscular and intermuscular increased signal
  - Contrast: Diffuse enhancement of affected area or ring enhancement of necrotic foci

---

The thigh, especially the vastus musculature, is involved most commonly (about 80%); the calf is next most frequently affected (about 20%). It may start in the calf and progress to the thigh. It is bilateral in more than one third of cases.

MRI shows diffuse enlargement of several muscles, and more than one compartment often is involved (Fig. 3–45). The intermuscular fatty septae may be obliterated, and subfascial edema often is evident. On T2W images, there is increased signal intensity diffusely in and between muscles. There may be foci of hemorrhage. Gadolinium administration shows diffuse enhancement, but there also may be focal areas of rim enhancement, probably from hyperemia about an area of infarcted or necrotic muscle.

The diagnosis is not specific by MRI alone, but in conjunction with the clinical history, often a specific diagnosis can be made. If there is any question as to the diagnosis, percutaneous biopsy for culture and histology easily can be performed.

Accessory Muscles

Accessory muscles may be an incidental finding on MRI examinations; they also may present clinically as a mass or cause compression of an adjacent nerve. Accessory muscles occur in many locations throughout the body. The diagnosis of an accessory muscle is easy with MRI because the signal intensity and feathery texture are identical to other adjacent muscles (Fig. 3–46).

Radiation/Surgery/Chemotherapy

Lesions in the extremities that are treated with surgery, local radiation therapy, or chemotherapy often develop diffuse high signal intensity in the muscle and subcutaneous fat with the typical feathery appearance in muscle on T2W images (Fig. 3–47). These findings are nonspecific, but they should not alert the radiologist to persistent or recurrent tumor, because it is a common "normal" finding

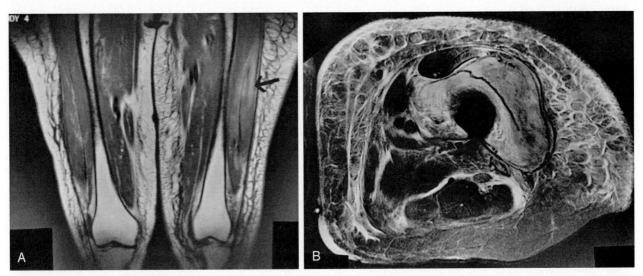

Figure 3–45. MUSCLE INFARCTION.
A, T1 coronal image, thighs. Both thighs are abnormal, but the findings are much more pronounced on the left. There is subcutaneous edema with a reticular pattern. The muscles are enlarged, and high signal in the left thigh muscle *(arrow)* indicates hemorrhage from the muscle infarction in this diabetic patient. *B*, STIR axial image, left thigh. Subcutaneous edema with reticular high signal is present diffusely. There is increased signal within the vastus musculature, and intermuscular septae show high signal as well.

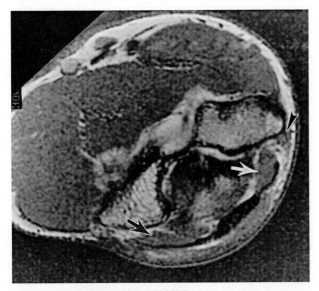

Figure 3–46. ANOMALOUS MUSCLE.
T1 axial image, elbow. This is a baseball player with ulnar neuropathy. The ulnar nerve *(arrowhead)* is subluxed medially on the medial epicondyle. The normal position for the nerve is occupied by a muscle (based on signal characteristics identical to adjacent muscles on all pulse sequences). This is an accessory or anomalous anconeus epitrochlearis muscle *(white arrow)*. The normal, laterally located anconeus is seen also *(black arrow)*.

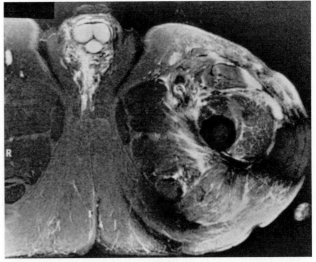

Figure 3–47. RADIATION CHANGES.
STIR axial image, proximal thigh. There is diffuse intramuscular and subcutaneous high signal. This man received radiation and surgery for a tumor in this region. These findings are expected after therapy. The lack of a round, high-signal mass essentially excludes recurrent tumor.

after treatment. Only the presence of a rounded mass should be of concern for persistent or recurrent tumor in the site of previous surgery or radiation. Often, a mass at a surgical site is a hematoma or seroma, rather than tumor; this can be determined by giving intravenous contrast material to determine if the mass is cystic or solid.

References

1. Zeiss J, Saddemi SR, Ebraheim NA. MR imaging of the quadriceps tendon: normal layered configuration and its importance in cases of tendon rupture. *AJR* 1992; 159:1031–1034.
2. Erickson SJ, Cox IH, Hyde JS, et al. Effect of tendon orientation on MR imaging signal intensity: a manifestation of the "magic angle" phenomenon. *Radiology* 1991; 181:389–392.
3. Kannus P, Józsa L. Histopathological changes preceding spontaneous rupture of a tendon. *J Bone Joint Surg [Am]* 1991; 73:1507–1524.
4. Chan TW, Dalinka MK, Kneeland JB, Chervrot A. Biceps tendon dislocation: evaluation with MR imaging. *Radiology* 1991; 179:649–652.
5. Bencardino J, Rosenberg ZS, Beltran J, et al. MR imaging of dislocation of the posterior tibial tendon. *AJR* 1997; 169:1109–1112.
6. Fleckenstein JL, Weatherall PT, Parkey RW, et al. Sports-related muscle injuries: evaluation with MR imaging. *Radiology* 1989; 172:793–798.
7. Shellock FG, Fukunaga T, Mink JH, Edgerton VR. Acute effects of exercise on MR imaging of skeletal muscle: concentric vs eccentric actions. *AJR* 1991; 156:765–768.
8. Shellock FG, Fukunaga T, Mink JH, Edgerton VR. Exertional muscle injury: evaluation of concentric versus eccentric actions with serial MR imaging. *Radiology* 1991; 179:659–664.
9. Nurenberg P, Giddings CJ, Stray-Gundersen J, et al. MR imaging—guided muscle biopsy for correlation of increased signal intensity with ultrastructural change and delayed-onset muscle soreness after exercise. *Radiology* 1992; 184:865–869.
10. De Smet AA. Magnetic resonance findings in skeletal tears. *Skeletal Radiol* 1993; 22:479–484.
11. El-Khoury GY, Brandser EA, Kathol MH, et al. Imaging of muscle injuries. *Skeletal Radiol* 1996; 25:3–11.
12. Kransdorf MJ, Meis JM, Jelinek JS. Myositis ossificans: MR appearance with radiologic-pathologic correlation. *AJR* 1991; 157:1243–1248.
13. Amendola A, Rorabeck CH, Vellette D, et al. The use of magnetic resonance imaging in exertional compartment syndromes. *Am J Sports Med* 1990; 18:29–34.
14. Gordon BA, Martinez S, Collins AJ. Pyomyositis: characteristics at CT and MR imaging. *Radiology* 1995; 197:279–286.
15. Schmid MR, Kossmann T, Duewell S. Differentiation of necrotizing fasciitis and cellulitis using MR imaging. *AJR* 1998; 170:615–620.
16. Rahmouni A, Chosidow O, Mathieu D, et al. MR imaging in acute infectious cellulitis. *Radiology* 1994; 192:493–496.
17. Hernandez RJ, Sullivan DB, Chenevert TL, Keim DR. MR imaging in children with dermatomyositis: musculoskletal findings and correlation with clinical and laboratory findings. *AJR* 1993; 161:359–366.
18. Schweitzer ME, Fort J. Cost-effectiveness of MR imaging in evaluating polymyositis. *AJR* 1995; 165:1469–1471.
19. Murphy WA, Totty WG, Carroll JE. MRI of normal and pathologic skeletal muscle. *AJR* 1986; 146:565–574.
20. Lie G-C, Jong Y-J, Chiang C-H, Jaw T-S. Duchenne muscular distrophy: MR grading system with functional correlation. *Radiology* 1993; 186:475–480.
21. Fleckenstein JL, Watumull D, Conner KE, et al. Denervated human skeletal muscle: MR imaging evaluation. *Radiology* 1993; 187:213–218.
22. Uetani M, Hayashi K, Matsunaga N, et al. Denervated skeletal muscle: MR imaging—work in progress. *Radiology* 1993; 189:511–515.
23. Williams JB, Youngberg RA, Bui-Mansfield LT, Pitcher JD. MR imaging of skeletal muscle metastases. *AJR* 1997; 168:555–557.
24. Chason DP, Fleckenstein JL, Burns DK, Rojas G. Diabetic muscle infarction: radiologic evaluation. *Skeletal Radiol* 1996; 25:127–132.
25. Jelinek JS, Murphey MD, Aboulafia AJ, et al. Muscle infarction in patients with diabetes mellitus: MR imaging findings. *Radiology* 1999; 211:241–247.

4 PERIPHERAL NERVES

HOW TO IMAGE NERVES
NORMAL AND ABNORMAL
Background
Anatomy and MRI Appearance
Abnormalities of Nerves
  Traumatic Nerve Injury

Nerve Tumors
  Neuromas
  Neurofibroma and neurilemoma
  Fibrolipomatous hamartoma
  Pseudotumors of nerves
Compression Neuropathy and
  Entrapment Syndromes

Miscellaneous Abnormalities
  Tumor encasement/radiation
    changes
  Inflammatory neuritis
  Unexplained neuropathy

HOW TO IMAGE NERVES

Coils/Patient Position. High-resolution images of the small peripheral nerves require the use of phased array surface coils. The large sciatic nerve can be evaluated without a surface coil, but better resolution will be possible if surface coils are used. Positioning of the patient is determined by which nerve is being evaluated. In general, the nerve can be imaged with the same surface coils, in the same position, and with the same field of view and section thickness as would be used for the nearby joint.

Image Orientation. If at all possible, images of nerves should be obtained in two orthogonal planes. Images that run parallel to the long axis of the nerve (in-plane or longitudinal images) are good for an overview of the course of the nerve and to detect displacement or enlargement. Partial volume artifacts may, however, complicate interpretation of these images. Images obtained with the nerve in cross-section (perpendicular to the long axis of the nerve) avoid partial volume averaging artifacts and allow for assessment of the size, configuration, signal intensity, and fascicular pattern of the nerve.

Pulse Sequences. T1W and some types of T2W fat-suppressed (turbo T2 with fat suppression or STIR) images are best to evaluate the peripheral nerves. T1 images show the anatomy adjacent to the nerve, and the T2W sequences are good for showing pathology of the nerve and the fascicular pattern.

Contrast. Contrast enhancement is generally of no added value in the evaluation of nerves. Only if there is a question as to whether a mass was cystic or solid is contrast important to differentiate between the two.

NORMAL AND ABNORMAL

Background

Electrophysiologic studies are a widely used invasive technique for detecting a conduction abnormality in peripheral nerves. These tests are sensitive, but they lack specificity and cannot show anatomic detail that would delineate the precise location of an abnormality, which often affects treatment planning. Microsurgery for repair of damaged nerves has gained acceptance, and a means of documenting the presence and extent of a nerve abnormality by direct visualization in a noninvasive way prior to surgery has value. MRI is the best imaging technique available to evaluate the nerves at this time, but so far very little work has been done in this area. Like it or not, nerves are present on every extremity MRI examination we evaluate, and it is necessary to be aware of the normal and abnormal appearances in order to be able to offer differential diagnoses for the findings.

Normal Anatomy and MRI Appearance

The fundamental unit of a peripheral nerve is the axon, which may be either myelinated or unmyelinated, and which carries efferent (motor) or afferent (sensory) electrical impulses. Peripheral nerves have a mixture of both myelinated and unmyelinated axons. A myelinated fiber exists when a single axon is encased by a single Schwann cell; unmyelinated fibers result if a single Schwann cell encases multiple axons. Thus, layers of Schwann cells form the myelin sheaths.[1, 2]

Large peripheral nerves have three connective tissue sheaths that support and protect the axons and myelin sheaths (Fig. 4–1). The innermost sheath is the *endoneurium*, which invests each individual myelinated axon. Several axons, along with their Schwann cells and endoneurial sheaths, are bundled together into fascicles that are each wrapped in a dense sheath of *perineurium*, which serves as a protective barrier to infectious agents or toxins. The third layer is the *epineurium*, which surrounds the entire peripheral nerve and protects the axons dur-

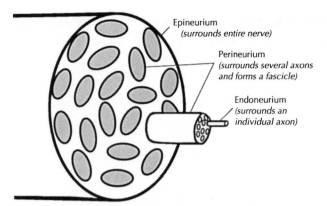

Figure 4–1. ANATOMY OF A PERIPHERAL NERVE.
Fascicles are the smallest unit of a nerve visible on MRI. Fascicles are composed of several axons wrapped in a layer of perineurium. Several fascicles form a nerve, which is surrounded by a layer of epineurium. Individual axons are covered by endoneurium, but are not visible on MRI.

ing stretching forces on the nerve. The connective tissue sheaths cannot be detected with MRI, but nerve fascicles are the smallest units of nerves that currently can be identified.

Variable amounts of fat are present between fascicles, more being present in nerves of the lower extremities than in those of the upper extremities. Large peripheral nerves contain about ten fascicles. Each fascicle is composed of motor, sensory, and sympathetic fibers.

MRI shows normal nerves as round or oval in cross section (Fig. 4–2). The rod-like fascicles in the nerves are seen end on in transverse images as a stippled or honeycomb-like appearance, called a fascicular pattern. The fascicles are uniform in size and similar to, or slightly hyperintense to, muscle on T2W images. On T1W images, the fascicles are similar in signal intensity to muscle with intervening areas of relatively high signal similar to fat (Fig. 4–2). The fascicular pattern is much easier to detect on T2W than on T1W images, especially in small nerves (Fig. 4–3).

Large nerves, like the sciatic nerve, may have a striated appearance when imaged longitudinally (resembling strands of hair or spaghetti), with signal intensity typical of fat separating the fascicles (Fig. 4–2). Nerves are relatively easy to identify if they are surrounded by fat; however, if they lie adjacent to muscle, without intervening fat, they can be very difficult to detect. T2W images in the axial plane give the best chance of identifying and following the nerve in the latter situation.

Abnormalities of Nerves

Peripheral nerves can be affected by trauma, compression or encasement by an adjacent mass or infiltrative process, nerve entrapment syndromes, nerve sheath tumors, inflammatory neuritis, radiation, hereditary hypertrophic neuropathies, and inflammatory pseudotumors. Nerve problems are evaluated on MRI by directly imaging the nerve and looking for abnormalities in position, size, or signal intensity and, secondly, by looking for abnormalities that would indicate denervation in the muscles supplied by the nerve (Fig. 4–4).

Nerves are abnormal if they have diffuse or focal enlargement or diffuse or focal high signal intensity

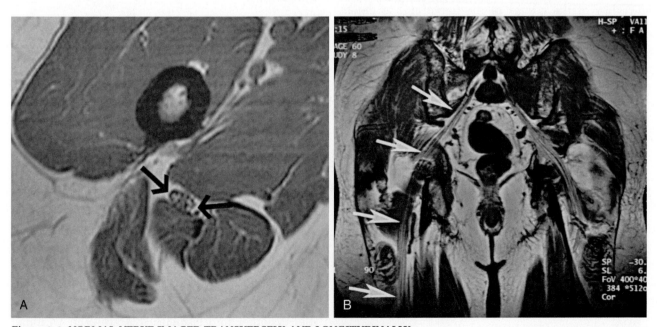

Figure 4–2. NORMAL NERVE IMAGED TRANSVERSELY AND LONGITUDINALLY.
A, Axial T1 image, proximal thigh. *Arrows* point to the sciatic nerve, which is oval in cross section. The uniform stippled appearance is the result of intermediate-signal fascicles separated by high-signal fat. **B,** Coronal T1 image, pelvis. Sciatic nerves imaged longitudinally are evident bilaterally (*white arrows* on the right) as striated structures (like spaghetti or strands of hair). The abnormal appearance in the marrow is from multiple myeloma.

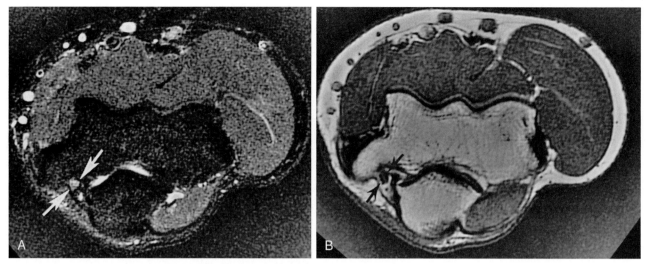

Figure 4–3. NORMAL NERVE WITH FASCICLES MORE EVIDENT ON T2 THAN T1.
A, Axial STIR image, elbow. The fascicles of the ulnar nerve *(white arrows)* are easier to identify with this sequence than the T1 sequence in *B. B,* Axial T1 image, elbow. The fascicles of the ulnar nerve *(black arrows)* are relatively more difficult to see on T1W images.

on T2W images. Determining if the signal intensity is too high is a very subjective exercise. Alteration in the fascicular pattern also may occur in an abnormal nerve (Fig. 4–4). Fascicles in an abnormal nerve may be difficult to identify, enlarged, or hyperintense. This results in a non-uniform pattern of fascicles, which is also virtually always accompanied by increased signal intensity in the nerve on T2W images. Obviously, nerves have limited ways to appear abnormal on MRI and the findings are usually

Figure 4–4. MR FEATURES OF AN ABNORMAL NERVE.
A, Axial T1 image, proximal calf. There is an osteochondroma (o) projecting from the posterior tibia (t). Streaks of high-signal fat infiltrate the soleus muscle *(arrows),* indicating atrophy secondary to denervation. *B,* Axial STIR image, calf (same patient and level as in *A*). An enlarged and high-signal posterior tibial nerve *(open arrows)* is being compressed and displaced by the osteochondroma. Fascicles are difficult to identify in the nerve. Edema in the soleus muscle from denervation is seen. *C,* Axial T2* image, carpal tunnel. Months after a carpal tunnel release, the patient had recurrent symptoms. The median nerve *(arrows)* is enlarged, high signal, and without intermediate signal fascicles.

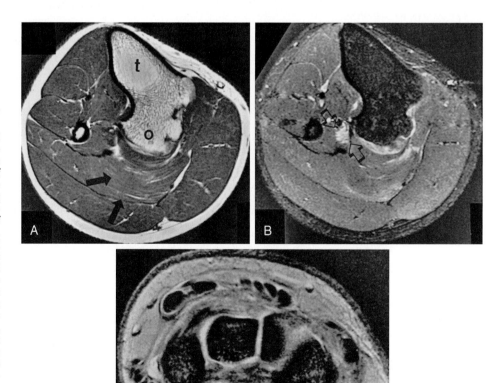

BOX 4–1: ABNORMAL PERIPHERAL NERVES

Primary Signs (nerve)
- Increased size
- Increased signal, T2
- Abnormal position (displacement) from mass, subluxation, osteophyte
- Fascicular pattern abnormal (non-uniform, enlarged)

Secondary Signs (muscle)
- Denervation of muscle supplied by nerve
    - < 1 year: high signal in muscle on T2 from intramuscular edema
    - > 1 year: high signal in muscle on T1 from fat infiltration

nonspecific, requiring a differential diagnosis, but MRI still adds significant information that can help in the management of patients (Box 4–1).

Traumatic Nerve Injury

Neurologic symptoms may be present after a nerve injury from disruption of axonal conduction, but the nerve remains intact (neurapraxia). MRI generally is not performed in this setting.

More severe trauma to nerves can result in partial or complete transection of the nerve. With an acute injury, MRI can show the precise location of the nerve abnormality because of the presence of high

signal intensity edema on T2W images, and it can show the site of nerve disruption. The nerve may respond by forming a neuroma within the first year after the injury, which is sometimes painful.

Blunt trauma to a nerve may result in a focal neuritis with nerve swelling and surrounding soft tissue edema in the acute setting. This will appear as focal nerve enlargement with intraneural and perineural high signal intensity on T2W MR images (Figs. 4–5 and 4–6). Enlargement of the nerve can be recognized by comparing the caliber from proximal to distal, because it should gradually decrease in size as images progress distally.

Nerves can sublux over an adjacent bone, the ulnar nerve relative to the medial epicondyle of the humerus being a classic example (Fig. 4–7). This may lead to stretching of the nerve, irritation from friction, and swelling of the nerve (neuritis) with increased nerve size and increased signal intensity seen on T2W images. Nerves in an abnormal location from subluxation or traumatic transection of a nerve must not be confused with surgical transposition of a nerve to a new anatomic location in order to avoid chronic irritation. Transfer of the ulnar nerve at the elbow is a standard surgical procedure that results in the nerve being positioned anterior to its usual location (Fig. 4–8).

Nerve Tumors

Neuromas. Neuromas frequently occur as a consequence of an injury with traumatic (or iatrogenic) transection of a nerve. These tumors may be painful and occur within one year of the injury. This phe-

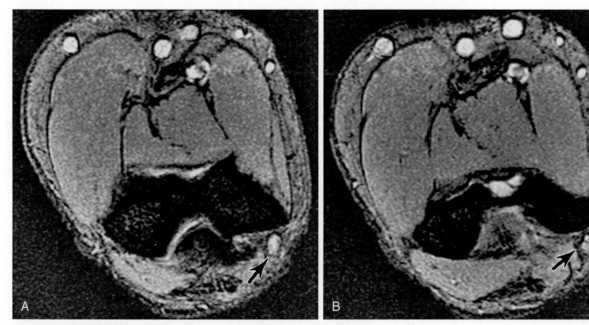

Figure 4–5. POSTTRAUMATIC NEURITIS.
A, Axial T2* image, elbow. Blunt trauma resulted in focal ulnar nerve *(arrow)* enlargement, increased signal, and lack of fascicular pattern. **B,** Axial T2* image, elbow. This cut was obtained immediately above that in *A,* and shows the ulnar nerve with a normal appearance, being smaller, slightly lower signal, and with fascicles. The nerve should be the same size or slightly larger on more proximal images as compared to more distal.

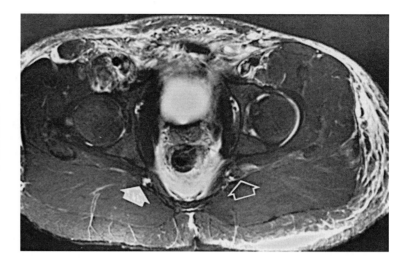

Figure 4–6. POSTTRAUMATIC NEURITIS.
Axial STIR image, pelvis. This was a polytrauma patient in a car accident. Focal enlargement of the left sciatic nerve *(open arrow)* with surrounding high-signal edema/hemorrhage accounted for his neurologic symptoms. The normal appearance of the sciatic nerve is seen on the right side for comparison *(solid arrow)*.

nomenon is well known in the setting of an amputation of an extremity, where a neuroma develops at the distal end of a severed nerve. There is no malignant potential for a traumatic neuroma, which simply represents the attempt of the nerve to repair by disorganized proliferation of cells in multiple directions.

A neuroma will appear as a fusiform or bulbous mass of the nerve end with heterogeneous signal intensity, and there may or may not be strand-like regions (disorganized fascicular appearance) of low signal intensity interspersed in the mass. The normal nerve proximal to the mass can be detected entering the mass; if the nerve has not been completely transected, an exiting nerve may be seen distal to the mass. Chronic friction or irritation of an intact nerve also can result in a neuroma with fusiform swelling in a nerve that is not disrupted. A neuroma has intermediate signal intensity on T1W images and intermediate to high signal on T2W images (Figs. 4–9 through 4–11). Diffuse enhancement

of the mass can be expected after intravenous contrast administration.

Neurofibroma and Neurilemoma (Box 4–2). Aside from post-traumatic neuromas, the tumors of significance that involve peripheral nerves are neurilemomas (also called Schwannomas) and neurofibromas. These are benign lesions that are usually difficult or impossible to distinguish from each other; they often are lumped together by referring to them as *nerve sheath tumors*. The major difference between the two is that neurilemomas arise from the surface of a nerve, whereas neurofibromas arise centrally, with the nerve coursing through the tumor. Both entities have an association with neurofibromatosis, but most lesions are solitary and unrelated to that disease. Patients with neurofibro-

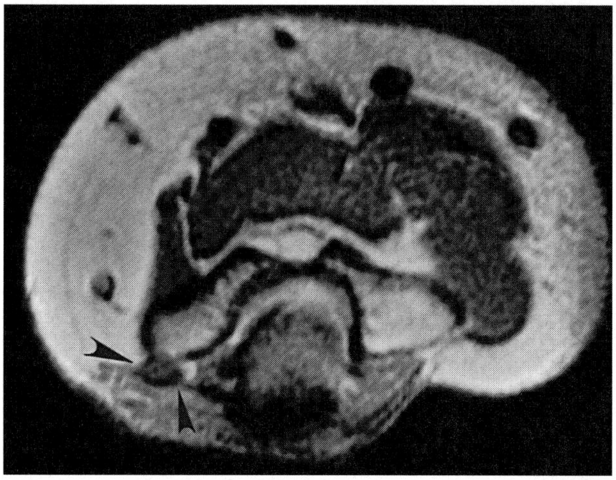

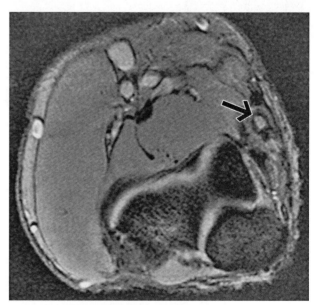

Figure 4–7. FOCAL NEURITIS FROM A CHRONICALLY SUBLUXED NERVE.
Axial proton density image, elbow. The ulnar nerve *(arrowheads)* is subluxed medially on the medial epicondyle. This has led to chronic irritation and a focal neuritis, as manifested by nerve enlargement.

Figure 4–8. ABNORMAL POSITION OF A NERVE FROM SURGICAL TRANSPOSITION.
Axial T2* image, elbow. The ulnar nerve *(arrow)* is located far anterior to its normal position on the back of the humerus. This is not from an injury or subluxation, but from surgical transfer of the nerve to prevent chronic irritation.

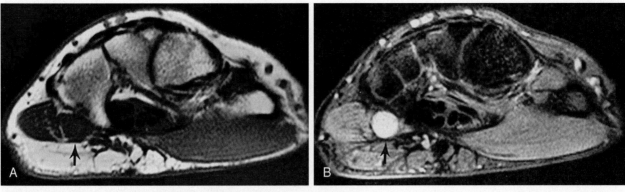

Figure 4–9. NEUROMA FROM CHRONIC IRRITATION.
A, Axial T1 image, wrist. There is an intermediate signal mass *(arrow)* adjacent to the hook of the hamate that blends with the adjacent muscle. *B,* Axial T2* image, wrist (same level as in *A*). A high-signal round mass *(arrow)* is obvious on this sequence. This was a neuroma of the deep branch of the ulnar nerve due to chronic irritation against the hook of the hamate.

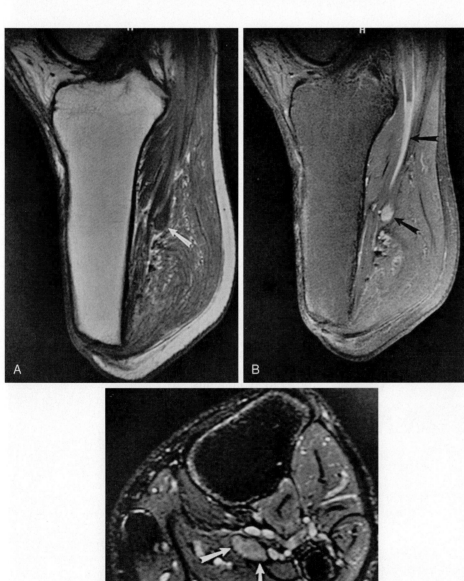

Figure 4–10. AMPUTATION NEUROMA.
A, T1 sagittal image, proximal calf. The *white arrow* points to an intermediate signal bulbous mass at the cut end of the posterior tibial nerve in this patient, who had a below-the-knee amputation 18 months previously and now has pain symptoms. *B,* Sagittal T1 fat saturation with contrast image, same location as in *A*. The nerve and distal bulbous neuroma enhance *(arrows)*. *C,* Axial STIR image, through neuroma of posterior tibial nerve. The nerve *(white arrows)* is markedly enlarged, high-signal intensity, and devoid of the normal fascicular pattern.

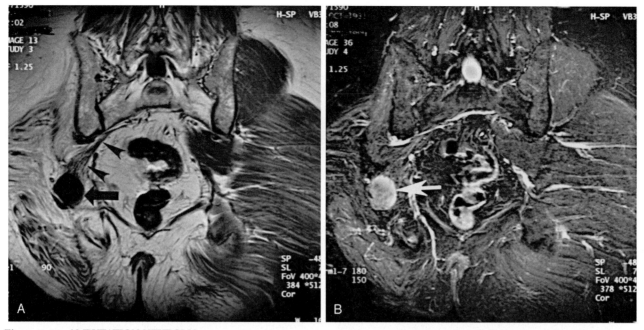

Figure 4–11. AMPUTATION NEUROMA.
A, T1 coronal image, pelvis. The sciatic nerve *(arrowheads)* with its striated appearance is leading directly to a low-signal mass *(arrow),* which is a neuroma that was discovered 20 years after a disarticulation of the hip for a soft tissue sarcoma. This patient was being treated for phantom limb pain. **B,** STIR coronal image, pelvis (same location as in *A*). The neuroma becomes high signal intensity *(white arrow),* whereas the sciatic nerve remains intermediate signal.

matosis tend to have multiple nerve sheath tumors or diffuse plexiform neurofibromas. Malignant degeneration rarely may occur; differentiation of benign from malignant nerve sheath tumors generally is not possible with MRI.

On MRI, both of these nerve sheath tumors appear as well-defined, smooth, fusiform-shaped masses. The mass is intermediate to low signal intensity on T1W images and generally shows a diffuse, increased signal intensity on T2W images (Fig. 4–12). Nerve sheath tumors may become necrotic, with a cystic or hemorrhagic appearance; this occurs much more commonly with schwannomas than with neurofibromas. Contrast enhancement is diffuse in the

---

BOX 4–2: NERVE SHEATH TUMORS

Suggestive MRI Features
• String Sign
    Fusiform mass with vertical, soft tissue "string" extending from either or both ends of the mass. The string represents normal entering or exiting nerve.
• Split Fat Sign
    Peripheral rim of fat surrounding mass, from displacement of fat in neurovascular bundle
• Target Pattern
    T2 and post-contrast T1 MRI with low signal-centrally and high signal in the periphery of the mass

---

tumor, unless it has a necrotic or cystic center, or if the target sign is present (see later) (Fig. 4–12).

Three additional signs on MRI may be present and help to limit the differential diagnosis of a mass to a nerve sheath tumor, if identified: (1) the string sign, (2) the split fat sign, and (3) the target sign.[2–4]

The string sign consists of the appearance of a fusiform mass with a "string" of vertically oriented soft tissue extending from one or both ends of the mass. The string represents the normal entering or exiting nerve that is in continuity with the nerve sheath tumor (Fig. 4–13). Masses that are not of neural origin may have features that mimic a nerve sheath tumor and must be carefully evaluated in order to avoid a mistake. Vessels adjacent to a mass may create an appearance similar to the string sign and lead to a misdiagnosis (Fig. 4–14).

The split fat sign describes the peripheral rim of fat that often is seen surrounding the margins of a nerve sheath tumor. This is thought to relate to the displacement of the fat that normally surrounds the neurovascular bundle, the site of origin of these lesions (Figs. 4–13 and 4–15).

The target sign consists of low signal intensity centrally and high signal intensity peripherally on T2W and post–contrast-enhanced T1W images (Fig. 4–12). The target pattern is probably a reflection of the histology of these lesions, with peripheral myxomatous tissue and central fibrous tissue creating the signal characteristics. This sign has been described in neurofibromas, but it probably can occur in other nerve tumors.

Fibrolipomatous Hamartoma. This is a rare lesion of major nerves and their branches. There is gradual

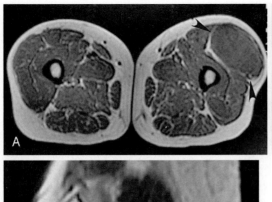

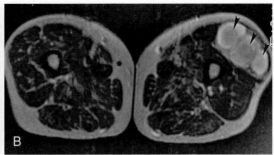

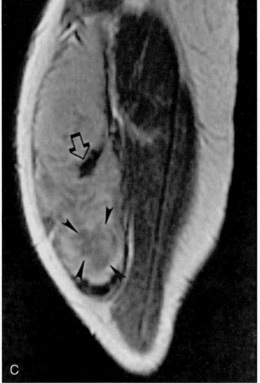

Figure 4–12. NEUROFIBROMA: Target Sign and Necrosis.
A, T1 axial image, mid-thighs. There is a large intermediate signal mass *(arrowheads)* interposed between the vastus intermedius and vastus lateralis; the latter muscle is thinned and stretched over the neurofibroma. *B,* Axial spin echo–T2 image (same location as in *A*). The mass becomes high signal and actually appears to be composed of three different masses, each with vague, lower-signal centers *(arrowheads),* known as the target sign. *C,* Sagittal T1 image with contrast, same patient as in *A* and *B*. There is near-complete high signal from contrast enhancement in the mass. There is a focal area of necrosis *(open arrow)* that did not take up contrast. In the lower portion of the mass, there is a vague, rounded area of intermediate signal *(arrowheads)* that does not show contrast enhancement that again represents the target sign typical of a neurofibroma.

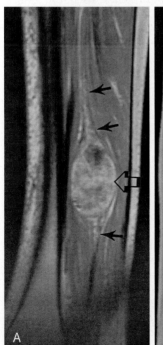
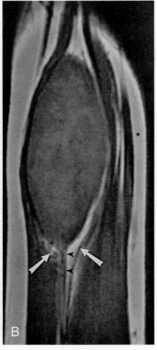

Figure 4–13. NERVE SHEATH TUMORS: String Sign.
A, T1 sagittal image with contrast, calf. There is a fusiform mass *(open arrow)* with strings of vertically oriented soft tissue *(solid arrows)* extending from both ends of the mass, representing the entering and exiting nerve related to this schwannoma. There is diffuse contrast enhancement with focal areas of low signal, which proved to be areas of hemorrhage and necrosis at surgery. *B,* T1 coronal image, forearm. A large fusiform mass in the forearm (hand is toward the top of this image) has a vertically oriented string of soft tissue extending proximal to the mass *(arrowheads),* and a peripheral rim of fat *(white arrows)* surrounding the mass, which represents the split fat sign in this neurofibroma.

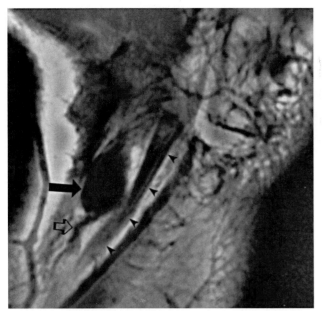

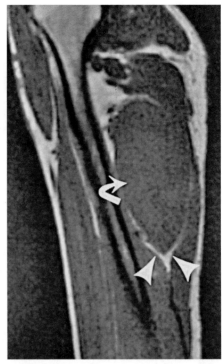

Figure 4–14. PSEUDO-STRING SIGN.
T1 coronal image, wrist. A low-signal fusiform mass *(solid arrow)* has a string of soft tissue extending proximal *(open arrow)* to it. The patient had symptoms of median neuritis. This was a ganglion cyst at surgery, and the string appearance is due to an adjacent blood vessel. The median nerve *(arrowheads)* is actually displaced by the mass and slightly enlarged from neuritis caused by chronic irritation.

Figure 4–15. NERVE SHEATH TUMOR: Split Fat Sign.
T1 coronal image, upper arm. A fusiform mass *(curved arrow)* has fat diverging around its distal end *(arrowheads)*, known as the split fat sign. This was a schwannoma.

infiltration of the nerve by fibrofatty tissue. These lesions occur in children or young adults. They can cause an enlarging mass, macrodactyly, and compression neuropathy. The hand is the site most commonly involved, especially the median nerve. MRI shows an enlarged nerve composed of tubular, serpentine-like, longitudinal low signal intensity structures, representing the fascicles with perineural fibrosis, coursing through a nerve that has signal characteristics typical of fat (Fig. 4–16).[5]

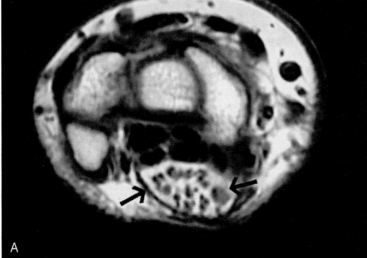

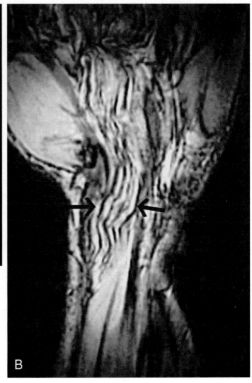

Figure 4–16. FIBROLIPOMATOUS HAMARTOMA.
A, T1 axial image, wrist. The median nerve *(arrows)* is gigantic in the carpal tunnel. The fascicles are larger than normal, but otherwise normal in appearance and surrounded by normal high-signal fat. This is typical of the appearance and location of a fibrolipomatous hamartoma. *B,* T1 coronal image, wrist. The enlarged low signal and wavy fascicles with intervening fat in the median nerve *(arrows)* are coursing longitudinally through the wrist.

Pseudotumors of Nerves. Ganglion cysts can develop in a nerve sheath and cause compression of the underlying nerve. The ganglion cyst has the same appearance as elsewhere, with low signal intensity on T1W images and high signal intensity on T2W images, frequently with lobulated margins and thin septations within the mass. If the ganglion follows a nerve, the diagnosis should be suggested. The peroneal nerve at the knee joint is most commonly affected (Fig. 4–17).

Morton's neuromas are not true neuromas or neoplasms of the nerve. Morton's neuromas cause severe pain between the toes in the second and third web spaces and occur as a reaction to the plantar digital nerves in the foot being compressed and irritated between metatarsal heads, resulting in perineural fibrosis, neural degeneration, and inflammatory changes surrounding the nerve. This presents as a teardrop-shaped mass that projects between and plantar to the metatarsal heads. The MRI appearance is delineated in detail in Chapter 16.

Compressive Neuropathy and Entrapment Syndromes

Compression or entrapment of a short segment of nerve at specific and predictable anatomic sites, as the nerves pass through openings in muscular or fibrous tissue or fibro-osseous tunnels, can cause symptoms that vary with the site involved. MRI

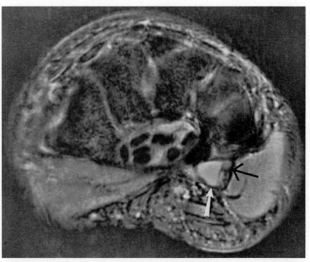

Figure 4–18. COMPRESSIVE NEUROPATHY FROM A MASS. T2* axial image, wrist. A high-signal ganglion cyst *(white arrow)* adjacent to the hook of the hamate resulted in a compressive neuropathy of the ulnar nerve in Guyon's canal. The ulnar nerve is significantly enlarged *(black arrow)* from the chronic irritation that caused neuritis.

can be used to detect objective findings of nerve compression. MRI may show alterations in the size, signal intensity, or position of a peripheral nerve (increased size and increased signal intensity on T2W images). Osseous or soft tissue lesions that cause the compression neuropathy can be depicted, if present (Fig. 4–18). Findings of muscle denervation may be evident; when acute, these consist of increased signal intensity on T2W images of the muscles innervated by the affected nerve. Denervation progresses to muscle atrophy with fatty infiltration on a more chronic basis, manifested by high signal intensity typical of fat infiltrating muscle on T1W images.[6]

Some of the more common sites of compression and entrapment neuropathies are listed here:

- *Brachial plexus* at insertion of anterior scalene muscle on first rib (scalenus anticus syndrome), or at the crossing of a cervical rib (cervical rib syndrome)
- *Suprascapular nerve* in the suprascapular or spinoglenoid notch of the scapula (suprascapular notch syndrome)
- *Axillary nerve* in the quadrilateral space of the axilla (quadrilateral space syndrome)
- *Radial nerve* in the axilla (sleep palsy), spiral groove of the distal humerus (from a fracture), or deep to the supinator muscle at the elbow (posterior interosseous nerve syndrome)
- *Median nerve* in the distal humerus deep to the ligament of Struthers, deep to the pronator teres muscle at the elbow (pronator syndrome), or in the carpal tunnel at the wrist (carpal tunnel syndrome)
- *Ulnar nerve* in the cubital tunnel of the elbow (cubital tunnel syndrome), or Guyon's canal in the wrist (ulnar tunnel syndrome)

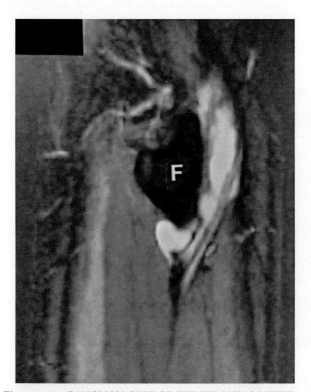

Figure 4–17. GANGLION CYST OF THE PERONEAL NERVE. STIR sagittal image at the knee shows a high-signal, lobulated, elongated mass wrapping around the neck of the fibula (F), following the distribution of the peroneal nerve. This is a ganglion cyst that caused compression of the nerve.

- *Sciatic nerve* at the greater sciatic foramen in the pelvis (piriformis syndrome)
- *Lateral femoral cutaneous nerve* at the attachment of the inguinal ligament to the anterior superior iliac spine (meralgia paresthetica)
- *Posterior tibial nerve* in the tarsal tunnel of the hindfoot and ankle (tarsal tunnel syndrome)

Miscellaneous Nerve Abnormalities

Tumor Encasement/Radiation Changes. Nerves may be encased or displaced by adjacent tumor, such as a primary carcinoma, lymphoma, or desmoid tumors, which can cause neurologic symptoms and pain. MRI can show the tumor and its relationship to nerves (Fig. 4–19). Patients who receive radiation therapy for a tumor may develop radiation-induced neuritis as an inflammatory reaction of the nerve to the radiation. The symptoms are not distinguishable from encasement by tumor. MRI will show if there is tumor present or not, and can show increased signal intensity and enlargement of the nerves in the radiation portal on T2W images from radiation neuritis unrelated to tumor.

Inflammatory Neuritis. Nerves may become inflamed and symptomatic for unknown reasons. It is believed that this often is the result of a viral infection, and it is referred to as idiopathic inflammatory neuritis. There is often a history of a recent flu-like syndrome that preceded the onset of neural symptoms. These acute neuromuscular disorders

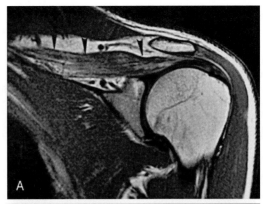
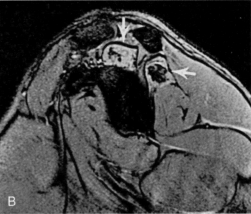

Figure 4–20. INFLAMMATORY NEURITIS.
A, T1 coronal image, shoulder. There is fatty infiltration of the supraspinatus muscle *(arrowheads)* without a tear of the rotator cuff, indicating a nerve abnormality. This patient had profound weakness and pain, and this was believed to be from a viral neuritis (Parsonage-Turner syndrome). *B,* T2* sagittal image, shoulder. Higher signal is present in both the supraspinatus and infraspinatus muscles *(white arrows),* rather than in the other musculature of the shoulder girdle, from muscle atrophy secondary to the brachial neuritis.

have not shown abnormalities of the nerves on MRI, but have shown abnormalities in the affected muscles.

Acute brachial neuritis, also called Parsonage-Turner syndrome, is a painful neuromuscular disorder that affects the shoulder with marked weakness and pain, and which probably is the result of a viral neuritis. The clinical symptoms may be similar to the many other causes of shoulder pain, and MRI may be helpful to make the diagnosis. The findings are those of muscle edema with high signal intensity on T2W images, or of muscle atrophy with high signal intensity on T1W images in the supraspinatus, infraspinatus, or deltoid muscles (Fig. 4–20).[7]

Unexplained Neuropathy. Focal or diffuse nerve abnormalities may be seen from an inflammatory pseudotumor of the nerve or from hereditary hypertrophic neuropathies (Charcot-Marie-Tooth disease, Dejerine-Sottas syndrome). The findings are nonspecific on MRI, consisting of nerve enlargement, heterogeneity in size of the fascicles, and hyperintense signal on T2W images.

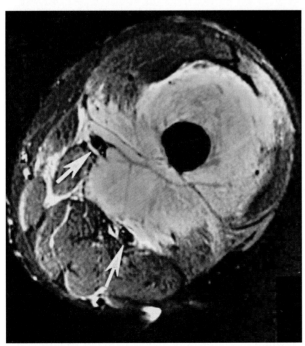

Figure 4–19. TUMOR ENCASING THE NEUROVASCULAR BUNDLE.
STIR axial image, mid-thigh. Diffuse high signal is seen in several muscles that are infiltrated with lymphoma. The *white arrows* point to the neurovascular bundles, which also are surrounded by tumor.

References

1. Maravilla KR, Bowen BC. Imaging of the peripheral nervous system: evaluation of peripheral neuropathy and plexopathy. *AJNR* 1998; 19:1011–1023.
2. Murphey MD, Smith WS, Smith SE, et al. Imaging of musculoskeletal neurogenic tumors: radiologic-pathologic correlation. *Radiographics* 1999; 19:1253–1280.
3. Kransdorf MJ, Murphey MD. *Imaging of Soft Tissue Tumors.* Philadelphia: W.B. Saunders; 1997.
4. Suh JS, Abenoza P, Galloway HR, et al. Peripheral (extracranial) nerve tumors: correlation of MR imaging and histologic findings. *Radiology* 1992; 183:341–346.
5. Cavallaro MC, Taylor JAM, Gorman JD, et al. Imaging findings in a patient with fibrolipomatous hamartoma of the median nerve. *AJR* 1993; 161:837–838.
6. Sallomi D, Janzen DL, Munk PL, et al. Muscle denervation patterns in upper limb nerve injuries: MR imaging findings and anatomic basis. *AJR* 1998; 171:779–784.
7. Helms CA, Martinez, S, Speer KP. Acute brachial neuritis (Parsonage-Turner syndrome): MR imaging appearance—report of three cases. *Radiology* 1998; 207:255–259.

HOW TO IMAGE INFECTION
OSTEOMYELITIS
Definition of Terms
Sequestrum
Involucrum
Cloaca
Sinus Tract
Abscess/Phlegmon
Routes of Contamination
Hematogenous Seeding
Contiguous Spread
Direct Implantation

MR Imaging of Osteomyelitis
Acute Osteomyelitis
Subacute Osteomyelitis
Chronic Osteomyelitis
SOFT TISSUE INFECTION
Cellulitis
Septic Tenosynovitis/Septic Bursitis
Infectious Myositis
Necrotizing Fasciitis

SEPTIC ARTHRITIS
MISCELLANEOUS
Foreign Bodies
Chronic Recurrent Multifocal Osteomyelitis
Acquired Immunodeficiency Syndrome (AIDS)
Diabetic Foot Infection

HOW TO IMAGE INFECTION
(Box 5–1)

Musculoskeletal infections affect bones, soft tissues, and joints. Infection often is considered a therapeutic emergency, and MR imaging is used to determine the presence or absence of disease and its extent. The MR study should be directed to the site of involvement based on clinical grounds or where abnormalities on other imaging studies have been found. Thus, the coil used, the patient's position, the planes of imaging, and the field of view will vary for each site.

Coils/Patient Position. The patient is usually supine in the magnet, unless the region affected involves mainly the posterior soft tissues, such as the buttocks or posterior thoracic cage. Spine phased array coils are used for any portion of the spine; the body coil for the thorax, pelvis, and femurs; and surface coils for the other extremities and joints.

BOX 5–1: MR FOR MUSCULOSKELETAL INFECTIONS

Sequences
- T1
- STIR or fast T2
- T1 postcontrast with fat saturation

Imaging Planes
- Spine: axial and sagittal
- Pelvis, hip, shoulder, wrist: axial and coronal
- Knee, ankle, elbow: axial and sagittal
- Foot: axial, sagittal, and coronal

Image Orientation. The best imaging planes for the spine are sagittal and axial; for the pelvis, coronal and axial images are preferred; in general, axial and coronal images are used for lesions near the hip, foot, shoulder, and wrist; and lesions near the knee, ankle, and elbow are evaluated best with axial and sagittal images.

Pulse Sequences/Regions of Interest. In the spine, sagittal and stacked axial T1W, fast T2W, and post-gadolinium T1W images of the region of interest are obtained. In the pelvis and extremities, our routine protocols include T1, STIR, and post-gadolinium T1W images.[1–4] Section thickness in the spine is 4 mm, in the pelvis 7 mm, and in the extremities 4 mm (or larger, depending on the volume to be covered).

Contrast. Intravenous gadolinium routinely is used for diagnosing musculoskeletal infections. It allows differentiation of an abscess from cellulitis or phlegmon in the soft tissues, or an abscess from bone marrow edema in the marrow space.[4] Gadolinium increases the conspicuity of sinus tracts and sequestra as well.

OSTEOMYELITIS

MR imaging allows for early detection of osteomyelitis, the extent of involvement, and the activity of the disease in cases of chronic osteomyelitis.

Definition of Terms (Box 5–2)

Sequestrum. A fragment of necrotic (dead) bone separated from living bone by surrounding granula-

BOX 5–2: DEFINITION OF TERMS

- *Cloaca:* Defect in the periosteum created by infection
- *Involucrum:* Thick sleeve of periosteal new bone surrounding dead cortical bone
- *Sequestrum:* Fragment of dead bone surrounded by granulation tissue
- *Sinus tract:* Channel extending from bone to skin surface, lined with granulation tissue
- *Fistula:* Channel between two internal organs

tion tissue is a sequestrum. This is seen on a radiograph as a dense bone fragment (the sequestrum) surrounded by a radiolucency (the granulation tissue); on MR images, the sequestrum is a low signal intensity structure on T1W and STIR sequences, whereas the surrounding granulation tissue is intermediate to low signal intensity on T1W images and high signal intensity with STIR or T2W sequences (Fig. 5–1). With gadolinium, the granulation tissue is enhanced, whereas the sequestrum remains low signal intensity.

Involucrum. An envelope of thick, wavy periosteal reaction formed around the cortex of an infected tubular bone is known as the involucrum. It commonly is found in bones of infants and children with osteomyelitis. As the infection is controlled, the dead cortical bone is incorporated with the involucrum, forming a thickened cortex (Fig. 5–1). On MRI, the ossified periosteal shell and the dead tubular cortical bone are low signal intensity on all pulse sequences; periosteal reaction and cortical bone are separated by linear intermediate to high signal intensity on T2W or STIR images (Fig. 5–2), until the periosteal reaction and cortical bone are incorporated.

Cloaca. An opening through the periosteum that permits pus from the infected bone to enter the soft tissues is called a cloaca. On MRI, the linear low signal intensity periosteum that is elevated from the cortical bone or the thickened cortex is interrupted by a high signal intensity gap (cloaca) on T2W images (Fig. 5–1). On T2W images, the high signal intensity pus can be seen extending into the soft tissues from the cloaca and may form a sinus tract or abscess.[5]

Sinus Tract. This is a channel between an infected bone and the skin surface, whereas a *fistula* represents a tract or channel between two internal organs. Both sinus tracts and fistulae are lined by vascular granulation tissue, and they function as conduits for pus to flow away from the infected bone. On MRI, a sinus tract or fistula is linear low signal intensity on T1W images, best seen if the subcutaneous fatty tissues are not infiltrated with edema. On T2W images, the channel demonstrates linear high signal intensity as a result of the granulation tissue and pus (Fig. 5–3). The granulation tissue is enhanced after intravenous injection of gadolinium, and the channel is most conspicuous with a fat-suppressed T1W sequence after contrast enhancement.

Abscess/Phlegmon. A cavity filled with pus that is surrounded by a capsule and lined with granulation

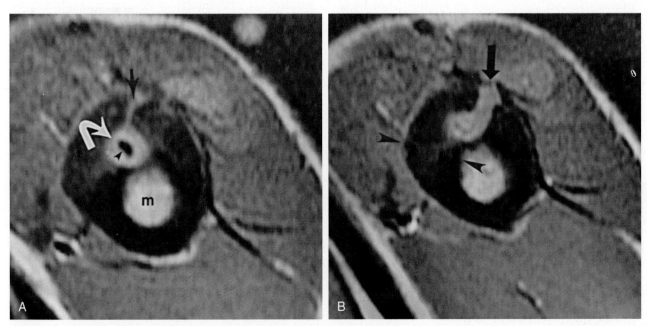

Figure 5–1. OSTEOMYELITIS: Sequestrum, Abscess, Cloaca, Periosteal New Bone.
A, Spin echo-T2 axial image, upper arm. There is high signal in the medullary cavity of the humerus (m) from osteomyelitis. A low-signal sequestrum *(arrowhead)* is surrounded by high-signal granulation tissue and pus *(curved arrow)*. A high-signal cloaca extends through the thickened cortex *(straight arrow)*. *B,* Spin echo-T2 axial image, upper arm. A cut adjacent to that in *A* shows the markedly thickened cortex (between *arrowheads*) formed by periosteal reaction/involucrum formation incorporated with the underlying cortex. A high-signal linear cloaca extends through the cortex as well *(arrow)*.

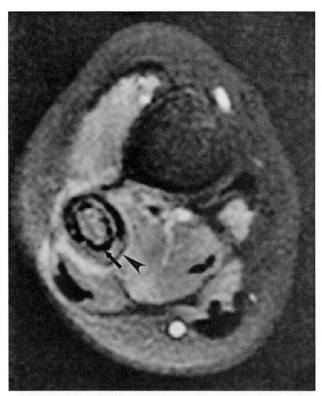

Figure 5–2. OSTEOMYELITIS: Involucrum.
Fast T2 with fat suppression image, axial calf. The low-signal linear periosteal reaction (involucrum) *(arrowhead)* and low-signal cortical bone *(arrow)* are separated by high-signal pus in this infected fibula in a child.

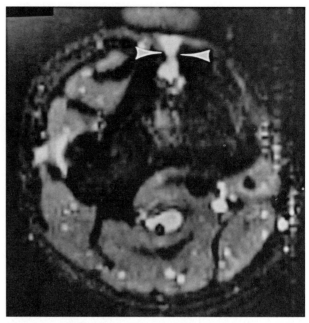

Figure 5–3. OSTEOMYELITIS: Sinus Tract.
STIR axial image, calf. There is a linear high-signal channel (between *arrowheads*) extending through the cortex of the tibia to the skin surface.

tissue is an *abscess,* whereas a *phlegmon* is a solid mass of inflammatory tissue. An abscess may be limited to the medullary bone, the cortex, the soft tissues, or more than one of these compartments (Fig. 5–4). On MRI, both the abscess and the phlegmon are intermediate to low signal intensity on T1W and high signal intensity on T2W images. After intravenous injection of gadolinium, the rim of an abscess is enhanced, whereas the center of the mass that contains the pus remains low signal intensity. A phlegmon enhances diffusely.

Routes of Contamination

(Box 5–3)

Osteomyelitis can develop via three routes: (1) hematogenous seeding, (2) contiguous spread from an adjacent infection, or (3) direct implantation of microorganisms.

Hematogenous Seeding. The location of lesions from hematogenous seeding is related to the vascular supply of tissues; in some patients, involvement may be multifocal. In hematogenous osteomyelitis, the contamination begins in the bone marrow and extends secondarily through the cortex and then to the adjacent soft tissues. In the spine, the common initial site of involvement is the subchondral bone of the vertebral body, which is supplied by nutrient

arterioles. This process eventually extends to the disk (spondylodiskitis). In children, vascular channels perforate the vertebral endplates, allowing direct access of microorganisms to the intervertebral disk (diskitis) without initial contamination of the vertebral bodies. In tubular bones, the vascular anat-

---

BOX 5–3: ROUTES OF BONE INFECTION

Hematogenous
- Infants (<1 year)
  — Metaphysis/epiphysis
- Children (1 year to growth plate closure)
  — Metaphysis
- Adults
  — Epiphysis

Direct Implantation
- Puncture wounds
- Human/animal bites
- Open fractures
- Surgery

Contiguous Spread
- Infection starts in soft tissues
  ↓
  Periostitis (periosteal involvement)
  ↓
  Osteitis (cortical involvement)
  ↓
  Osteomyelitis (marrow involvement)
- Reverse sequence from hematogenous spread

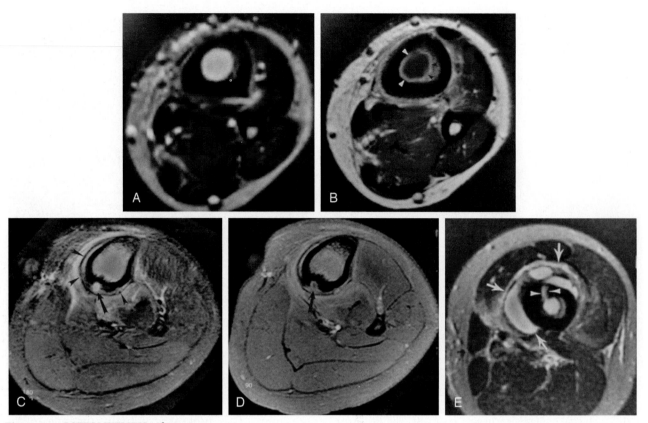

Figure 5–4. OSTEOMYELITIS: Abscess.
Medullary abscess. A, Spin echo-T2 image, axial calf. The medullary canal of the tibia is diffusely high signal. *B,* T1 contrast-enhanced axial image, calf. There is a thin line of enhancing tissue *(arrowheads)* surrounding a low-signal collection of pus in this abscess of the medullary bone. *Cortical abscess. C,* STIR axial image, calf. A round area of high signal is present in the posterior cortex of the tibia *(arrow)*, representing a cortical abscess. The medullary canal is also diffusely high signal from inflammation. The periosteum is elevated *(arrowheads)* from the cortical bone. *D,* T1 contrast-enhanced with fat suppression axial image, calf. The cortical abscess is high signal peripherally with a low-signal center that contains pus. The medullary canal and soft tissues surrounding bone all show enhancement, indicating there is no abscess in these locations, only inflammatory hyperemia. *Soft tissue abscess. E,* Spin echo-T2 axial image, thigh. There is a focal area of high signal in the medullary canal of the femur from an abscess with a cloaca in the lateral femoral cortex (between *arrowheads*). A fluid collection surrounding a large portion of the femur *(arrows)* caused by a soft tissue abscess also is present.

omy changes with age and is different for the infant, the child, and the adult.[5, 6] This particular vascular distribution explains the location of lesions for the different age groups.

Infantile pattern (0 to 1 year) is related to the fetal vascular arrangement that persists up to the age of one year. The metaphyseal and diaphyseal vessels penetrate the growthplate and extend into the epiphysis. In infants, infection affects primarily the epiphysis and the growthplate because of this vascular anatomy. Profuse involucrum formation is characteristic, reflecting the ease with which the periosteum is lifted from the underlying bone in infants and the presence of a rich vascularity. Development of soft tissue abscesses and extension into the joint are also common. Group A streptococcus is the commonest organism affecting infants with osteomyelitis.

Childhood pattern is between one year of age to closure of the growthplates (Fig. 5–5). The metaphyseal vessels become terminal ramifications of nutrient arteries, with the capillaries forming large sinus-oidal lakes in the metaphysis. The slow blood flow in this area contributes to the increased incidence of osteomyelitis that affects the metaphysis in the child. Later, extension into the epiphysis may occur from contiguous spread. Involucrum, sequestrum, and abscess formation are common. Articular extension (septic arthritis) occurs at sites where the growth plate is intraarticular, such as in the hip, elbow, and shoulder. In flat bones, such as the pelvis, childhood osteomyelitis shows a predilection for metaphyseal-equivalent locations adjacent to apophyses (eg, the iliac crests), and for epiphyseal-equivalent locations adjacent to articular cartilage (eg, around the triradiate cartilage). *Staphylococcus aureus* (80%) and group A *Streptococcus* are the most frequent organisms that affect children.

Adult pattern of hematogenous seeding of osteomyelitis is seen when growthplate closure has occurred. The diaphyseal and metaphyseal vessels penetrate the fused growthplate, which allows infection to localize in the subchondral bone regions (epiphyses). Septic arthritis may complicate this

Figure 5–5. OSTEOMYELITIS: Hematogenous Spread.
A, T1 sagittal image, ankle. Low signal in the distal tibial metaphysis is from hematogenous spread of infection to the region of terminal arterial ramifications in this child with open growth-plates. There is elevation of the periosteum anterior to the tibial cortex. *B,* STIR sagittal image, ankle (different patient than in *A*). Heterogeneous high signal from hematogenous spread of infection is present in the distal fibular metaphysis. This infection has been present long enough that it has extended by contiguous spread through the growth plate into the epiphysis *(arrow).*

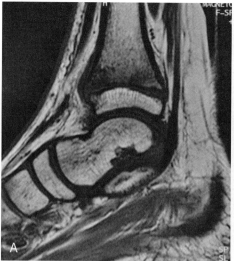
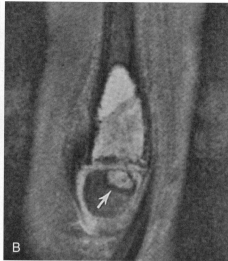

epiphyseal location. The spine, the pelvis, and the small bones of the hands and feet are the most common sites of infection.

Contiguous Spread. When soft tissues initially are infected, and the noncontained infection extends to adjacent osseous structures, it is considered contamination by contiguous spread (Fig. 5–6). Contamination of bone by contiguous spread most commonly is seen in debilitated patients, in diabetics, and in

patients treated with corticosteroids. The soft tissue infection invades bone marrow by progressing in sequence from cellulitis in the soft tissues to periostitis to osteitis to osteomyelitis. Osteitis indicates involvement of cortical bone; extension of the cortical infection into the marrow cavity produces osteomyelitis. The direction of contamination in contiguous spread of infection is the reverse of that which occurs with hematogenous osteomyelitis. With hematogenous osteomyelitis, marrow is affected initially, followed by cortical destruction, then periosteal contamination, and finally soft tissue cellulitis, phlegmon, or abscess.

Direct Implantation. Contamination of tissues by direct implantation of infectious agents is usually the result of puncture wounds, foreign bodies, open fractures, and surgery. Human bites (*S. aureus, Bacillus funformis*) and animal bites (*Pasteurella multocida, S. aureus,* and *S. epidermidis*) are also common causes of infection from direct implantation.[7] The infection starts at the site of implantation, which may be in the soft tissues, the periosteum, or the cortical or medullary bone; soft tissue involvement almost always is present (Fig. 5–7).

MR Imaging of Osteomyelitis
(Box 5–4)

Osteomyelitis classically is divided into three stages: acute, subacute, and chronic. These stages are based on the patient's clinical picture, on the duration of the disease, and on imaging findings.[8–16]

Acute Osteomyelitis

Acute osteomyelitis of hematogenous origin has normal radiographs in the first week, followed in the next 7 to 14 days by osteoporosis, fine linear periosteal reaction, and eventually permeative or moth-eaten bone destruction.[17] Prior to radiographic manifestations of infection, MRI demonstrates oblit-

Figure 5–6. OSTEOMYELITIS: Contiguous Spread.
T1 coronal image, knee. This patient had a below-the-knee amputation in the remote past. An ulcer developed in the distal soft tissues over the tibia. Infection spread from the soft tissue abscess *(arrowheads)* through the periosteum and cortex into the medullary canal, where there is now osteomyelitis *(arrow).*

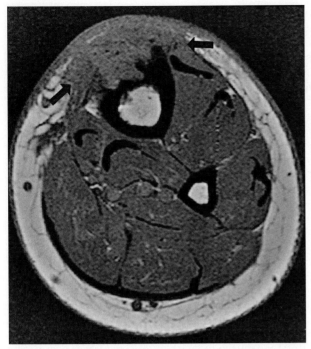

Figure 5–7. OSTEOMYELITIS: Direct Implantation.
T1 axial image, calf. There is a soft tissue and cortical abscess in the anterior and medial aspect of the tibia with cortical destruction and a soft tissue mass *(arrows)*. This occurred from direct implantation of bacteria when a shovel went through the skin and into the bone.

eration of the medullary fat by bone marrow edema, which is high signal intensity on STIR images and low to intermediate signal intensity on T1W images (Fig. 5–8). These MR features are not specific. MR is highly sensitive but not specific for diagnosing infection, with reported specificities for osteomyelitis ranging from 53% to 94%; however, MR has a negative predictive value for osteomyelitis close to 100%. As the disease progresses, MR demonstrates elevation of the periosteum, which is a low signal intensity line on all pulse sequences. The space between the periosteum and cortical bone has intermediate signal intensity on T1W and high signal intensity on STIR images; this usually is accompanied by adjacent soft tissue edema. Cortical destruction is a later finding and is depicted initially by blurring and eventually focal interruption of the cortical line that is normally completely devoid of signal (low signal intensity) on all pulse sequences. The infection may transgress the periosteum with formation of a cloaca. This is seen best on STIR images as a high signal intensity defect traversing the black periosteal line. This may then evolve into an abscess cavity or a sinus tract.[18–21] An abscess cavity is usually oval in shape, low signal intensity on T1W, and high signal intensity on T2W images. It may blend in with, and be obscured by, diffuse surrounding edema. The use of gadolinium helps in distinguishing an abscess from surrounding edema. The abscess demonstrates high signal intensity enhancement of its capsule, whereas the cavity re-

mains low signal intensity. Cellulitis shows diffuse contrast enhancement.

Osteomyelitis from contiguous spread presents with the reverse sequence of events as hematogenous osteomyelitis. The soft tissues are affected initially with diffuse edema. There may be associated soft tissue ulcers and abscesses. Ulcers are identified as low signal intensity cutaneous defects. With soft tissue infection, there may be adjacent periosteal reaction and bone marrow edema, but these findings do not necessarily indicate osteomyelitis. Both joints and bone marrow may develop sympathetic effusions or marrow edema, respectively, from an adjacent inflammatory process. Distinguishing this sympathetic inflammatory reaction from true infection of these tissues is not always possible by MRI. Only if certain other characteristic MR features of osteomyelitis are present can these areas of marrow abnormality be strongly considered to represent infection. The diagnosis of osteomyelitis can be made with confidence when the previously described findings are associated with one of the following: (1) sinus tract, (2) cortical destruction, or (3) pro-

---

BOX 5–4: OSTEOMYELITIS: MRI FINDINGS

- Bone Marrow Inflammation
  - T1: low signal intensity
  - T2: high signal intensity
  - T1 with contrast: high signal intensity
- Intraosseous Abscess
  - T1: low signal intensity
  - T2: high signal intensity
  - T1 with contrast: high signal intensity only in periphery
- Sequestrum
  - T1: low signal intensity
  - T2: low signal intensity
  - T1 with contrast: high signal intensity surrounding sequestrum, which remains low signal
- Cortical Destruction
  - T1: intermediate signal intensity
  - T2: intermediate or high signal intensity
  - T1 with contrast: intermediate signal intensity
- Cloaca
  - T1: hard to see
  - T2: high signal intensity defect in low signal periosteum
  - T1 with contrast: not seen
- Sinus Tract
  - T1: not seen, or linear low signal intensity
  - T2: high signal intensity
  - T1 with contrast: high signal intensity in peripheral lining of low signal intensity tract

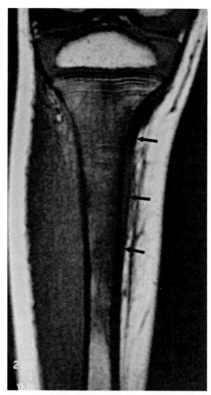

Figure 5–8. OSTEOMYELITIS: Acute.
T1 coronal image, proximal lower leg. There is diffuse intermediate signal in the proximal metaphysis and diametaphysis of the tibia in this child. This represents acute hematogenous osteomyelitis with pus and bone marrow edema. The medial cortex still appears intact, but the adjacent periosteum (the low signal line) *(arrows)* is elevated, caused by infection transgressing the cortex.

found high signal intensity of the marrow on T2W images.

Subacute Osteomyelitis

Subacute osteomyelitis is characterized on a radiograph by a geographic osteolytic lesion with or without sclerosis, often presenting as a lucent serpiginous channel within the medullary cavity. There may be an associated periosteal reaction. Brodie's abscess is one form of subacute osteomyelitis that is especially common in children. Radiographic features of a Brodie's abscess are those of a well-circumscribed lytic lesion with sclerotic borders in the metaphysis of a long bone. Periosteal reaction and a sequestrum may sometimes be present. The most frequent sites of involvement are the tibia and femur.

MR images demonstrate a well-circumscribed, serpiginous or oval lesion of low to intermediate signal intensity on T1W images and high signal intensity on T2W images (Fig. 5–9). A focus of subacute osteomyelitis is surrounded by a low signal intensity rim of variable thickness, representing fibrous tissue and reactive bone. There is usually associated bone marrow edema surrounding the lesion. These MR findings may be seen before any

characteristic radiographic changes are demonstrated. Periosteal reaction and adjacent soft tissue edema also may be present. Joint effusion may be seen, which may be sympathetic in origin or represent a true septic arthritis. When epiphyses or apophyses are involved with a Brodie's abscess, the findings may resemble a chondroblastoma, both on radiographs and MR imaging. The use of intravenous gadolinium may help distinguish these two entities. Only the periphery of a Brodie's abscess will enhance, whereas a chondroblastoma will demonstrate heterogenous enhancement of the entire lesion.

Chronic Osteomyelitis

Chronic osteomyelitis consists of an infection of more than 6 weeks' duration. In its florid state, it shows abundant sclerosis as manifested by periosteal and endosteal thickening, thickened and disorganized trabeculae, and cystic changes, with or without a sequestrum on radiographs. Chronic osteomyelitis of long duration with draining sinus tracts may develop squamous cell carcinoma.[22, 23] The most specific sign of active chronic osteomyelitis is the presence of a sequestrum, best demonstrated with computed tomography (CT). Other radiographic signs include the presence of poorly defined areas of osteolysis, osteolysis in areas of previous sclerosis, and development of a new, thin, linear periosteal reaction.

The MR findings that indicate an active chronic osteomyelitis are (1) identification of a sequestrum (Fig. 5–10) that is low signal intensity on all pulse sequences. Injection of intravenous gadolinium will increase its conspicuity because granulation tissue surrounding the sequestrum will enhance, but the sequestrum will remain low signal intensity; (2) intramedullary abscess cavity, which will be an oblong, relatively well-delineated mass of low signal intensity on T1W and high signal intensity on T2W images (after intravenous injection of gadolinium, the rim of the intraosseous abscess will enhance with high signal intensity, whereas the pus-filled cavity will remain low signal intensity on T1W images); (3) cloaca, which is seen on T2W images as a high signal intensity gap through the cortex and periosteum; (4) subperiosteal fluid collection (representing either pus or edema), seen on T2W images as a high signal intensity linear fluid collection elevating the periosteum and paralleling the cortex; and (5) sinus tract, identified on T2W images as a high signal intensity channel extending from bone into the soft tissues, or on contrast-enhanced T1W images as enhancement along its borders.[19, 24] Demonstration of increased signal intensity of the bone marrow on T2W images may represent postsurgical or postinfectious granulation tissue and not necessarily persistent infection. However, serial MR studies showing progression of this process in the marrow indicates the presence of active osteomyelitis.

The MR diagnosis of healed osteomyelitis is based

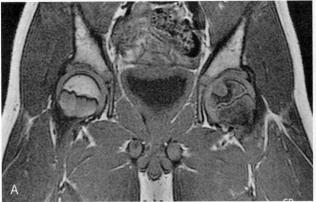
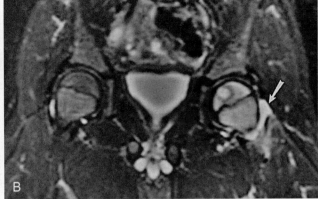

Figure 5–9. OSTEOMYELITIS: Subacute.
A, T1 coronal image, pelvis. There is a focal intermediate signal lesion (abscess) in the left femoral head surrounded by a rim of low signal (fibrosis or reactive new bone). The surrounding marrow is intermediate signal secondary to reactive marrow edema that surrounds the subacute osteomyelitis. *B,* STIR coronal image, pelvis. The focal abscess becomes high signal, the thin line of surrounding reactive bone remains low signal, and the diffuse surrounding reactive marrow edema is high signal. In addition, there is a high-signal joint effusion *(arrow),* which represents either a reaction to the adjacent inflammatory process or a septic joint.

on the absence of the above signs and on the return of normal fatty marrow in the medullary cavity, seen as high signal intensity marrow on T1W and low signal intensity on T2W images.

SOFT TISSUE INFECTION

Soft tissue infections include cellulitis, septic tenosynovitis, septic bursitis, infectious myositis, and necrotizing fasciitis. Despite the fact that MRI findings are not specific, MR is the best imaging modality to detect any soft tissue abnormality. It is used to evaluate the presence or absence of disease, evaluate its extent, and identify possible sites for biopsy.

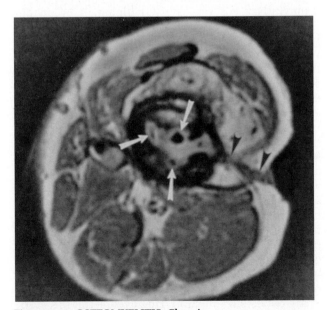

Figure 5–10. OSTEOMYELITIS: Chronic.
Proton density axial image, thigh. Several features of chronic infection are evident: sequestra *(arrows),* cloaca, sinus tract *(arrowheads),* and an abscess in the medullary canal (high signal diffusely, except for the sequestra).

Cellulitis (Box 5–5)

Cellulitis represents diffuse inflammation of subcutaneous fat and skin. On MRI, cellulitis is seen as diffuse areas of low signal intensity on T1W and high signal intensity on T2W images, with a reticular (lace-like) pattern in the subcutaneous fat and skin thickening (Fig. 5–11). After injection of intravenous gadolinium contrast, diffuse increased signal intensity is present in the same areas that are abnormal on the unenhanced T1W and T2W sequences.[25]

Septic Tenosynovitis/Septic Bursitis

Septic tenosynovitis and septic bursitis usually result from penetrating trauma or may be a manifestation of tuberculosis.[26] Septic and aseptic causes of bursitis and tenosynovitis cannot be distinguished by imaging features. Fluid surrounding a tendon (Fig. 5–12) or within a bursa will be low signal intensity on T1W and high signal intensity on any type of T2W images, and it will demonstrate enhancement of the synovial lining of these structures after intravenous contrast injection. These abnormalities usually are accompanied by adjacent cellulitis.

Infectious Myositis

Infectious myositis is very rare, but it can result from penetrating trauma or from hematogenous

---

BOX 5–5: CELLULITIS

- Abnormal signal limited to subcutaneous fat
  — Reticulated pattern: low signal on T1, high signal on T2 and enhancement with contrast
- No abnormality of deep fascial planes

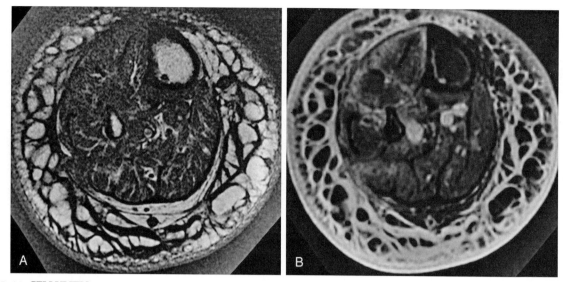

Figure 5–11. CELLULITIS.
A, T1 axial image, lower leg. There is diffuse skin thickening and a reticular pattern of low-signal edema in the subcutaneous fat. *B,* STIR axial image, lower leg. The reticular pattern of edema and skin thickening become high signal on this sequence. There is no abnormal high signal in the intermuscular fascial planes, allowing distinction of cellulitis from necrotizing fasciitis.

seeding in intravenous drug abusers or immunocompromised patients. *S. aureus* is the most common causative agent. Lesions are multifocal in about half the patients. Usually, abnormal findings are limited to the muscles or intermuscular fascia. MRI shows muscle enlargement with intermediate signal intensity on T1W images and increased signal intensity on T2W images. There occasionally may be associated changes of cellulitis. In some cases, solitary or multiple abscesses may be present.[27–30] Abscesses may be surrounded by a high signal intensity rim on T1W images with contrast administration. A high signal intensity rim also has been described on T1W images without contrast in muscle abscesses. These findings are not specific, and the precise diagnosis usually is obtained by aspiration or biopsy and culture of the abnormal muscle.

Necrotizing Fasciitis (Box 5–6)

Necrotizing fasciitis is associated with a high mortality rate and represents a surgical emergency. Early diagnosis and extensive debridement are associated with improved prognosis.[31] MRI is used to distinguish cellulitis from necrotizing fasciitis. In cellulitis, abnormal signal intensity is seen only in the subcutaneous fat.[25] With necrotizing fasciitis, the abnormal signal intensity extends into the deep fasciae between muscles, and occasionally into muscles. The abnormal signal intensity is best demonstrated on STIR images. Linear high signal intensity is seen within both the superficial and deep fasciae from fascial necrosis. The associated muscle involvement, when present, is identified as poorly defined areas of high signal intensity on T2W or STIR images within the muscles, with or without hyperintense fluid collections representing abscesses. Muscle involvement is not required to make the diagnosis, but fascial involvement is.[32] Postcontrast T1W images show enhancement in the fascial planes, focal enhancement of the affected muscles, and peripheral enhancement of the abscess cavities, corresponding to the findings seen on STIR images. Contrast administration is not necessary to make the

Figure 5–12. INFECTED TENOSYNOVITIS.
T2* axial image, hand. There is a focal high-signal mass *(arrow)* immediately adjacent to a flexor tendon. There also is diffuse high signal surrounding the flexor tendons from tenosynovitis *(arrowheads).* This was purulent fluid at surgery, and a wood foreign body was found in the focal fluid collection.

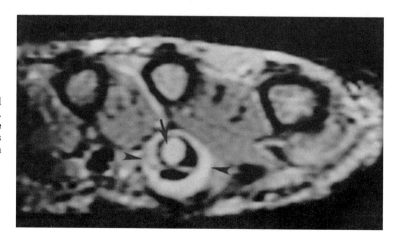

BOX 5–6: NECROTIZING FASCIITIS

- Deep fasciae
  — T2: high signal intensity
  — T1 with contrast: high signal intensity
- Subcutaneous fat
  — Diffuse reticulations
  — T2 and T1 with contrast: increased
    signal intensity
- Muscle
  — T2 and T1 with contrast: increased
    signal intensity
- Abscess in msucle
  — T2: increased signal intensity
  — T1 postcontrast: rim enhancement with
    decreased signal intensity center

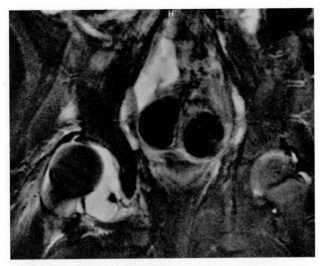

Figure 5–14. SEPTIC ARTHRITIS.
STIR coronal image, pelvis. This is a child with a large, high-signal joint effusion in the right hip that causes the femoral head to sublux laterally from the acetabulum. No bone erosion or marrow edema is evident.

diagnosis in suspected cases of necrotizing fasciitis (Fig. 5–13).

SEPTIC ARTHRITIS

In the presence of a monoarticular inflammatory process, the diagnosis of a septic joint should always be considered as a possibility (Fig. 5–14). Predisposing factors include diabetes, corticosteroid therapy, debilitating diseases, and intravenous drug abuse.[33–35] In intravenous drug abusers, the sites of predilection are the acromioclavicular, sternoclavicular, and sacroiliac joints, as well as the spine (Fig. 5–15). Whenever the diagnosis of septic arthritis is entertained clinically, the joint should be aspirated for culture and sensitivity. In some instances, such as tuberculous arthritis, a synovial biopsy may be necessary to establish the diagnosis.

MR findings of septic arthritis are not specific and are the same as for any inflammatory arthritis. Initially, there is a joint effusion and synovitis; later on, joint space narrowing and erosions may appear. The joint effusion and synovitis are low signal intensity on T1W images and high signal intensity on T2W images, although synovitis will be slightly higher signal intensity than joint fluid on T1W images. After intravenous contrast, the joint effusion

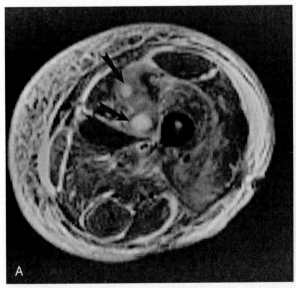
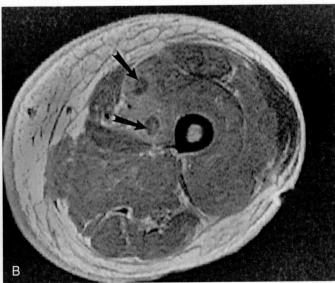

Figure 5–13. NECROTIZING FASCIITIS.
A, STIR axial image, thigh. There is intermuscular fascial edema, subcutaneous edema, and intramuscular diffuse edema, all manifested as high signal intensity. In addition, there are two focal areas of high signal within muscle *(arrows)* from abscesses. Only intermuscular and subcutaneous high signal are required to make the diagnosis. *B,* T1 contrast-enhanced axial image, thigh. There is mild diffuse enhancement of the muscle surrounding the two low-signal abscesses *(arrows).* The other manifestations of this inflammatory process are masked with this sequence.

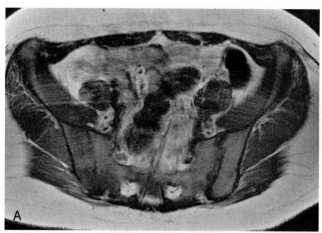

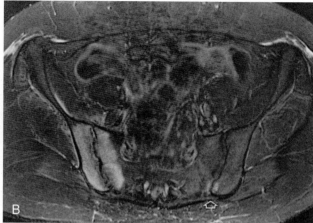

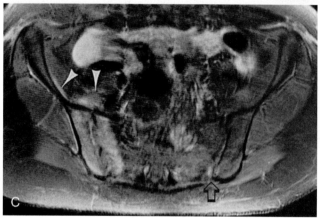

Figure 5–15. SEPTIC ARTHRITIS.
A, T1 axial image, pelvis. The black cortical lines in the right sacroiliac joint are obliterated (compare to left joint). *B,* STIR axial image, pelvis. Large bands of marrow edema are present on either side of the right sacroiliac joint. There is high signal within the joint and cortical destruction. Also, high signal is present in the soft tissues anterior to the joint and right iliac wing. Small areas of marrow edema are present on the posterior aspect of the left sacroiliac joint *(open arrow)* in this drug abuser with septic joints. *C,* T1 contrast-enhanced with fat suppression axial image, pelvis. Almost identical features to the STIR image are seen, indicating hyperemia from infection, but no abscess formation. The high signal seen in the anterior soft tissues *(arrowheads)* is from either cellulitis or reactive hyperemia. There is bone marrow edema, granulation tissue, or synovitis in the joint, as well as cortical erosions and early changes of infection in the left sacroiliac joint *(open arrow).*

remains low signal intensity, whereas synovitis becomes high signal intensity. Erosions are seen as marginal subchondral defects, low signal intensity on T1W and high signal intensity on T2W images. Adjacent soft tissue and bone marrow edema may be seen with a septic joint; these findings generally indicate a sympathetic hyperemia with edema, but occasionally the bone or soft tissues adjacent to the infected joint also may be infected.

MISCELLANEOUS

A number of situations deserve special consideration. These include infection associated with foreign bodies, chronic recurrent multifocal osteomyelitis, acquired immunodeficiency syndrome (AIDS), and the diabetic foot.

Foreign Bodies

Soft tissue or intraarticular foreign bodies may cause an infection. These foreign bodies are most often wood, thorns, or glass and are usually not radioopaque. Their sites of predilection are the feet and hands. Foreign bodies in the soft tissues create an inflammatory reaction (cellulitis), and eventually

may lead to the formation of an abscess cavity or a sinus tract to permit the extrusion of the foreign body. The foreign body ultimately may cause osteomyelitis.

On MR images, foreign bodies are low signal intensity on all sequences and can be very subtle in appearance. In general, they are linear in shape, which is a very helpful criterion for identification. On T2W images, foreign bodies are surrounded by high signal intensity, representing granulation tissue, cellulitis, or abscess (Fig. 5–16). Intravenous contrast may increase the conspicuity of foreign bodies, which remain low signal intensity, surrounded by diffuse increased signal intensity in the case of granulation tissue or cellulitis, or abscess cavity that remains low signal intensity except in its periphery.

Intraarticular foreign bodies are not as common as soft tissue foreign bodies, but they generate a marked reactive synovitis. On T1W images, the foreign bodies, synovitis, and joint effusion will be low signal intensity, although the foreign bodies may be even lower signal intensity than the surrounding fluid. On T2W images, foreign bodies remain low signal intensity, whereas the joint effusion and the synovitis become high signal intensity. A high index of suspicion is necessary to identify foreign bodies, and again their linear shape is a very helpful clue for their identification (Fig. 5–17).

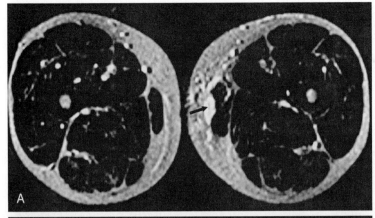

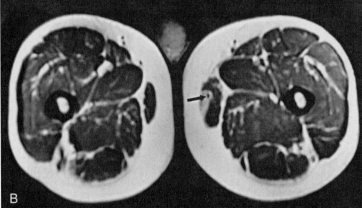

Figure 5–16. FOREIGN BODY: Soft Tissues.
A, Spin echo-T2 axial image, thighs. There is a focal region of high-signal intensity adjacent to muscle in the medial aspect of the left thigh at the site of clinical pain and swelling. A vague, linear low-signal structure representing a foreign body (wood) is present in the center of the lesion *(arrow)*. The high signal may be from focal cellulitis, abscess, or granulation tissue. **B,** T1 contrast-enhanced axial image, thighs. The low-signal wood foreign body is more visible *(arrow)*. The enhancement of the tissue surrounding the foreign body indicates that it is not from abscess, and either represents granulation tissue or focal cellulitis.

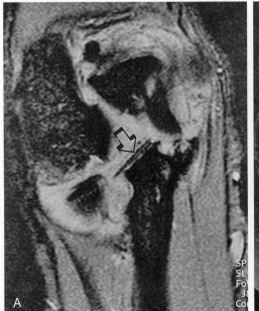

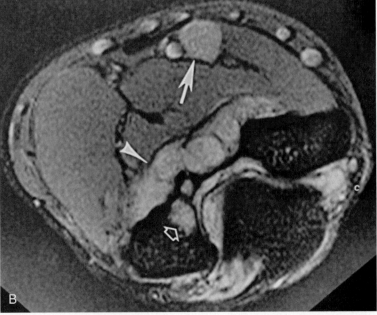

Figure 5–17. FOREIGN BODY: Articular.
A, T2* coronal image, elbow. A linear foreign body *(open arrow)* is seen adjacent to the posterior ulna within the elbow joint. This was a thorn from a rose bush. High-signal synovitis/joint effusion is present, as well as bone erosion in the ulna from the inflammatory articular process. **B,** T2* axial image, elbow. The tremendous synovitis and joint effusion are evident *(arrowhead)*. An enlarged lymph node is noted *(arrow)*, and bone erosions in the humerus *(open arrow)* are obvious.

BOX 5–7: FEATURES OF OSTEOMYELITIS IN DIABETIC FEET

Virtual Requirements
- Abnormal marrow signal on *both* T1 and T2
- Soft tissue ulcer or sinus tract overlying the abnormal bone and usually located at predictable pressure points (1st and 5th metatarsal heads, calcaneal tuberosity, distal phalanges of toes, malleoli of ankles)

Other Possible Findings
- Cortical destruction (loss of the black cortical line)
- Intraosseous fluid collection (abscess)
- Sequestrum
- Soft tissue cellulitis, abscesses
- Adjacent joint effusion

Chronic Recurrent Multifocal Osteomyelitis

Chronic recurrent multifocal osteomyelitis is a chronic osteomyelitis, usually affecting children and young adults. Any skeletal site can be involved, but there is a predilection for the metaphyses of the lower extremity, for the medial ends of the clavicles, and for a symmetrical presentation. Patients complain of pain and swelling in the affected areas, and up to 40% of patients have palmoplantar pustulosis.[36–39] This entity is included in the group of disorders designated as SAPHO (Synovitis, Acne, Pustulosis, Hyperostosis, and Osteitis) syndrome. Laboratory findings are not specific, and blood and bone cultures are usually negative. Histologically, the osteolytic portion of the lesion contains a predominance of plasma cells, and the term *plasma cell osteomyelitis* has been used for this condition. The dominant radiographic feature is sclerosis, in combination with a variable amount of osteolysis and periostitis. No characteristic MR findings have been described. The entity should be considered in the presence of multifocal involvement or when the medial end of the clavicle is affected.

Acquired Immunodeficiency Syndrome

Patients with human immunodeficiency virus (HIV) infection are immunocompromised and have a susceptibility for bacterial and fungal infections. These patients are predisposed to osteomyelitis, septic arthritis, and pyomyositis with MR changes as described previously.[40–42] A rare form of osteomyelitis that has a higher incidence in AIDS patients is bacillary angiomatosis,[43] caused by a gram-negative microorganism. Patients usually present with skin lesions characterized by multiple angiomatous papules. The bone lesions consist of multiple osteolytic foci involving both cortex and medullary cavity, associated with soft tissue masses. The tubular bones of the extremities, in particular the tibia, are the sites of predilection.

Radiographic findings of bacillary angiomatosis consist of poorly and well-defined cortical osteolytic defects associated with a variable amount of medullary osteolysis, sclerosis, and periosteal reaction. On MR images, lobulated soft tissue masses adjacent to cortical defects can be identified. These masses are intermediate signal intensity (higher than muscle) on T1W images and high signal intensity on T2W images. In addition to the cortical destruction and soft tissue masses, changes consistent with osteomyelitis in the adjacent marrow are evident.

Diabetic Foot Infection
(Boxes 5–7 through 5–9)

Foot disease in diabetics is a common problem and usually is related to one or more of the following: vascular disease, infection, neuroarthropathy,

BOX 5–8: MARROW SIGNAL ABNORMALITIES IN DIABETIC FEET

T1 MARROW SIGNAL	T2 (STIR) MARROW SIGNAL	DIAGNOSIS
↑ (fat)	↓	Definitely no osteomyelitis
↑ (fat)	↑	Mild reactive marrow edema, no osteomyelitis
↓	↑	Differential diagnosis • Osteomyelitis • Reactive marrow edema (marked) • Acute neuropathic changes (use location of lesions, etc., to help distinguish and sharpen your biopsy needles to prove)

and tendon rupture. Infection in diabetics is usually the result of a soft tissue injury, usually followed by cellulitis; the infection may remain limited to the soft tissues or extend to adjacent bone. Soft tissue ulcerations usually are found under pressure areas of the foot, such as the plantar soft tissues beneath or adjacent to the first and fifth metatarsal heads, the calcaneal tuberosity, the distal phalanges, and the malleoli. These ulcers are seen in most diabetic patients with foot infections, and osteomyelitis rarely is present without associated soft tissue ulcers (Fig. 5–18).[3]

Ulcers can be identified on MRI as soft tissue defects of low signal intensity on both T1W and T2W images. Cellulitis usually is associated with the soft tissue ulcers and is identified on MRI as diffuse areas of low signal intensity on T1W and high signal intensity on T2W images, with enhancement after gadolinium administration. Osteitis can be identified on MR images as blurring or destruction of the black cortical line on all pulse sequences, and osteomyelitis as abnormal low signal intensity marrow on T1W and high signal intensity on STIR images, with enhancement after gadolinium administration. Abnormal signal intensity in the bone marrow is not specific for infection and also can be seen with neuroarthropathy or from aseptic marrow edema (sympathetic reaction) secondary to hyper-

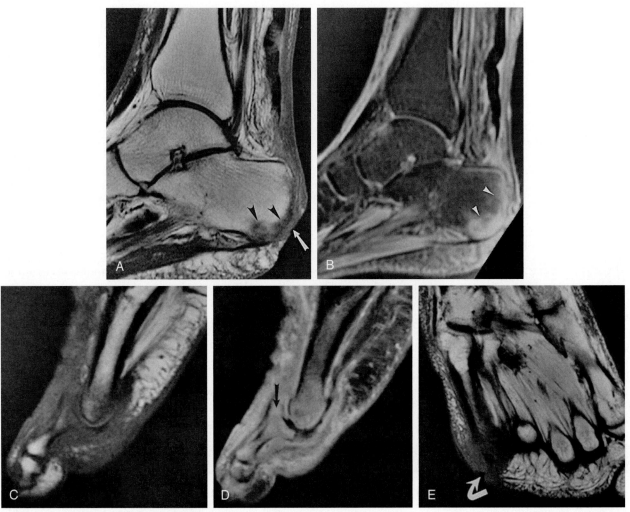

Figure 5–18. DIABETIC FOOT INFECTION.
A, T1 sagittal image, hindfoot. There is a large soft tissue defect (ulcer) over the calcaneal tuberosity *(arrow)*. Abnormal low signal is present in the adjacent calcaneal bone marrow *(arrowheads)*. Incidentally, the Achilles tendon is ruptured distally, and retracted proximally with undulation of the tendon. *B*, STIR sagittal image, hindfoot. The ulcer has been cut off in this photograph. The abnormal marrow signal is more obvious on this sequence than on T1. Although the signal in the calcaneus could be from reactive marrow edema, it is much more likely to be osteomyelitis, based on the presence of the overlying ulcer as well as cortical destruction. *C*, T1 sagittal image, fifth metatarsophalangeal joint (different patient than in *A* and *B*). There is intermediate signal in the metatarsal head and the base of the proximal phalanx. The subcutaneous fat surrounding the joint is replaced by intermediate signal inflammatory tissue that is either cellulitis or abscess. *D*, T1 contrast-enhanced with fat suppression sagittal image, fifth toe. Everything that was abnormal intermediate signal on the T1W image in *C* enhances. In addition, a focal area of cortical destruction on the dorsum of the base of the proximal phalanx is more obvious *(arrow)*. The findings are compatible with osteomyelitis and adjacent cellulitis without abscess formation. *E*, T1 coronal image, forefoot (same patient as in *C* and *D*). The ulcer *(curved arrow)* overlying the area of abnormal marrow signal and the cortical destruction make osteomyelitis a virtual certainty.

BOX 5–9: DIABETIC DILEMMA		
	OSTEOMYELITIS	**NEUROARTHROPATHY**
Location	Adjacent to ulcers at pressure points • Metatarsal heads (1st & 5th) • Calcaneal tuberosity • Distal phalanges of toes • Malleoli of ankle May or may not involve joints	Always involves joints • Tarsometatarsal (Lisfranc) joints and adjacent bones • Talonavicular and calcaneocuboid (Chopart) joints and adjacent bones • Ankle and subtalar joints and adjacent bones
Other Features	Cortical destruction Sequestrum Intraosseous fluid collection (abscess)	Bone fragmentation Malalignment
Nondiscriminatory Features	Joint effusion Soft tissue edema Bone marrow edema Periosteal reaction	Joint effusion Soft tissue edema Bone marrow edema Periosteal reaction

emia from the adjacent soft tissue inflammatory process. In addition to abnormal bone marrow signal intensity, one or more of the following changes significantly increases the diagnostic confidence of osteomyelitis in a diabetic foot: (1) cutaneous ulcer overlying the bone abnormality, (2) sinus tract extending to bone, (3) cortical destruction (4) intramedullary abscess, and (5) sequestrum formation. Absence of bone marrow changes on STIR images excludes the diagnosis of osteomyelitis.[44–50]

Certain features help distinguish acute neuropathic changes from diabetic foot infections. Neuroarthropathy always affects joints. It often is associated with bone fragmentation and subluxation. The commonest sites of involvement are the tarsometatarsal joints (Lisfranc joint), the talonavicular and calcaneocuboid joints (Chopart joint), and the subtalar joints. A biopsy is indicated whenever imaging features are not conclusive for either osteomyelitis or neuroarthropathy.

References

1. Jones KM, Unger EC, Granstrom P, et al. Bone marrow imaging using STIR at 0.5 and 1.5T. *Magn Reson Imaging* 1992; 10:169–176.
2. Morrison WB, Schweitzer ME, Bock H, et al. Diagnosis of osteomyelitis: utility of fat-suppressed contrast-enhanced MR imaging. *Radiology* 1993; 189:251–257.
3. Morrison WB, Schweitzer ME, Batte WG, et al. Osteomyelitis of the foot: relative importance of primary and secondary MR imaging signs. *Radiology* 1998; 207:625–632.
4. Hopkins KL, Li KCP, Bergman G. Gadolinium-DTPA-enhanced magnetic resonance imaging of musculoskeletal infectious processes. *Skeletal Radiol* 1995; 24:325–330.
5. Resnick D, Niwayama G. Osteomyelitis, septic arthritis, and soft tissue infection: mechanisms and situations. In Resnick D (ed): *Diagnosis of Bone and Joint Disorders*, edn 3. Philadelphia: W.B. Saunders; 1995.
6. Trueta J. The three types of acute hematogenous osteomyelitis: a clinical and vascular study. *J Bone Joint Surg [Br]* 1959; 41:671–680.
7. Marcy SM. Infections due to dog and cat bites. *Pediatr Infect Dis* 1982; 1:351–356.
8. Beltran J, Noto AM, McGhee RB, et al. Infections of the musculoskeletal system: high-field strength MR imaging. *Radiology* 1987; 164:449–454.
9. Tumeh SS, Aliabadi P, Weissman BN, et al. Disease activity in osteomyelitis: role of radiography. *Radiology* 1987; 165:781–784.
10. Tang, JS, Gold RH, Bassett LW, et al. Musculoskeletal infection of the extremities: evaluation with MR imaging. *Radiology* 1988; 166:205–209.
11. Unger E, Moldofsky P, Gatenby R, et al. Diagnosis of osteomyelitis by MR imaging. *AJR* 1988; 150:605–610.
12. Wegener WA, Alavi A. Diagnostic imaging of musculoskeletal infection: roentgenography; gallium; indium-labeled white blood cell, gammaglobulin bone scintigraphy; and MRI. *Orthop Clin North Am* 1991; 22:401–418.
13. Gold RH, Hawkins RA, Katz RD. Bacterial osteomyelitis: findings on plain radiography, CT, MR, and scintigraphy. *AJR* 1991; 12:292–297.
14. Tehranzadeh J, Wang F, Mesqarzadeh M. Magnetic resonance imaging of osteomyelitis. *Crit Rev Diagn Imaging* 1992; 33:495–534.
15. Crim JR, Seeger LL. Imaging evaluation of osteomyelitis. *Crit Rev Diagn Imaging* 1994; 35:201–256.
16. Chew FS, Schulze ES, Mattia AR. Osteomyelitis. *AJR* 1994; 162:942.
17. Capitanio MA, Kirkpatrick JA. Early roentgen observations in acute osteomyelitis. *AJR* 1970; 108:488–496.
18. Chandnani VP, Beltran J, Morris DS, et al. Acute experimental osteomyelitis and abscesses: detection with MR imaging versus CT. *Radiology* 1990; 174:233–236.
19. Cohen MD, Cory DA, Kleiman M, et al. Magnetic resonance differentiation of acute and chronic osteomyelitis in children. *Clin Radiol* 1990; 41:53–56.
20. Dangman BC, Hoffer FA, Rand FF, et al. Osteomyelitis in children: gadolinium-enhanced MR imaging. *Radiology* 1992; 182:743–747.
21. Mazur JM, Ross G, Cummings RJ, et al. Usefulness of magnetic resonance imaging for the diagnosis of acute musculoskeletal infections in children. *J Pediatr Orthop* 1995; 15:144–147.
22. Fitzgerald RH, Brewer NS, Dahlin DC. Squamous-cell carcinoma complicating chronic osteomyelitis. *J Bone Joint Surg [Am]* 1976; 58:1146–1148.
23. Mason MD, Zlatkin MB, Esterhai JL, et al. Chronic complicated osteomyelitis of the lower extremity: evaluation with MR imaging. *Radiology* 1989; 173:355–359.
24. Quinn SF, Murray W, Clark RA, Cockran C. MR imaging of

chronic osteomyelitis. *J Comput Assist Tomogr* 1988; 12:113–117.

25. Rahmouni A, Chosidow O, Mathieu D, et al. MR imaging in acute infectious cellulitis. *Radiology* 1994; 192:493–496.

26. Jaovisidha S, Chen C, Ryu KN, et al. Tuberculous tenosynovitis and bursitis: imaging findings in 21 cases. *Radiology* 1996; 201:507–513.

27. Yuh WTC, Schreiber AE, Montgomery WJ, et al. Magnetic resonance imaging of pyomyositis. *Skeletal Radiol* 1988; 17:190–193.

28. Fleckenstein JL, Burns DK, Murphy FK, et al. Differential diagnosis of bacterial myositis in AIDS: evaluation with MR imaging. *Radiology* 1991; 179:653–658.

29. Applegate GR, Cohen AJ. Pyomyositis: Early detection utilizing multiple imaging modalities. *Magn Reson Imaging* 1991; 9:187–193.

30. Gordon BA, Martinez S, Collins AJ. Pyomyositis: characteristics at CT and MR imaging. *Radiology* 1995; 197:279–286.

31. Freischlag JA, Ajalat G, Bussutil RW. Treatment of necrotizing soft tissue infections. *Am J Surg* 1985; 149:751–755.

32. Schmid MR, Kossmann T, Duewell S. Differentiation of ncrotizing fasciitis and cellulitis using MR imaging. *AJR* 1998; 170:615–620.

33. Roca RP, Yoshikawa TT. Primary skeletal infections in heroin users. *Clin Orthop* 1979; 144:238–248.

34. Firooznia H, Golimbu C, Rafii M, et al. Radiology of musculoskeletal complications of drug addiction. *Semin Roentgenol* 1983; 18:198–206.

35. Zimmerman B III, Erickson AD, Mikolich DJ. Septic acromioclavicular arthritis and osteomyelitis in a patient with acquired immunodeficiency syndrome. *Arthritis Rheum* 1989; 32:1175–1178.

36. Kahn M-F, Chamot A-M. SAPHO syndrome. *Rheum Dis Clin North Am* 1992; 18:225–246.

37. Carr AJ, Cole WG, Robertson DM, et al. Chronic multifocal osteomyelitis. *J Bone Joint Surg [Br]* 1993; 75:582–591.

38. Kasperczyk A, Freyschmidt J. Pustulotic arthroosteitis: spectrum of bone lesions with palmoplantar pustulosis. *Radiology* 1994; 191:207–211.

39. Sundaram M, McDonald D, Engel E, et al. Chronic recurrent multifocal osteomyelitis: an evolving clinical and radiological spectrum. *Skeletal Radiol* 1996; 25:333–336.

40. Steinbach LS, Tehranzadeh J, Fleckenstein JL, et al. Human immunodeficiency virus infection: musculoskeletal manifestations. *Radiology* 1993; 186:833–838.

41. Lee DJ, Sartoris DJ. Musculoskeletal manifestations of human immunodeficiency virus infection: review of imaging characteristics. *Radiol Clin North Am* 1994; 32:399–411.

42. Wyatt SH, Fishman EK. CT/MRI of musculoskeletal complications of AIDS. *Skeletal Radiol* 1995; 24:481–488.

43. Baron AL, Steinbach LS, LeBoit PE, et al. Osteolytic lesions and bacillary angiomatosis in HIV infection: radiologic differentiation from AIDS-related Kaposi sarcoma. *Radiology* 1990; 177:77–81.

44. Yuh WTC, Corson JD, Baraniewski HM, et al. Osteomyelitis of the foot in diabetic patients: evaluation with plain film, 99mTc-MDP bone scintigraphy, and MR imaging. *AJR* 1989; 152:795–800.

45. Wang A, Weinstein D, Greenfield L, et al. MRI and diabetic foot infections. *Magn Reson Imaging* 1990; 8:805–809.

46. Beltran J, Campanini DS, Knight C, et al. The diabetic foot: magnetic resonance imaging evaluation. *Skeletal Radiol* 1990; 19:37–41.

47. Durham JR, Lukens ML, Campanini DS, et al. Impact of magnetic resonance imaging on the management of diabetic foot infections. *Am J Surg* 1991; 162:150–153.

48. Eckman MH, Greenfield S, Mackey WC, et al. Foot infections in diabetic patients: decision and cost-effectiveness analyses. *JAMA* 1995; 273:712–720.

49. Gold RH, Tong DJ, Crim JR, et al. Imaging the diabetic foot. *Skeletal Radiol* 1995; 24:563–571.

50. Craig JG, Amin MB, Wu K, et al. Osteomyelitis of the diabetic foot: MR imaging-pathologic correlation. *Radiology* 1997; 203:849–855.

6 ARTHRITIS

HOW TO IMAGE ARTHRITIS AND
  CARTILAGE
RHEUMATOID ARTHRITIS
GOUT
CALCIUM PYROPHOSPHATE
  DIHYDRATE DEPOSITION

HEMOPHILIA
AMYLOID
TUMORS
SYNOVIAL CHONDROMATOSIS

PIGMENTED VILLONODULAR
  SYNOVITIS
LOOSE BODIES
CARTILAGE

HOW TO IMAGE ARTHRITIS AND CARTILAGE

Coils/Patient Position. Which joint is being imaged will determine which coil and which position will be used. For instance, in the knee the standard extremity coil is used in the same manner as imaging for a torn meniscus. The same would hold for the wrist, elbow, and so forth.

Image Orientation. Joints imaged for arthritis and for cartilage are best seen with the standard planes of imaging discussed in the other chapters. For example, in the knee three planes (axial, coronal, and sagittal) should be used to evaluate the cartilage adequately.

Pulse Sequences/Regions of Interest. For most entities involving the joints as an arthritis, it is recommended that both T1W and some type of T2W sequence be used in each plane of imaging. Cartilage-sensitive sequences are discussed in greater detail later in this chapter.

Contrast. There is no need to use contrast for evaluating arthritis or cartilage, although it markedly increases the conspicuity of pannus.

Most joint abnormalities are discussed in the chapters under the specific joints (eg, avascular necrosis in the marrow or hip chapters). This short chapter discusses a few additional abnormalities that can affect any joint, such as pigmented villonodular synovitis (PVNS), synovial chondromatosis, and a few common arthritides; it also provides an overview of cartilage imaging.

MRI has little role in most cases of arthritis. Plain films seem to suffice for initial diagnosis, as well as in follow up to determine progression. Although MRI can certainly depict erosive changes and cartilage loss in small joints in various arthritides, it currently does not seem to offer additional information over plain films, and therefore is not recommended for routine use in arthritis. It is important to recognize, however, the changes encountered in the more common arthritides, because these changes occasionally are seen in patients imaged for other reasons.

RHEUMATOID ARTHRITIS

The erosive changes in rheumatoid arthritis (RA) virtually mirror those seen on conventional radiographs (Fig. 6–1). MRI does not seem to show them to better advantage, and therefore is not recommended as a useful clinical tool for showing the extent of disease. Pannus cannot be reliably differentiated from synovium and joint fluid; however, with gadolinium some investigators have reported that pannus can be easily identified because of the intense enhancement that occurs in the highly vascular pannus. If one cares to look at unenhanced images of joints very closely, pannus has a slightly higher signal than joint fluid on T1W images, allowing it to be identified even without the expense and hassle of contrast administration. Because treatment currently is not predicated on the amount of pannus present, this does not justify routine use of gadolinium in these patients.

Occasionally, a swollen joint in a patient with RA shows multiple small loose bodies, called rice bodies (Fig. 6–2). They are so called because of their resemblance at surgery to white rice. On MRI, they can mimic another cause of multiple loose bodies such as synovial chondromatosis, but typically rice bodies are much smaller than the loose bodies of synovial chondromatosis and remain low signal on T2W images. Most, but not all, patients already carry a diagnosis of RA, so the entity is easily recognized as rice bodies if the radiologist is familiar with this process. Rice bodies can easily be removed by a surgeon if they cause mechanical symptoms, but otherwise the treatment is the same as for any joint inflamed by RA.

GOUT

As with RA, the radiographic findings in gout are sufficient for diagnosis, and MRI has little to offer in this disease. However, it is important to appreciate that gouty tophi occasionally are seen in patients not known to have gout, in which case they can

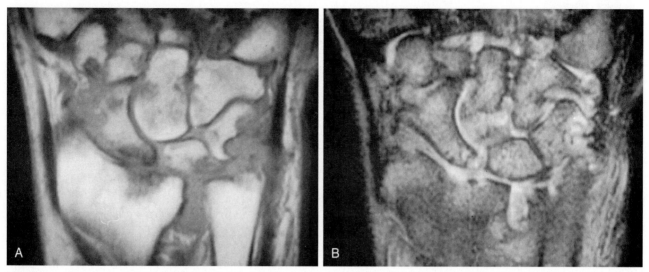

Figure 6–1. These coronal T1W *(A)* and gradient echo *(B)* images in a patient with advanced rheumatoid arthritis show the distended joints and multiple erosions throughout the wrist.

cause diagnostic confusion. Gouty tophi can occur in almost any soft tissue location, including intraarticularly. They can erode bones or can begin within bones (intraosseous tophi). In cases where the tophus is large and the diagnosis of gout is unknown, the tophus can be misdiagnosed as a tumor with resultant biopsy. Tophi are typically low in signal on both T1 and T2W images (Fig. 6–3), which distinguishes them from most other joint problems and from most tumors (with the exception of fibrous tumors, PVNS, and amyloid).

CALCIUM PYROPHOSPHATE DIHYDRATE DEPOSITION

As with the aforementioned arthritides, MR imaging has little to offer in the diagnosis of calcium pyrophosphate dihydrate deposition (CPPD), or pseudogout. The appearance of chondrocalcinosis in the menisci of the knee has been reported to have linear high signal that can mimic a meniscal tear (Fig. 6–4), but this has not been a significant pitfall in our experience. One might intuitively think that calcification would produce low signal on MR images; however, in many cases, such as in the lumbar spine, calcification paradoxically causes intermediate to high signal on T1W images. The reason for this has not been explained, but several theories have been discussed in the literature.[1,2]

Chondrocalcinosis also can appear as linear or punctate areas of low signal in hyaline cartilage, particularly noticeable on T2* sequences because of the blooming artifact.

HEMOPHILIA

Although not imaged with MR very frequently, some of the findings seen in hemophilia are worth

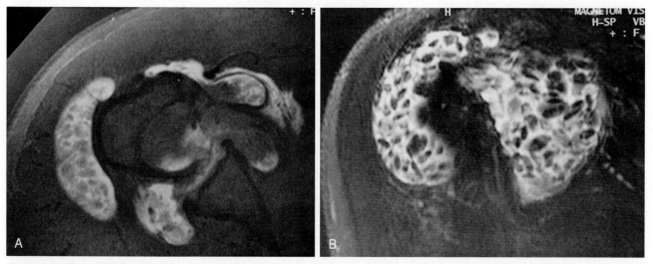

Figure 6–2. These T1W images with fat suppression following a gadolinium arthrogram in the *(A)* axial and *(B)* oblique coronal planes through the shoulder show multiple small filling defects or loose bodies. At surgery, these were found to be rice bodies.

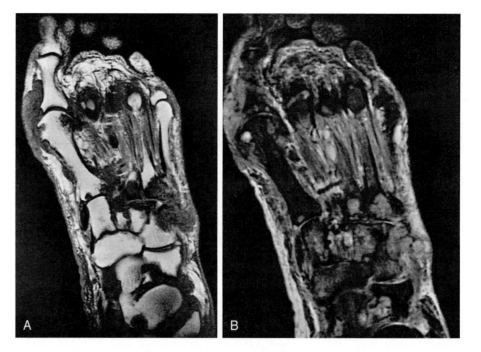

Figure 6–3. Coronal *(A)* T1W and *(B)* STIR images in the foot of a patient with advanced gout reveal multiple erosions and tophi, most of which are low in signal on both sequences.

mentioning. The joint destruction and cartilage loss seen on MR imaging are pretty much what one would expect from the conventional radiographs. However, chronic joint hemorrhages leave deposits of hemosiderin, which is seen on MR images as clumps of low signal lining the synovium on both T1W and T2W images (Fig. 6–5). This has been termed hemosiderotic arthritis. The amount of hemosiderin seen varies from none to moderate, with it almost never being as prominent as that seen in PVNS. In joints with a lot of hemosiderin, there typically is advanced joint destruction, something that is uncommon in PVNS. It is virtually never a diagnostic dilemma to differentiate hemophilia from PVNS, because patients with hemophilia are well aware of their diagnosis long before a joint is imaged. The main indications for imaging a hemophil-

iac joint are to determine the extent of cartilage destruction and the thickness of the synovium; these features help determine how to manage the joint abnormality.

AMYLOID

Amyloid deposits tend to occur in and around large joints and can cause significant joint swelling and pain (Fig. 6–6). Bony erosion can be prominent.[3] Amyloid also can occur in the spine (where it is much more common), where it may resemble a disc infection (Fig. 6–7). In the spine, the deposits can be either amyloid or an amyloid-like entity called β-2-microglobulin.[4] In a patient with suspected disc infection, it is imperative to inquire as

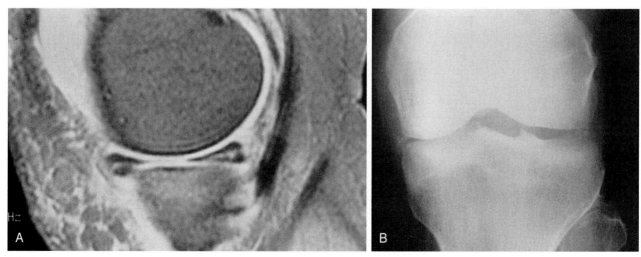

Figure 6–4. *A,* A sagittal proton-density image with fat suppression shows high signal in the anterior and posterior horns of the medial meniscus that resemble tears. *B,* However, a plain film shows chondrocalcinosis, which was responsible for the high signal.

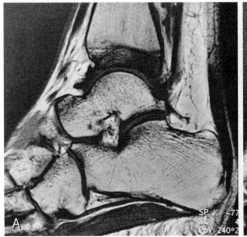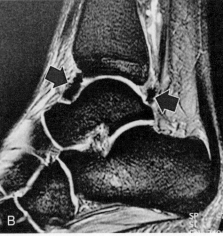

Figure 6–5. These sagittal T1W *(A)* and gradient echo *(B)* images in the ankle of a patient with hemophilia show a large joint effusion that is low in signal on the T2* sequence *(arrows)*, consistent with hemosiderin deposition.

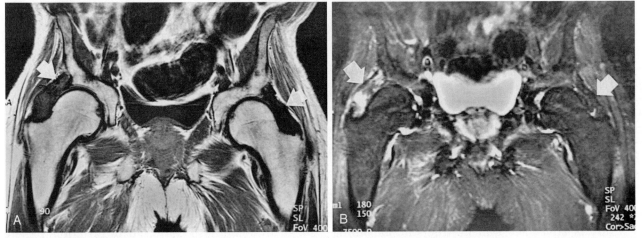

Figure 6–6. Coronal *(A)* T1W and *(B)* STIR images in a patient with renal disease reveal bilateral hip joint swelling *(arrows)*, which is predominantly low in signal on both sequences. These were masses of amyloid deposits around both hips.

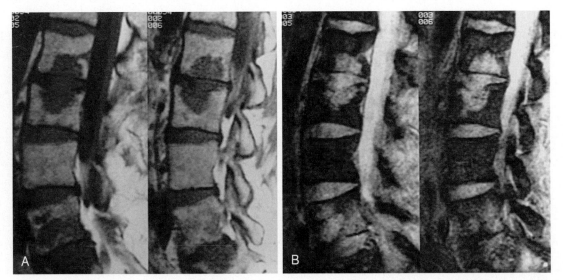

Figure 6–7. Sagittal T1W *(A)* and gradient echo *(B)* images of the spine in a patient on dialysis for renal failure show abnormalities at the L2–L3 and L5–S1 disks that resemble disc infection. This was not infection; it was amyloid or β-2-microglobulin deposition.

to whether the patient has renal failure or is on dialysis, because amyloid or β-2-microglobulin deposits from renal disease can perfectly mimic infection on both radiographs and MRI, resulting in an unnecessary biopsy. It is the only entity described that mimics a disk infection. Amyloid deposits have been reported to be low in signal on both T1W and T2W images, which is distinctly unusual for most pathologic processes. Most examples we have seen in the spine have demonstrated high signal on T2W images.

TUMORS

There are no tumors that originate in joints, but there are a few entities that are tumor-like and present as joint swelling. The most common of these are synovial chondromatosis and PVNS. Uncommon entities that can present similarly are synovial hemangiomas and lipoma arborescens; these are rare enough that they will not be mentioned further in this book.

SYNOVIAL CHONDROMATOSIS

There are two forms of synovial chondromatosis: primary and secondary. Primary synovial chondromatosis is an uncommon entity that is caused by metaplasia of the synovium, which produces multiple loose bodies within a joint. Initially, these are cartilagenous bodies that are not calcified; they generally progress to calcified loose bodies, all of which are the same size. They may cause mechanical symptoms, as with any loose body in a joint, or they may merely cause a feeling of swelling or fullness in the joint. Eventually, they will imbed in the synovium and not float freely in the joint. Cartilage erosion from these loose bodies is a late finding if it occurs at all. Treatment is removal of the loose bodies and a synovectomy.

Secondary synovial chondromatosis is a much more common disorder. It is believed to be secondary to trauma, which causes shedding of bits of articular cartilage resulting in loose bodies in the joint. These bodies may or may not calcify. These loose bodies, unlike in primary synovial chondromatosis, are of all different sizes and generally are fewer in number. Osteoarthritis typically is present because of the cartilage damage. Treatment is removal of the loose bodies and smoothing of the articular cartilage defects. A synovectomy is not necessary, because this condition is not caused by metaplasia of the synovium.

Synovial chondromatosis typically is an easy radiographic diagnosis, with the presence of multiple calcified loose bodies being virtually pathognomonic. However, its not always that straightforward. Up to 20% of cases do not have the loose bodies calcified, in which case the radiograph shows only joint swelling, if anything. MRI can show multiple loose bodies (Fig. 6–8), but occasionally has a second appearance that is not as easily recognized as synovial chondromatosis. In these cases, the MR examination shows a confluent mass of tissue that is high in signal on T2W images and looks more like a tumor than multiple loose bodies (Fig. 6–9). We have seen biopsy in several of these cases incorrectly called chondrosarcoma, with extensive, radical surgery performed before the benign nature of the process was recognized. Therefore, it is critical that the radiologist recognize this benign disorder rather than allow the pathologist to sort it out. Remember, there are no malignant tumors that begin in a joint, so a mass in a joint should raise the concern for synovial chondromatosis and PVNS.

PIGMENTED VILLONODULAR SYNOVITIS

PVNS is a disorder of unknown cause that can affect any joint, bursa, or tendon sheath (when it affects a tendon sheath, it is called giant cell tumor of tendon sheath). It results in synovial hypertrophy with diffuse hemosiderin deposits within the joint. It virtually never calcifies and only causes joint space narrowing late in its course; therefore, radiographs simply show a swollen joint, if anything at all. When a large joint is affected, the hemosiderin

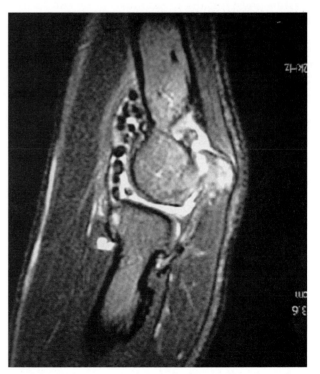

Figure 6–8. This sagittal T2W image through the elbow shows multiple loose bodies in the anterior compartment of the joint. These were visible on a plain film. This is synovial osteochondromatosis.

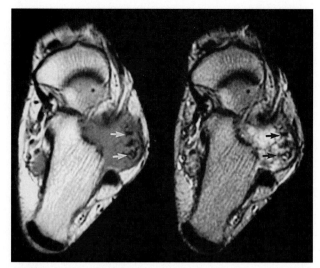

Figure 6–9. Axial T1W *(left)* and T2W *(right)* images of the ankle show a soft tissue mass in the ankle joint, which is low signal on T1W images and high on the T2W images, yet has some low-signal areas on both sequences *(arrows)*. This is synovial osteochondromatosis, which is not as obvious as in Figure 6–8, because no discrete loose bodies are identified. This appearance frequently is misdiagnosed as a tumor.

can produce a dense effusion that can be seen radiographically.

MRI is virtually pathognomonic. A joint effusion with diffuse low signal lining hypertrophied synovium on T2W images is characteristic (Fig. 6–10). The process can erode into bone, making large cystic cavities, but typically is confined to the soft tissues within a joint.

PVNS has two presentations in joints: diffuse and focal. When it is diffuse, it requires a total synovectomy for treatment, which is difficult to perform. Recurrence is common after attempted resection for diffuse PVNS. In focal PVNS (also called focal nodular PVNS), resection is considerably easier and more effective.

LOOSE BODIES

Loose bodies in joints can be difficult to find with any imaging modality, but MRI seems to be better than almost any other technique.[5] MR arthrography is superior to plain MRI unless a large joint effusion is present. Loose bodies can be made of cartilage, cortical bone (Fig. 6–11), or cancellous bone (usually with some cortical bone attached). We try to include a gradient echo sequence in at least one plane when looking for loose bodies in the hope that, if they have cortical bone attached to them, they will "bloom" and be more easily seen. We often receive requests to image a patient for a loose body in the elbow, and occasionally in the ankle, but we have never been asked to image a knee for a loose body, even though we often see them in the knee. We occasionally see loose bodies in the shoulder and in the hip.

CARTILAGE

Many articles have been published on MR imaging of cartilage with multiple comparisons of various imaging sequences for their utility in diagnosing cartilage abnormalities.[6–9] For the most part, they advocate several sequences, all of which seem superior to standard spin echo sequences. Which sequence is really the best is debatable, but thus far no single sequence is indisputably better than all the others, so it seems for now one can pick one of several available sequences that perform well at

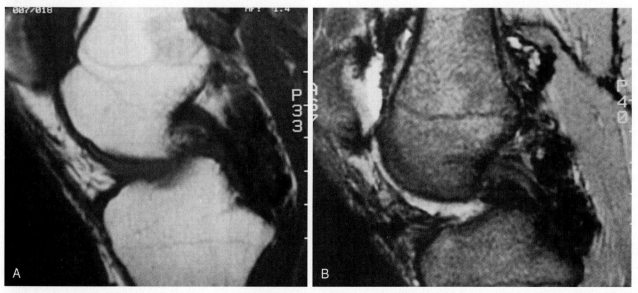

Figure 6–10. Sagittal T1W *(A)* and gradient echo *(B)* images through the knee in a patient with painful swelling show low signal lining the joint synovium in the suprapatellar pouch and mass-like low signal posterior to the posterior cruciate ligament. This represents hemosiderin deposits in pigmented villonodular synovitis.

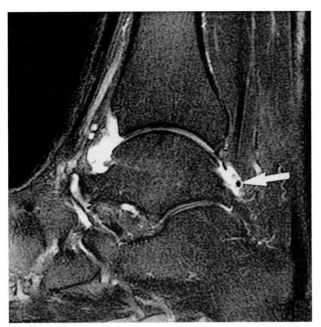

Figure 6–11. A sagittal fast spin echo-T2W image with fat suppression in the ankle of a patient with locking shows a loose body in the posterior compartment *(arrow)*. Without fluid in the joint, loose bodies can be very difficult to identify.

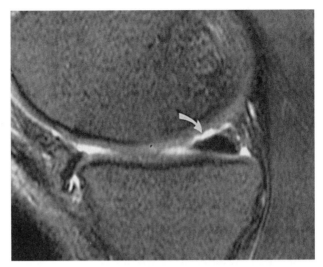

Figure 6–12. A sagittal fast spin echo-T2W image with fat suppression through the medial compartment of the knee shows surface irregularity of the femoral cartilage *(arrow)*.

showing hyaline articular cartilage. It is imperative that every knee MR examination have a cartilage-sensitive sequence. Some of the cartilage sequences promulgated in the literature are not readily available on commercial magnets, and others require inordinate imaging times, so that they are rendered useless for routine use. Some authors recommend their use only when cartilage abnormalities are suspected. You had better suspect a cartilage abnormality in every knee and have a sequence that shows the cartilage to good advantage, or your orthopedic surgeon will look elsewhere for an imaging diagnosis. Cartilage treatment has become important in orthopedic surgery and MRI is known to be useful in demonstrating abnormal cartilage in the knee, ankle, and elbow.

Multiple grading systems for cartilage abnormalities have been described, both in the radiology and the orthopedic surgery literature. One radiologist's grade 2 lesion is another's grade 3. Simply saying there is a grade 2 or 3 cartilage abnormality leaves one wondering which grading scale is being employed. It can get very confusing and often is misleading. No single grading system seems to enjoy a majority of proponents; hence, we do not recommend a description of the cartilage using a grading system, except for research papers, unless everyone involved with that patient's care is using the same grading system—something that would be very unlikely, because one cannot predict where a patient might next go for treatment. A simple description of the MRI appearance will give the surgeon all he or she needs to treat the abnormality. Also, a description of the abnormality allows anyone who desires to place the lesion in his or her particular grading scale.

Descriptions of the cartilage should tell if there is focal abnormal signal, surface fibrillation or irregularity (Fig. 6–12), a partial-thickness defect, a full-thickness defect (Fig. 6–13), and if the underlying bone has abnormal signal (Fig. 6–14). We refrain

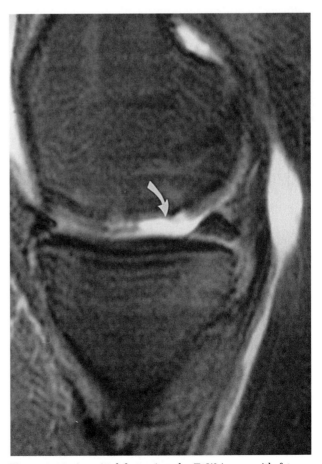

Figure 6–13. A sagittal fast spin echo-T2W image with fat suppression through the medial compartment of the knee shows a full-thickness cartilage defect on the femoral condyle *(arrow)*.

from commenting on generalized thinning of the cartilage, because it is virtually impossible to document at arthroscopy, is age and activity dependent, is not relevant to any symptoms or therapy that has been described, and probably has a better than even chance of being inaccurate.

The easiest part of diagnosing cartilage abnormalities is picking an appropriate MRI sequence. Almost any sequence other than conventional spin echo T1W and T2W images will suffice. This includes fast spin echo-T2 (not proton density), STIR, and gradient echo (either two- or three-dimensional). One sequence that is being strongly advocated in the radiology literature is a 3D volume-spoiled GRASS (gradient-recalled acquisition—the steady state) with fat suppression.[6] Although it does provide elegant images of cartilage (Fig. 6–15), it has two drawbacks: first, it takes over 10 minutes to acquire, which is entirely too long for routine use; secondly, it produces 60 images that need to be inspected. For most of us, that is information overload. One cannot examine all of the images with the diligence needed to have a high accuracy. We added this sequence to our standard knee protocol for about 6 months, and in hundreds of cases never found a single example in which a cartilage abnormality was seen on the GRASS images that we did not see on the fast spin echo-T2 images.

The hard part about diagnosing cartilage abnormalities is simply looking at all the cartilage surfaces. We have found that it is preferable to have a cartilage-sensitive sequence in all three planes, because the conspicuity of the abnormality often is prominent in one of the planes and very subtle in the other two. It is dependent on the location of the abnormality. We probably spend as much time inspecting the knee for cartilage abnormalities as we do looking at the remainder of the entire knee.

In summary, MRI has little utility in routine imaging for arthritis; however, radiologists need to be familiar with the more common appearances of the arthritides, because they occasionally will be en-

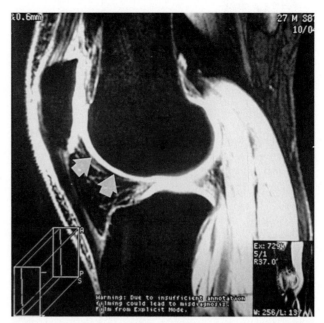

Figure 6–15. A sagittal 3D volume-spoiled GRASS image with fat suppression shows the articular cartilage to be very high in signal *(arrows)*. Although the cartilage is elegantly depicted, this image takes over 10 minutes to acquire.

countered. Cartilage imaging is considered an essential part of the imaging of the knee, ankle, and elbow. An appropriate sequence will afford a good look at the cartilage, and a full description of the abnormality should be made rather than placing it in some grading system.

References

1. Major N, Helms C, Genant H. Calcification demonstrated as high signal intensity on T1-weighted MR images of the disks of the lumbar spine. *Radiology* 1993; 189:494–496.
2. Bangert B, Modic M, Ross J, et al. Hyperintense disks on T1-weighted MR images: correlation with calcification. *Radiology* 1995; 195:437–444.
3. Kurer M, Baillod R, Madgwick J. Musculoskeletal manifestations of amyloidosis. *J Bone Joint Surg [Br]* 1991; 73:271–276.
4. Naidich JB, Mossey RT, McHeffey AB, et al. Spondyloarthropathy from long-term hemodialysis. *Radiology* 1988; 167:761–764.
5. Brossmann J, Preidler KW, Daenen B, et al. Imaging of osseous and cartilaginous intraarticular bodies in the knee—comparison of MR imaging and MR arthrography with CT and CT arthrography in cadavers. *Radiology* 1996; 200:509–517.
6. Disler DG, Mccauley TR, Kelman CG, et al. Fat-suppressed three-dimensional spoiled gradient-echo MR imaging of hyaline cartilage defects in the knee—comparison with standard MR imaging and arthroscopy. *AJR* 1996; 167:127–132.
7. Gagliardi JA, Chung EM, Chandnani VP, et al. Detection and staging of chondromalacia patellae: relative efficacies of conventional MR imaging, MR arthrography, and CT arthrography. *AJR* 1994; 163:629–636.
8. Hodler J, Resnick D. Current status of imaging of articular cartilage [review]. *Skeletal Radiol* 1996; 25:703–709.
9. Recht MP, Piraino DW, Paletta GA, Schils JP, Belhobek GH. Accuracy of fat-suppressed three-dimensional spoiled gradient-echo flash MR imaging in the detection of patellofemoral articular cartilage abnormalities. *Radiology* 1996; 198:209–212.

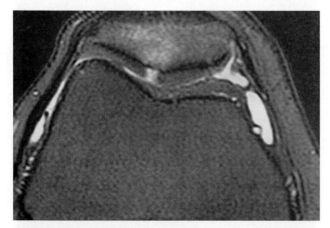

Figure 6–14. An axial fast spin echo-T2W image with fat suppression through the patella shows a focal, full-thickness defect near the apex of the patella with high signal in the underlying bone.

7 TUMORS

STAGING OF MUSCULOSKELETAL
   TUMORS
Principles of Staging
   Grade
   Local Extent
   Metastases
Principles of Imaging
   Bone Tumors
   Soft Tissue Tumors
   Important MRI Features
      Intraosseous tumor extent
      Extraosseous tumor extent
      Neurovascular or joint
         involvement
      Nodes
Evaluation of Tumor After Therapy
   Postchemotherapy
   Post-surgery/Radiation
HOW TO IMAGE TUMORS
APPROACH TO IMAGE
   INTERPRETATION
General Principles

Bone Lesions
   Differential Features
      Increased signal: T1W images
         Intraosseous lipoma
         Intraosseous hemangioma
         Medullary bone infarct
         Paget's disease
      Decreased signal: T2W images
         Sclerosis/calcification/matrix
         Fibrous lesions
         Primary lymphoma of bone
      Fluid/fluid levels
      Cartilaginous tumors
         Enchondroma/chondrosarcoma
         *Chondroid tumor vs. medullary
            bone infarct*
         Osteochondroma
Soft Tissue Tumors
   General Principles
   Differential Features

High signal on T1W images
   Lipomatous masses
   Vascular malformations
   Hematoma
   Melanoma
Low signal on T2W images
   Pigmented villonodular synovitis
   *Giant cell tumor of the tendon
      sheath*
   Fibrous lesions
   Amyloid
   Gout
   Melanoma
Cystic-appearing masses
   Cyst
   Intramuscular myxoma
   *Cystic-appearing malignant
      tumors*
   Nerve sheath tumors

MRI plays a central role in the work-up of a patient presenting with a suspected musculoskeletal tumor. MRI can confirm the presence of a lesion, allow for a specific diagnosis in some cases, define the extent of tumor spread, provide biopsy guidance, and assist in the evaluation of recurrent disease after therapy.

Therapeutic planning at the time of presentation is based primarily on the stage of the lesion. Local staging of a tumor depends on which anatomic structures and spaces (compartments) are involved, and this is best demonstrated with MRI.[1,2] Because an understanding of tumor staging is an important precursor to designing an optimal MRI protocol for evaluating these lesions, this chapter begins with a section briefly describing the principles of tumor staging. Despite your understandable natural instinct to skip over this material, we strongly urge you to read it in order to better understand how to set up and interpret MRI studies for this important indication.

STAGING OF MUSCULOSKELETAL TUMORS

Principles of Staging

The primary goal of the oncologic surgeon is to provide local control of disease by obtaining ade-quate tumor margins at the time of resection. If possible, this is achieved through a limb-sparing procedure; but if the lesion is too advanced, an amputation or disarticulation is required. The decision to amputate or perform a limb-sparing procedure depends on many factors, including tumor size, its relationship to adjacent structures such as nerves, vessels, and joints, and the overall stage of the tumor at the time of presentation.[3]

Although there are different staging systems, they are based on three components: (1) the grade of the tumor, (2) its local extent, and (3) the presence or absence of metastases.[3,4] The Enneking staging system,[3] which has been adopted by the Musculoskeletal Tumor Society, is outlined in Box 7–1.

Grade

The grade of the tumor is a measure of its potential to metastasize.[4] It is based primarily on histologic features and therefore requires a preoperative biopsy. A sarcoma is classified as either low grade or high grade. In general, a low-grade lesion is less biologically active and requires a relatively conservative surgical procedure. Conversely, a high-grade lesion usually necessitates a more radical procedure, because of its more aggressive nature.

BOX 7–1: SARCOMA STAGING			
STAGE	**GRADE (G)**	**SITE (T)**	**METASTASES (M)**
IA	Low (G1)	Intracompartmental (T1)	No (M0)
IB	Low (G1)	Extracompartmental (T2)	No (M0)
IIA	High (G2)	Intracompartmental (T1)	No (M0)
IIB	High (G2)	Extracompartmental (T2)	No (M0)
III	Any (G)	Any (T)	Yes (M1)
			Regional or distant

Local Extent

Factors related to the local extent of the tumor include its size and degree of involvement of adjacent tissues. Sarcomas tend to grow centrifugally along pathways of least resistance and are contained in part by a pseudocapsule as they extend into adjacent tissues.[5] A malignant lesion may remain confined within the pseudocapsule (intracapsular); in general, however, malignant cells often extend beyond these capsular boundaries. If a lesion extends through its capsule but is still confined within a single anatomic compartment, it is considered extracapsular and intracompartmental. If the tumor extends into an adjacent compartment, it is classified as extracompartmental. Extracompartmental spread may occur via direct tumor invasion of an adjacent compartment or by contamination resulting from fracture, hemorrhage, or an operative procedure such as an unplanned resection or poorly planned biopsy.[4] In general, lesions with more advanced local extension, including involvement of neurovascular structures or joints, require excision of more adjacent tissue than smaller tumors.

Metastases

The third component of the staging system is the presence or absence of nodal or distant metastases. Regional lymph node involvement is much less common with musculoskeletal sarcomas than are pulmonary metastases, but both are equally poor prognostic factors.

PRINCIPLES OF IMAGING

Bone Tumors

MRI is the most sensitive imaging modality for detecting and delineating bone tumors, especially those involving the marrow cavity. However, the MR appearance of most osseous lesions is very nonspecific, and conventional radiographs are absolutely essential for evaluating a primary bone tumor. They should be obtained early in the work-up of a symptomatic patient, because they are inexpensive and provide the most specific information of any modality regarding the true nature of a lesion. The radiographic findings and degree of clinical suspicion will dictate further work-up. If an aggressive osseous lesion is identified on conventional radiographs, MRI is useful in the preoperative assessment of these patients, because it is the best modality for local staging.[6] If a bone lesion is clearly benign radiographically, MRI generally is not necessary.

For the patient with normal radiographs, a radionuclide bone scan often is the next study obtained; if a focal abnormality is detected, MRI is useful for further characterization.[7] Even with a negative bone scan, MRI can detect occult intramedullary lesions and should be obtained in the patient with a known primary tumor and focal symptoms or laboratory abnormalities that suggest osseous metastases (Fig. 7–1).

Soft Tissue Tumors

In the patient with a suspected soft tissue mass, conventional radiographs still should be obtained because they may reveal bone involvement or soft tissue calcifications that might be missed with MRI. In some cases, the MR appearance of a soft tissue mass is so characteristic that a confident, specific diagnosis can be provided, obviating further work-up. Even if the MR features do not allow a specific diagnosis to be made, MRI is still useful for staging these lesions.

Important MRI Features (Box 7–2)

For both osseous and soft tissue lesions, the critical factors influencing respectability that should be addressed in the MRI report include intra- and extraosseous tumor extent, neurovascular or joint involvement, and nodes.

Intraosseous Tumor Extent

This is best determined with T1W or STIR imaging (Fig. 7–2). The intraosseous extent of tumor may be overestimated with STIR, because it can be very difficult to separate intraosseous tumor from peritumoral edema on these images.[8] MRI also is able to detect skip lesions (foci of tumor that are not

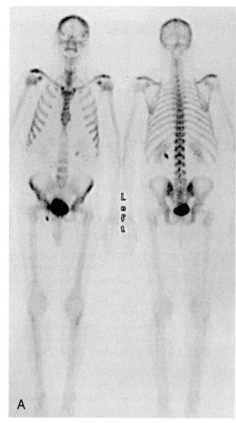

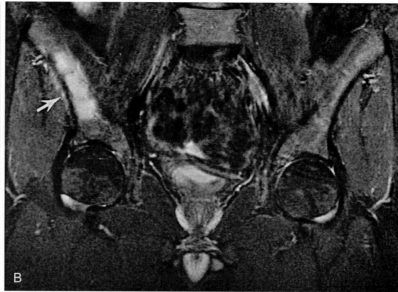

Figure 7–1. RIGHT ILIAC METASTASIS NOT DETECTED ON BONE SCAN.
A, Whole-body bone scan image. There is no scintigraphic evidence of metastasis in this 54-year-old man with a history of colon cancer and recent right hip pain. **B,** STIR coronal image, pelvis. There is abnormal signal intensity within the right iliac bone *(arrow)* at the site of an osseous metastasis.

contiguous with the primary lesion) missed with scintigraphy.[9]

Extraosseous Tumor Extent

This is best evaluated with T2W or STIR imaging (Fig. 7–2). Most tumors become hyperintense to fat on these sequences, and it may be difficult to separate tumor from adjacent edema. MR features of edema that help to differentiate it from neoplasm include feathery margins, an absence of mass effect, and no distortion of muscle planes (Fig. 7–2).[10]

Because a 5-cm "cuff" of normal tissue beyond the tumor margins usually is desired at surgery, exact measurements of the intra- and extraosseous components should be provided with reference to an osseous landmark (eg, the articular surface of the

medial femoral condyle for a lesion involving the femoral shaft).

Neurovascular or Joint Involvement

Identification of neurovascular involvement is critical (Fig. 7–3). It may preclude the possibility of a limb-sparing procedure, because the functional status of a patient with a denervated limb after surgery may be worse than that achieved with an amputation. MRI is highly accurate in demonstrating a lack of neurovascular involvement when a clear plane of normal tissue is demonstrated between nerves or vessels and tumor. Gross tumor invasion usually is easily diagnosed, but if there is equivocal tumor involvement, this should be reported as such. The structures can be reassessed at the time of surgery.[11] On a practical note, an anatomic atlas should be consulted in most cases to determine the expected position of pertinent nerves and vessels. Otherwise, neurovascular involvement might be overlooked if these structures are completely obliterated by a tumor.

Because each joint is a distinct compartment, articular invasion changes the stage of a tumor and should be critically evaluated on every scan (Fig. 7–4). MRI is very accurate for excluding joint involvement when the joint margins appear free of tumor, but is less accurate when the tumor is in close proximity to the joint. This results in a tendency to overcall joint invasion, which could result in an unnecessarily radical surgical procedure.[12]

BOX 7–2: CHECKLIST FOR STAGING MUSCULOSKELETAL TUMOR ON MRI

- Intraosseous extent
- Extraosseous extent
- Neurovascular involvement
- Joint invasion
- Skip metastases in same bone
- Local adenopathy

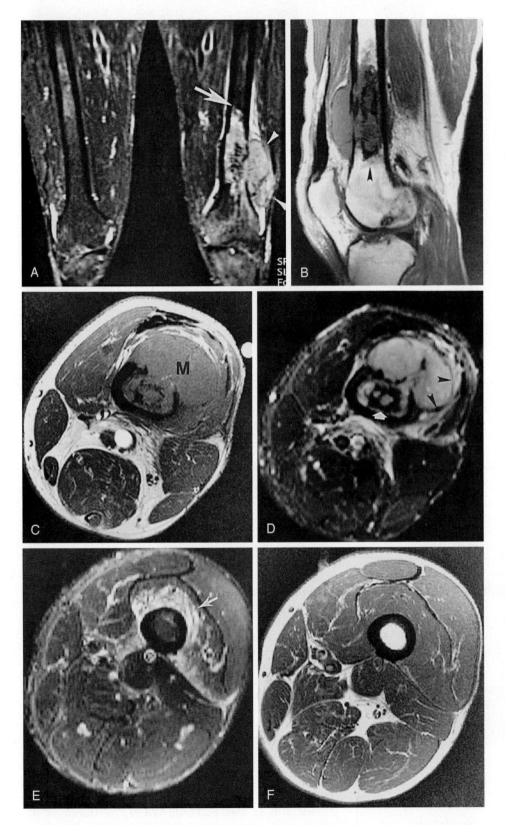

Figure 7–2. LOCAL EXTENT OF TUMOR, MR EVALUATION.
A, STIR coronal image, distal femora. A large tumor (chondrosarcoma) is seen in the distal left femur with both intraosseous and extraosseous *(arrowheads)* components. The proximal intraosseous tumor margin is easily distinguished *(arrow)*; however, note the difficulty in separating the distal margin from high signal–intensity edema in the femoral condyles. *B,* Sagittal T1 image, distal left femur. The intra and extraosseous components of the tumor are well demonstrated. Note the better delineation of the distal intraosseous margin *(arrowhead).* *C,* T1 axial image, distal left femur. The extraosseous tumor mass (M) is difficult to separate from adjacent muscle. *D,* STIR axial image, distal left femur. The margins of the extraosseous component *(arrowheads)* are easier to delineate from adjacent edema and muscles. Low signal intensity within the intraosseous portion of the tumor is related to calcified chondroid matrix *(white arrow).* *E,* STIR axial image, mid left femur. There is high signal intensity within the vastus intermedius muscle along the more proximal portion of the left femur *(arrow).* *F,* T1 axial image, mid left femur. Note the normal architecture of the vastus intermedius with preservation of the intramuscular fat and lack of mass effect, indicating that high signal intensity represents tumor related edema.

Nodes

Local and, when possible, regional lymph nodes should be assessed because nodal involvement carries the same poor prognosis as distant metastases in a patient with a musculoskeletal sarcoma.

Evaluation of Tumor After Therapy

Postchemotherapy

Survival of patients with musculoskeletal sarcomas has improved with the development of better adjuvant chemotherapeutic regimens. Assessing the degree of tumor response to chemotherapy is important for establishing the patient's prognosis and for planning further therapy.[13] If viable tumor cells make up less than 10% of a lesion after therapy, this indicates a good response (a "responder"), whereas more than 10% represents a poor response (a "nonresponder"). Currently this is determined after resection of the tumor, but several series have evaluated the use of MRI in this setting with conflicting results.

Changes in tumor size, signal intensity, or adjacent edema on conventional sequences are not sufficiently predictive to separate responders from nonresponders.[13] Similarly, because both tumor and non-neoplastic reactive tissue enhances on standard, postgadolinium T1W images, this technique also is unreliable for this purpose.[13] Dynamic enhancement patterns on gadolinium-enhanced, rapid

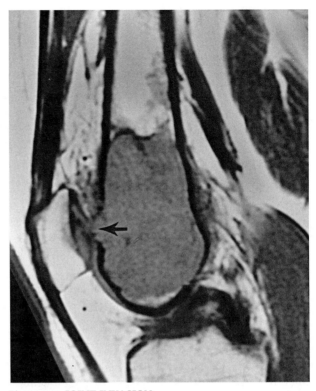

Figure 7–4. JOINT INVASION.
T1 sagittal image, distal femur. There is direct invasion of the patellofemoral compartment of the knee *(arrow)* by this giant cell tumor.

gradient echo-T1W sequences have shown a high degree of correlation with response or nonresponse, because residual tumor enhances earlier than reactive tissue.[13,14] However, we do not use these methods because they are time consuming, technically challenging, and still not reliable enough to replace biopsy and histology.[15]

Post-surgery/Radiation

MRI is valuable for detecting tumor recurrence after surgical or radiation therapy, primarily because of its superb soft tissue contrast. Unfortunately, it is sometimes too sensitive in this regard, because postsurgical and post-radiation changes in tissues can produce signal intensity that may be mistaken for neoplasm. Careful analysis of T1W, T2W, and STIR images, combined with an understanding of a few basic principles, can markedly improve the diagnostic accuracy of MRI in this setting.

A lack of increased signal intensity on T2W or STIR images is a strong predictor of no tumor recurrence, because recurrent tumor usually demonstrates high signal intensity on these images. However, there are other, non-neoplastic causes of increased signal intensity in these patients that can mimic tumor. These include radiation-induced edema, as well as postoperative fluid collections such as hematoma, seroma, or abscess.[16] Certain features help to separate these entities.

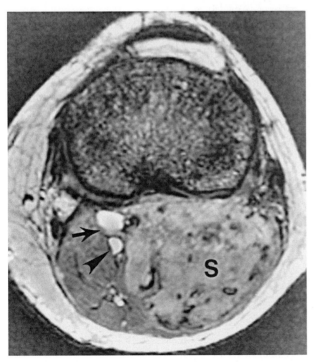

Figure 7–3. VASCULAR INVOLVEMENT.
T2* (gradient echo) axial image, knee. This large synovial sarcoma (S) in the popliteal fossa abuts the popliteal artery *(arrowhead)* and partially encases the popliteal vein *(arrow)*.

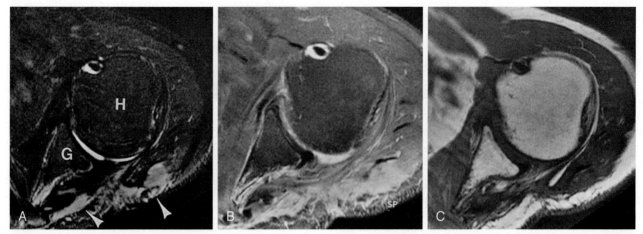

Figure 7–5. POSTSURGICAL CHANGES.
A, STIR axial image, left shoulder. There is high signal intensity infiltrating the posterior soft tissues *(arrowheads)* in this patient, who had undergone prior sarcoma resection in this region. (H—humeral head; G—glenoid). *B,* T1 axial image, with fat saturation, left shoulder after intravenous gadolinium administration. There is diffuse enhancement within the posterior soft tissues. *C,* T1 axial image, left shoulder. There is no evidence of focal mass effect or distortion of muscle architecture in the areas of abnormal signal and enhancement, indicating that these findings do not represent tumor recurrence.

Surgery and radiation therapy often result in edema or hemorrhage within tissues, but the absence of a discrete mass is strong evidence against tumor recurrence. This can be evaluated on T1W images by looking for loss of the normal fatty marbling within muscle or distortion of the intermuscular fascial planes. The presence of normal skeletal muscle architecture in these regions on T1W images (normal texture sign) is highly predictive of no tumor recurrence, despite the presence of increased signal intensity on T2W images or enhancement after gadolinium administration (Fig. 7–5).[17]

If a mass is discovered, administration of intravenous gadolinium may be helpful for further characterization. For example, a postoperative lymphocele, seroma, or abscess appears as a high signal–intensity mass on T2W images, but will not demonstrate internal enhancement on postgadolinium T1W images (Fig. 7–6). If an enhancing mass is identified, biopsy is indicated because recurrent tumor is likely (Fig. 7–7); however, post-therapy granulation tissue also can enhance and produce an identical appearance.

HOW TO IMAGE TUMORS

Based on these principles, an imaging protocol can be designed that provides the information needed for accurate staging or post-therapy follow-up.

Coils and Patient Position. In most cases, the patient is scanned in a supine position. Rarely, a prone position may allow for improved comfort and less motion artifact (such as when scanning the sternum). We typically begin with a sequence using the body coil and a large field of view to ensure that all portions of the primary tumor are identified. This is important for surgical planning, identifying skip or metastatic lesions, and for designing additional sequences. Once the extent of the tumor has been documented, higher-resolution images should be ob-

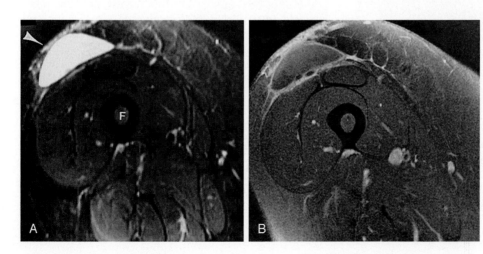

Figure 7–6. POSTOPERATIVE SEROMA.
A, STIR axial image, proximal right thigh. There is a well-marginated, lenticular-shaped mass *(arrowhead)* demonstrating homogeneous high signal intensity within the subcutaneous fat at the site of prior sarcoma resection. (F—femur.) *B,* T1 axial image with fat saturation, proximal right thigh after the administration of intravenous gadolinium. There is enhancement of the periphery of the mass without central enhancement, confirming that this represents a postoperative fluid collection.

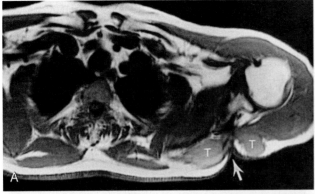
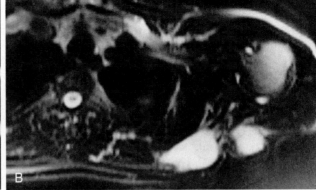
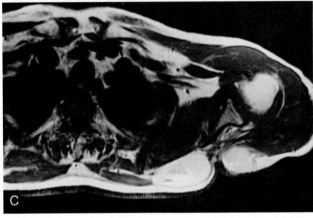

Figure 7–7. RECURRENT TUMOR.
A, T1 axial image, left chest. There is a scar *(arrow)* and postoperative deformity at the site of prior leiomyosarcoma resection. Additionally, there are two subcutaneous nodules at the operative site (T) demonstrating intermediate signal intensity. *B,* STIR axial image, left chest. Both masses demonstrate diffusely increased signal intensity. *C,* Axial T1 image, left chest after the intravenous administration of gadolinium. Both masses demonstrate relatively diffuse enhancement and were shown to represent recurrent sarcoma at subsequent surgery.

tained, using a surface coil whenever possible. This provides for optimal assessment of tumor margins and involvement of neurovascular or joint structures.

Image Orientation. The initial large field of view sequence should be performed in a coronal or sagittal plane to best display the entire length of the lesion. Axial images are then obtained with a smaller field of view to delineate tumor margins and neurovascular or articular involvement. These should be supplemented with additional longitudinal images to produce images that are tangential, rather than en face, to the lesion. Therefore, sagittal images are most helpful for a mass involving the anterior or posterior tissues of an extremity, whereas coronal images are used for lesions that are primarily medial or lateral in location.

Pulse Sequences/Regions of Interest/Contrast Enhancement. A skin marker should be placed over the suspected mass to confirm that the tissues of interest have been covered. In a postoperative patient, the entire length of the scar should be imaged. STIR imaging is most helpful for the initial large field of view sequence because it is very sensitive to both neoplastic tissue and associated edema or hemorrhage. It is also superb for detecting any skip or metastatic lesions. It may be difficult to differentiate tumor from edema in the medullary canal on STIR images alone, and an additional body coil coronal or sagittal T1W sequence is a useful adjunct because of the sharp contrast between tumor and fat on this sequence. T1W images also are useful for

defining anatomy and detecting high-signal fat or hemorrhage within a lesion.

Axial T1W and STIR images are then obtained, followed by T1 and fast spin echo-T2W or STIR images in a longitudinal plane, using a surface coil, if possible, to better resolve tumor margins and involvement of adjacent structures. A word of caution regarding fast spin echo-T2W sequences: the relatively bright signal intensity of fat on these images is similar to that of most pathologic processes, and this may mask an intramedullary lesion. Fat saturation should be used routinely with this sequence to improve lesion detection.

Gradient echo sequences are not a part of our routine tumor protocol, although these can be used for evaluating flow within a lesion or adjacent vessels.

We do not administer intravenous gadolinium as part of our standard tumor protocol, but use it when attempting to differentiate cystic from cystic-appearing solid lesions.

After surgical or radiation therapy, we use T1W and STIR sequences to image the area of interest, and use gadolinium only if a cystic-appearing mass is identified.

APPROACH TO IMAGE INTERPRETATION

General Principles

In general, many benign lesions demonstrate smooth margins, homogeneous signal intensity, and a lack of involvement of neurovascular structures. Conversely, malignant masses tend to display heterogeneous signal, irregular margins, associated edema, and invasion of neurovascular or osseous structures.

Unfortunately, there is a large amount of overlap in the appearances of benign and malignant lesions using these characteristics, and it can be dangerous to attempt to conclusively determine whether a mass is benign or malignant based on its MRI appearance.[18] Most lesions need to be classified as indeterminate and undergo biopsy for accurate characterization.

Contrast enhancement using standard, T1W sequences has not been helpful in differentiating benign from malignant lesions, although gadolinium-enhanced imaging using rapid T1W gradient echo sequences can provide some information regarding the malignant potential of a tumor based on the rate of enhancement.[19] Benign tumors tend to enhance more slowly than malignant lesions, but in a given patient, we prefer to biopsy the lesion, rather than rely on statistical probability, because of the large amount of overlap between benign and malignant lesions.

Bone Lesions

A reasonable differential diagnosis can be developed for most osseous lesions using the patient's age and the location of the lesion (within the skeleton and within the particular bone) and its radiographic appearance. For most bone tumors, MRI is used for staging, rather than for arriving at a specific diagnosis, because the true nature and aggressiveness of a lesion are much more accurately determined with conventional radiographs. Consequently, recent radiographs always should be viewed in conjunction with the MRI. This is also important because some benign osseous lesions display a very aggressive, potentially misleading appearance on MRI. These include osteoid osteoma, chondroblastoma, osteoblastoma, eosinophilic granuloma, and stress fracture. The edema associated with these lesions often results in extensive signal abnormality in the medullary cavity and adjacent soft tissues, mimicking more aggressive lesions such as osteomyelitis or malignant tumor.[20]

An osteoid osteoma is a cortically based lesion. The key to its diagnosis is the demonstration of a focal tumor nidus within the area of cortical/periosteal reaction. The tumor nidus typically demonstrates low to intermediate signal intensity on T1W images, low or high signal on T2W images, and a variable degree of enhancement after gadolinium administration.[21] There is usually a significant amount of surrounding marrow or soft tissue edema that can obscure the nidus and lead to an erroneous diagnosis (Fig. 7–8). In many cases, the nidus is more readily identified with computed tomography (CT) scanning through the lesion.

Chondroblastoma should be suspected when a le-

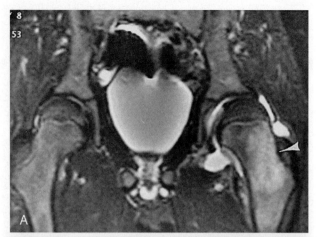
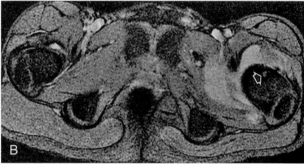

Figure 7–8. MARROW EDEMA RELATED TO AN OSTEOID OSTEOMA.
A, STIR coronal image, pelvis. There is a geographic area of increased signal intensity within the left femoral neck *(arrowhead),* along with a moderate sized left hip effusion. *B,* T2* (gradient echo) axial image, proximal left femurs. The tumor nidus is seen along the anterior left femoral neck as a small subcortical focus of increased signal intensity *(open arrow).*

sion is found in a skeletally immature patient with its epicenter in the epiphysis. Striking signal abnormality, corresponding to edema, often extends into the adjacent medullary cavity and overlying soft tissues.

In the case of a stress fracture, the presence of a linear fracture line within an area of marrow edema or cortical bone is diagnostic. In the absence of a fracture line, follow-up radiographs obtained 2 to 3 weeks later may be diagnostic. Biopsy should be avoided, because the immature osteoid related to the healing process may be mistaken for malignancy at histology.

Differential Features: Bone Lesions

Although conventional radiographs provide the most specific information regarding the true nature of a bone tumor, there are some MRI features that can help to limit the differential diagnosis.

Increased Signal: T1W Images (Box 7–3)

Intraosseous Lipoma. These lesions most commonly occur in the calcaneus, proximal femur, and humerus. They sometimes are difficult to differentiate from other lytic lesions on conventional radiographs, but are easily recognized on MR images due to their predominantly fat signal on all sequences.

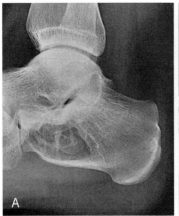
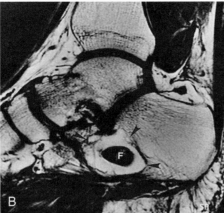
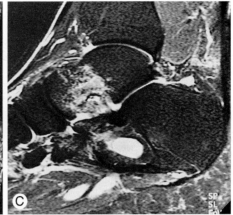

Figure 7–9. HIGH SIGNAL INTENSITY, T1: Intraosseous Lipoma, Calcaneus.
A, Lateral radiograph, calcaneus. A well-circumscribed, geographic lytic lesion is seen in the mid to anterior calcaneus with central calcification. **B,** T1 sagittal image, calcaneus. Extensive high signal–intensity fat is seen within the lesion *(arrowheads),* along with low signal–intensity fluid (F) centrally. **C,** STIR sagittal image, calcaneus. The extensive fat within the lesion is suppressed, whereas the central cystic change demonstrates homogenously increased signal.

An intraosseous lipoma also may contain areas of increased or decreased signal intensity on T2W images, reflecting cystic degeneration or calcification, respectively (Fig. 7–9).

Intraosseous Hemangioma. These lesions are common in the spine. Simple hemangiomas display increased signal intensity on T2W images, but are differentiated from other lesions by high signal intensity on T1W images caused by their fat content (Fig. 7–10). Alternatively, hypervascular (aggressive) intraosseous hemangiomas typically do not contain fat and are therefore indistinguishable from other tumors.[22]

Medullary Bone Infarct. A medullary bone infarct is a geographic lesion with a serpentine, low signal intensity margin on T1 and T2W MR images. These usually contain fat centrally, interspersed with foci of mixed signal intensity, corresponding to areas of fibrosis, calcification, or edema (Fig. 7–11).

Paget's Disease. The MRI appearance of Paget's disease is variable. Areas of fat commonly are found within involved areas, but more heterogeneous signal intensity, corresponding to hypervascular marrow, may be seen in the active stage of the disease (Fig. 7–12).[23] Other findings, such as cortical thickening, bone enlargement, and prominent, coarse trabeculae, often are better demonstrated on conventional radiographs.

Decreased Signal: T2W Images (Box 7–4)

Sclerosis/Calcification/Matrix. The presence of extremely low signal intensity within an osseous lesion on T2W images suggests sclerotic bone, calcification, or osteoid/chondroid tumor matrix. Once again, these are better characterized with conventional radiographs or CT (Fig. 7–13).

Fibrous Lesions. Fibrous tissue is usually of low to intermediate signal intensity on T2W images, but fibrous lesions of bone often demonstrate variable MR features.

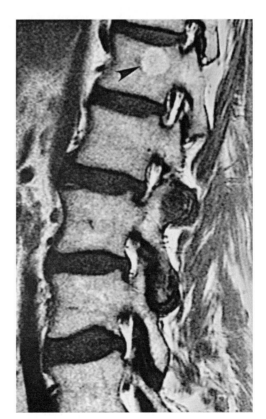

Figure 7–10. HIGH SIGNAL INTENSITY, T1: Intraosseous Hemangioma.
T1 sagittal image, lumbar spine. A rounded focus of high signal intensity is present in the L1 vertebra *(arrowhead),* indicating fat within this small hemangioma.

BOX 7–3: OSSEOUS LESIONS CONTAINING HIGH SIGNAL ON T1W IMAGES

- Intraosseous lipoma
- Hemangioma
- Bone infarct
- Paget's disease

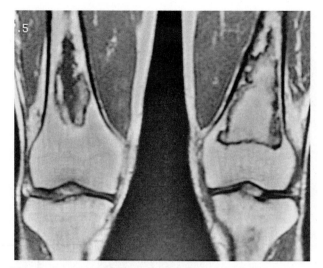

Figure 7–11. HIGH SIGNAL INTENSITY, T1: Medullary Bone Infarcts.
T1 coronal image, knees. Geographic areas of abnormal signal intensity are seen within the medullary cavities of both distal femurs. Note the low signal–intensity serpentine margins, confirming that these represent medullary infarcts, as well as the extensive fat signal intensity within the left femoral lesion.

A xanthofibroma (fibrous cortical defect, nonossifying fibroma) is a benign osseous lesion found in adolescents and young adults. These are readily diagnosed on conventional radiographs, but may be incidentally detected on MR images. They display intermediate to low signal intensity on T1W images, and often demonstrate low to intermediate signal on T2W images because of their fibrous nature. However, increased signal also may be seen on T2W images, along with variable degrees of enhancement

> ### BOX 7–4: OSSEOUS LESIONS CONTAINING LOW SIGNAL ON T2W IMAGES
>
> - Sclerosis/calcification/matrix
> - Some fibrous lesions
> - Primary lymphoma of bone

after gadolinium administration. Their lobular contour, eccentric location, low signal intensity, and sclerotic margin are helpful distinguishing features.[24]

Similarly, it was suggested in the early MRI literature that fibrous dysplasia displays decreased signal intensity on both T1 and T2W images due to its predominantly fibrous nature. However, this lesion does not have a characteristic appearance on MR images and often demonstrates heterogeneous signal intensity that may be high, low, or mixed on T2W images (Fig. 7–14).[25]

Primary Lymphoma of Bone. Primary lymphoma of bone is often of low signal intensity on T2W images, although its appearance is variable.[26–28] Some investigators have found that the low signal–intensity tissue corresponds to areas of fibrosis on pathologic analysis.

Fluid/Fluid Levels
The classic MR appearance of an aneurysmal bone cyst (ABC) is that of an expansile, lobular mass that contains multiple cyst-like collections and demonstrates high signal intensity on T2W images. Fluid/fluid levels usually are present within these cavities and correspond to stagnant blood products within

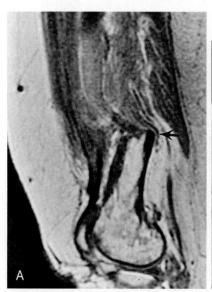
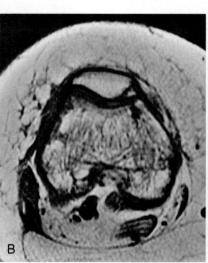
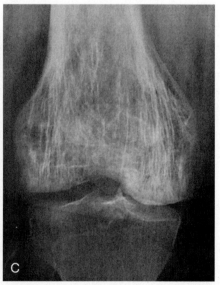

Figure 7–12. HIGH SIGNAL INTENSITY, T1: Paget's Disease with Pathologic Fracture.
A, T1 sagittal image, left femur. There is a fracture of the distal left femoral shaft *(arrow),* with mildly mottled but predominately fat signal intensity within the distal femoral fragment. *B,* T1 axial image, distal femur. There is predominantly fat signal intensity within the distal femur but also note the accentuated, thickened low signal–intensity trabeculae. (Compare to normal marrow in the patella.) *C,* Anteroposterior radiograph, distal femur. The classic features of coarse cortical, and trabecular thickening confirm the diagnosis of Paget's disease.

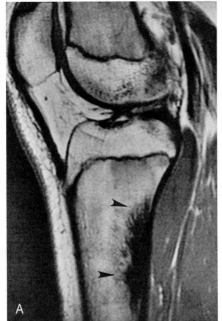

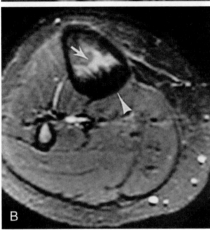

Figure 7–13. LOW SIGNAL INTENSITY, T2: Large Bone Island (Enostosis).
A, T1 sagittal image, proximal tibia. An eccentric, geographic focus of extremely low signal intensity is seen in the posterior left tibia *(arrowheads).* Note the spiculated margins. *B,* STIR axial image, proximal tibia. The lesion remains of extremely low signal intensity, confirming its sclerotic nature *(arrowhead).* Note also the high signal–intensity edema in the adjacent marrow *(arrow).* Subsequent biopsy revealed this to be a large bone island.

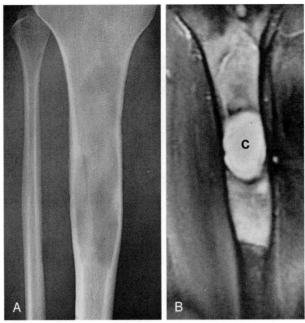

Figure 7–14. FIBROUS DYSPLASIA.
A, Anteroposterior radiograph demonstrates typical findings of fibrous dysplasia in the proximal tibia, with a long, mildly expansile lytic lesion that demonstrates hazy internal matrix. *B,* STIR coronal image, proximal tibia. Most of the lesion demonstrates relatively homogeneous, mildly increased signal intensity, with a focus of higher signal–intensity cystic change centrally (C). (From Higgins CB, Hricak H, Helms CA (eds). *Magnetic Resonance Imaging of the Body,* 3rd ed. Philadelphia, Lippincott-Raven, 1997.)

the cavernous spaces that make up these lesions (Fig. 7–15).[29] Initially, fluid/fluid levels were thought to be specific for an ABC, but they are a nonspecific feature of many entities that contain collections of blood, including telangiectatic osteosarcoma, chondroblastoma, giant cell tumor of bone, fibrous dysplasia, malignant fibrous histiocytoma of bone, and others.[30] Also, because an ABC may arise within some of these lesions, such as telangectatic osteosarcoma or giant cell tumor (secondary ABC), unless these cystic, nonenhancing spaces are seen to fill the entire mass, one of these other tumors must be suspected and biopsy is indicated.

Cartilaginous Tumors (Box 7–5)

Enchondroma/Chondrosarcoma. An enchondroma displays a distinctive MR appearance. This benign tumor is composed of multiple lobules that demonstrate homogeneously high signal intensity on T2W or STIR images, usually separated by thin, low signal intensity septae (Fig. 7–16). The increased signal–intensity corresponds to the high water content of the hyaline cartilage lobules that make up these lesions. Low signal–intensity foci corresponding to calcified cartilage matrix may also be apparent. A pattern of enhancing rings and arcs is seen in cartilaginous tumors on postcontrast images,

---

BOX 7–5: CARTILAGE TUMORS: MR FEATURES

- High-signal lobules (cartilage) on T2 separated by thin, low-signal septae
- Low signal–intensity foci on T1W and T2W images (calcified cartilage matrix)
- Arcs and rings enhancement pattern
- Often impossible to distinguish enchondroma from low-grade chondrosarcoma
- Watch out for features suggesting chondrosarcoma:
    —Endosteal scalloping greater than 2/3 of cortex
    —Cortical destruction and soft tissue mass
    —Edema in adjacent marrow or soft tissues

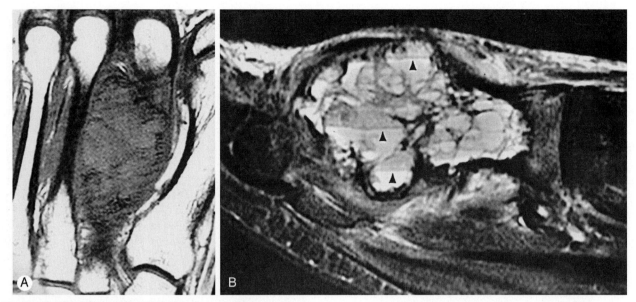

Figure 7–15. FLUID–FLUID LEVELS: Aneurysmal Bone Cyst.
A, T1 long axis image, midfoot. There is a large, lobular mass arising from the shaft of the second metacarpal. *B,* STIR sagittal image, midfoot. The mass demonstrates multiple high signal–intensity loculations with numerous fluid–fluid levels *(arrowheads).*

presumably caused by the presence of vessels within the fibrous septae and lack of cartilage enhancement. Unfortunately, this MR appearance, including the enhancement pattern, can be seen in both enchondromas and low-grade chondrosarcomas.[31, 32]

Imaging findings suggestive of chondrosarcoma rather than a benign enchondroma include deep

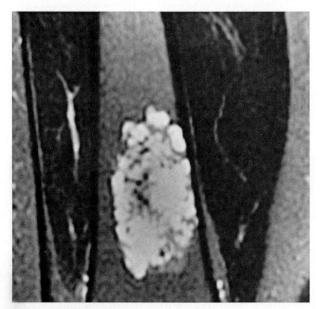

Figure 7–16. ENCHONDROMA.
T2 coronal image, distal femur. This intramedullary lesion in the distal femur demonstrates typical features of an enchondroma, including predominantly high signal intensity, lobular margins, thin internal septations, and low signal foci related to chondroid matrix. Note also the lack of surrounding marrow edema. (From Higgins CB, Hricak H, Helms CA (eds). *Magnetic Resonance Imaging of the Body,* 3rd ed. Philadelphia, Lippincott-Raven, 1997.)

endosteal scalloping (greater than two thirds of the cortex), cortical destruction with or without an associated soft tissue mass, and edema-like signal intensity in the adjacent marrow cavity and overlying soft tissues on STIR images.[33, 34] Even so, it is often difficult, if not impossible, to distinguish between benign and low-grade malignant cartilaginous tumors based on MRI features alone.

Chondroid Tumor versus Medullary Bone Infarct. Differentiation of a cartilaginous tumor from a medullary bone infarct can be challenging on conventional radiographs, because chondroid matrix can appear quite similar to the dystrophic calcifications present within an area of infarction. These can be distinguished easily using MRI. As opposed to the cartilaginous lobules that make up the chondroid tumor, a medullary infarct is seen as a flame-shaped region of heterogeneous signal intensity, often containing fat, that is surrounded by a serpentine margin of low signal intensity on all sequences.

Osteochondroma. This is the most common benign tumor of bone and usually is diagnosed on conventional radiographs. MR can differentiate an osteochondroma from other juxtacortical lesions by demonstrating contiguity of the lesion's medullary cavity and cortex with those of the bone of origin. The marrow fat within the lesion should be isointense with the medullary fat of the host bone on all sequences. The cartilage cap of the lesion is detected easily because of its high signal intensity on T2W or STIR images (Fig. 7–17). Although the relationship between the thickness of the cap and malignancy is controversial, a thickness of greater than 2 cm should be viewed as suspicious for neoplastic degeneration.[35]

MRI also can demonstrate other symptomatic complications of these tumors, such as neurovascular impingement, bursal formation, or fracture (Fig. 7–17).[36]

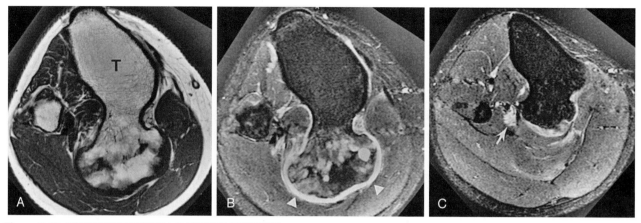

Figure 7–17. OSTEOCHONDROMA CAUSING NEURITIS.
A, T1 axial image, proximal tibia. A large, pedunculated osteochondroma arises from the posterior tibia (T). Note the continuity of cortical margins and medullary cavities of the lesion and parent bone, as well as the normal marrow signal intensity within the proximal lesion and tibia. *B,* STIR axial image, proximal tibia. The high signal–intensity, thin cartilage cap is well demonstrated *(arrowheads),* as are high signal cartilagenous foci within the lesion. *C,* STIR axial image, tibia (4 cm distal to *B*). The tibial nerve is focally enlarged *(arrow)* and demonstrates increased signal intensity where it abuts the osteochondroma. Mechanical irritation resulted in a focal neuritis.

Soft Tissue Tumors

General Principles

Some soft tissue tumors can be diagnosed with certainty based on their MR signal characteristics; helpful differential MR features are discussed below. For those soft tissue masses that demonstrate a nonspecific, indeterminate MR appearance, a differential diagnosis can be generated using the patient's age, the location of the mass, and the information found in Tables 7–1 and 7–2.[37, 38] For most lesions, a reasonable differential would include the top three benign and malignant tumors listed in Tables 7–1 and 7–2 for a given age and location, but again, most indeterminate soft tissue masses should be biopsied.

Differential Features: Soft Tissue Lesions

High Signal on T1W Images (Box 7–6)
The differential diagnosis for lesions that contain areas of high signal intensity on T1W images is relatively limited. This finding usually indicates fat or subacute blood products within the mass.

Lipomatous Masses. A lipoma is a benign fatty tumor that displays a characteristic MR appearance, allowing for a confident diagnosis. These generally are well-defined, lobular masses that demonstrate homogeneous signal intensity that parallels subcutaneous fat on all sequences (high signal intensity on T1W images and intermediate to high signal intensity on T2W images) (Fig. 7–18). Thin, curvilinear septations often course through the fatty mass and may enhance mildly after gadolinium administration.[39] Most superficial lesions are relatively well circumscribed, whereas deeper lesions may arise within muscle and appear more infiltrative.[40]

An atypical lipoma (well-differentiated liposarcoma) is considered a low-grade malignant tumor that tends to recur locally after surgery but does not metastasize.[41] Histologically, these are composed of mature adipose tissue and other nonfatty elements, often contained in thick, irregular septa. The MR appearance of these lesions parallels their histology. They typically demonstrate predominantly fat signal with coarse, thickened septae or scattered areas of nonfatty tissue. The nonlipomatous elements demonstrate low signal intensity on T1W images and high signal or enhancement on T2W or postgadolinium T1W images, respectively (Fig. 7–19).

There are several subtypes of liposarcomas. Myxoid liposarcoma is the most common and may appear quite benign on MR images. These gelatinous lesions often demonstrate a cystic appearance that is indistinguishable from other myxomatous tumors or even a simple cyst (Fig. 7–20). High-grade liposarcomas often contain no recognizable fat and are therefore indistinguishable from other malignant soft tissue tumors.[42]

Vascular Malformations. These benign vascular lesions lie along a pathologic spectrum from the capillary and cavernous hemangiomas (containing variable amounts of nonvascular tissue such as fat, smooth muscle, fibrous tissue, etc.) to true arteriovenous malformations that are made up of larger vessels. Regardless of the specific type of malformation, it is most important to recognize these as benign

---

BOX 7–6: SOFT TISSUE MASSES CONTAINING HIGH SIGNAL ON T1W IMAGES

- Lipoma
- Liposarcoma
- Hematoma (subacute)
- Hemangioma
- Melanoma

Text continued on page 142

TABLE 7-1. DISTRIBUTION OF COMMON BENIGN SOFT TISSUE TUMORS BY ANATOMIC LOCATION AND AGE
(Based on an Analysis of 18,677 Cases Seen in Consultation by the Department of Soft Tissue Pathology, AFIP, over 10 Years)

AGES (y)	HAND AND WRIST	NO (%)	UPPER EXTREMITY	NO (%)	AXILLA AND SHOULDER	NO (%)	FOOT AND ANKLE	NO (%)	LOWER EXTREMITY	NO (%)
0–5	Hemangioma	15(15)[1]	Fibrous hamartoma infancy	15(16)	Fibrous hamartoma infancy	23(29)	Granuloma annulare	23(30)	Granuloma annulare	42(23)
	Granuloma annulare	14(14)	Granuloma annulare	15(16)	Hemangioma	12(15)	Infantile fibromatosis	11(14)	Hemangioma	26(14)
	Infantile fibromatosis	13(13)	Hemangioma	14(15)	Lipoblastoma	11(14)	Hemangioma	8(11)	Myofibromatosis	16(9)
	Infantile digital fibroma	8(8)	Infantile fibromatosis	12(13)	Fibrous hemartoma	7(9)	Fibromatosis	8(11)	Fibrous histiocytoma	15(8)
	Fibromatosis	8(8)	Fibrous histiocytoma	6(6)	Myofibromatosis	6(8)	Infantile digital fibroma	7(9)	Lipoblastoma	13(7)
	Aponeurotic fibroma	7(7)	Juvenile xanthogranuloma	6(6)	Lymphangioma	5(6)	Lipoblastoma	6(8)	Lymphangioma	10(6)
	Fibrous histiocytoma	5(5)	Myofibromatosis	6(6)	Nodular fasciitis	4(5)	Lipoma	4(5)	Juvenile xanthogranuloma	10(6)
	Other	27(28)	Other	20(21)	Other	12(15)	Other	9(12)	Other	48(27)
6–15	Fibrous histiocytoma	32(14)	Fibrous histiocytoma	41(23)	Fibrous histiocytoma	25(34)	Fibromatosis	35(22)	Hemangioma	47(22)
	Hemangioma	31(13)	Nodular fasciitis	39(21)	Nodular fasciitis	18(25)	Granuloma annulare	21(13)	Fibrous histiocytoma	34(16)
	Aponeurotic fibroma	25(11)	Hemangioma	24(13)	Hemangioma	7(10)	Hemangioma	21(13)	Nodular fasciitis	22(10)
	Fibroma tendon sheath	22(9)	Granuloma annulare	12(7)	Granular cell tumor	3(4)	Fibrous histiocytoma	14(9)	Granuloma annulare	20(9)
	GCT tendon sheath[2]	17(7)	Fibromatosis	11(6)	Neurofibroma	2(3)	GCT tendon sheath	13(8)	Fibromatosis	14(6)
	Fibromatosis	13(6)	Neurofibroma	7(4)	Lymphangioma	2(3)	Chondroma	11(7)	Lipoma	13(6)
	Neurothekeoma	9(4)	Neurothekeoma	6(3)	Myofibromatosis		Lipoma	9(6)	Neurofibroma	8(4)
	Other	86(37)	Other	42(23)	Other	12(16)	Other	37(23)	Other	58(27)
16–25	GCT tendon sheath	84(20)	Nodular fasciitis	130(35)	Fibrous histiocytoma	62(36)	Fibromatosis	46(22)	Fibrous histiocytoma	118(24)
	Fibrous histiocytoma	57(14)	Fibrous histiocytoma	87(23)	Nodular fasciitis	35(20)	GCT tendon sheath	29(14)	Nodular fasciitis	61(13)
	Hemangioma	40(10)	Hemangioma	36(10)	Fibromatosis	16(9)	Granuloma annulare	25(12)	Hemangioma	55(11)
	Fibroma tendon sheath	40(10)	Neurofibroma	24(6)	Lipoma	14(8)	Fibrous histiocytoma	24(12)	Neurofibroma	48(10)
	Nodular fasciitis	26(6)	Granuloma annulare	20(5)	Neurofibroma	12(7)	Hemangioma	13(6)	Fibromatosis	38(8)
	Granuloma annulare	21(5)	Granular cell tumor	17(5)	Hemangioma	4(2)	PVNS[3]	12(6)	Lipoma	22(5)
	Ganglion	20(5)	Schwannoma	11(3)	Schwannoma	4(2)	Neurofibroma	11(5)	Schwannoma	20(4)
	Other	132(31)	Other	51(14)	Other	25(15)	Other	45(22)	Other	122(25)
26–45	Fibrous histiocytoma	167(18)	Nodular fasciitis	309(38)	Lipoma	105(28)	Fibromatosis	99(21)	Fibrous histiocytoma	245(25)
	GCT tendon sheath	148(16)	Fibrous histiocytoma	145(18)	Fibrous histiocytoma	92(24)	Fibrous histiocytoma	74(16)	Nodular fasciitis	229(23)
	Fibroma tendon sheath	106(11)	Angiolipoma	48(6)	Nodular fasciitis	55(14)	GCT tendon sheath	41(9)	Lipoma	101(10)
	Hemangioma	86(10)	Hemangioma	43(5)	Fibromatosis	29(8)	Hemangioma	36(8)	Neurofibroma	71(7)
	Nodular fasciitis	79(8)	Schwannoma	43(5)	Hemangioma	17(4)	Schwannoma	30(6)	Schwannoma	59(6)
	Fibromatosis	46(5)	Neurofibroma	37(5)	Neurofibroma	13(3)	Neurofibroma	24(5)	Myxoma	53(5)
	Chondroma	42(4)	Lipoma	32(4)	Schwannoma	12(3)	Chondroma	23(5)	Hemangioma	52(5)
	Other	269(29)	Other	153(19)	Other	57(15)	Other	135(29)	Other	185(19)
46–65	GCT tendon sheath	143(23)	Nodular fasciitis	86(20)	Lipoma	189(58)	Fibromatosis	83(25)	Lipoma	157(23)
	Fibrous histiocytoma	63(10)	Lipoma	80(19)	Fibrous histiocytoma	28(9)	Fibrous histiocytoma	43(13)	Myxoma	109(16)
	Hemangioma	61(10)	Fibrous histiocytoma	44(10)	Myxoma	16(5)	Lipoma	35(11)	Fibrous histiocytoma	93(14)
	Lipoma	59(9)	Schwannoma	30(7)	Fibromatosis	14(4)	Schwannoma	25(8)	Nodular fasciitis	40(6)
	Chondroma	52(8)	Chondroma	24(6)	Nodular fasciitis	13(4)	GCT tendon sheath	21(6)	Schwannoma	39(6)
	Fibromatosis	43(7)	Myxoma	24(6)	Schwannoma	12(4)	Chondroma	21(6)	Neurofibroma	31(5)
	Fibroma tendon sheath	37(6)	Hemangioma	19(4)	Granular cell tumor	12(4)	Hemangioma	16(5)	Proliferative fasciitis	28(4)
	Other	172(27)	Other	125(29)	Other	44(13)	Other	89(27)	Other	186(27)
66 & Up	GCT tendon sheath	51(21)	Lipoma	39(22)	Lipoma	83(58)	Fibromatosis	16(14)	Lipoma	68(26)
	Hemangioma	24(10)	Myxoma	19(11)	Myxoma	14(10)	Schwannoma	15(13)	Myxoma	44(17)
	Schwannoma	24(10)	Nodular fasciitis	18(10)	Schwannoma	6(4)	Fibrous histiocytoma	13(11)	Fibrous histiocytoma	33(13)
	Chondroma	21(9)	Schwannoma	12(7)	Fibromatosis	5(3)	Chondroma	11(9)	Schwannoma	31(12)
	Neurofibroma	14(6)	Glomus tumor	10(6)	Fibrous histiocytoma	5(3)	Lipoma	10(8)	Hemangiopericytoma	10(4)
	Fibromatosis	13(5)	Neurofibroma	10(6)	Proliferative fasciitis	5(3)	Granuloma annulare	8(7)	Neurofibroma	9(4)
	Lipoma		Angiolipoma		Hemangioma	4(3)	GCT tendon sheath	6(5)	Hemangioma	8(3)
	Other	71(29)	Other	55(31)	Other	22(15)	Other	39(33)	Other	56(22)

138

AGES (y)	HIP, GROIN, & BUTTOCKS	NO (%)	HEAD AND NECK	NO (%)	TRUNK	NO (%)	RETROPERITONEUM	NO (%)
0–5	Fibrous hamartoma infancy	14(20)	Nodular fasciitis	47(20)	Hemangioma	36(18)	Lipoblastoma	7(37)
	Lipoblastoma	14(20)	Hemangioma	43(18)	Juvenile xanthogranuloma	24(12)	Lymphangioma	5(26)
	Myofibromatosis	8(11)	Myofibromatosis	27(11)	Myofibromatosis	24(12)	Hemangioma	4(21)
	Lymphangioma	7(10)	Fibromatosis	17(7)	Nodular fasciitis	17(8)	Ganglioneuroma	2(11)
	Fibrous histiocytoma	5(7)	Granuloma annulare	14(6)	Lipoblastoma	17(8)	Fibrous hemartoma infancy	1(5)
	Nodular fasciitis	4(6)	Fibrous histiocytoma	13(5)	Infantile fibromatosis	15(7)		
	Infantile fibromatosis	4(6)	Infantile fibromatosis	13(5)	Fibrous hamartoma infancy	15(7)		
	Other	14(20)	Other	63(27)	Other	55(27)		
6–15	Nodular fasciitis	15(27)	Nodular fasciitis	75(33)	Nodular fasciitis	54(28)	Lymphangioma	7(37)
	Fibroma	7(13)	Fibrous histiocytoma	34(15)	Fibrous histiocytoma	43(22)	Ganglioneuroma	4(21)
	Fibrous histiocytoma	6(11)	Neurofibroma	23(10)	Hemangioma	25(13)	Schwannoma	2(11)
	Fibromatosis	5(9)	Hemangioma	21(9)	Lipoma	9(5)	Fibromatosis	2(11)
	Lipoma	5(9)	Myofibromatosis	14(6)	Neurofibroma	7(4)	Paraganglioma	1(5)
	Lipoblastoma	3(5)	Fibromatosis	12(5)	Fibromatosis	6(3)	Hemangioma	1(5)
	Neurofibroma	3(5)	Lipoma	6(3)	Granular cell tumor	6(3)	Inflammatory pseudotumor	1(5)
	Other	11(20)	Other	43(19)	Other	45(23)	Other	1(5)
16–25	Neurofibroma	20(16)	Nodular fasciitis	61(21)	Nodular fasciitis	112(24)	Fibromatosis	14(20)
	Fibromatosis	18(15)	Hemangioma	48(17)	Fibromatosis	72(16)	Schwannoma	10(14)
	Fibrous histiocytoma	18(15)	Fibrous histiocytoma	45(16)	Fibrous histiocytoma	71(15)	Neurofibroma	9(13)
	Nodular fasciitis	12(10)	Neurofibroma	37(13)	Hemangioma	52(11)	Hemangiopericytoma	8(11)
	Hemangioma	9(7)	Schwannoma	19(7)	Neurofibroma	38(8)	Lymphangioma	8(11)
	Lipoma	8(7)	Fibromatosis	11(4)	Lipoma	21(5)	Ganglioneuroma	6(8)
	Hemangiopericytoma	8(7)	Lipoma	10(4)	Schwannoma	17(4)	Hemangioma	4(6)
	Other	29(24)	Other	56(19)	Other	79(17)	Other	12(17)
26–45	Lipoma	57(17)	Lipoma	168(22)	Lipoma	178(19)	Schwannoma	38(23)
	Neurofibroma	38(12)	Nodular fasciitis	145(19)	Nodular fasciitis	150(16)	Fibromatosis	30(18)
	Fibrous histiocytoma	37(11)	Fibrous histiocytoma	137(18)	Fibromatosis	148(16)	Hemangiopericytoma	25(15)
	Fibromatosis	36(11)	Hemangioma	97(13)	Fibrous histiocytoma	98(10)	Neurofibroma	13(8)
	Nodular fasciitis	31(9)	Neurofibroma	57(8)	Hemangioma	78(8)	Angiomyolipoma	10(6)
	Hemangiopericytoma	24(7)	Hemangiopericytoma	37(5)	Neurofibroma	65(7)	Hemangioma	9(5)
	Myxoma	22(7)	Schwannoma	27(4)	Schwannoma	51(5)	Sclerosing retroperitonitis	7(4)
	Other	83(25)	Other	91(12)	Other	180(19)	Other	34(20)
46–65	Lipoma	76(35)	Lipoma	306(46)	Lipoma	290(44)	Schwannoma	33(19)
	Myxoma	36(17)	Nodular fasciitis	66(10)	Fibromatosis	63(9)	Fibromatosis	25(14)
	Fibrous histiocytoma	17(8)	Hemangioma	55(8)	Nodular fasciitis	44(7)	Sclerosing retroperitonitis	25(14)
	Schwannoma	17(8)	Fibrous histiocytoma	42(6)	Hemangioma	31(5)	Hemangiopericytoma	21(12)
	Nodular fasciitis	11(5)	Neurofibroma	30(4)	Fibrous histiocytoma	29(4)	Angiomyolipoma	12(7)
	Hemangiopericytoma	11(5)	Schwannoma	25(4)	Neurofibroma	28(4)	Lipoma	10(6)
	Hemangioma	9(4)	Myxoma	23(3)	Schwannoma	28(4)	Paraganglioma	9(5)
	Other	40(18)	Other	120(18)	Other	151(23)	Other	40(23)
66 & Up	Lipoma	22(21)	Lipoma	158(50)	Lipoma	124(42)	Schwannoma	19(26)
	Myxoma	16(15)	Hemangioma	22(7)	Fibromatosis	26(9)	Hemangiopericytoma	14(19)
	Neurofibroma	13(12)	Schwannoma	18(6)	Neurofibroma	20(7)	Lipoma	6(8)
	Schwannoma	10(9)	Fibrous histiocytoma	17(5)	Schwannoma	18(6)	Mesothelioma	6(8)
	Hemangiopericytoma	10(9)	Neurofibroma	16(5)	Elastofibroma	17(6)	Sclerosing retroperitonitis	5(7)
	Hemangioma	8(8)	Nodular fasciitis	13(4)	Myxoma	16(5)	Fibromatosis	4(6)
	Nodular fasciitis	4(4)	Myxoma	12(4)	Hemangioma	14(5)	Paraganglioma	4(6)
	Other	23(22)	Other	58(18)	Other	61(21)	Other	14(19)

[1]15(15) indicates there were 15 hemangiomas in the hand and wrist of patients 0–5 years, and this represents 15% of all benign tumors in this location and age group.
[2]Giant cell tumor of tendon sheath.
[3]Pigmented villonodular synovitis.
From Kransdorf MJ. Benign soft-tissue tumors in a large referral population: distribution of specific diagnoses by age, sex, and location. AJR 1995; 164:395–402.

TABLE 7-2. DISTRIBUTION OF COMMON MALIGNANT SOFT TISSUE TUMORS BY ANATOMIC LOCATION AND AGE
(Based on an Analysis of 12,370 Cases Seen in Consultation by the Department of Soft Tissue Pathology, AFIP, over 10 Years)

AGES (y)	HAND AND WRIST	NO (%)	UPPER EXTREMITY	NO (%)	AXILLA AND SHOULDER	NO (%)	FOOT AND ANKLE	NO (%)	LOWER EXTREMITY	NO (%)
0–5	Fibrosarcoma	5(45)[1]	Fibrosarcoma	9(29)	Fibrosarcoma	9(56)	Fibrosarcoma	5(45)	Fibrosarcoma	24(45)
	Angiosarcoma	1(9)	Rhabdomyosarcoma	7(23)	Rhabdomyosarcoma	4(25)	DFSP	2(18)	Rhabdomyosarcoma	8(15)
	Epithelioid sarcoma	1(9)	Angiomatoid MFH	3(10)	Angiomatoid MFH	1(6)	MPNST	2(18)	Giant cell fibroblastoma	5(9)
	Malig GCT tendon sheath[2]	1(9)	DFSP	2(6)	Chondrosarcoma	1(6)	Rhabdomyosarcoma	2(18)	MPNST	5(9)
	DFSP[3]	1(9)	Giant cell fibroblastoma	2(6)	MPNST	1(6)			Angiomatoid MFH	3(6)
	MPNST[4]	1(9)	MPNST	2(6)					DFSP	3(6)
	Rhabdomyosarcoma	1(9)	MFH	2(6)					Angiosarcoma	2(4)
			Other	4(13)					Other	3(6)
6–15	Epithelioid sarcoma	9(21)	Angiomatoid MFH	30(33)	Angiomatoid MFH	8(21)	Synovial sarcoma	11(21)	Synovial sarcoma	28(22)
	Angiomatoid MFH	7(16)	Synovial sarcoma	14(15)	MFH	5(13)	DFSP	9(17)	Angiomatoid MFH	22(17)
	Synovial sarcoma	5(12)	Fibrosarcoma	8(9)	Ewing sarcoma	4(10)	Rhabdomyosarcoma	5(9)	MFH	13(10)
	MFH	4(9)	MPNST	7(8)	MPNST	4(10)	Angiosarcoma	4(8)	Liposarcoma	11(9)
	Angiosarcoma	3(7)	MFH	7(8)	Rhabdomyosarcoma	3(8)	Clear cell sarcoma	4(8)	MPNST	9(7)
	Rhabdomyosarcoma	3(7)	Rhabdomyosarcoma	7(8)	Fibrosarcoma	3(8)	Fibrosarcoma	3(6)	DFSP	8(6)
	Clear cell sarcoma	2(5)	Epithelioid sarcoma	4(4)	Synovial sarcoma		Chondrosarcoma		Rhabdomyosarcoma	6(5)
	Other	10(23)	Other	15(16)	Other	8(21)	Other	13(25)	Other	31(24)
16–25	Epithelioid sarcoma	25(29)	Synovial sarcoma	32(23)	Synovial sarcoma	13(18)	Synovial sarcoma	27(30)	Synovial sarcoma	76(22)
	MFH	11(13)	MFH	19(14)	DFSP	12(16)	Clear cell sarcoma	10(11)	Liposarcoma	45(13)
	DFSP	7(8)	MPNST	16(12)	MPNST	11(15)	Fibrosarcoma	7(8)	MPNST	44(13)
	Synovial sarcoma	7(8)	Fibrosarcoma	12(9)	Fibrosarcoma	8(11)	DFSP	7(8)	MFH	36(11)
	Rhabdomyosarcoma	7(8)	Angiomatoid MFH	10(7)	MFH	8(11)	MFH	6(7)	Fibrosarcoma	24(7)
	Angiomatoid MFH	5(6)	Epithelioid sarcoma	9(7)	Rhabdomyosarcoma	3(4)	Hemangioendothelioma	6(7)	DFSP	18(5)
	Hemangioendothelioma	5(6)	Hemangioendothelioma	6(4)	Angiomatoid MFH		MPNST	5(6)	Angiomatoid MFH	15(4)
	Other	19(22)	Other	34(25)	Other	15(20)	Other	22(24)	Other	80(24)
26–45	MFH	26(18)	MFH	65(28)	DFSP	55(33)	Synovial sarcoma	50(26)	Liposarcoma	196(28)
	Epithelioid sarcoma	24(16)	MPNST	29(12)	MFH	30(18)	Clear cell sarcoma	25(13)	MFH	151(21)
	Synovial sarcoma	21(14)	Fibrosarcoma	25(11)	Liposarcoma	22(13)	MFH	25(13)	Synovial sarcoma	78(11)
	Fibrosarcoma	17(12)	Synovial sarcoma	23(10)	MPNST	21(12)	Hemangioendothelioma	14(7)	MPNST	70(10)
	Clear cell sarcoma	9(6)	Liposarcoma	20(8)	Fibrosarcoma	10(6)	DFSP	13(7)	DFSP	47(7)
	Liposarcoma	7(5)	DFSP	18(8)	Synovial sarcoma	7(4)	Liposarcoma	11(6)	Leiomyosarcoma	35(5)
	MPNST		Epithelioid sarcoma	13(6)	Chondrosarcoma	6(4)	MPNST		Fibrosarcoma	33(5)
	Other	33(23)	Other	43(18)	Other	18(11)	Other	38(20)	Other	98(14)
46–65	MFH	16(19)	MFH	133(46)	MFH	66(35)	MFH	39(25)	MFH	399(43)
	Synovial sarcoma	12(14)	Liposarcoma	34(12)	Liposarcoma	39(21)	Synovial sarcoma	27(17)	Liposarcoma	232(25)
	Fibrosarcoma	8(10)	Leiomyosarcoma	22(8)	DFSP	20(11)	Leiomyosarcoma	19(12)	Leiomyosarcoma	63(7)
	Epithelioid sarcoma	7(8)	Fibrosarcoma	18(6)	MPNST	14(7)	Kaposi sarcoma	14(9)	Synovial sarcoma	40(4)
	Liposarcoma	7(8)	MPNST	17(6)	Leiomyosarcoma	8(4)	Liposarcoma	9(6)	MPNST	38(4)
	Chondrosarcoma	5(6)	Synovial sarcoma	16(5)	Fibrosarcoma	4(2)	Fibrosarcoma	8(5)	Chondrosarcoma	37(4)
	Clear cell sarcoma		Hemangioendothelioma	9(3)	Synovial sarcoma		Clear cell sarcoma	7(5)	Fibrosarcoma	24(3)
	Other	22(26)	Other	43(15)	Other	15(8)	Other	32(21)	Other	87(9)
66 & Up	MFH	28(35)	MFH	183(60)	MFH	67(50)	Kaposi sarcoma	49(37)	MFH	455(55)
	Leiomyosarcoma	8(10)	Liposarcoma	25(8)	Liposarcoma	30(23)	MFH	26(19)	Liposarcoma	178(22)
	Synovial sarcoma	6(8)	Leiomyosarcoma	23(8)	MPNST	12(9)	Leiomyosarcoma	20(15)	Leiomyosarcoma	86(10)
	Kaposi sarcoma	5(6)	MPNST	20(7)	DFSP	6(5)	Fibrosarcoma	9(7)	Fibrosarcoma	22(3)
	DFSP	4(5)	Kaposi sarcoma	10(3)	Fibrosarcoma	4(3)	Chondrosarcoma	6(4)	Chondrosarcoma	16(2)
	MPNST	4(5)	Fibrosarcoma	8(3)	Leiomyosarcoma	3(2)	MPNST	5(4)	MPNST	15(2)
	Clear cell sarcoma	3(4)	Angiosarcoma	6(2)	Chondrosarcoma	2(2)	Liposarcoma	3(2)	Synovial sarcoma	11(1)
	Other	21(27)	Other	29(10)	Other	9(7)	Other	16(12)	Other	43(5)

AGES (y)	HIP, GROIN, & BUTTOCKS	NO (%)	HEAD AND NECK	NO (%)	TRUNK	NO (%)	RETROPERITONEUM	NO (%)
0–5	Fibrosarcoma	7(32)	Fibrosarcoma	22(37)	Fibrosarcoma	13(26)	Fibrosarcoma	4(20)
	Giant cell fibroblastoma	3(14)	Rhabdomyosarcoma	20(33)	Giant cell fibroblastoma	8(16)	Neuroblastoma	4(20)
	Rhabdomyosarcoma	3(14)	Malig hemangiopericytoma	3(5)	Rhabdomyosarcoma	8(16)	Rhabdomyosarcoma	4(20)
	DFSP	2(9)	Alveolar soft part sarcoma	2(3)	Angiomatoid MFH	6(12)	Ganglioneuroblastoma	3(15)
	MFH	2(9)	DFSP	2(3)	DFSP	4(8)	Angiosarcoma	2(10)
	Leiomyosarcoma	1(5)	MPNST	2(3)	Ewing sarcoma	3(6)	Leiomyosarcoma	2(10)
	Synovial sarcoma	1(5)	Giant cell fibroblastoma	2(3)	Neuroblastoma	3(6)	Alveolar soft part sarcoma	1(5)
	Other	3(14)	Other	7(12)	Other	5(10)		
6–15	Angiomatoid MFH	8(21)	Rhabdomyosarcoma	17(26)	Angiomatoid MFH	14(15)	Rhabdomyosarcoma	9(31)
	Synovial sarcoma	7(19)	Fibrosarcoma	13(20)	Fibrosarcoma	13(14)	MPNST	5(17)
	Rhabdomyosarcoma	6(16)	Synovial sarcoma	7(11)	Ewing sarcoma	12(13)	Neuroblastoma	4(14)
	MFH	4(11)	MPNST	6(9)	DFSP	12(13)	Ewing sarcoma	2(7)
	Epithelioid sarcoma	2(5)	MFH	6(9)	MPNST	9(10)	Fibrosarcoma	2(7)
	Fibrosarcoma	2(5)	Angiomatoid MFH	4(6)	Rhabdomyosarcoma	8(9)	MFH	2(7)
	MPNST	2(5)	DFSP	2(3)	MFH	3(3)	Malig hemangiopericytoma	2(7)
	Other	7(18)	Other	10(15)	Other	20(22)	Other	3(10)
16–25	Synovial sarcoma	15(18)	Fibrosarcoma	15(17)	DFSP	37(23)	MPNST	9(20)
	MPNST	13(16)	DFSP	14(16)	MFH	21(13)	Ewing sarcoma	8(18)
	Liposarcoma	8(10)	MPNST	8(9)	MPNST	19(12)	Leiomyosarcoma	6(14)
	DFSP	6(7)	Synovial sarcoma	8(9)	Fibrosarcoma	15(9)	Ganglioneuroblastoma	4(9)
	MFH	6(7)	Rhabdomyosarcoma	7(8)	Synovial sarcoma	13(8)	Neuroblastoma	4(9)
	Rhabdomyosarcoma	5(6)	MFH	6(7)	Ewing sarcoma	12(7)	Rhabdomyosarcoma	3(7)
	Leiomyosarcoma	4(5)	Angiomatoid MFH	6(7)	Angiomatoid MFH	6(4)	Malig hemangiopericytoma	2(5)
	Other	26(31)	Other	23(26)	Other	38(24)	Other	8(18)
26–45	Liposarcoma	45(18)	DFSP	59(30)	DFSP	129(30)	Leiomyosarcoma	57(32)
	DFSP	42(17)	MPNST	27(14)	MFH	77(18)	Liposarcoma	52(29)
	MFH	38(16)	Liposarcoma	18(9)	MPNST	45(10)	MFH	22(12)
	MPNST	26(11)	MFH	15(8)	Liposarcoma	41(9)	MPNST	11(6)
	Synovial sarcoma	15(6)	Fibrosarcoma	14(7)	Fibrosarcoma	36(8)	Fibrosarcoma	7(4)
	Leiomyosarcoma	13(5)	Synovial sarcoma	10(5)	Synovial sarcoma	20(5)	Malig hemangiopericytoma	7(4)
	Fibrosarcoma	12(5)	Angiosarcoma	9(4)	Angiosarcoma	15(3)	Ewing sarcoma	3(2)
	Other	53(22)	Other	42(22)	Other	70(16)	Other	20(11)
46–65	Liposarcoma	67(24)	MFH	54(28)	MFH	131(31)	Liposarcoma	170(33)
	MFH	66(23)	DFSP	28(15)	Liposarcoma	80(19)	Leiomyosarcoma	154(30)
	Leiomyosarcoma	40(14)	MPNST	23(12)	DFSP	60(14)	MFH	111(22)
	DFSP	20(7)	Liposarcoma	22(12)	MPNST	35(8)	MPNST	23(5)
	Fibrosarcoma	16(6)	Angiosarcoma	16(8)	Leiomyosarcoma	27(6)	Malignant mesenchymoma	10(2)
	Synovial sarcoma	14(5)	Atypical fibroxanthoma	12(6)	Fibrosarcoma	24(6)	Fibrosarcoma	9(2)
	Chondrosarcoma	14(5)	Leiomyosarcoma	11(6)	Angiosarcoma	15(4)	Malign hemangiopericytoma	7(1)
	Other	46(16)	Other	24(13)	Other	50(12)	Other	27(5)
66 & Up	MFH	111(46)	MFH	82(34)	MFH	137(44)	Liposarcoma	164(39)
	Liposarcoma	49(20)	Atypical fibroxanthoma	41(17)	Liposarcoma	56(18)	Leiomyosarcoma	118(28)
	Leiomyosarcoma	24(10)	Angiosarcoma	27(11)	Leiomyosarcoma	23(7)	MFH	93(22)
	Angiosarcoma	11(5)	Liposarcoma	20(8)	MPNST	20(6)	MPNST	13(3)
	MPNST	11(5)	MPNST	16(7)	DFSP	17(5)	Fibrosarcoma	8(2)
	Fibrosarcoma	10(4)	Leiomyosarcoma	13(5)	Chondrosarcoma	11(4)	Osteosarcoma	6(1)
	Chondrosarcoma	7(3)	Fibrosarcoma	10(4)	Other	35(11)	Malignant mesenchymoma	5(1)
	Other	20(8)	Other	31(13)			Other	9(2)

[1] 15(45) indicates there were 5 fibrosarcomas in the hand and wrist of patients 0–5 years, and this represents 45% of all malignant tumors in this location and age group.
[2] Malignant giant cell tumor of tendon sheath.
[3] Dermatofibrosarcoma protuberans.
[4] Malignant peripheral nerve sheath tumor.
From Kransdorf MJ. Malignant soft-tissue tumors in a large referral population: distribution by age, sex, and location. AJR 1995; 164:129–134.

141

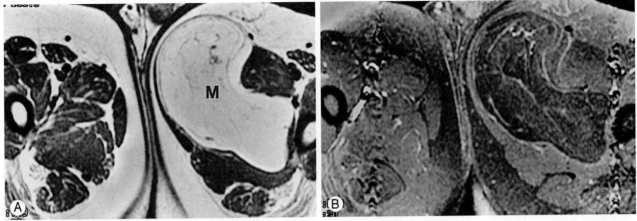

Figure 7–18. HIGH SIGNAL INTENSITY, T1: Soft Tissue Lipoma.
A, Axial T1 weighted image demonstrates a large, high signal–intensity mass (M) with thin internal septations extending between the proximal adductor muscles of the left thigh. *B,* T1 axial image with fat suppression, proximal thighs. With the exception of the thin internal septations, there is excellent suppression of the signal intensity from this mass, confirming its lipomatous nature. (From Higgins CB, Hricak H, Helms CA (eds). *Magnetic Resonance Imaging of the Body,* 3rd ed. Philadelphia, Lippincott-Raven, 1997.)

vascular lesions and to describe their extent, as well as what anatomic structures they involve.

Cavernous hemangiomas usually display relatively well-defined, lobular contours, although they

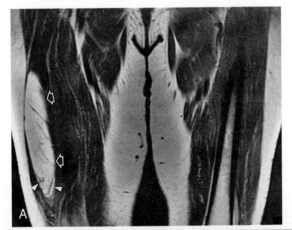

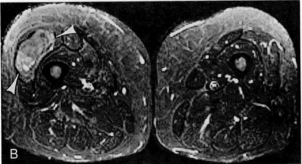

Figure 7–19. HIGH SIGNAL INTENSITY, T1: Atypical Lipoma (Well-Differentiated Liposarcoma).
A, T1 coronal image, thighs. There is a lenticular-shaped mass of fat signal intensity within the anterior compartment of the right thigh *(open arrows).* Note the mildly thickened septae in the distal portion of the mass *(arrowheads). B,* STIR axial image, thighs. There is heterogeneously increased signal intensity within the distal portion of the mass, indicating nonlipomatous tissue *(arrowheads).* Subsequent biopsy of this portion of the mass revealed an atypical lipoma.

may appear infiltrative. On T1W images, they are predominantly isointense to muscle, but often demonstrate variable amounts of increased signal intensity related to fat content. Their very high signal intensity on T2W images reflects the stagnant blood within their cavernous spaces (Fig. 7–21). Scattered foci of decreased signal intensity corresponding to calcified phleboliths, thrombosed channels, or septae seen on end also may be seen on T2W images.[43]

Arteriovenous malformations are composed of large, high flow vessels, which result in dark intraluminal flow voids on T1W and T2W images and increased signal intensity on "flow-sensitive" gradient echo images (Fig. 7–22).[44] Large feeding arteries and draining veins also may be evident in the adjacent soft tissues.

Hematoma. Hemorrhage into soft tissues usually displays a heterogeneous, often laminated appearance. The signal characteristics of extracranial hemorrhage are less predictable than with intracranial bleeding, but an acute hematoma (roughly up to 1 week old) is typically isointense to skeletal muscle on T1W images and of lower signal intensity than muscle on T2W images. In subacute and chronic hematomas, areas of high signal intensity usually are evident on T1W images somewhere within the mass (Fig. 7–23). These areas may display increased or decreased signal intensity on T2W images. In more chronic hematomas, areas of hemosiderin deposition, typically along the periphery, demonstrate decreased signal intensity on both T1W and T2W images.[45]

It must be remembered that a hemorrhagic neoplasm can be indistinguishable from a hematoma related to other causes (Fig. 7–24). At a minimum, any hematoma detected with MRI must be followed to resolution, either clinically or with serial imaging. Gadolinium administration may reveal an enhancing tumor mass; however, this must be interpreted with caution, because fibrovascular tissue within an organizing hematoma may also enhance.[15]

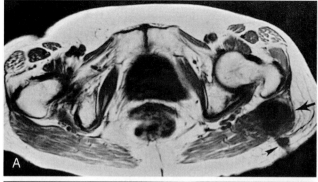

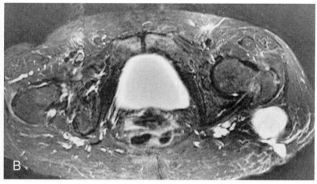

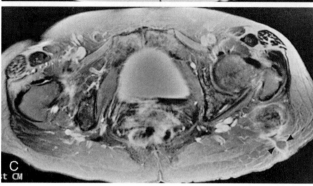

Figure 7–20. LIPOSARCOMA WITHOUT FAT EVIDENT.
A, T1 axial image, pelvis. There is a very low signal–intensity, rounded mass in the left gluteal musculature *(arrow).* The low signal intensity within the subcutaneous fat *(arrowhead)* is related to a prior biopsy. *B,* STIR axial image, pelvis. The mass demonstrates homogeneously increased signal intensity and relatively smooth margins. *C,* T1 axial image, with fat saturation, pelvis, after the administration of intravenous gadolinium. The mass demonstrates poorly defined, heterogeneous enhancement. Note the enhancement along the margins of the biopsy track and lack of enhancement of the central fluid within it *(arrowheads).*

In questionable cases, image-guided biopsy should be considered.

Melanoma. Malignant melanoma may demonstrate increased signal intensity on T1W images, presumably caused by the presence of paramagnetic compounds within the lesion. For the same reason, these tumors may display low signal intensity on T2W images (Fig. 7–25).

Low Signal on T2W Images (Box 7–7)

Pigmented Villonodular Synovitis. Pigmented villonodular synovitis (PVNS) is a synovial disease of unknown cause that most commonly affects the knee and results in an abnormal proliferation of histiocytes and giant cells, which usually contain hemosiderin. The most distinctive MR features of this entity are mass-like areas of synovial proliferation that demonstrate foci of low signal intensity on T1W and T2W images, related to the hemosiderin (Fig. 7–26).[46] A similar appearance may be seen with chronic hemarthrosis, chronic rheumatoid arthritis, chronic infectious arthritis (such as tuberculosis), amyloidosis, or gout.

Giant Cell Tumor of the Tendon Sheath. An extraarticular form of PVNS is called giant cell tumor of the tendon sheath. This is typically a focal mass arising in proximity to a tendon and most commonly is found in the hand and wrist. Because of their similar histology to PVNS, these lesions dis-

Figure 7–21. HIGH SIGNAL INTENSITY, T1: Soft Tissue Hemangioma.
A, T1 coronal image, foot. There is a large mass in the plantar medial soft tissues of the foot *(arrows),* which demonstrates scattered areas of fat signal intensity internally. T—talus; C—calcaneus. *B,* STIR coronal image, foot. The mass is better demonstrated as it infiltrates between the flexor tendons. The extensive high signal intensity and lobular margins are typical of soft tissue hemangioma. P—posterior tibial tendon; D—flexor digitorum tendon; H—flexor hallucis longus tendon.

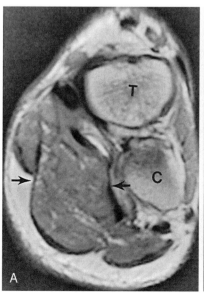

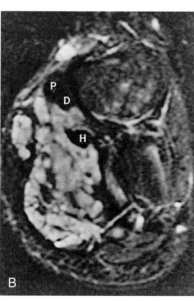

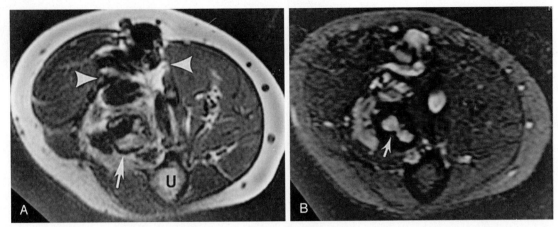

Figure 7–22. HIGH SIGNAL INTENSITY, T1: Arteriovenous Malformation.
A, T1 axial image, proximal forearm. A palpable mass in the volar soft tissues of the proximal forearm *(arrowheads)* is shown to be made up of large, low signal–intensity tubular structures interspersed with high signal–intensity fat. U—ulna; *arrow*—radius. *B,* T2* (gradient echo) axial image, proximal forearm. Flow-related high signal–intensity is seen within the large vessels making up this anteriovenous malformation on this "flow-sensitive" sequence. Note the direct extension into the proximal radius *(arrow).* (From Higgins CB, Hricak H, Helms CA (eds). *Magnetic Resonance Imaging of the Body,* 3rd ed. Philadelphia, Lippincott-Raven, 1997.)

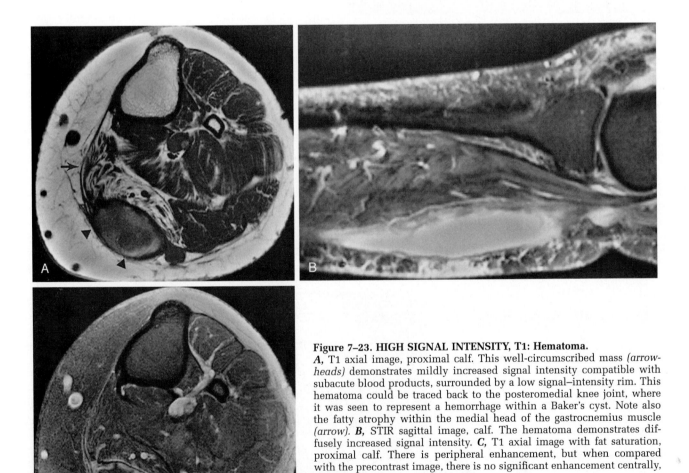

Figure 7–23. HIGH SIGNAL INTENSITY, T1: Hematoma.
A, T1 axial image, proximal calf. This well-circumscribed mass *(arrowheads)* demonstrates mildly increased signal intensity compatible with subacute blood products, surrounded by a low signal–intensity rim. This hematoma could be traced back to the posteromedial knee joint, where it was seen to represent a hemorrhage within a Baker's cyst. Note also the fatty atrophy within the medial head of the gastrocnemius muscle *(arrow).* *B,* STIR sagittal image, calf. The hematoma demonstrates diffusely increased signal intensity. *C,* T1 axial image with fat saturation, proximal calf. There is peripheral enhancement, but when compared with the precontrast image, there is no significant enhancement centrally, indicating its cystic nature.

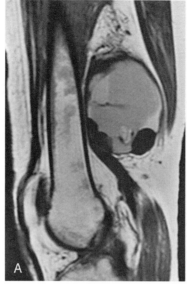
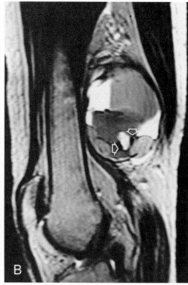

Figure 7–24. HIGH SIGNAL INTENSITY, T1: Hemorrhagic Tumor.
A, T1 sagittal image, distal thigh. A large, heterogeneous mass is seen in the posterior compartment of the distal thigh. Note the multiple fluid–fluid levels and areas of high signal intensity compatible with subacute hemorrhage. *B,* T2 sagittal image, distal thigh. The peripheral rim and internal foci *(open arrows)* of persistent low signal intensity are compatible with hemosiderin. Biopsy revealed hemorrhagic synovial sarcoma.

play intermediate to low signal intensity on T1W images and heterogenous signal intensity on T2W images, with areas of decreased signal related to hemosiderin.[47]

Fibrous Lesions. Soft tissue lesions containing predominantly fibrous tissue often demonstrate intermediate to low signal intensity on T2W images, at least in some portion of the mass (Fig. 7–27). Common entities include: plantar fibroma (arising within the plantar aponeurosis), Morton neuroma (a mass of perineural fibrosis surrounding a plantar digital nerve, most commonly between the third and fourth metatarsal heads), and desmoid tumors (benign but locally aggressive fibrotic lesions).

Amyloid. Amyloid is a protein-like substance that is deposited throughout musculoskeletal tissues as part of a primary disorder or related to other chronic diseases (secondary amyoloidosis). The secondary form is most common in patients with endstage renal disease who are undergoing hemodialysis. Amyloid deposition can occur in bone, intervertebral disc, or other soft tissues, with the hip and shoulder being the most commonly affected joints (Fig. 7–28). The tissue demonstrates low to intermediate signal intensity on T1W and T2W images, probably caused by its collagen-like make up.[48]

Gout. Gouty tophi may also demonstrate low to intermediate signal intensity on T1W and T2W images, with or without associated bone erosions. These signal characteristics may be related to fibrous tissue, hemosiderin deposition, or calcification.[49]

Melanoma. Malignant melanoma demonstrates variable signal intensities on MRI, but may display low signal intensity on T2W images, probably be-

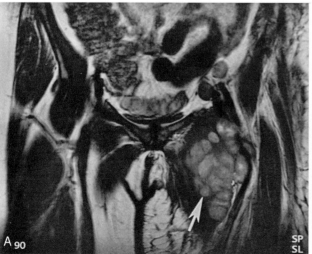
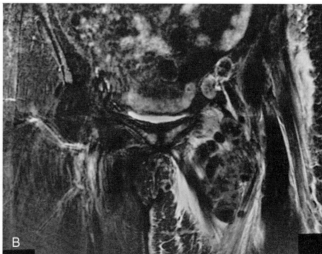

Figure 7–25. HIGH SIGNAL INTENSITY, T1: Melanoma.
A, T1 coronal image, pelvis. There is a large, lobular melanoma metastasis in the proximal adductor muscles of the left thigh, demonstrating rather extensive, increased signal intensity *(arrow).* *B,* STIR coronal image, pelvis. Note the large foci of low signal intensity within the mass, presumably related to paramagnetic compounds.

BOX 7–7: SOFT TISSUE MASSES CONTAINING LOW SIGNAL ON T2W IMAGES

- Pigmented villonodular synovitis/giant cell tumor of the tendon sheath
- Fibrous lesions
- Hematoma (chronic → hemosiderin)
- Amyloid
- Gout
- Melanoma

BOX 7–8: CYSTIC-APPEARING MASSES

- Cyst/ganglion
- Intramuscular myxoma
- Myxoid malignancy
  —Liposarcoma
  —Chondrosarcoma
  —Malignant fibrous histiocytoma
- Synovial sarcoma
- Nerve sheath tumor
- Intravenous gadolinium can differentiate cystic/solid lesions

cause of paramagnetic compounds within the tumor (see Fig. 7–25).

Cystic-Appearing Masses (Box 7–8)

Cyst. Cystic lesions, such as fluid-filled bursae, synovial cysts, or ganglia, are common musculoskeletal masses. These often occur in typical locations such as the popliteal fossa or along the dorsum of the wrist, but may arise in unusual locations. A purely cystic mass demonstrates homogeneous low signal intensity, hypointense to muscle, on T1W images, and diffusely high signal on T2W images. Thin, low signal intensity septae commonly are present within ganglion cysts on T2W images. After intravenous gadolinium administration, there is enhancement of the thin, peripheral wall and internal septae, if present, with a lack of central enhancement otherwise (Fig. 7–29).

Intramuscular Myxoma. These tumors are related to ganglion cysts and contain thick, gelatinous material that accounts for their cystic appearance on MRI. They are typically well-circumscribed lesions that are homogeneously hypointense to muscle on T1W images and diffusely hyperintense to fat on T2W images (Fig. 7–30). After gadolinium administration, these usually demonstrate some peripheral or septal enhancement, although heterogeneous internal enhancement may be seen.[50]

Cystic-Appearing Malignant Tumors. Solid tumors that contain myxoid elements (myxoid liposarcoma, chondrosarcoma, malignant fibrous histiocytoma) or synovial sarcoma may demonstrate a cystic, or predominantly cystic, appearance (Fig. 7–31).[51, 52] Therefore, when a cystic-appearing lesion is identified in an atypical location, evaluation with contrast enhancement is indicated. Unless the classic MR features of a pure cyst are identified (thin wall, homogeneous low signal intensity on T1W images, high signal on T2W images, lack of central enhancement), aspiration or biopsy should be per-

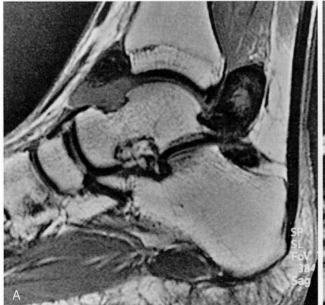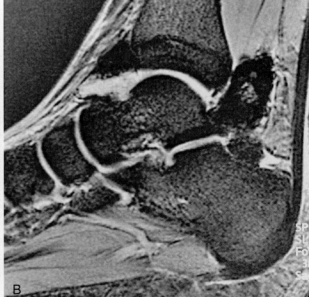

Figure 7–26. LOW SIGNAL INTENSITY, T2: Pigmented Villonodular Synovitis.
A, T1 sagittal image, ankle. Large, low signal–intensity masses are seen within the anterior and posterior recesses of the ankle joint. *B,* T2*-gradient echo sagittal image, ankle. The masses remain of low signal intensity and demonstrate slight blooming secondary to susceptibility effects of hemosiderin.

Figure 7–27. LOW SIGNAL INTENSITY, T2: Fibromatosis.
A, Sagittal T1 image, knee. Large, lobular, low signal–intensity masses are seen in the soft tissues of the posterior distal thigh and proximal calf *(open arrows). B,* STIR sagittal image, knee. The masses remain of diffusely low signal intensity and were shown on subsequent biopsy to represent fibromatosis.

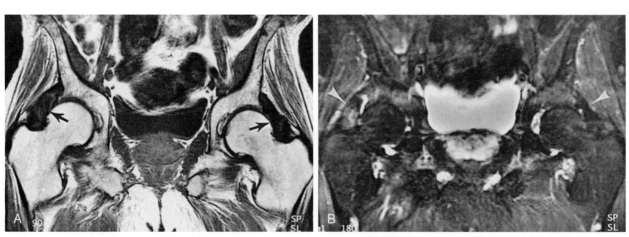

Figure 7–28. LOW SIGNAL INTENSITY, T2: Amyloid.
A, T1 coronal image, pelvis. Prominent low signal–intensity tissue is seen within both hip joints *(arrows). B,* STIR coronal image, pelvis. The tissue remains of relatively low signal intensity and is outlined by small bilateral joint effusions *(arrowheads).* The patient has a history of end stage renal disease.

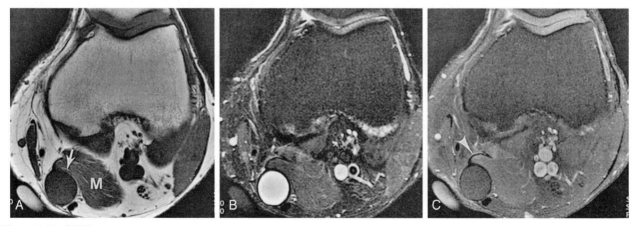

Figure 7–29. CYST.
A, T1 axial image, knee. There is a well-circumscribed mass in the posteromedial soft tissues *(arrow),* distorting the adjacent semimembranosus muscle (M). Note the homogeneous internal signal intensity, which is lower than that of the adjacent muscle. *B,* STIR axial image, knee. The mass demonstrates homogeneously increased signal intensity. *C,* T1 fat suppressed axial image, knee, after the administration of intravenous gadolinium. There is no enhancement of the mass, confirming the cystic nature of this ganglion, which appears to arise from the semimembranosus tendon *(arrowhead).*

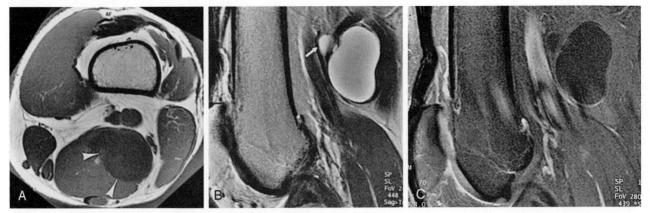

Figure 7–30. CYSTIC-APPEARING LESION: Myxoma.
A, T1 axial image, distal thigh. There is a low signal–intensity mass *(arrowheads)* arising within the semimembranosus muscle. Note that its internal signal intensity is lower than that of the surrounding muscle. *B,* Sagittal turbo spin echo-T2 image, distal thigh. The mass demonstrates homogeneously increased signal intensity. Note the anterior lobulation *(small arrow).* *C,* T1 fat-suppressed sagittal image, knee, after the administration of intravenous gadolinium. There is no internal enhancement within this intramuscular myxoma.

formed to differentiate a benign cyst or intramuscular myxoma from a malignant lesion.

Nerve Sheath Tumors. Peripheral nerve sheath tumors (schwannoma, neurofibroma) may demonstrate a cystic appearance because of their well-circumscribed margins and homogeneous high signal intensity on T2W images. MR features suggesting the diagnosis of a nerve sheath tumor rather than a cyst include identification of the tubular-shaped nerve entering and exiting the mass (best seen on longitudinal images), the split-fat sign (a peripheral rim of fat surrounding the lesion), multiple small nerve fascicles within the lesion on T2W images, and the target sign on T2W images (higher signal in the periphery surrounding central lower signal intensity) (Fig. 7–32).[51,53,54] These also typically demonstrate diffuse enhancement after the intravenous administration of gadolinium.

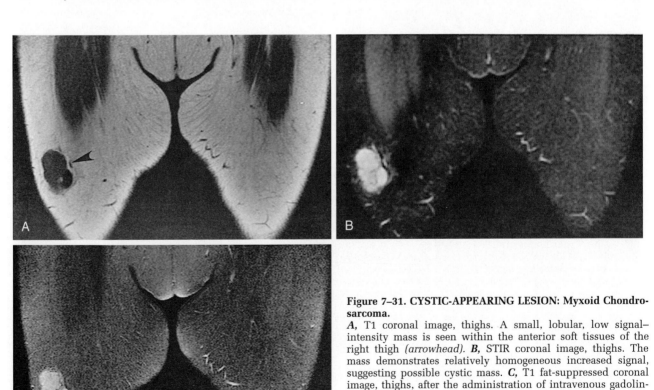

Figure 7–31. CYSTIC-APPEARING LESION: Myxoid Chondrosarcoma.
A, T1 coronal image, thighs. A small, lobular, low signal–intensity mass is seen within the anterior soft tissues of the right thigh *(arrowhead).* *B,* STIR coronal image, thighs. The mass demonstrates relatively homogeneous increased signal, suggesting possible cystic mass. *C,* T1 fat-suppressed coronal image, thighs, after the administration of intravenous gadolinium. The mass demonstrates diffuse enhancement, confirming its noncystic nature. Subsequent biopsy showed this to be an extraskeletal myxoid chondrosarcoma.

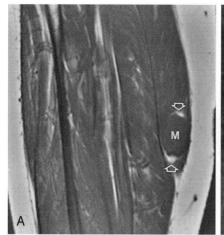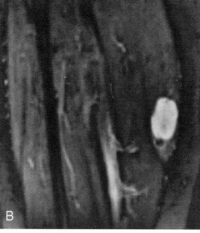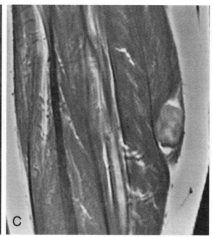

Figure 7–32. CYSTIC-APPEARING LESION: Nerve Sheath Tumor.
A, T1 sagittal image. There is an ovoid, low signal–intensity mass (M) within the gastrocnemius muscle *(open arrows). B,* STIR sagittal image, proximal calf. The mass demonstrates mildly heterogeneous, increased signal intensity with low signal intensity centrally (target sign). *C,* T1 sagittal image after the administration of intravenous gadolinium, proximal calf. The mass demonstrates heterogeneous enhancement, proving it is not a cystic lesion.

References

1. Bloem JL, Taminiau AHM, Eulderink F, Hermans J, Pauwels EK. Radiologic staging of primary bone sarcoma: MR imaging, scintigraphy, angiography and CT correlated with pathologic examination. *Radiology* 1988; 169:805–810.
2. Massengill AD, Seeger LL, Eckardt JJ. The role of plain radiography, computed tomography and magnetic resonance imaging in sarcoma evaluation. *Hematol Oncol Clin North Am* 1995; 9:571–604.
3. Enneking WF. Staging of musculoskeletal neoplasms. *Skeletal Radiol* 1985; 13:183–194.
4. Peabody TD, Gibbs CP, Simon MA. Current concepts review: evaluation and staging of musculoskeletal neoplasms. *J Bone Joint Surg [Am]* 1998; 80:1204–1218.
5. Peabody TD, Simon MA. Principles of staging of soft-tissue sarcomas. *Clin Orthop* 1993; 289:19–31.
6. Sundaram M, McGuire MH, Herbold DR, Wolverson MK, Heiberg E. Magnetic resonance imaging in planning limb-salvage surgery for primary malignant tumors of bone. *J Bone Joint Surg [Am]* 1986; 68:809–819.
7. Frank JA, Ling A, Patronas NJ, et al. Detection of malignant bone tumors: MR imaging vs scintigraphy. *AJR* 1990; 155:1043–1048.
8. Onikul E, Fletcher BD, Parham DM, Chen G. Accuracy of MR imaging for estimating intraosseous extent of osteosarcoma. *AJR* 1996; 167:1211–1215.
9. Wetzel LH, Schweiger GD, Levine E. MR imaging of transarticular skip metastases from distal femoral osteosarcoma. *J Comput Assist Tomogr* 1990; 14:315–317.
10. Hanna SL, Fletcher BD, Parham DM, Bugg MF. Muscle edema in musculoskeletal tumors: MR imaging characteristics and clinical significance. *J Magn Reson Imaging* 1991; 1:441–449.
11. van Trommel MF, Kroon HM, Bloem JL, Hogendoorn PCW, Taminiau AHM. MR imaging based strategies in limb salvage surgery for osteosarcoma of the distal femur. *Skeletal Radiol* 1997; 26:636–641.
12. Schima W, Amann G, Stiglbauer R, et al. Preoperative staging of osteosarcoma: efficacy of MR iamging in detecting joint involvement. *AJR* 1994; 163:1171–1175.
13. Fletcher BD. Response of osteosarcoma and Ewing sarcoma to chemotherapy: imaging evaluation. *AJR* 1991; 157:825–833.
14. Hanna SL, Parham DM, Fairclough DL, et al. Assessment of osteosarcoma response to preoperative chemotherapy using dynamic FLASH gadolinium-DTPA magnetic resonance mapping. *Invest Radiol* 1992; 27:367–373.
15. Kransdorf MJ, Murphey MD. The use of gadolinium in the MR evaluation of soft tissue tumors. *Semin Ultrasound CT MRI* 1997; 18:251–268.
16. Vanel D, Shapeero LG, DeBaere T, et al. MR imaging in the follow-up of malignant and aggressive soft-tissue tumors: results of 511 examinations. *Radiology* 1994; 190:263–268.
17. Biondetti PR, Ehman RL. Soft-tissue sarcomas: use of textural patterns in skeletal muscle as a diagnostic feature in postoperative MR imaging. *Radiology* 1992; 183:845–848.
18. Crim JR, Seeger LL, Yoo L, Chancnani V, Eckardt JJ. Diagnosis of soft-tissue masses with MR imaging: can benign masses be differentiated from malignant ones? *Radiology* 1992; 185:581–586.
19. Erlemann R, Reiser MF, Peters PE, et al. Musculoskeletal neoplasms: static and dynamic Gd-DTPA-enhanced MR imaging. *Radiology* 1989; 171:767–773.
20. Hayes CW, Conway WF, Sundaram M. Misleading aggressive MR imaging appearance of some benign musculoskeletal lesions. *Radiographics* 1992; 12:1119–1134.
21. Assoun J, Richardi G, Railhac JJ, et al. Osteoid osteoma: MR imaging versus CT. *Radiology* 1994; 191:217–223.
22. Laredo J-D, Assouline E, Gelbert F, et al. Vertebral hemangiomas: fat content as a sign of aggressiveness. *Radiology* 1990; 177:467–472.
23. Roberts MC, Kressel HY, Fallon MD, Zlatkin MB, Dalinka MK. Paget disease: MR imaging findings. *Radiology* 1989; 173:341–345.
24. Jee WH, Choe BY, Kang HS, et al. Nonossifying fibroma: characteristics at MR imaging with pathologic correlation. *Radiology* 1998; 209:197–202.
25. Norris MA, Kaplan PA, Pathria M, Greenway G. Fibrous dysplasia: magnetic resonance imaging appearance at 1.5 Tesla. *Clin Imaging* 1990; 14:211–215.
26. Vincent JM, Ng YY, Norton AJ, Armstrong P. Case report: primary lymphoma of bone—MRI appearances with pathological correlation. *Clin Radiol* 1992; 45:407–409.
27. Stiglbauer R, Augustin I, Kramer J, et al. MRI in the diagnosis of primary lymphoma of bone: correlation with histopathology. *J Comput Assist Tomogr* 1992; 16:248–253.
28. White LM, Schweitzer ME, Khalili K, et al. MR imaging of primary lymphoma of bone: Variability of T2-weighted signal intensity. *AJR* 1998; 170:1243–1247.
29. Beltran J, Simon DC, Levey M, et al. Aneurysmal bone cysts: MR imaging at 1.5T. *Radiology* 1986; 158:689–690.
30. Tsai JC, Dalinka MK, Fallon MD, Zlatkin MB, Kressel HY. Fluid-fluid level: a nonspecific finding in tumors of bone and soft tissue. Radiology 1990; 175:779–782.
31. Cohen EK, Kressel HY, Frank TS, et al. Hyaline cartilage-origin bone and soft tissue neoplasms: MR appearance and histologic correlation. *Radiology* 1988; 167:477–481.

32. Aoki J, Sone S, Fujioka F, et al. MR of enchondroma and chondrosarcoma: rings and arcs of Gd-DTPA enhancement. *J Comput Assist Tomogr* 1991; 15:1011–1016.

33. Janzen L, Logan PM, O'Connell JX, Connell DG, Munk PL. Intramedullary chondroid tumors of bone: correlation of abnormal peritumoral marrow and soft tissue MRI signal with tumor type. *Skeletal Radiol* 1997; 26:100–106.

34. Murphey MD, Flemming DJ, Boyea SR, et al. Enchondroma versus chondrosarcoma in the appendicular skeleton: differentiating features. *Radiographics* 1998; 18:1213–1237.

35. Lee JK, Yao L, Wirth CR. MR imaging of solitary osteochondromas: report of eight cases. *AJR* 1987; 149:557–560.

36. Mehta M, White LM, Knapp T, et al. MR imaging of symptomatic osteochondromas with pathological correlation. *Skeletal Radiol* 1998; 27:427–433.

37. Kransdorf MJ. Benign soft-tissue tumors in a large referral population: distribution of specific diagnoses by age, sex and location. *AJR* 1995; 164:395–402.

38. Kransdorf MJ. Malignant soft-tissue tumors in a large referral population: distribution of diagnoses by age, sex, and location. *AJR* 1995; 164:129–134.

39. Hosono M, Kobayashi H, Fujimoto R, et al. Septum-like structures in lipoma and liposarcoma: MR imaging and pathologic correlation. *Skeletal Radiol* 1997; 26:150–154.

40. Matsumoto K, Hukuda S, Ishizawa M, Chano T, Okabe H. MRI findings in intramuscular lipomas. *Skeletal Radiol* 1999; 28:145–152.

41. Bush CH, Spanier SS, Gillespy T III. Imaging of atypical lipomas of the extremities: report of three cases. *Skeletal Radiol* 1988; 17:472–475.

42. Einarsdottir H, Soderlund V, Larson O, Jenner G, Bauer CF. MR imaging of lipoma and liposarcoma. *Acta Radiol* 1999; 40:64–68.

43. Cohen EK, Kressel HY, Perosio T, et al. MR imaging of soft-tissue hemangiomas: correlation with pathologic findings. *AJR* 1988; 150:1079–1081.

44. Cohen JM, Weinreb JC, Redman HC. Arteriovenous malformations of the extremities: MR imaging. *Radiology* 1986; 158:475–479.

45. Rubin JI, Gomori JM, Grossman RI, et al. High-field MR imaging of extracranial hematomas. *AJR* 1987; 148:813–817.

46. Hughes TH, Sartoris DJ, Schweitzer ME, Resnick DL. Pigmented villonodular synovitis: MRI characteristics. *Skeletal Radiol* 1995; 24:7–12.

47. Jelinek JS, Kransdorf MJ, Shmookler BM, Aboulafia AA, Malawer MM. Giant cell tumor of the tendon sheath: MR findings in nine cases. *AJR* 1994; 162:919–922.

48. Otake S, Tsuruta Y, Yamana D, Mizutani H, Ohba S. Amyloid arthropathy of the hip joint: MR demonstration of presumed amyloid lesions in 152 patients with long-term hemodialysis. *Eur Radiol* 1998; 8:1352–1356.

49. Chen KHC, Yeh LR, Pan B-H, et al. Intra-articular gouty tophi of the knee: CT and MR imaging in 12 patients. *Skeletal Radiol* 1999; 28:75–80.

50. Peterson KK, Renfrew DL, Feddersen RM, Buckwalter JA, El-Khoury GY. Magnetic resonance imaging of myxoid containing tumors. *Skeletal Radiol* 1991; 20:245–250.

51. Kransdorf MJ, Murphey MD. *Imaging of Soft Tissue Tumors.* Philadelphia: W.B. Saunders; 1997.

52. Morton MJ, Berquist TH, McLeod RA, Unni KK, Si FH. MR imaging of synovial sarcoma. *AJR* 1991; 156:337–340.

53. Stull M, Moser RP, Kransdorf MJ, et al. Magnetic resonance appearance of peripheral nerve sheath tumors. *Skeletal Radiol* 1991; 20:9–14.

54. Suh JS, Abernoza P, Galloway HR, et al. Peripheral (extracranial) nerve tumors: correlation of MR imaging and histologic findings. *Radiology* 1992; 183:341–346.

8 OSSEOUS TRAUMA

HOW TO IMAGE OSSEOUS TRAUMA
Anatomy
Overview of Osseous Trauma
Imaging Options
ACUTE TRAUMA
Impaction injuries
  Contusion
  Contusion Patterns
    Anterior cruciate ligament tear
    Lateral patellar dislocation
  Radiographically Occult Fracture

Avulsion Injuries
  Common Sites
  MR Appearance
REPETITIVE TRAUMA
Insufficiency Fractures
  MR Appearance
Fatigue Fractures
  MR Appearance
  MR Grading System
Chronic Avulsive Injuries
  Chronic Avulsive Injury
  Shin Splints

  Thigh Splints
  Posttraumatic Osteolysis
Trauma to the Immature Skeleton
  Epiphysiolysis
  Posttraumatic Physeal Bridges
  Avulsion Fractures
DIFFERENTIAL DIAGNOSIS
Epiphyseal Marrow Edema
Fatigue Fracture Versus Tumor
OSTEOCHONDRITIS DISSECANS

HOW TO IMAGE OSSEOUS TRAUMA

Coils and Patient Position. The patient should be placed in a comfortable position with passive restraints, such as tape or Velcro straps, applied to the region of interest to minimize motion. Pain medication also may be required in cases of acute trauma to improve patient comfort. The body coil is used to image the pelvis and hips. An appropriate surface coil should be used elsewhere, as if the nearest joint were being imaged.

Image Orientation. Images should be obtained in the axial plane as well as the sagittal or coronal planes, depending on the area of interest. For example, the coronal plane is best for imaging the hips and proximal femora; sagittal images are most useful for the spine.

Pulse Sequences. Inversion recovery (STIR) sequences are the most sensitive for detecting abnormal marrow signal intensity that results from skeletal trauma, and should be used in all cases. A fast spin echo-T2W sequence with fat saturation is also quite sensitive, but the incomplete fat saturation that sometimes occurs with this technique can produce areas of artifactually increased signal intensity. This can mimic marrow edema when none is present.

T1W images should be obtained in at least one plane, because they provide an excellent depiction of overall anatomy and are reasonably sensitive for detecting osseous injuries, although they are less sensitive than STIR sequences. Gradient echo sequences should not be used when imaging osseous trauma with a high–field-strength magnet (greater than 1.0 Tesla), because marrow pathology is ob-

scured by susceptibility artifacts related to trabecular bone. With mid– and low–field-strength magnets, however, some gradient echo sequences are quite sensitive for detecting traumatic injuries, because susceptibility artifacts are less pronounced at these field strengths.

Because of the exquisite sensitivity of MRI for detecting osseous injuries, a streamlined screening protocol may be used to provide a rapid diagnosis, minimize costs, and enhance patient throughput. For this purpose, we employ a three-sequence trauma protocol using T1 and STIR sequences to optimally demonstrate osseous abnormalities.

Contrast. We do not use intravenous contrast in cases of trauma.

Anatomy

A familiarity with basic skeletal anatomy helps in understanding the MRI findings in osseous trauma. Cortical (compact) bone is found along the periphery of flat and tubular bones. The subchondral plate, the layer of cortical bone at the articular end of a long bone, plays an important role in providing support for the overlying articular cartilage.

Trabecular (cancellous) bone is composed of a meshwork of osseous struts that support the overlying cortex. Trabecular bone is found primarily in the axial skeleton and near the ends of long bones, where it plays an important role in absorbing dynamic stresses. Because of its elastic compliance, cancellous bone has a load-bearing capacity ten times that of compact, cortical bone.[1] This shock-absorbing capability is especially important around joints, where the trabecular bone dissipates axial forces away from the subchondral plate and overlying articular cartilage.

In a developing long bone, the physis (growthplate) allows for lengthening of the bone through enchondral ossification. Prior to closure, the growthplate constitutes the weak link in the muscle–tendon–bone and bone–ligament–bone units.[2] As such, it is particularly vulnerable to traumatic injuries at epiphyses (at the ends of long bones) and apophyses (growth centers not involved in longitudinal bone growth, such as the trochanter of the hip.)

Overview of Osseous Trauma

Osseous injury may result from a single traumatic event, or may occur over a period of time due to repetitive stresses that lead to the gradual breakdown and ultimate mechanical failure of the bone. Acute trauma may result in impaction injuries (ranging from bone contusions to complete fractures) or avulsion fractures in which a tendon or ligament pulls off a piece of bone, cartilage, or both. Chronic injuries, resulting from less intense, repetitive trauma, range from a focal stress reaction to a frank fatigue or insufficiency fracture.

Imaging Options

Conventional radiographs still should be the first modality used for evaluating osseous trauma, but many acute and chronic osseous injuries are not detectable on radiographs. Most of these radiographically occult injuries can be detected with radionuclide bone scanning, but this technique suffers from several limitations. The examination requires 4 to 6 hours, thereby delaying diagnosis in these patients, who often are awaiting triage in the emergency department; the scan may be falsely negative for up to 24 to 72 hours after the injury, especially in elderly patients.[3] Finally, a positive scan is quite nonspecific, because the images are of extremely low spatial resolution, and a wide variety of osseous pathology can result in abnormal uptake.[4] This can be especially problematic in older patients, in whom insufficiency fractures and neoplasm are common.

MRI is exquisitely sensitive for detecting osseous injuries that result from either acute or chronic, repetitive trauma. By using streamlined protocols, MRI can be cost-competitive with a bone scan while providing a more rapid and specific diagnosis.[5] As a result, we use MRI as the next study in a patient who has normal radiographs and a suspected osseous injury. A normal MRI essentially excludes the presence of an osseous injury. An additional strength of MRI is its ability to demonstrate soft tissue injuries that may mimic a fracture clinically in cases where no osseous injury is present[6] (Fig. 8–1).

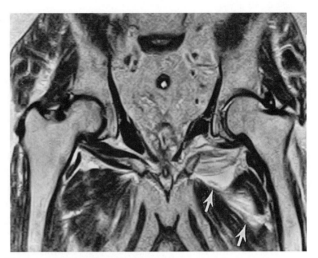

Figure 8–1. SOFT TISSUE INJURY.
Coronal T2 image, pelvis. This patient presented with left hip pain after a fall. Note the high signal edema or hemorrhage within the adductor muscles of the left hip *(arrows)* and lack of marrow edema or fracture line in the proximal left femur.

ACUTE OSSEOUS TRAUMA

Impaction Injuries

Contusion

Trabecular injuries that result from impaction forces are known as bone contusions, bone bruises, or microtrabecular fractures. Pathologic studies of these injuries reveal trabecular fractures, as well as edema and hemorrhage in the adjacent marrow fat.[7] Their detection is important for several reasons. Demonstration of an isolated bone contusion with MRI may explain a patient's symptoms and thereby avoid an unnecessary arthroscopic procedure. The sites of contusion also may provide clues about the mechanism of injury and associated soft tissue abnormalities that may be present.

Additionally, although most contusions resolve without complications, there is evidence that focal contusions involving the subchondral bone are associated with damage to the overlying cartilage.[8] Some investigators believe that this may place the patient at increased risk for collapse of the articular surface in the short term, or the development of osteoarthritis later.[9, 10] Therefore, detection of a subchondral contusion may result in a more conservative treatment plan, including a longer delay before returning to a normal activity level, to allow for trabecular healing and to minimize the potential for collapse of the overlying articular surface.

Bone contusions are most conspicuous on STIR or fat-saturated T2W images, where they appear as focal areas of increased signal intensity, presumably secondary to the hemorrhage and edema related to the trabecular fractures (Fig. 8–2).[11, 12] They often display poorly defined, reticular margins. On T1W images, these are usually of intermediate signal intensity (lower than fat, higher than muscle), because

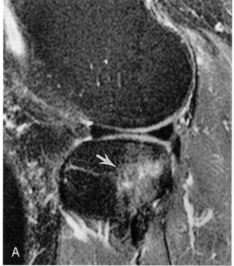
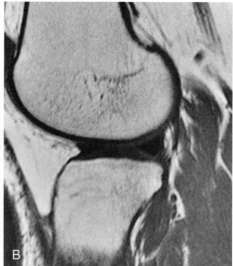

Figure 8–2. BONE CONTUSION. *A,* STIR sagittal image, knee. High signal–intensity reticular contusion within the lateral tibial plateau *(arrow)*. *B,* T1 sagittal image, knee. Note that the low signal–intensity contusion is much less conspicuous on the T1W than on the STIR image.

marrow fat is intermixed with the hemorrhage and edema. Contusions are easily missed on non–fat-saturated fast spin echo–T2W images because the trauma-related edema and surrounding marrow fat display similar signal intensities.[12]

Contusion Patterns

By analyzing the locations of osseous contusions, the mechanism of injury often can be inferred, and associated soft tissue abnormalities can be predicted and carefully searched for. Two commonly encountered patterns are discussed here (Box 8–1).

Anterior Cruciate Ligament (ACL) Tear. Osseous contusions are evident on MRI studies in approximately 80% of patients with acute ACL tears.[13] The most common mechanism of injury that results in a complete tear of the ACL involves a twisting force combined with a valgus stress. The ensuing impaction of the mid to anterior aspect of the lateral femoral condyle against the posterolateral tibial plateau results in typical contusions at these sites (Fig. 8–3).[14] Another contusion pattern often is seen concurrently in the medial compartment of the knee after an ACL tear.[15] These contusions involve the mid to anterior medial femoral condyle and posteromedial tibial plateau. These probably arise from a medial impaction force that results from the unstable knee rebounding after the ACL tear and lateral injuries have occurred (Fig. 8–3).

Lateral Patellar Dislocation. The typical contusions that result from patellar dislocation involve the medial patellar facet and the lateral femoral condyle, and are explained by the mechanism of injury. The patella dislocates in a lateral direction. As it relocates, the medial facet of the patella impacts against the anterolateral margin of the lateral femoral condyle, resulting in contusions at these sites (Fig. 8–4). Typical associated findings include a tear of the medial patellar retinaculum, a large joint effusion, and/or chondral or osteochondral injury to the medial patella.[16]

Radiographically Occult Fracture

In the case of a radiographically occult fracture, in addition to marrow edema, a fracture line is present. The fracture line occasionally may be obscured by adjacent marrow edema, but usually is identified as a linear or curvilinear focus of low signal intensity on T1W images that may demonstrate either low or high signal intensity on STIR images (Figs. 8–5 through 8–7).[17] Marrow signal intensity returns to normal with healing.

It has been well established that MRI is able to demonstrate radiographically occult fractures in a rapid, cost-effective manner, thereby allowing for optimal patient management.[18, 19] This is possible because the associated marrow edema and hemorrhage are present on MR images from the time of injury.

Even if a fracture is evident on conventional radiographs, MRI may provide additional useful information regarding the true extent of the fracture, the presence of additional fractures or contusions, and associated soft tissue injuries.

Avulsion Injuries

Avulsion fractures occur when excessive tensile forces result in a piece of bone or cartilage being

---

BOX 8–1: CONTUSION PATTERNS: Knee

Anterior Cruciate Ligament Tear
   Lateral Compartment
      — Mid-anterior lateral femoral condyle
      — Posterior-lateral tibial plateau
   Medial Compartment
      — Mid-anterior medial femoral condyle
      — Posterior-medial tibial plateau
Patellar Dislocation
   Medial facet of the patella
   Anterior lateral femoral condyle

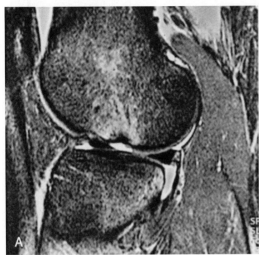
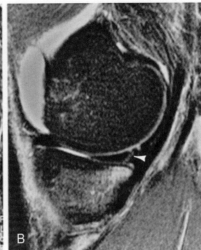

Figure 8–3. BONE CONTUSIONS ASSOCIATED WITH ANTERIOR CRUCIATE LIGAMENT TEAR.
A, STIR sagittal image, knee. Focal contusions are present in the lateral femoral condyle and posterolateral tibial plateau in this patient who sustained an anterior cruciate ligament tear. *B,* STIR sagittal image, knee. A concomitant contusion is seen in the posteromedial tibial plateau along with a vertical, peripheral tear at the posterior horn, medial meniscus *(arrowhead).*

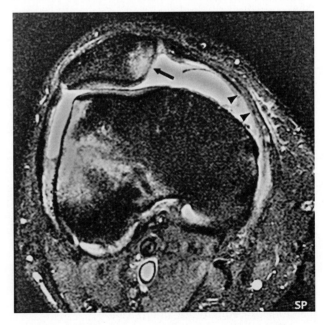

Figure 8–4. BONE CONTUSIONS ASSOCIATED WITH PATELLAR DISOCATION.
STIR axial image, knee. There are focal contusions in the lateral femoral condyle and medial patella. Note also the large joint effusion and tear of the medial retinaculum *(arrowheads).* Also, note the loss of cartilage on the medial facet of the patella *(arrow).*

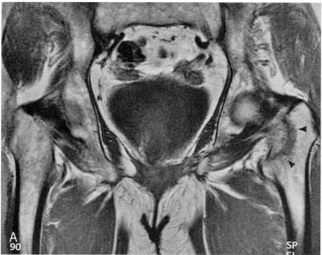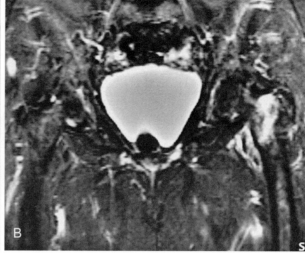

Figure 8–5. RADIOGRAPHICALLY OCCULT LEFT HIP FRACTURE.
A, T1 coronal image, pelvis. The nondisplaced left intertrochanteric fracture is identified by the low signal–intensity fracture line *(arrowheads). B,* STIR coronal image, pelvis. Note the high signal–intensity fracture line and adjacent edema.

pulled away from the host bone by ligament, tendon, or capsular structures. These injuries may occur with a single, acute event or may result from repetitive avulsive stresses.

Although these injuries can occur at any age, they are most common in the developing skeleton (children, and especially adolescents) because of the imbalance between muscle strength and the relatively weak, unfused apophysis. Avulsion fractures occur less frequently in adults, in whom the musculotendinous junction is the site that is most vulnerable to injuries from excessive tensile forces.

Common Sites (Box 8–2)

Avulsion fractures are most common in the pelvis. Frequent sites include the anterior superior iliac spine (sartorius and tensor fascia lata tendons), the anterior inferior iliac spine (rectus femoris tendon) (Fig. 8–8), ischial tuberosity (hamstring tendon), iliac crest (abdominal muscles), symphysis pubis, and inferior pubic rami (adductor muscles and gracilis tendon). In the proximal femur, the greater trochanter may be affected (hip rotators, including the gluteus minimus and medius tendons).[20] The lesser

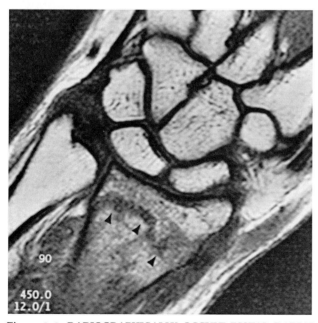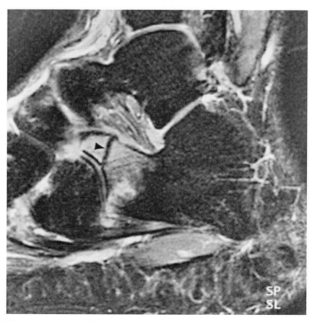

Figure 8–6. RADIOGRAPHICALLY OCCULT DISTAL RADIAL FRACTURE.
T1 coronal image, wrist. There is diffuse, low signal–intensity edema within the distal radius surrounding the curvilinear, low intensity fracture line *(arrowheads).*

Figure 8–7. RADIOGRAPHICALLY OCCULT FRACTURE, ANTERIOR PROCESS OF THE CALCANEUS.
STIR sagittal image, hindfoot. There is high signal–intensity edema surrounding the low–intensity fracture line across the anterior process of the calcaneus *(arrowhead).*

BOX 8–2: AVULSION INJURIES: Common Sites

	SITE	TENDON OR LIGAMENT
Pelvis	Ischial tuberosity	Hamstrings
	Anterior superior iliac spine	Sartorius/tensor fascia lata
	Anterior inferior iliac spine	Rectus femoris
	Symphysis/inferior pubic ramus	Adductors/gracilis
Femur	Greater trochanter	Gluteus medius, minimus/hip rotators
	Lesser trochanter	Iliopsoas (young person) (older patient = metastasis)
Knee	Lateral tibial pleateau (Segond fracture)	Lateral capsular ligament (mid ⅓)
	Fibular head	Lateral collateral ligament
		Biceps femoris—long head
	Tibial eminence	Anterior cruciate ligament
	Posterior tibial plateau	Posterior cruciate ligament
	Inferior pole of patella	Patellar tendon (Sinding-Larsen-Johansson syndrome)
	Tibial tubercle	Patellar tendon (Osgood Schlatter)
Ankle/foot	Calcaneus	Achilles
	Posterior margin—distal tibia	Posterior ankle joint capsule
	Dorsal margin, neck of talus	Anterior ankle joint capsule
	Base 5th metatarsal	Peroneus brevis
Humerus	Greater tubercle	Supraspinatus, infraspinatus, teres minor
	Lesser tubercle	Subscapularis
	Proximal shaft	Pectoralis major or latissimus dorsi
Elbow	Medial epicondyle	Flexor/pronator tendon
	Ulnar (sublime) tubercle	Ulnar collateral ligament

trochanter may rarely avulse in a young patient (iliopsoas tendon), but in an adult this injury is virtually always secondary to metastatic disease in the trochanter.

Common sites for avulsion fractures around the knee include the lateral tibial plateau (Segond fracture at the attachment of the lateral capsular ligament), the fibular head (biceps femoris tendon, lateral collateral ligament) (Fig. 8–9), the tibial eminence (anterior cruciate ligament), posterior tibial plateau (posterior cruciate ligament) (Fig. 8–10),

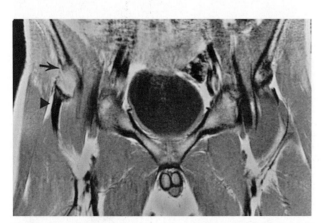

Figure 8–8. AVULSION FRACTURE, RIGHT ANTERIOR INFERIOR ILIAC SPINE.
T1 coronal image, pelvis. The right rectus femoris tendon *(arrowhead)* has avulsed a portion of the anterior inferior iliac spine *(arrow)*.

and tibial tubercle (patellar tendon).[20] Avulsion of the inferior pole of the patella can occur in children secondary to chronic avulsive forces (Sinding-Larsen-Johansson syndrome)[21] or as an acute cartilaginous avulsion fracture (patellar sleeve fracture).[22]

Avulsion of the posterior tuberosity of the calcaneus by the Achilles tendon (calcaneal insufficiency avulsion [CIA] fracture) is seen almost exclusively in diabetic patients. Avulsion fractures also may be seen along the dorsal surface of the neck of the talus or posterior margin of the distal tibia secondary to pull of the anterior and posterior portions of the ankle joint capsule, respectively. The base of the fifth metatarsal is another common site for an avulsion fracture (peroneus brevis tendon).[20]

The most common avulsion fracture in the upper limb involves the medial epicondyle apophysis (common flexor/pronator tendon) in children (Little Leaguer's elbow). The avulsed fragment may become entrapped in the humeral-ulnar joint space. Other sites in the upper extremity include the greater and lesser tuberosities (rotator cuff tendons), deltoid insertion on the lateral humeral shaft, and the insertion sites of the pectoralis major and latissimus dorsi tendons along the intertubercular sulcus.[20]

MR Appearance

Avulsion fractures typically demonstrate abnormal marrow signal at the site of the injury, but

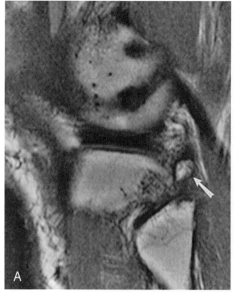
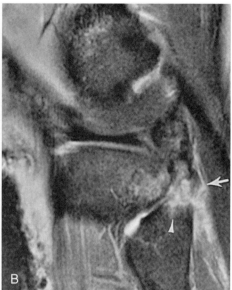

Figure 8–9. AVULSION FRACTURE, FIBULAR HEAD.
A, T1 sagittal image, knee. A small portion of the fibular head *(arrow)* has been avulsed by the biceps femoris tendon. *B,* STIR sagittal image, knee. There is high signal–intensity edema within the adjacent soft tissues *(arrow),* but note the relative lack of adjacent marrow edema *(arrowhead).*

the extent of the marrow abnormality generally is limited, and significantly less than what is seen with an impaction mechanism of injury. Prominent signal abnormality often is seen in the adjacent soft tissues, and the appearance may mimic a neoplasm or infection if a history of trauma is not obtained.[20] In these cases, correlation with conventional radiographs generally is useful because the injuries often demonstrate a typical radiographic appearance.

REPETITIVE TRAUMA

Stress injuries of bone typically are divided into two categories: insufficiency and fatigue fractures. Insufficiency fractures result from normal stresses applied to abnormal bone, whereas fatigue fractures occur when abnormal or unaccustomed stresses are applied to normal bone (Box 8–3).

Insufficiency Fractures

Several conditions weaken the elastic resistance of bone and predispose it to insufficiency fractures.

The most common is osteoporosis, but others include Paget disease, osteomalacia, and irradiation. Clinical diagnosis often is challenging, because the onset of symptoms may be insidious.

MR Appearance

Radiographic findings of insufficiency fractures often are subtle and difficult to appreciate because of the osteopenia associated with most of these conditions. However, MRI is able to detect these injuries with a very high degree of sensitivity. Insufficiency fractures appear as amorphous or linear foci of decreased signal intensity on T1W images. High signal–intensity edema is seen on STIR sequences, classically surrounding a low signal–intensity fracture line (Fig. 8–11).[23] Their appearance may mimic neoplasm, but a specific diagnosis of insufficiency fracture usually can be provided based on the MR morphology and location of the lesions.

With regard to morphology, demonstration of a linear component (corresponding to a fracture line) within the area of marrow signal abnormality indi-

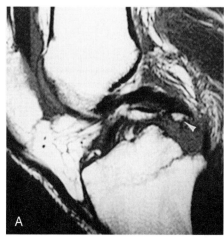
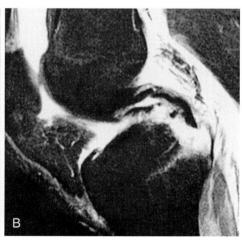

Figure 8–10. AVULSION FRACTURE, POSTERIOR TIBIAL PLATEAU.
A, T1 sagittal image, knee. A small portion of the posterior tibial plateau has been avulsed by the posterior cruciate ligament *(arrowhead).* *B,* STIR sagittal image, knee. Note the extensive soft tissue signal abnormality at the site of the avulsion and relative lack of marrow edema.

BOX 8–3: CHRONIC REPETITIVE INJURIES (STRESS FRACTURES)

INSUFFICIENCY FRACTURE
Normal Stresses → Abnormal Bone
Causes:
    Osteoporosis
    Osteomalacia
    Steroids
    Paget disease
    Hyperparathyroidism
    Rheumatoid arthritis
    Radiation
FATIGUE FRACTURE
Abnormal Stresses → Normal Bone
Causes:
    New activity
    ↑ Activity level (↑ exertion or duration)
    Poor equipment (eg, worn-out shoes)
    Abnormal biomechanics (eg, excessive
      pronation)

cates an insufficiency fracture (Fig. 8–12).[23] In many locations, the orientation of the fracture line is also typical. For example, in the sacrum, the fracture lines usually extend vertically through the sacral alae,[24] whereas in the supraacetabular region, they often parallel the curvature of the acetabular roof, forming the "arched eyebrow" appearance (Fig. 8–13).[25] As a general rule, insufficiency fractures typically lie perpendicular to the long axis and major trabeculae of the affected bone (with the exception of the uncommon longitudinal fractures of the tibial and femoral shafts).

Any bone can be affected, but most insufficiency fractures occur in certain predictable locations (Box 8–4). In the pelvis, common sites include the sacrum, pubic rami, symphysis, and supraacetabular regions. Pelvic insufficiency fractures frequently develop in patients who have undergone prior radiation therapy for pelvic neoplasm, often within twelve months of completing the therapy.[26]

Common sites in the lower extremity include the femoral head and neck, the supracondylar region of the distal femur, the proximal and distal tibial metaphyses, the distal fibular shaft, the calcaneus, and the talus.

Amorphous foci of edema-like signal intensity, presumably representing insufficiency fractures, have been observed in the epiphyseal bone marrow of renal transplant recipients. These transient lesions all resolved within one year, and could be distinguished from foci of avascular necrosis on the basis of their MR imaging appearance, because truly necrotic areas demonstrated more sharply circum-

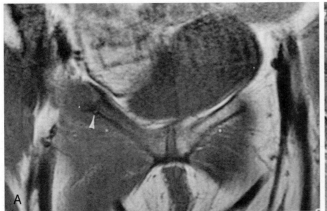
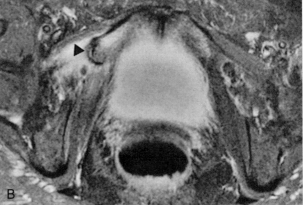
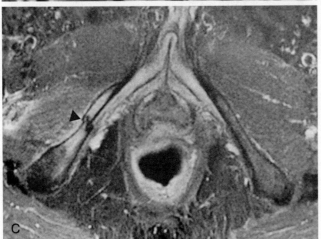

Figure 8–11. PELVIC INSUFFICIENCY FRACTURES.
A, Coronal T1 image, anterior pelvis. There is low signal–intensity edema within the right superior pubic ramus, where a linear fracture is also evident *(arrowhead).* *B,* STIR axial image, pelvis. High signal–intensity edema is seen within the marrow of the superior pubic ramus and adjacent soft tissue surrounding the curvilinear fracture line *(arrowhead).* *C,* STIR axial image, a more caudal level of the pelvis. High signal edema also is seen within the inferior pubic ramus, where there is a minimally displaced fracture *(arrowhead).*

Figure 8–12. PELVIC INSUFFI-CIENCY FRACTURES.
A, T1 coronal image, posterior pelvis. Low signal–intensity linear edema is seen in the sacral ala bilaterally, as well as in the left ischium *(arrow)*. Note the vertical orientation of the low signal–intensity fracture lines within the sacral ala *(arrowheads)*. *B,* STIR coronal image, posterior pelvis. High signal–intensity marrow edema within the sacral ala obscures the fracture lines *(arrowheads)*. Note the low signal–intensity fracture line in the left ischium surrounded by high signal edema *(arrow)*.

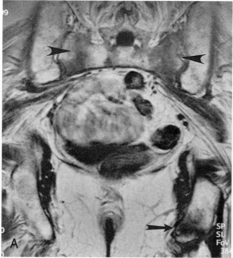 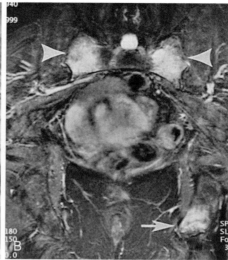

scribed, low signal–intensity margins, usually surrounding a focus of normal marrow fat.[27]

The upper extremities are not usually affected by insufficiency fractures.

Insufficiency fractures are very common in the spine. With an acute insufficiency fracture, the compressed vertebral body demonstrates intermediate to low signal intensity on T1W images and increased signal on T2W or STIR images, reflecting the associated marrow edema or hemorrhage. A fracture line usually is seen also (Fig. 8–14). An old, healed compression fracture displays normal marrow signal intensity on all sequences.

It often is difficult to differentiate an acute osteoporotic compression fracture in the spine from a pathologic fracture related to underlying tumor. Features that suggest a benign insufficiency fracture include abnormal signal intensity involving only a portion of the vertebral body marrow, a sharp linear margin between normal and abnormal marrow, lack of pedicle involvement, presence of a fluid-filled cleft within the vertebra on T2W images, the lack of a paraspinous mass, and a return to normal marrow signal intensity after gadolinium injection.[28, 29] In indeterminate cases, an immediate biopsy or follow-up MR examination in six to eight weeks is indicated. With a benign compression fracture, there usually is some evidence of healing in that time, with vertebral marrow signal intensity returning to normal.

Fatigue Fractures

Bone remodeling occurs in response to the mechanical stresses of normal, daily activities. Bone initially is resorbed in areas of activity-related microdamage, in preparation for reparative bone formation. However, because bone formation is slower than resorption, this leaves the bone in a temporarily weakened state. This process usually is maintained in a physiologic balance, but becomes patho-

Figure 8–13. SUPRAACETABULAR FRACTURES.
Low signal–intensity fracture lines are seen in the supraacetabular regions bilaterally. Note the curvilinear "arched eyebrow" morphology on the left *(arrow)*.

BOX 8–4: INSUFFICIENCY FRACTURES:
Common Sites

Spine	Vertebral body (compression)
Pelvis	Parasymphyseal
	Pubic rami
	Supraacetabular
	Sacrum
Proximal femur	Head
	Neck
	Basicervical region
Distal femur	Supracondylar region
Tibia	Proximal metaphysis
	Distal metaphysis
Fibula	Distal shaft
Calcaneus	Tuberosity

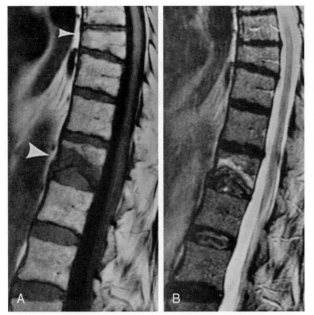

Figure 8–14. BENIGN, OSTEOPOROTIC COMPRESSION FRACTURE OF THE SPINE.
A, T1 sagittal image, thoracolumbar junction. There is a compression fracture of the inferior endplate of T12 with bandlike, low signal–intensity edema in the lower two thirds of the vertebra *(large arrowhead)*. Note the normal fat within the superior third of the T12 vertebra as well as the old, healed compression fracture at T9 *(small arrowhead)*. *B,* T2 sagittal image, thoracolumbar junction. High signal edema clearly demarcates the fracture line in the T12 vertebra.

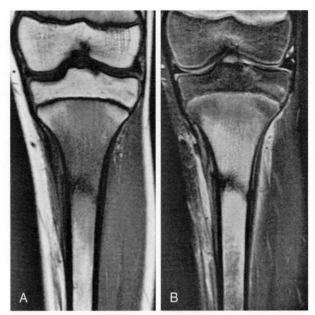

Figure 8–15. TIBIAL STRESS FRACTURE.
A, T1 coronal image, tibia. There is a horizontal, low-intensity fracture line surrounded by diffuse marrow edema. *B,* STIR coronal image, tibia. The low-intensity fracture line is more conspicuous because of the high signal intensity of the adjacent edema. Elevation of the low signal periosteum is also present medially and laterally.

logic when the development of microdamage greatly exceeds the reparative capacity of the bone, such as when a new activity is attempted, or there is an abrupt increase in the level of activity or intensity of exertion.[30]

Accurate diagnosis is important, because these injuries may progress to a displaced fracture if not treated promptly. The patient usually describes activity-related pain that abates with rest, but the symptoms may be quite insidious. If the activity is curtailed, the damage often heals prior to the development of a true fracture, and this probably explains why many stress-related bone injuries are never radiographically apparent. The sensitivity of early radiographs may be as low as 15%, and follow-up films are positive in only 50% of cases.[31, 32] Even so, radiographs should always be obtained in a patient with a suspected fatigue fracture, because classic radiographic findings, if present, will allow for a specific diagnosis.

MR Appearance

MRI is exquisitely sensitive for detecting fatigue injuries in bone and is more specific than a radionuclide bone scan. In areas of osseous stress reaction, MR findings include marrow edema on T1 and STIR images. Increased signal intensity may be observed on STIR images in the juxtacortical/subperiosteal region, which likely corresponds to periosteal but-

tressing, and a fracture line eventually may be detectable within the marrow or overlying cortex (Fig. 8–15).[19, 30] The abnormal signal intensity resolves as the injury heals, usually within six months. Persistence of signal abnormality beyond this point most likely represents recurrent injury.[33]

Common sites of fatigue fractures include the posterior aspect of the proximal tibia (running), the anterior midshaft of the tibia (jumping sports, dancing), the metatarsals (running, marching), the distal fibular shaft (running), the femoral neck (running, ballet) (Fig. 8–16), the sacrum (running, aerobics), and the pars interarticularis in the vertebrae (ballet, running, gymnastics) (Box 8–5). Fatigue fractures are uncommon in the upper extremities but can involve the humerus, ulna, clavicle, and first ribs.[34]

BOX 8–5: FATIGUE FRACTURES:
Common Sites

Lower Extremity	Tibia (especially posterior cortex, proximal shaft)
	Fibula (distal shaft)
	Metatarsal
	Calcaneus
	Navicular
	Femoral (neck and shaft)
Pelvis	Sacrum
Spine	Pars interarticularis

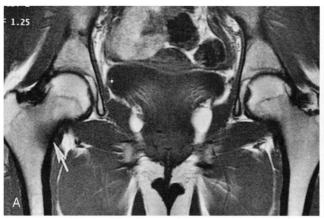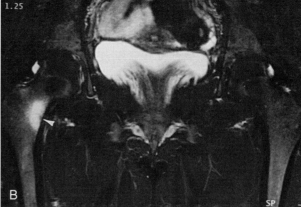

Figure 8–16. STRESS FRACTURE, RIGHT FEMORAL NECK.
A, T1 coronal image, hips. Low signal–intensity edema is seen along the medial basicervical region of the right femoral neck *(arrow).*
B, STIR coronal image, hips. A small, low signal fracture line is seen within the area of edema *(arrowhead).*

MR Grading System

Because fatigue damage occurs along a spectrum from accelerated remodeling to frank fracture, the degree of signal abnormality on MRI also is variable. A grading system has been established to help quantitate the degree of injury (Box 8–6). Grade 0 is a normal MRI study; grade 1 consists of periosteal edema/fluid on STIR images; grade 2 is high signal intensity within the marrow on STIR images, but normal-appearing marrow on T1W images; grade 3 is marrow signal abnormality on both T1 and STIR images; and grade 4 consists of either cortical signal abnormality or a discrete fracture line.[35]

Chronic Avulsive Injuries

Chronic Avulsive Injury

Chronic avulsive injuries of bone and periosteum result from repetitive forces at the sites of tendon insertions. These injuries tend to occur at the usual sites of avulsion fractures described previously. Radiographic findings include periosteal reaction and cortical irregularity that may mimic a malignancy. MRI can assist in arriving at a correct diagnosis (and avoiding a potentially confusing biopsy) by localizing the abnormality to the site of a tendon insertion, where it demonstrates cortical thickening, a lack of abnormal marrow signal intensity, and the

absence of an associated soft tissue mass (Fig. 8–17).[36]

Shin Splints

Shin splints is a term used to describe pain and tenderness in the lower leg that worsens with activity and abates with rest. The symptoms typically are localized along the posteromedial aspect of the tibia in the region of the soleus muscle origin. The pain is thought to be secondary to tears of Sharpey's fibers at the interface between muscle and bone, resulting in a traction periostitis, but the exact cause of this syndrome is unclear. In some cases, the pain also may be related to osseous fatigue damage. MR findings in patients with clinical evidence of acute shin splints include periosteal fluid/edema along the anteromedial or posteromedial aspects of the tibia, abnormal marrow signal intensity within the tibia and, in some cases, discrete fractures (Fig. 8–18).[37]

Thigh Splints

Similar to shin spints in the lower leg, a clinical syndrome has been described in the thigh known as thigh splints. A group of short, female military trainees who presented with nonspecific thigh pain, were found to have abnormal, linear activity on bone scans at the insertions of the adductor muscles along the anteromedial borders of the femurs.[38] Increased signal intensity on STIR images along the medial periosteum and within the femoral marrow in these regions allows for the diagnosis to be made with MRI (Fig. 8–19).

Posttraumatic Osteolysis

Posttraumatic osteolysis affects joints that sustain vertical stresses such as the symphysis pubis, acromio-clavicular, and sacroiliac joints. These stresses result in hyperemia, synovitis, and subchondral bone resorption in the affected joint. MR

BOX 8–6: CHRONIC STRESS INJURIES:
MR Grading System

	T1	STIR
Grade 0	Normal	Normal
Grade 1	Normal	↑ SI (periosteum)
Grade 2	Normal	↑ SI (marrow)
Grade 3	↓ SI (marrow)	↑ SI (marrow)
Grade 4	Fracture line	Fracture line

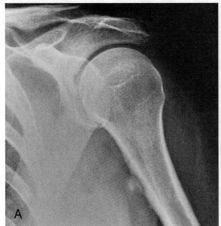 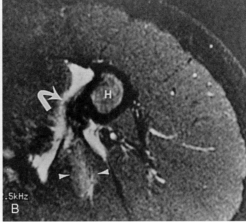

Figure 8–17. CHRONIC AVULSION INJURY, PROXIMAL HUMERUS.
A, Anteroposterior radiograph of the left humerus in internal rotation. A rounded calcific focus along the anteromedial surface of the proximal humeral shaft was thought to represent a possible surface tumor. B, STIR axial image, proximal upper arm. Extensive fluid or hemorrhage is seen around the avulsion injury at the origin of the latissimus dorsi (curved arrow) along the proximal humerus (H). Note also the edema/hemorrhage within the muscle compatible with strain or partial tear (arrowheads).

Figure 8–18. SHIN SPLINTS.
A, STIR axial image, mid-tibia. There is high signal–intensity periosteal edema/fluid along the anterior tibia (arrows), with some extension medially along the insertion of the soleus (arrowhead). This appearance is analogous to a grade I stress reaction. B, STIR axial image, mid-tibia (different patient than in A). In addition to high signal intensity–periosteal edema/fluid along the anterior tibia, there is focal intramedullary edema (arrowhead) in this patient who presented with symptoms of acute shin splints.

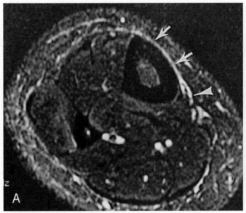 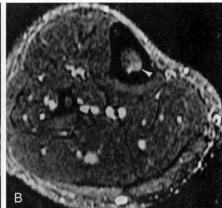

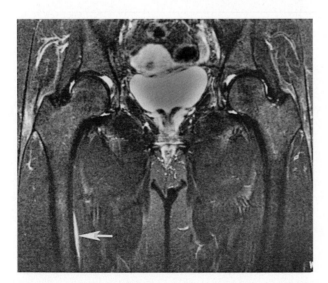

Figure 8–19. THIGH SPLINTS.
STIR coronal image, proximal femurs. Note the high signal–intensity periosteal edema/fluid along the proximal, medial femoral cortex (arrow).

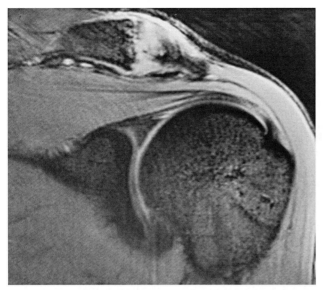

Figure 8–20. STRESS-RELATED OSTEOLYSIS IN THE LEFT ACROMIOCLAVICULAR JOINT.
Gradient echo-T2* coronal image, left shoulder. There is high signal–intensity edema and fluid in and around the left acromioclavicular joint with osteolysis of the anterior acromion and, to a lesser degree, distal clavicle.

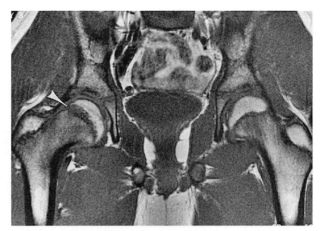

Figure 8–21. EPIPHYSIOLYSIS, RIGHT HIP.
T1 coronal image, hips. There is low signal–intensity edema within the right femoral neck, with widening of the lateral capital femoral physis *(arrowhead)* and malalignment of the capital femoral epiphysis.

findings include erosions and marrow edema related to the osteolysis, as well as joint fluid and synovial hypertrophy caused by the synovitis (Fig. 8–20).[39]

Trauma to the Immature Skeleton

Epiphysiolysis

Epiphysiolysis refers to traumatic injury to the growthplate secondary to compression and shear forces that result in a Salter I injury. This most commonly occurs in the proximal femur (slipped capital femoral epiphysis), distal radius (gymnasts), and proximal humerus (baseball pitchers).[40, 41] The MR findings in epiphysiolysis include joint effusion; physeal widening; bone marrow edema, mainly involving the metaphysis; metaphyseal fractures; and abnormal angulation of the epiphysis relative to the metaphysis (Figs. 8–21 and 8–22).[42] Cartilaginous growth into the metaphysis or premature closure of the epiphysis may occur later.

Posttraumatic Physeal Bridges

Fractures involving the developing growthplate may result in premature closure of a portion of the physis. These osseous bridges cause differential growth across the physis with resulting angular deformities. Diagnosis on conventional radiographs can be challenging; however, these bridges are readily diagnosed with MR images.[43] Gradient echo T2*W images are excellent for identifying the presence, extent, and location of the osseous bridge. The low-signal bone bridge is easily seen as it crosses the bright cartilage in the normal portions of the

growthplate. On T1W images, these are seen as areas of bridging marrow fat across the dark physis (Fig. 8–23).

Avulsion Fractures

Prior to closure of the physis, tendons and ligaments are stronger than the growthplate. This accounts for the high incidence of apophyseal avulsions in skeletally immature patients. This is

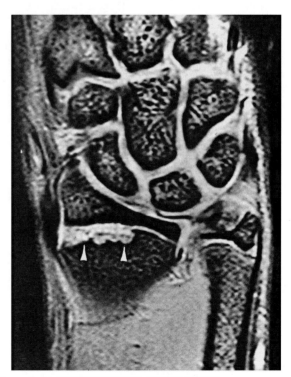

Figure 8–22. EPIPHYSIOLYSIS, RIGHT WRIST.
Gradient echo-T2* coronal image, right wrist. This demonstrates widening of the radial aspect of the distal radial physis, with high signal–intensity cartilage extending into the metaphysis *(arrowheads)*.

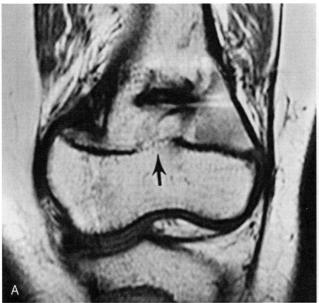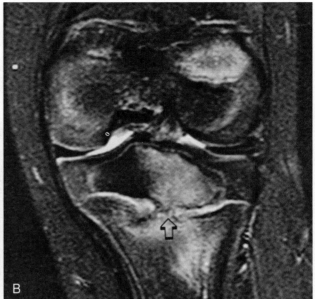

Figure 8–23. PHYSEAL BRIDGES.
A, T1 coronal image, distal femur. There is an osseous bridge with normal marrow fat *(arrow)* across the low signal–intensity distal femoral physis in this patient, who had sustained prior Salter-Harris II fracture. Note also the signal artifact in the distal femoral metaphysis, relating to prior fixation hardware. **B,** STIR coronal image, proximal tibia (different patient than in *A*). A low signal–intensity osseous bar *(open arrow)* is seen crossing the high signal–intensity proximal tibial physis in this patient who had sustained a prior physeal fracture. Marrow edema is present in the epiphysis and metaphysis on either side of the bar.

discussed more fully in the section in this chapter entitled "Avulsion Injuries."

DIFFERENTIAL DIAGNOSIS

Epiphyseal Marrow Edema (Box 8–7)

Other conditions can cause marrow signal abnormalities that may be indistinguishable from trauma-related changes, especially in the epiphysis. These include degenerative arthritis, transient osteoporosis, early avascular necrosis, spontaneous osteonecrosis, infection, altered weight-bearing, and fatigue/insufficiency fracture.

Degenerative arthritis can result in chronic subchondral edema, but other signs of osteoarthritis, such as articular cartilage loss and osteophytes, also will be present.

In the hip, transient osteoporosis (transient bone marrow edema) may mimic contusion, but its typi-

cal involvement of the entire femoral head and neck, combined with a history of a gradual onset of symptoms, aid in its diagnosis. Early avascular necrosis initially may result in MR findings of epiphyseal marrow edema. Spontaneous osteonecrosis of the knee results in striking epiphyseal bone marrow edema, but the typical history of abrupt onset of atraumatic pain in an elderly individual and flattening of the articular surface usually allow for an accurate diagnosis. Infection can mimic traumatic marrow edema, but usually can be differentiated on the basis of the clinical presentation.

Edema-like signal intensity may be present within the marrow of asymptomatic individuals, secondary to altered weight-bearing or a recent change in activity level.[44]

Fatigue Fracture Versus Tumor

Perhaps the most difficult problem is differentiating a developing fatigue fracture from tumor, because early radiographic and MR changes may mimic a neoplasm. Caution should be exercised, because biopsy of a stress fracture may result in a mistaken diagnosis of neoplasm, caused by the immature osteoid formed as part of the healing process. If a stress fracture is suspected, follow-up radiographs in 1 to 2 weeks or a repeat MR examination may reveal signs of healing or a discrete fracture line, thereby allowing for accurate diagnosis (Fig. 8–24).

OSTEOCHONDRITIS DISSECANS

Osteochondritis dissecans (OCD) refers to fragmentation or separation of a portion of subchondral

---

BOX 8–7: EPIPHYSEAL MARROW EDEMA: Differential Diagnosis

Traumatic contusion
Radiographically occult fracture
Degenerative arthritis
Transient osteoporosis
Early avascular necrosis
Spontaneous osteonecrosis
Infection
Altered weight-bearing
Fatigue/insufficiency fracture

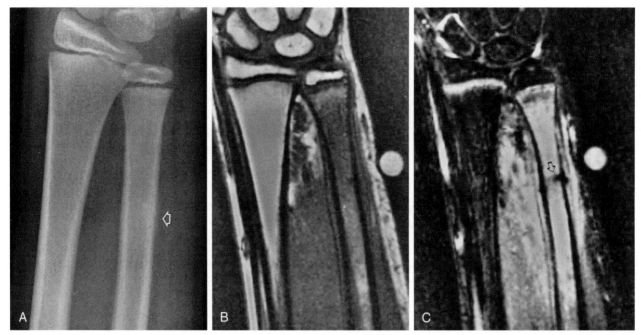

Figure 8–24. STRESS FRACTURE MIMICKING TUMOR.
A, Anteroposterior radiograph, forearm. Poorly defined periosteal reaction is seen along the medial aspect of the distal ulnar shaft *(open arrow)* in this 11-year-old patient who presented with right arm pain. *B,* Coronal T1 image, forearm. Diffuse, abnormal low signal intensity is seen throughout the marrow of the distal ulnar shaft. Periosteal elevation also is present. *C,* STIR coronal image, forearm. A linear stress fracture line is seen *(open arrow)* within the marrow edema in the distal ulnar shaft.

bone along an articular surface. The exact cause is not known, but repetitive trauma or acute shear forces are likely involved in most cases. Two forms of OCD have been described: juvenile, occurring before physeal closure, and adult. Most juvenile lesions heal with conservative therapy, whereas there is a poorer prognosis for adult OCD. The knee, ankle, and elbow joints most frequently are involved, but the shoulder and hip also may be affected (Box 8–8).[45]

In the knee, the most common site of involvement is the lateral aspect of the medial femoral condyle, along its non–weight-bearing surface. In the elbow, the lesion involves the capitellum along its convex anterior surface, and in the ankle, lesions are found in the anterolateral or posteromedial aspects of the talar dome.

Noninvasive assessment of the stability of the fragment is important, because it may help direct further therapy. Fragments are considered stable if they are attached to the host bone, and generally are

treated nonoperatively. If the fragment is unstable (loose) or displaced from its bed, operative therapy is indicated.

Conventional radiographs may demonstrate a displaced osseous fragment, but are otherwise unreliable for assessing lesion stability. MRI is able to demonstrate the fragment, overlying cartilage, and the interface between the fragment and parent bone. MRI signs of an unstable fragment include one or more of the following findings on T2W or STIR images: (1) linear high signal intensity surrounding the fragment (Fig. 8–25), (2) 5 mm or larger cystic changes between the fragment and host bone, (3) a high signal intensity linear defect in the overlying cartilage, or (4) a focal, 5 mm or larger, cartilage defect (Box 8–9).[46]

BOX 8–8: OSTEOCHONDRITIS DISSECANS: Common Locations

Knee	Medial femoral condyle (non–weight-bearing surface)
Elbow	Capitellum
Ankle	Talar dome (anterolateral or posteromedial

BOX 8–9: OSTEOCHONDRITIS DISSECANS: MR Signs of an Unstable Fragment

On STIR or T2W images:
• Linear high signal intensity surrounding the fragment
• 5 mm or larger cystic foci between fragment and host bone
• High signal–intensity linear focus in overlying cartilage
• 5 mm or larger defect in overlying cartilage

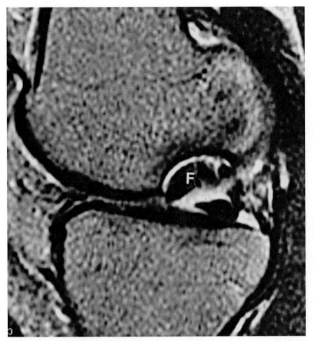

Figure 8–25. OSTEOCHONDRITIS DISSECANS OF THE KNEE, UNSTABLE FRAGMENT.
T2 sagittal image, knee. Note the high signal–intensity fluid that surrounds the in situ fragment (F) of osteochondritis dissecans involving the medial femoral condyle.

References

1. Radin E, Paul I, Lowy M. A comparison of the dynamic force transmitting properties of subchondral bone and articular cartilage. *J Bone Joint Surg [AM]* 1970; 52:444–456.
2. El-Khoury GY, Brandser EA, Kathol MH, et al. Imaging of muscle injuries. *Skeletal Radiol* 1996; 25: 3–11.
3. Rizzo PF, Gould ES, Lyden JP, Asnis SE. Diagnosis of occult fractures about the hip: magnetic resonance imaging compared with bone-scanning. *J Bone Joint Surg AM* 1993; 75:395–401.
4. Shin AY, Morin WD, Gorman JD, et al. The superiority of magnetic resonance imaging in differentiating the cause of hip pain in endurance athletes. *Am J Sports Med* 1996; 24:168–176.
5. Rubin SJ, Marquardt JD, Gottlieb RH, et al. Magnetic resonance imaging: a cost-effective alternative to bone scintigraphy in the evaluation of patients with suspected hip fractures. *Skeletal Radiol* 1998; 27: 199–204.
6. Bogost GA, Lizerbram EK, Crues JV III. MR imaging in evaluation of suspected hip fracture: frequency of unsuspected bone and soft-tissue injury. *Radiology* 1995; 197:263–267.
7. Rangger C, Kathrein A, Freund MC, et al. Bone bruise of the knee: histology and cryosections in 5 cases. *Acta Orthop Scand* 1998; 69:291–294.
8. Johnson DL, Urban WP, Caborn DNM, et al. Articular cartilage changes seen with magnetic resonance imaging—detected bone bruises associated with acute anterior cruciate ligament rupture. *Am J Sports Med* 1998; 26:409–414.
9. Blum GM, Crues JV III, Sheehan W. MR of occult bony trauma: the missing link. *Appl Radiol* 1993; March:15–21.
10. Faber K, Dill J, Thain L, et al. Intermediate follow-up of occult osteochondral lesions following ACL reconstruction [abstr.]. *Arthroscopy* 1996; 12:370–371.
11. Vellet AD, Marks PH, Fowler PJ, Munro TG. Occult posttraumatic osteochondral lesions of the knee: prevalence, classification and short-term sequelae evaluated with MR imaging. *Radiology* 1991; 178:271–276.
12. Kapelov SR, Teresi LM, Bradley WG, et al. Bone contusions of the knee: increased lesion detection with fast spin-echo MR imaging with spectroscopic fat saturation. Radiology 1993; 189:901–904.
13. Spindler KP, Schils P, Bergfled JA, et al. Prospective study of osseous, articular, and meniscal lesions in recent anterior cruciate ligament tears by magnetic resonance imaging and arthroscopy. *Am J Sports Med* 1993; 21:551–557.
14. Kaplan PA, Walker CW, Kilcoyne RF, et al. Occult fracture patterns of the knee associated with anterior cruciate ligament tears: assessment with MR imaging. *Radiology* 1992; 183:835–838.
15. Kaplan PA, Gehl RH, Dussault, RG, et al. Bone contusions of the posterior lip of the medial tibial plateau (contrecoup injury) and associated internal derangements of the knee at MR imaging. *Radiology* 1999; 211:747–753.
16. Kirsch MD, Fitzgerald SW, Friedman H, Rogers LF. Transient lateral patellar dislocation: diagnosis with MR imaging. *AJR* 1993; 161:109–113.
17. Meyers SP, Wiener SN. Magnetic resonance imaging features of fractures using the short tau inversion (STIR) sequence: correlation with radiographic findings. *Skeletal Radiol* 1991; 20:499–507.
18. Fowler C, Sullivan B, Williams LA, et al. A comparison of bone scintigraphy and MRI in the early diagnosis of the occult scaphoid waist fracture. *Skeletal Radiol* 1998; 27:683–687.
19. Haramati N, Staron RB, Barax C, Feldman F. Magnetic resonance imaging of occult fractures of the proximal femur. *Skeletal Radiol* 1994; 23:19–22.
20. Stevens MA, El-Khoury GY, Kathol MH, et al. Imaging features of avulsion injuries. *Radiographics* 1999; 19:655–672.
21. Donnelly LF, Bisset GS, Helms CA, Squire DL. Chronic avulsive injuries of childhood. *Skeletal Radiol* 1999; 28:138–144.
22. Bates GD, Hresko MT, Jaramillo D. Patellar sleeve fracture: demonstration with MR imaging. *Radiology* 1994; 193:825–827.
23. Crangier C, Garcia J, Howarth NR, et al. Role of MRI in the diagnosis of insufficiency fractures of the sacrum and acetabular roof. *Skeletal Radiol* 1997; 26:517–524.
24. Brahme SK, Cervilla V, Vint V, et al. Magnetic resonance appearance of sacral insufficiency fractures. *Skeletal Radiol* 1990; 19:489–493.
25. Otte MT, Helms CA, Fritz RC. MR imaging of supra-acetabular insufficiency fractures. *Skeletal Radiol* 1997; 26:279–283.
26. Blomlie V, Rofstad EK, Talle K, et al. Incidence of radiation-induced insufficiency fractures of the female pelvis: evaluation with MR imaging. *AJR* 1996;167:1205–1210.
27. Van de Berg BC, Malghem J, Goffin EJ, et al. Transient epiphyseal lesions in renal transplant recipients: presumed insufficiency stress fractures. *Radiology* 1994; 191:403–407.
28. An HS, Andershak TG, Nguyen C, et al. Can we distinguish between benign versus malignant compression fractures of the spine by magnetic resonance imaging? *Spine* 1995; 20:1776–1782.
29. Moulopoulos LA, Yoshimitsu K, Johnston DA, et al. MR prediction of benign and malignant vertebral compression fractures. *J Magn Reson Imaging* 1996; 6:667–674.
30. Anderson MW, Greenspan A. Stress fractures. *Radiology* 1996; 199:1–12.
31. Greaney RB, Gerber FH, Laughlin RL, et al. Distribution and natural history of stress fractures in U.S. Marine recruits. *Radiology* 1983; 146:339–346.
32. Nielsen MB, Hansen K, Holmes P, Dyrbye M. Tibial periosteal reactions in soldiers: a scintigraphic study of 29 cases of lower leg pain. *Acta Orthop Scand* 1991; 62:531–534.
33. Slocum KA, Gorman JD, Puckett ML, Jones SB. Resolution of abnormal MR signal intensity in patients with stress fractures of the femoral neck. *AJR* 1997; 168:1295–1299.
34. Daffner RH, Pavlov H. Stress fractures: current concepts. *AJR* 1992; 159:245–252.
35. Fredericson M, Bergman AG, Hoffman KL, Dillingham MS. Tibial stress reaction in runners: correlation of clinical symptoms and scintigraphy with a new magnetic resonance grading system. *Am J Sports Med* 1995; 23:472–481.
36. Donnelly LF, Helms CA, Bisset GS III. Chronic avulsive injury of the deltoid insertion in adolescents: imaging findings in three cases. *Radiology* 1999; 211:233–236.
37. Anderson MW, Ugalde V, Batt ME, Gaycayan J. Shin splints: MR appearance in a preliminary study. Radiology 1997; 204:177–180.

38. Charkes ND, Siddhivarn N, Schneck CD. Bone scanning in the adductor insertion avulsion syndrome ("thigh splints"). *J Nucl Med* 1987; 28:1835–1838.
39. De la Puente R, Boutin RD, Theodorou DJ, et al. Post-traumatic and stress-induced osteolysis of the distal clavicle: MR imaging findings in 17 patients. *Skeletal Radiol* 1999; 28:202–208.
40. Umans H, Liebling MS, Moy L, et al. Slipped capital femoral epiphysis: a physeal lesion diagnosed by MRI with radiographic and CT correlation. *Skeletal Radiol* 1998; 27:139–144.
41. Shih C, Chang C-Y, Penn I-W, et al. Chronically stressed wrists in adolescent gymnasts: MR imaging appearance. *Radiology* 1995; 195:855–859.
42. Laor T, Hartman AL, Jamarillo D. Local physeal widening on MR imaging: an incidental finding suggesting prior metaphyseal insult. *Pediatr Radiol* 1997; 27:654–662.
43. Craig JG, Cramer KE, Cody DD, et al. Premature partial closure and other deformities of the growth plate: MR imaging and three-dimensional modeling. *Radiology* 1999; 210:835–843.
44. Schweitzer ME, White LM. Does altered biomechanics cause marrow edema? *Radiology* 1996; 198:851–853.
45. Schenck RC, Goodnight JM. Osteochondritis dissecans. *J Bone Joint Surg [Am]* 1996; 78:439–456.
46. DeSmet AA, Ilahi OA, Graf BK. Reassessment of the MR criteria for stability of osteochondiritis dissecans in the knee and ankle. *Skeletal Radiol* 1996; 25:159–163.

9

TEMPOROMANDIBULAR JOINT

HOW TO IMAGE THE
  TEMPOROMANDIBULAR JOINT
NORMAL TMJ
Osseous Structures
Disk

ABNORMAL TMJ
Internal Derangements
MRI of Internal Derangements/
  Degeneration
TMJ PROTOCOLS

HOW TO IMAGE THE TEMPOROMANDIBULAR JOINT

See the temporomandibular joint (TMJ) protocols at the end of the chapter.

Coils/Patient Position. Small surface coils are used, generally with a diameter of about 3 inches. Bilateral simultaneous examinations of the TMJs can be done with coupled surface coils.

The patient is supine in the bore of the magnet, with the coils centered over the TMJs by centering the coils just anterior to the tragus of the ear.

Images are obtained through the joints with the mouth closed. Images also can be obtained with the mouth open, which is done with a special device that holds the mouth open, or for the more innovative (cheap) among us, gauze can be wrapped around a syringe and placed in the mouth for the patient to bite down on. The size of the syringe is determined by the extent that the mouth can open.

Image Orientation. An axial localizer image through the TMJ condyles is obtained first. Using the axial scout image, a line is drawn between the anterior aspects of the two condyles, then sagittal images are obtained perpendicular to this line. This is essentially always the sagittal plane relative to the bore of the magnet, but is a sagittal oblique image of the TMJs. These images are obtained first with the mouth closed, and then the sagittal sequence can be repeated with the mouth open if one wishes to know if the TMJ disk reduces with mouth opening.

Coronal oblique images through the TMJs are obtained as an optional sequence in some patients, in order to show the condyles well in another plane and to demonstrate the disk in the rare event that it may displace in exclusively a medial or lateral direction relative to the condyle. These are done by obtaining images parallel to the long axis of the condyles based on the axial scout view. Coronal oblique images are done only with the mouth closed. Our only indication for obtaining coronal oblique images is that the referring physician asked for them.

Pulse Sequences/Regions of Interest. T1W images demonstrate the pertinent anatomy well. The section thickness is 3 mm with no gap; a 6-cm field of view is used. Both TMJs are imaged as a general rule, mainly because we have the coupled coils that allow it to be done easily, and also because bilateral abnormalities are common. However, it is only necessary to image the symptomatic joint.

T2W images are not necessary for evaluation of routine internal derangement but may be valuable in patients who have had recent trauma to the joint, because they may show abnormalities in the muscles surrounding the joint.

Contrast. Contrast enhancement is of no value for diagnosing routine internal derangements of the TMJ.

NORMAL TMJ

Osseous Structures

The osseous components of the TMJ are the mandibular condyle and the temporal bone at the base of the skull (Figs. 9–1 and 9–2). The relevant portions of the temporal bone that articulate with the condyle are the glenoid fossa and the articular eminence. The condyle should be concentrically positioned in the glenoid fossa with the mouth closed. With the mouth open, the condyle translates anteriorly so that the condyle is positioned directly underneath the apex of the articular eminence. The articular surfaces of the TMJ are covered with a thin layer of fibrocartilage.[1]

Disk

The soft tissue structure of interest in the TMJ is the articular meniscus or disk. The disk is interposed between the condyle and the temporal bone, completely separating the joint into superior and inferior recesses. The TMJ disk is made of fibrous tissue and has an asymmetric biconcave configura-

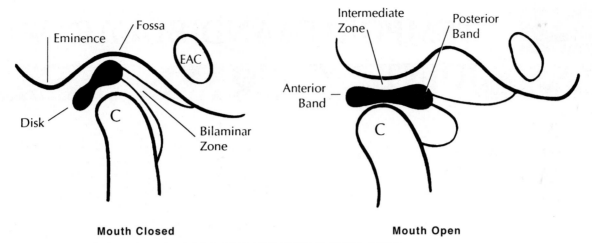

Figure 9–1. NORMAL TEMPOROMANDIBULAR JOINT ANATOMY (SAGITTAL VIEW).
Mouth closed (left) and open (right); anterior is to the left of each figure. The relationship of the disk to the osseous structures is depicted, with the intermediate zone interposed between the eminence and condyle wherever they are closest to each other. The posterior band is located at the 12 o'clock position on the condyle. EAC—external auditory canal; C—condyle.

tion. The disk is thicker peripherally than it is centrally. The thin central portion of the disk is called the intermediate zone. The thicker periphery of the disk is divided into anterior and posterior bands (Figs. 9–1 and 9–2). The anterior band of the disk is usually smaller than the posterior band. The disk attaches to the joint capsule, pterygoid muscle, and bone. Posteriorly, the disk is continuous with collagen fibers and loose fibroelastic tissue known as the bilaminar zone or posterior attachment. The bilaminar zone functions as a rubber band, allowing the meniscus to move forward with the condyle during mouth opening, and then recoils back to its original

position, bringing the disk with it, as the mouth closes.

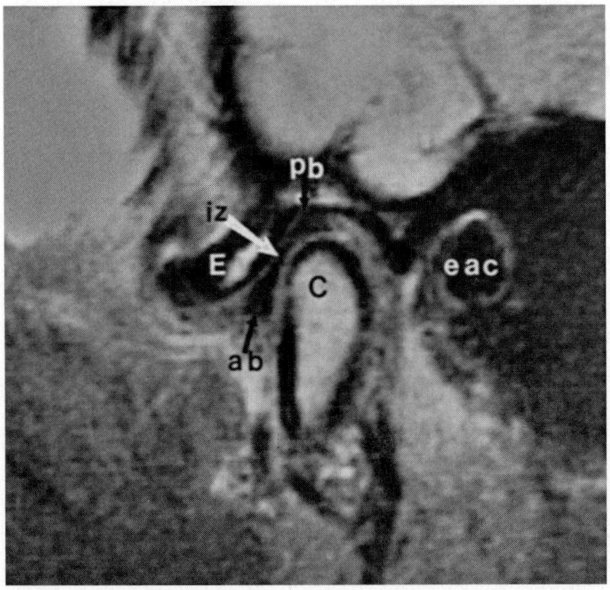

The normal position of the TMJ disk, regardless of whether or not the mouth is open or closed, is with the thin intermediate zone interposed between the condyle and the adjacent temporal bone, wherever the two bones are most closely apposed to one another.[1]

MRI of the normal TMJ in the sagittal plane shows the biconcave disk as an asymmetric bow-tie configuration. The thin intermediate zone can be seen between the two most closely apposed cortical bone surfaces of the condyle and eminence with any degree of mouth opening, as well as with the mouth completely closed. Normally, the posterior band is located at the 12 o'clock position, directly on top of the condyle, with the mouth closed. The posterior band may not always be evident when the mouth is closed, because its signal blends with the adjacent low signal intensity cortical bone of the condyle and glenoid fossa. The posterior band becomes more obvious with the mouth open, as it displaces away from adjacent bone (Fig. 9–3).

The disk is overall low signal intensity on all pulse sequences, but careful scrutiny shows intermediate signal intensity centrally in the anterior or posterior bands.

ABNORMAL TMJ (Box 9–1)

The TMJ is undoubtedly the dullest joint radiologists image. It performs only two tricks that relate to MRI diagnosis: the disk can become displaced (internal derangement), and degenerative joint disease can occur as a consequence of chronic disk displacement. Trauma and inflammatory arthritides also affect the TMJ, but we essentially never image with MRI for those indications. To spice things up, some people believe that avascular necrosis of the mandibular condyle occurs. With such a limited

Figure 9–2. NORMAL TEMPOROMANDIBULAR JOINT.
Mouth closed (sagittal T1 image). Osseous structures: EAC—external auditory canal, E—articular eminence; C—condyle. Disk: ab—anterior band; pb—posterior band; iz—intermediate zone. Note the posterior band at the 12 o'clock position relative to the condyle, and the intermediate zone between the condyle and eminence, where they are most closely apposed.

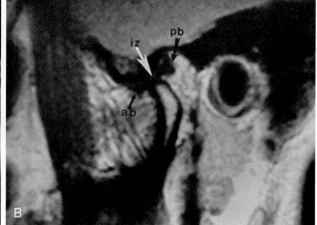

Figure 9–3. NORMAL TEMPOROMANDIBULAR JOINT.
A, Mouth closed (sagittal T1 image). Disk is in normal position, but the posterior band is difficult to identify because it blends with adjacent cortical bone. The intermediate zone (iz) and anterior band (ab) are easy to see and confirm the normal disk position. *B,* Mouth partially open (sagittal T1 image). The entire disk, including the posterior band (pb), becomes obvious as it displaces away from adjacent bones. The intermediate zone (iz) remains in its normal position, interposed between the condyle and eminence wherever they are closest together, and the anterior band (ab) remains obvious.

repertoire, it is hard for clinicians to misdiagnose a patient with TMJ symptoms. Yet, we are asked a few times a year to image the TMJ in order to look for internal derangements in patients who do not respond to therapy as expected, or who have unusual symptoms. Thus, we must know how to evaluate the images.

Internal Derangements

Internal derangements of the TMJ occur in women more often than men, and a young adult population generally is affected. Symptoms may be those of headache, earache, pain and tenderness over the joint, joint noise (snap, crackle, pop), and a limited ability to open the mouth.

Internal derangements of the TMJ may be classified into three different categories, and frequently a patient will progress in sequence from one category to the next.[1] The forms of internal derangement, in increasing order of severity, are:

• Anterior displacement of the disk, *with* reduction to normal position with mouth opening;
• Anterior displacement of the disk, *without* reduction to normal position with mouth opening; and
• Anterior displacement of the disk with a perforation.

An internally deranged disk is always in an abnormal position when the mouth is closed, but may or may not be in an abnormal position when the mouth is open (Fig. 9–4). Although we evaluate as to whether or not the disk reduces to normal position with mouth opening, this can change from day to day, is usually an easy clinical diagnosis, and generally does not contribute to the type of therapy chosen. Limited mouth opening occurs with internal derangements as the result of a displaced disk that does not reduce to normal position with mouth opening; the disk acts as a physical barrier to anterior translation of the condyle (Fig. 9–4). The disk is less likely to reduce to a normal position as the bilaminar zone becomes progressively stretched and dysfunctional.

BOX 9–1: TMJ: All You Really Need to Know

Normal Disk
Biconcave structure with thin intermediate zone articulating between the condyle and eminence
  wherever they are most closely apposed on sagittal images
Abnormal Disk
• Disk displaced anteriorly from position described above when mouth is closed. Intermediate zone
  no longer interposed between the closest contact point of condyle and eminence
• Disk may reduce to normal position with mouth opening *(anterior displacement with reduction)*
• Disk may remain displaced with mouth opening *(anterior displacement without reduction)*
• Disk degenerates with loss of internal intermediate signal and biconcave shape
• Joint degenerates
  — Subchondral cyst, subchondral sclerosis, osteophytes of condyle
  — ? Osteonecrosis

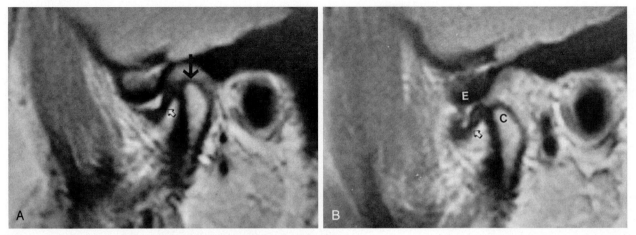

Figure 9–4. ANTERIOR DISK DISPLACEMENT WITHOUT REDUCTION.
A, Closed mouth (sagittal T1 image) shows the posterior band located anterior to the 12 o'clock position *(solid arrow)* of the condyle. The intermediate zone *(open arrow)* is not positioned between the condyle and eminence, where they are closest together. *B,* Open mouth image (sagittal T1 image) demonstrates limited anterior translation, with the condyle (C) not reaching the apex of the articular eminence (E). The disk remains anteriorly displaced and folded at the intermediate zone *(open arrow).*

Finally, a disk perforation can occur, or the disk may become thickened and fibrotic. Degenerative joint disease generally occurs with this most advanced stage of internal derangement.

MRI of Internal Derangements/ Degeneration

Sagittal MRI images of internal derangements of the TMJ show the disk in an abnormal anterior position relative to the condyle with the mouth closed. The posterior band will not be positioned directly on top of the condyle, and the intermediate zone will not articulate directly between the condyle and eminence where they are most closely apposed to one another. Perforations of the disk cannot be detected by MRI. A thickened disk that has lost its biconcave configuration and intermediate signal intensity should be mentioned, because it may affect treatment.

Sagittal images with the mouth open either will show the disk in normal position (anterior displacement with reduction), or the disk will remain displaced anterior to the condyle (anterior displacement without reduction). The key to diagnosis remains the position of the thin intermediate zone relative to the adjacent osseous structures. The displaced disk may have a crumpled, folded, or globular appearance (Fig. 9–4). The joint demonstrates limited anterior translation if the apex of the con-

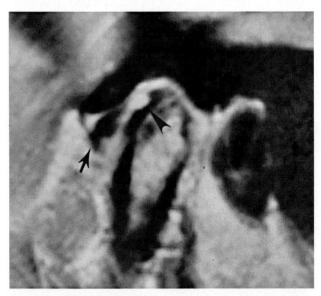

Figure 9–5. DEGENERATIVE EROSION OF THE TEMPORO-MANDIBULAR JOINT.
Closed mouth (sagittal T1 image). Erosion of the condyle *(arrowhead)* from degenerative joint disease secondary to a chronically displaced disk *(arrow).*

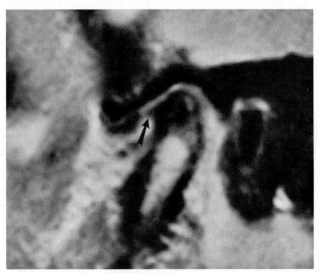

Figure 9–6. DEGENERATIVE SCLEROSIS AND OSTEOPHYTES OF CONDYLE.
Mouth open (sagittal T1 image). Severe degenerative joint disease with low-signal sclerosis of the condyle and an anterior osteophyte (hammer-and-nail deformity) *(arrow),* along with limited anterior translation of the condyle from long-standing internal derangement of the joint with disk displacement.

dyle does not progress as far anterior as the apex of the articular eminence of the temporal bone.

Degenerative changes of the TMJ may be manifested as an erosion of the condyle as the earliest osseous manifestation (Fig. 9–5). This has the appearance of a subchondral, rounded area of low signal intensity on the T1W sagittal images. More advanced degenerative changes may be seen as areas of low signal intensity sclerosis in the subchondral medullary bone of the condyle; anterior osteophytes also may be present, resembling a "hammer-and-nail" deformity (especially for those of us who are not accurate with the hammer) (Fig. 9–6).

Certain abnormalities in signal intensity in the marrow of the condyle are considered by some to be the result of avascular necrosis; others believe they are simply degenerative changes. Biopsy or surgical specimens of subchondral bone obtained from patients with degenerative joint disease show areas of osteonecrosis histologically, so the differentiation is probably impossible to make with certainty, and it probably makes no difference to the treatment or outcome of the TMJ patient.

Reference

1. Kaplan PA, Helms CA. Current status of temporomandibular joint imaging for diagnosis of internal derangements. *AJR* 1989; 152:697–705.

TMJ PROTOCOLS
This is one set of suggested protocols; there are many variations that would work equally well.

Sequence #	1	2	3
Sequence Type	T1	T1	Optional T1
Orientation	Closed mouth sagittal	Open mouth sagittal	Coronal
Field of View (cm)	6	6	6
Slice Thickness (mm)	3	3	3
Contrast	No	No	No

Scout

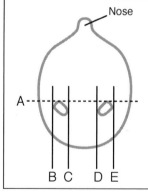

- Axial scout
- Obtain sagittal images perpendicular to a line connecting mandibular condyles (line A)
- Cover entire mandibular condyle between lines B & C and lines D & E

Final Image

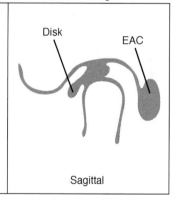

Sagittal

- Image both joints

Scout

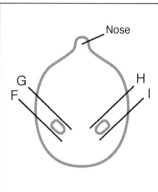

- Axial scout
- Obtain coronal oblique images parallel to long axis of mandibular condyles
- Cover between lines F & G and lines H & I

Final Image

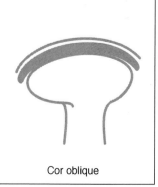

Cor oblique

- Image both joints

HOW TO IMAGE THE SHOULDER
TENDONS AND THE
  CORACOACROMIAL ARCH
Normal Anatomy
  Tendons
  Coracoacromial Arch
Shoulder Impingement
  Causes
  Effects of Impingement
Tendon Tears, Degeneration,
  Dislocation
  Supraspinatus
  Long Head of the Biceps
  Infraspinatus
  Subscapularis
  Massive Cuff Tears
Rotator Interval Abnormalities
INSTABILITY
Anatomy Relating to Instability
  Capsule
  Glenohumeral Ligaments
  Labrum

Instability Lesions
  Capsule
  Glenohumeral Ligaments
  Bones
  Labrum
Non-Instability Labral Lesions
  SLAP Lesions
  Paralabral Cysts
  GLAD Lesions
POSTOPERATIVE SHOULDER
Impingement and Rotator Cuff
  Surgery
Surgery for Instability
MISCELLANEOUS CAPSULAR,
  BURSAL, AND TENDON
  ABNORMALITIES
Adhesive Capsulitis
Synovial Cysts
Calcific Tendinitis and Bursitis
Subcoracoid Bursitis

NERVE ABNORMALITIES
Suprascapular Nerve Entrapment
Quadrilateral Space Syndrome
Parsonage-Turner Syndrome
BONE ABNORMALITIES
Posttraumatic Osteolysis of the
  Clavicle
Occult Fractures
Avascular Necrosis
Tumors
SOFT TISSUE ABNORMALITIES
Benign and Malignant Tumors
Pectoralis Muscle Injuries
SHOULDER PROTOCOLS

HOW TO IMAGE THE SHOULDER

See the shoulder protocols at the end of the chapter.

Coils/Patient Position. A surface coil is required in order to obtain high-resolution, detailed images. The patient is positioned supine with the arm at his or her side in neutral position or slight external rotation for a standard examination. The arm position influences how well different structures can be identified on MR images.[1, 2]

Image Orientation (Box 10–1). A small field of view (12 cm), and 3- to 4- mm-thick slices are obtained in three imaging planes: (1) coronal oblique, (2) axial, and (3) sagittal oblique.

The coronal oblique images are acquired with cuts made parallel to the supraspinatus tendon, which is seen on an axial cut, through the superior portion of the shoulder; alternatively, they may be acquired in a plane perpendicular to the articular surface of the glenoid, as seen on axial images. The axial images are obtained from the top of the acromion to the bottom of the glenohumeral joint using a coronal scout image as a localizer. The sagittal oblique images are acquired with cuts parallel to the articular surface of the glenoid as seen on axial images, from the scapular neck through the lateral margin of the humerus.

Pulse Sequences/Regions of Interest. Several different pulse sequences are used for the evaluation of internal derangements of the shoulder joint. They depend on whether the shoulder is imaged with or without intraarticular gadolinium.

The pulse sequences we use for standard shoulder MR are (1) coronal oblique T1W, T2*, and T2W with fat saturation; (2) axial T2*; and (3) sagittal T2*.

The pulse sequences for shoulder MR arthrography consist of T1W images with fat saturation in coronal oblique and sagittal oblique planes, T2W coronal oblique images with fat saturation (to detect subacromial/subdeltoid bursal fluid or other extraarticular fluid collections or masses), T1W axials with or without fat suppression for labral lesions, and T1W sagittal oblique images without fat saturation (to detect muscle atrophy).

Contrast. We previously did standard shoulder MR routinely without intraarticular gadolinium. We found ourselves struggling to be certain in many cases, and our correlation with arthroscopic or surgical findings were less than desirable. For these

---

BOX 10–1: SHOULDER STRUCTURES TO EVALUATE IN DIFFERENT PLANES

Coronal oblique
Infraspinatus muscle and tendon ⎤
Supraspinatus muscle and tendon ⎦ – longitudinally
Acromioclavicular joint
Acromion
Glenohumeral joint
Subacromial/subdeltoid bursa
Labrum (superior and inferior portions)
Sagittal oblique
Supraspinatus muscle and tendon ⎤
Infraspinatus muscle and tendon │
Teres minor muscle and tendon │
Long head of biceps tendon (proximal portion) ⎬ – in cross section
Subscapularis muscle and tendon │
Rotator interval
Acromion ⎦
Coracoacromial ligament
Coracoacromial arch
Glenohumeral ligaments
Axial
Long head of biceps tendon (in cross section through bicipital groove)
Subscapularis muscle and tendon (longitudinally)
Labrum (anterior and posterior portions)
Capsule
Glenohumeral joint
Glenohumeral ligaments

---

reasons, we now do shoulder MR arthrography on all patients, unless the referring physician specifically asks for a shoulder MR examination without arthrography. This has resulted in a considerable increase in our referrals for MR evaluation of the shoulder joint. Shoulder MR arthrography is a must in the evaluation of patients with instability. In our experience, it is also extremely useful in demonstrating subtle and sometimes not so subtle full-thickness tears of the rotator cuff.

Shoulder MR arthrography is performed after intraarticular injection of gadopentetate dimeglumine (gadolinium). The solution used for the arthrogram consists of 0.1 mL of gadolinium mixed with 10 mL of normal saline and 3 mL of iodinated contrast. About 10 to 12 mL of that mixture is injected into the shoulder joint prior to MRI using fluoroscopic guidance and the same approach as for a conventional shoulder arthrogram.

TENDONS AND THE CORACOACROMIAL ARCH

Normal Anatomy

Tendons

The rotator cuff typically is considered to be composed of four tendons: the supraspinatus, infraspinatus, teres minor, and subscapularis. In fact, the rotator cuff is a laminated structure formed by the joint capsule and the ligaments, as well as the four tendons listed above. The four tendons of the rotator cuff have cylindrical and flat portions that fan out and interdigitate with each other in order to form a continuous tendinous hood at their insertions onto the tuberosities of the humerus. There are no synovial tendon sheaths or surrounding paratenon investing the rotator cuff tendons. The coracohumeral ligament extends from the coracoid process to insert onto the lesser and greater tuberosities and the intervening transverse humeral ligament on the humerus. The coracohumeral ligament is located superficial to the joint capsule and the supraspinatus and infraspinatus tendons. These structures comprise the multiple layers to the rotator cuff.[3]

The supraspinatus tendon runs between the undersurface of the acromion and the top of the humeral head. It inserts into fibrocartilage (not hyaline cartilage) on top of the greater tuberosity of the humerus. Located posteriorly on the greater tuberosity, from a superior to an inferior position, are the infraspinatus and the teres minor tendons; running anterior to the shoulder joint is the subscapularis tendon, which attaches to the lesser tuberosity.[4] The supraspinatus muscle acts with the deltoid muscle to abduct the arm. The infraspinatus muscle and the teres minor muscle externally rotate the humerus, and contraction of the subscapularis muscle results in internal rotation of the humerus.

The entire length of two of the rotator cuff ten-

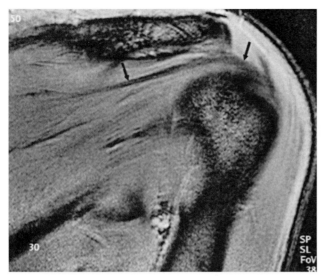

Figure 10–1. NORMAL INFRASPINATUS TENDON.
T2* coronal oblique image, shoulder. The low-signal infraspinatus tendon runs obliquely *(arrows)* in a craniocaudal direction, attaching to the posterior and superior aspect of the greater tuberosity of the humerus.

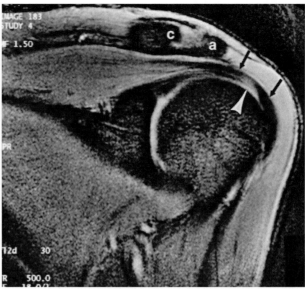

Figure 10–2. NORMAL SUPRASPINATUS TENDON.
T2* coronal oblique image, shoulder. The cigar-shaped supraspinatus muscle runs horizontally. The musculotendinous junction is located just lateral to the acromioclavicular joint (c—clavicle; a—acromion). The tendon *(arrows)* is located between the acromion and humerus, attaches to the top of the greater tuberosity, and is low signal except for a focal region of intermediate signal *(arrowhead)* from the magic-angle phenomenon.

dons, the supraspinatus and infraspinatus, can be seen well in the coronal oblique plane. Posterior to the humeral head, the infraspinatus tendon can be seen coursing obliquely in a craniocaudal direction at about a 45-degree angle to attach to the posterior portion of the greater tuberosity (Fig. 10–1). On more anterior slices, the horizontally oriented supraspinatus muscle and tendon are always seen on the same cuts that best demonstrate the acromioclavicular joint. The musculotendinous junction of the supraspinatus normally is located just lateral to the acromioclavicular joint (Fig. 10–2). The supraspinatus runs at an angle of approximately 45 degrees relative to the coronal plane.

Other tendons that also can be evaluated well on the coronal oblique images are the deltoid tendon slips that attach to the superior and inferior margins of the acromion (Fig. 10–3) and portions of the long head of the biceps tendon. The coracoacromial ligament is another low signal intensity structure that inserts on the lateral and inferior aspect of the acromion, appearing similar to the deltoid tendon attachment. The long head of the biceps tendon can be seen on far anterior cuts through the shoulder, from its origin at the superior labrum (the "biceps anchor") (Fig. 10–4), and inferiorly into the bicipital groove.[5]

The subscapularis muscle runs anterior to the shoulder and its tendon attaches to the lesser tuberosity. The length of the subscapularis tendon and muscle can be demonstrated best on axial images (Fig. 10–5). Its attachment blends with the transverse humeral ligament, which bridges the lesser and greater tuberosities and holds the long head of the biceps tendon in the bicipital groove.

The portion of the long head of the biceps tendon that is located within the bicipital groove is cut transversely on axial images and is a round or oval

structure. In some cases, it blends with the low signal intensity cortex of the humerus and may be difficult to identify. A small amount of fluid is seen in the dependent side of the long head of the biceps

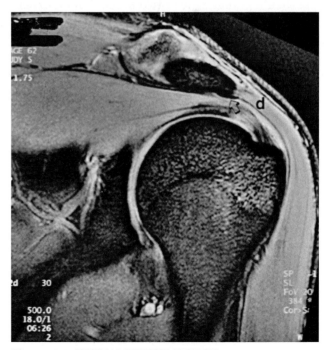

Figure 10–3. NORMAL DELTOID TENDON.
T2* coronal oblique image, shoulder. There is horizontal linear low signal *(open arrow)* that represents the tendon slip of the deltoid attaching to the acromion. This must not be confused with a subacromial spur. The deltoid muscle (d) is intermediate signal and located just lateral to the acromion and humerus.

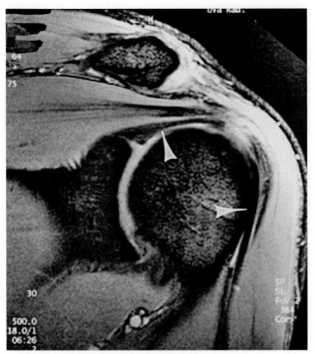

Figure 10–4. NORMAL BICEPS TENDON.
T2* coronal oblique image, shoulder. The long head of the biceps tendon *(arrowheads)* runs vertically in the bicipital groove, and attaches to the superior labrum (the biceps–labral anchor). The biceps is located far anterior in the shoulder and runs underneath the supraspinatus tendon.

tions may be seen lateral to the biceps tendon, which represent the anterolateral branch of the anterior circumflex artery and vein (Fig. 10–6).

On sagittal oblique images, the tendons of the supraspinatus, infraspinatus, teres minor, most proximal portion of the long head of the biceps, and the multiple tendon slips of the subscapularis all are imaged in cross section, surrounded by their associated muscles (Fig. 10–7). This plane of imaging is valuable for confirming the status of tendons when abnormalities are seen or suspected in the other planes of imaging, where the tendons are viewed longitudinally. The space between the supraspinatus tendon and the subscapularis tendon, which also is seen well on sagittal oblique images, is known as the rotator interval.

Tendons are normally low signal intensity on all pulse sequences; however, increased signal intensity in normal tendons may be caused by the magic-angle phenomenon.[6, 7] The magic-angle phenomenon occurs when collagen fibers are oriented at about 55 degrees to the constant magnetic induction field.[8] This results in an intermediate signal intensity within the otherwise low signal intensity tendon on short echo time (TE) sequences such as T1W, proton density, and gradient echo (T2*) images. In the shoulder, this phenomenon happens to occur commonly about 1 cm proximal to the insertion of the supraspinatus tendon on the greater tuberosity, which is the hypovascular region of the tendon, also known as the critical zone (Fig. 10–2).[6, 7] The intermediate signal intensity from the magic-angle

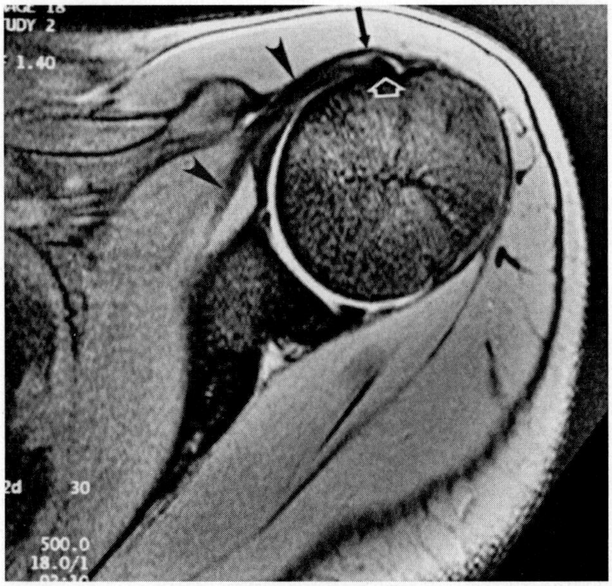

tendon sheath normally; with a shoulder joint effusion, fluid may encircle the biceps tendon, because the tendon sheath is in direct communication with the shoulder joint. One or two rounded fluid collec-

Figure 10–5. NORMAL SUBSCAPULARIS TENDON.
T2* axial image, shoulder. The subscapularis tendon *(arrowheads)* runs anterior to the shoulder beneath the coracoid process and blends with the transverse humeral ligament *(arrow)* that spans the bicipital groove and holds the biceps tendon *(open arrow)* in place.

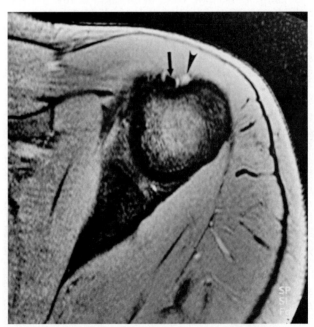

Figure 10–6. BICEPS TENDON AND ADJACENT VESSELS.
T2* axial image, shoulder. The biceps tendon *(arrow)* is imaged transversely in the bicipital groove. A small amount of fluid is seen on either side of the tendon in its sheath. The round, high-signal structure lateral to the tendon is the anterior circumflex humeral artery/vein *(arrowhead)* and does not represent tenosynovitis.

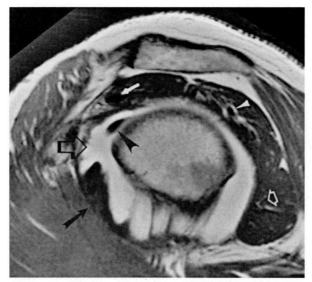

Figure 10–7. NORMAL SHOULDER, SAGITTAL PLANE.
T1 sagittal oblique, shoulder MR arthrogram. Beneath the acromion is the supraspinatus tendon *(white arrow)* and infraspinatus tendon *(white arrowhead)* with their surrounding muscles. Posteroinferiorly is the teres minor tendon *(open white arrow)* and muscle. The biceps tendon *(black arrowhead)* is located inferior to the supraspinatus tendon. The multiple slips of the subscapularis are seen anteriorly *(black arrow)*. The space between the supraspinatus and subscapularis tendons is the rotator interval *(open black arrow)*. The acromion is flat (type I acromion).

Coracoacromial Arch

The coracoacromial arch is formed by the humeral head posteriorly, the acromion superiorly, and by the coracoid process and the intervening coracoacromial ligament anteriorly.[9] Located within the coracoacromial arch, from superior to inferior, are the subacromial/subdeltoid bursa, the supraspinatus tendon and muscle, and the long head of the biceps tendon. The coracoacromial ligament restricts anterior and superior motion of the humeral head and overlying tendons (Figs. 10–7 and 10–8). Anything that decreases the space within the coracoacromial arch could lead to symptoms of impingement. Structures that form or are contained by the coracoacromial arch must be carefully evaluated in the different planes of imaging.

On sagittal oblique images, the coracoacromial ligament is seen as a taut, thin band with parallel margins. Typical of all ligaments, it demonstrates low signal intensity on all pulse sequences (Fig. 10–9).

The configuration and the orientation of the acromion are evaluated in both the coronal and sagittal oblique planes. Normally, the anterior and the most posterior aspects of the inferior black cortical line of the acromion on a sagittal oblique view should be nearly horizontal or else curved, paralleling the humeral head (Fig. 10–9). On coronal oblique images, the anterior aspect of the acromion should be horizontal and at the same level as the clavicle (Fig. 10–10). The normal acromioclavicular joint has a smooth undersurface, with both bones running in a smooth horizontal plane. Similarly, the undersurface of the acromion should be smooth and without spurs.

A boomerang-shaped fat plane surrounding the subacromial/subdeltoid bursa is evident between the acromioclavicular joint and the underlying supraspinatus tendon and muscle on coronal oblique images (Fig. 10–11). The subacromial/subdeltoid bursa normally is evident only because it is outlined by fat. The bursa should have no fluid, or only a

phenomenon disappears with long TE sequences, such as T2W images, making it possible to differentiate magic angle from an abnormal tendon.[8] A good rule to distinguish the magic-angle phenomenon from a tear on T2* images is that the signal intensity within the tendon is never higher than the signal intensity within the adjacent muscle if it is from the magic-angle phenomenon (Fig. 10–2), whereas with a tendon tear the signal intensity is higher than that of muscle.

Other potential causes of increased signal intensity in a normal supraspinatus tendon (besides the magic-angle phenomenon) include the presence of connective tissue between tendon fascicles, partial volume averaging effect, and overlap of the supraspinatus and infraspinatus tendons from imaging with the arm in internal rotation (Box 10–2).

BOX 10–2: ↑ SIGNAL IN DISTAL SUPRASPINATUS TENDON

- Magic angle (short TE sequences only)
- Overlap of supraspinatus and infraspinatus tendons (internal rotation)
- Connective tissue between tendon fibers
- Partial volume averaging
- Tendon degeneration
- Tendon tears (high signal on long TE sequences)

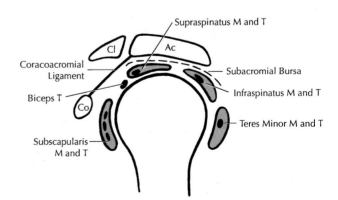

Figure 10–8. CORACOACROMIAL ARCH.
Diagram of the coracoacromial arch in the sagittal plane. The tendons of the rotator cuff with their surrounding muscles are arranged around the humeral head. The biceps tendon is inferior to the supraspinatus tendon. The coracoacromial ligament forms the anterior margin of the arch. Co—coracoid process; Cl—clavicle; Ac—acromion; T—tendon; M—muscle.

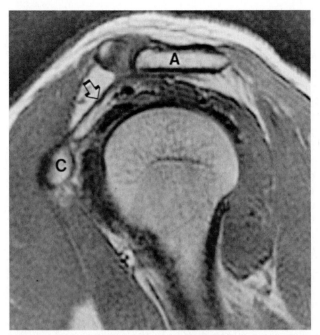

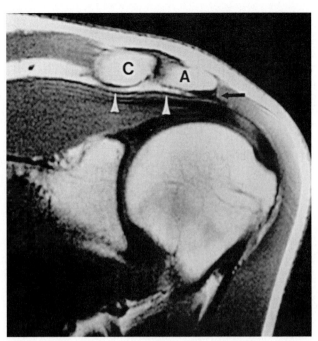

Figure 10–9. CORACOACROMIAL ARCH; TYPE I ACROMION.
T1 sagittal oblique image, shoulder. The coracoacromial ligament *(open arrow)* anterior to the shoulder is a taut, low-signal band between its attachments on the acromion (A) and the coracoid process (C). The muscles and tendons of the rotator cuff, as well as the long head of the biceps, are seen well in cross section. The undersurface of the acromion is flat (type I acromion).

Figure 10–10. NORMAL ACROMIOHUMERAL INTERVAL.
T1 coronal oblique image, shoulder. There is a normal orientation of the acromion (A) with the clavicle (C), with a flat undersurface oriented horizontally. The intact fat plane *(arrowheads)* between the acromioclavicular joint and the underlying supraspinatus tendon indicates no signs of impingement. The linear low signal *(arrow)* on the undersurface of the acromion is the deltoid tendon slip/coracoacromial ligament attachment and not a subacromial spur.

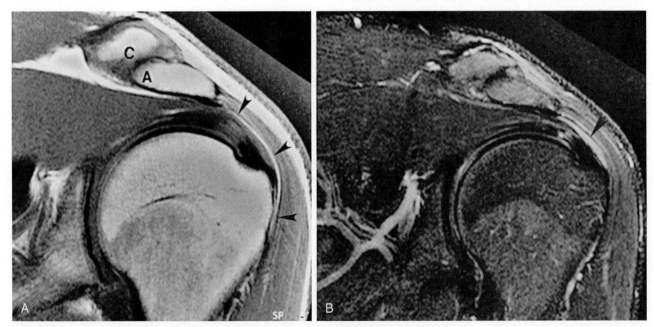

Figure 10–11. SUBACROMIAL/SUBDELTOID BURSAL FAT; LOW-LYING ACROMION.
A, T1 coronal oblique image, shoulder. The boomerang-shaped, thin, high-signal fat *(arrowheads)* is associated with the subacromial/subdeltoid bursa. The fat of the bursa may appear normal on T1W images, even in the presence of bursitis. The acromion (A) is low-lying compared to the clavicle (C), which predisposes to impingement syndrome. *B,* Fast T2 with fat suppression coronal oblique image, shoulder. There is a small amount of fluid in the subacromial/subdeltoid bursa *(arrowhead)* from bursitis.

small wisp of fluid, but certainly should not be distended with fluid. Another fat plane that is separate from that of the subacromial/subdeltoid bursa normally is evident, separating the supraspinatus muscle and tendon from the undersurfaces of the overlying acromion and acromioclavicular joint (Fig. 10–10).

Shoulder Impingement

In 1972, an orthopedic surgeon, Neer, proposed the concept that tears of the supraspinatus tendon are related to impingement on the tendon by the structures that form the coracoacromial arch. Any condition that limits the space within the coracoacromial arch can produce impingement on the subacromial bursa, the supraspinatus tendon, and the long head of the biceps tendon. Neer proposed surgical decompression to treat this impingement syndrome, consisting of an anteroinferior acromioplasty and resection of the coracoacromial ligament, thus decompressing and creating more room for the supraspinatus tendon and other affected structures.[10] Abnormalities from impingement that affect the supraspinatus tendon and surrounding structures range from edema to full-thickness tendon tears. All of these abnormalities are associated with symptoms of pain and collectively are referred to as the impingement syndrome. It is characterized clinically by acute or chronic shoulder pain induced by movements of abduction and external rotation or by elevation and internal rotation of the shoulder. It can occur in young athletes involved with repetitive movements of elevation and abduction of the shoulder, or in the elderly population from degenerative changes of the acromioclavicular joint and formation of subacromial spurs. In general, impingement is more common with increasing age (Box 10–3).

Causes

The supraspinatus tendon is predisposed to impingement from several sources that can be identified with MRI: (1) abnormal configuration of the anterior acromion, (2) anterior downsloping of the acromion, (3) low-lying acromion, (4) inferolateral tilt of the acromion, (5) os acromiale, (6) acromioclavicular degenerative joint disease, (7) thickening of the coracoacromial ligament, (8) posttraumatic osseous deformity, (9) instability, and (10) muscle overdevelopment.[11, 12]

Acromial Configuration. Bigliani et al.[13] described three predominant shapes of the acromion (Fig. 10–12) based on scapular Y view radiographs of the shoulder, and believed the shape was an important factor contributing to impingement. A type I acromion has a flat undersurface. Type II has a concave undersurface with the inferior acromial cortex parallel to the cortex of the underlying humeral head. A type III acromion has an interiorly projecting anterior hook that narrows the space between the acro-

BOX 10–3: SHOULDER IMPINGEMENT SYNDROME

Symptoms
• Pain
— Abduction and external rotation
— Elevation and internal rotation
Causes (anything ↓ size of coracoacromial arch)
• Acromial shape
— Type III: inferiorly projecting hook (sagittal oblique)
• Acromial orientation
— Anterior down-sloping (sagittal oblique)
— Inferolateral tilt (coronal oblique)
— Low-lying (coronal oblique)
• Acromioclavicular degenerative joint disease
• Os acromiale
• Thick coracoacromial ligament
• Posttraumatic osseous deformity
• Instability
• Muscle overdevelopment
Potential consequences
Tendons
• Supraspinatus tendon
— Degeneration, partial tear, complete tear
• Proximal long head, biceps brachii tendon
— Degeneration, partial tear, complete tear
Bones
• Degenerative cysts, sclerosis of greater tuberosity and/or humeral head
Bursa
• Subacromial/subdeltoid bursitis

mion and the humerus.[13] This hook may either be from an acquired traction spur at the site of attachment of the coracoacromial ligament or may be a congenital configuration of the acromion. A fourth type of acromion has also been described, which consists of a convex undersurface of the acromion

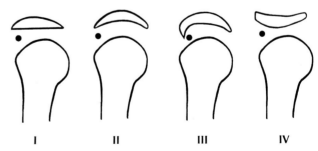

Figure 10–12. ACROMIAL SHAPES.
Diagram of the different acromial shapes from the sagittal perspective. The round black dot represents the supraspinatus tendon in the anterior portion of the shoulder. A type I acromion has a flat undersurface; type II has a curved undersurface that parallels the humeral head; type III has an inferiorly projecting spur anteriorly; and type IV has a convex undersurface. Types III and IV have increased incidences of impingement and cuff tears.

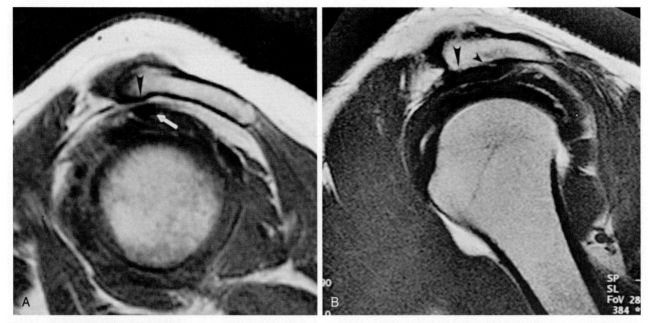

Figure 10–13. TYPE III ACROMION.
A, T1 sagittal oblique image, shoulder. The acromion parallels the curve of the humeral head except anteriorly, where it projects inferiorly *(arrowhead).* This is probably a congenital acromial configuration (type III). There is still an intact fat plane between the acromion and the underlying supraspinatus tendon *(arrow).* *B,* T1 sagittal oblique image, shoulder (different patient than in *A*). The anterior acromion projects inferiorly *(large arrowhead)* and there is a high-signal, marrow-filled subacromial spur seen more posteriorly *(small arrowhead).* The fat plane between the acromion and the rotator cuff is obliterated by these acquired spurs.

in its lateral portion.[14] The type III acromion has a significantly higher incidence of impingement and rotator cuff tears than do the other acromial shapes.[15]

The shape of the acromion can be determined on sagittal oblique MR images on the slice lateral to the acromioclavicular joint (Figs. 10–9 and 10–13), although there is poor interobserver agreement as to the acromial shape. The anterior inferior acromion is located immediately above the critical zone (hypovascular area) of the supraspinatus tendon. This relationship of the supraspinatus tendon to the anterior inferior acromion is obvious in the sagittal oblique plane of imaging, and it is clear that a spur or hook could irritate the adjacent distal supraspinatus tendon, which is the region of the tendon particularly susceptible to degeneration and tears. Subacromial spurs have fatty marrow within them (high signal on T1W images), even when very small, and can be distinguished from the low signal intensity deltoid tendon or coracoacromial ligament insertions on the lateral portion of the acromion that have an otherwise similar configuration and location as a spur.

Acromial Slope. The slope of the acromion can be evaluated on sagittal and coronal oblique images. Normally, the lateral aspect of the acromion is oriented nearly horizontal on sagittal oblique images. An anterior, down-sloping acromion occurs when the inferior cortex of the anterior acromion is located more caudally than the inferior cortex of the posterior aspect of the acromion. Another abnormal slope to the acromion consists of an inferolateral

tilt, which can be detected on coronal oblique images. An inferolateral tilt or slope occurs when the most lateral portion of the acromion is tilted inferiorly relative to the clavicle (Fig. 10–14). Sloping of the acromion in either direction increases the risk

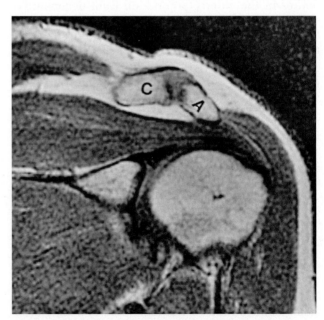

Figure 10–14. ACROMIAL SLOPE: Inferolateral tilt.
T1 coronal oblique image, shoulder. The acromion (A) tilts inferiorly relative to the horizontal clavicle (C). This narrows the space between the humeral head and the acromion where the supraspinatus tendon and the subacromial/subdeltoid bursa exist, increasing the risk of impingement.

for impingement from mechanical trauma to the underlying distal supraspinatus tendon (Fig. 10–15).

Acromial Position. Normally, the inferior cortex of the acromion is in line with the inferior cortex of the clavicle on coronal oblique views. A low-lying acromion exists when its inferior cortex is positioned below the inferior cortex of the clavicle (Fig. 10–11). This causes narrowing of the acromiohumeral space, which may predispose to impingement.

Os Acromiale. This is an accessory ossification center of the acromion that is normally fused by 25 years of age. An unfused os acromiale after this age is seen in up to 15% of the population, and its presence is associated with an increased incidence of impingement and rotator cuff tears, presumably because the os is mobile and thus decreases the space in the coracoacromial arch with motion.[16] The os acromiale is best identified on axial images, although it can be seen in all imaging planes (Fig. 10–16).

Acromial-Clavicular Joint Degenerative Changes. Degenerative joint disease of the acromioclavicular joint may manifest as inferiorly projecting osteophytes, fibrous overgrowth of the capsule, or both (Fig. 10–17).[17, 18] On radiographs, osteophytes are underestimated and fibrous overgrowth is not depicted at all; MR directly demonstrates the presence, severity, and extent of these structures that may cause impingement. Obliteration of the fat between the supraspinatus muscle or tendon and the overlying acromioclavicular joint, or indentation of the supraspinatus tendon or muscle by abnormalities of the acromioclavicular joint, are indications that the degenerative changes are considerable and may well contribute to impingement.

Coracoacromial Ligament. Focal thickening of the coracoacromial ligament may be observed on sagittal oblique MR images and is considered a sign of impingement (Fig. 10–18). Chronic anterior shoulder instability may cause thickening of the ligament, and may or may not be associated with concomitant impingement.

Posttraumatic Deformity. As a result of hypertro-

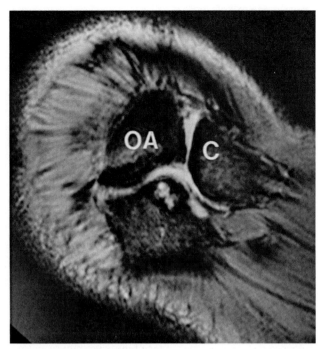

Figure 10–16. OS ACROMIALE.
T2* axial image, shoulder. A cut through the level of the acromioclavicular joint shows a separate os acromiale (OA) that did not fuse in this patient. This predisposes to impingement. There are degenerative, high-signal cysts between the os and the adjacent scapula.

phic callous formation or malalignment of fracture fragments that involve the bones adjacent to the coracoacromial arch, there may be narrowing of the coracoacromial arch with resultant impingement.

Instability. Glenohumeral degenerative changes can be caused by shoulder instability, and instability can be a contributing factor to impingement. Instability and impingement are two conditions that often coexist; this is discussed later in this chapter.

Muscle Overdevelopment. Supraspinatus muscle enlargement, as seen in weightlifters, swimmers, and other athletes (radiologists going through piles of x-rays) may induce impingement even if the coracoacromial arch and acromiohumeral intervals are normal, because the large muscle decreases the space available for the tendon to glide between the structures of the coracoacromial arch. A deformity (indentation) of the superior surface of the supraspinatus muscle caused by the acromioclavicular joint will be the only abnormality seen with MRI.

Effects of Impingement (Box 10–4)

Tendons. The supraspinatus tendon is affected far more commonly than other tendons in the shoulder. Impingement on the supraspinatus tendon from any source can cause tendon degeneration and partial or full-thickness tears. Conversely, the same tendon abnormalities may exist without evidence of structural or mechanical causes of impingement. It is interesting to note that most partial thickness tears of the supraspinatus tendon occur on the undersur-

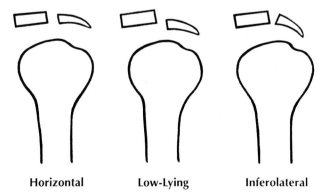

Horizontal	Low-Lying	Inferolateral

Figure 10–15. ACROMIAL ORIENTATION. ✳
Diagram of the relationship of the acromion to the clavicle and humerus. The horizontal orientation is normal and without an increased risk of impingement. The low-lying and the inferolateral sloping acromions are both associated with impingement.

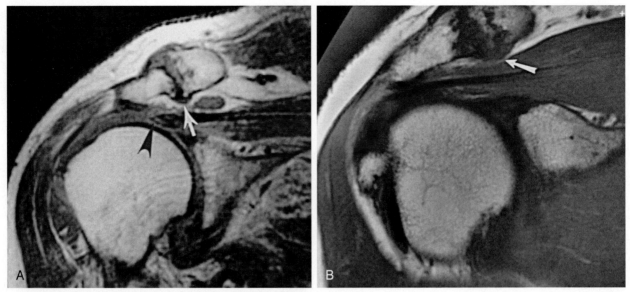

Figure 10–17. ACROMIOCLAVICULAR JOINT DEGENERATIVE CHANGES.
A, T1 coronal oblique image, shoulder. There is degenerative joint disease of the acromioclavicular joint with osteophytes projecting inferiorly *(arrow).* The supraspinatus is completely torn, with the tendon *(arrowhead)* retracted medially. *B,* T1 coronal oblique image, shoulder (different patient than in *A*). There is fibrous overgrowth of the capsule and osteophytes of the acromioclavicular joint, impinging on and indenting the top of the supraspinatus muscle and tendon *(arrow).* The distal tendon is mildly abnormal with high signal and thickening from degeneration/partial tears.

face (articular) aspect of the tendon, rather than on the superior (bursal) surface, where abnormalities in the coracoacromial arch would logically be expected to cause early partial tears. The proximal long head of the biceps tendon may be affected by impingement in the same ways as the supraspinatus tendon because of its similar location and course

just beneath the supraspinatus tendon within the shoulder joint.

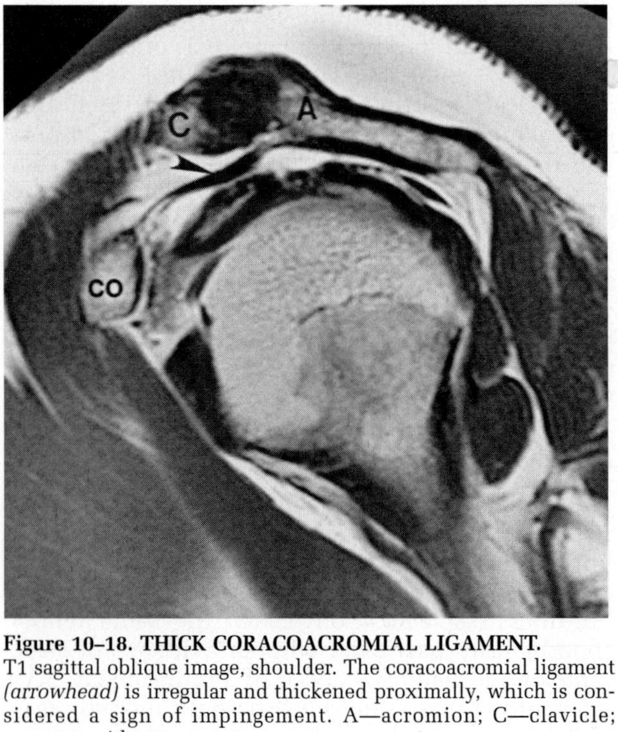

Degenerative Osseous Cysts. Although the supraspinatus tendon is the structure most often affected by impingement, certain associated osseous findings are very common as well. Small degenerative cysts in the lateral humeral head and cortical hypertrophy, sclerosis, and small degenerative cysts in the greater tuberosity often are present and may precede MRI evidence of abnormalities within the tendons. The osseous degenerative changes have been found histologically to be associated with microtears of the adjacent tendon.

Subacromial/Subdeltoid Bursitis. Irritation of the subacromial/subdeltoid bursa can occur from impingement. When this occurs, it becomes distended with fluid and is painful (Fig. 10–11). Normally there is no fluid, or only a trace of detectable fluid, in this bursa. Bursal fluid is common in the pres-

Figure 10–18. THICK CORACOACROMIAL LIGAMENT.
T1 sagittal oblique image, shoulder. The coracoacromial ligament *(arrowhead)* is irregular and thickened proximally, which is considered a sign of impingement. A—acromion; C—clavicle; co—coracoid process.

BOX 10–4: MR OF SHOULDER IMPINGEMENT

Identification of mechanical causes
Evaluation of tendon integrity
— Abnormal high signal intensity (degeneration/partial tears)
— Abnormal shape: thin, thick, irregular (partial tears)
— Discontinuity (complete tears)
Subacromial/subdeltoid bursal fluid
Glenohumeral degenerative joint disease

ence of rotator cuff tears. Bursal fluid cannot be seen without a T2W sequence, thus the need for this sequence even when an MR arthrogram is performed.

Tendon Tears, Degeneration, Dislocation

Supraspinatus (Box 10–5)

Degeneration and Partial Tendon Tears. These two entities generally are indistinguishable from one another on T1W images, where they appear as focal or diffuse regions of intratendinous intermediate signal intensity (Fig. 10–19). If these areas maintain the same signal intensity as muscle on T2W images, they are most consistent with tendon degeneration; if these areas become high signal intensity, like fluid on T2W images, they represent partial tendon tears. It frequently is difficult to make the distinction between degeneration or partial tendon tears, and then the general terms tendinosis or tendinopathy may be used to describe the abnormalities. Conversely, it is just as acceptable to state that abnormal signal in the tendon that is not clearly from tears on T1 and T2W images represents tendon degeneration or partial tears. Tendon degeneration and partial tears usually coexist.

Magic-angle phenomenon has similar signal characteristics as tendon partial tears or degeneration on short TE images. However, the findings are focal instead of diffuse, are at a specific location (one cm from the insertion of the supraspinatus tendon on the greater tuberosity) and, most importantly, disappear on long TE images.[19, 20] In addition, the signal changes are not associated with thinning, thickening, or irregularity of the tendon.

BOX 10–5: ROTATOR CUFF TENDON PATHOLOGY

Full-thickness tear
- Direct signs
  — Tendon discontinuity
  — Fluid signal in tendon gap
  — Retraction of musculotendinous junction
- Associated findings
  — Subacromial/subdeltoid bursal fluid
  — Muscle atrophy

Partial thickness tear
- ↑ signal T1 and T2, joint or bursal surface
  — Higher signal than muscle on T2 (similar to joint fluid)

Degeneration
- Intrasubstance ↑ signal, T1 and T2
  — Not as high signal as joint fluid

A partial tear on the undersurface (joint surface) of the tendon fills with high signal intensity gadolinium solution on MR arthrograms (Fig. 10–20). Partial thickness tears on the upper (bursal) surface of the tendon need to be evaluated just like a regular shoulder MRI without arthrography, because gadolinium cannot enter the tear in that location. Partial tears generally start on the undersurface of the distal end of the supraspinatus tendon, and the inferior layer(s) may retract medially, whereas the superior layers remain intact (Fig. 10–20).

Detection of tendon abnormalities prior to the development of a full-thickness tear is important, because the process may be arrested with conservative therapy, debridement, and decompression surgery.

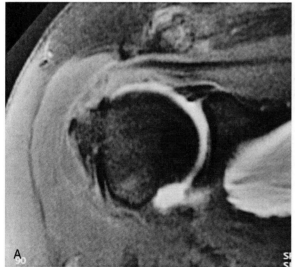 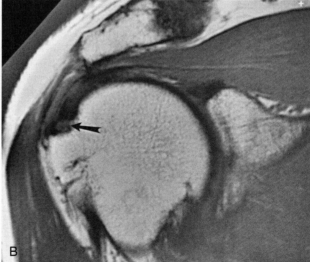

Figure 10–19. DEGENERATION/PARTIAL SUPRASPINATUS TEARS.
A, T1 with fat suppression, coronal oblique shoulder MR arthrogram. The distal 3 cm of the supraspinatus tendon is diffusely thickened and high signal, compatible with degeneration and partial tears. *B,* T1 coronal oblique image, shoulder (different patient than in *A*). There is linear intermediate signal *(arrow)* between a large portion of the distal supraspinatus tendon and the adjacent greater tuberosity from a partial tear.

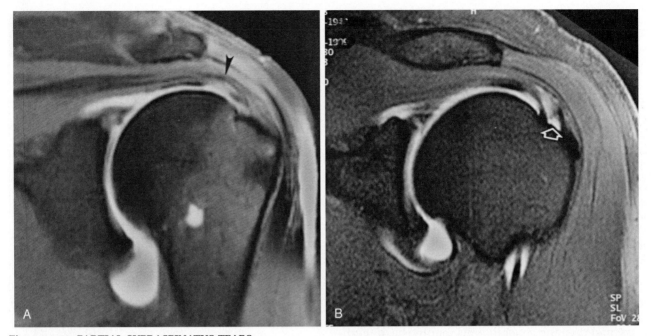

Figure 10–20. PARTIAL SUPRASPINATUS TEARS.
A, T1 fat-suppressed, coronal oblique shoulder MR arthrogram. There is a focal defect in the undersurface of the distal supraspinatus tendon *(arrowhead)* that is filled with high-signal contrast, making the abnormality conspicuous. The superior labrum has high signal from a tear also. *B,* T1 fat-suppressed, coronal oblique shoulder MR arthrogram (different patient than in *A*). High-signal contrast fills a longitudinal tear of the distal supraspinatus tendon *(open arrow)*. The inferior portion of the tendon has torn off of the tuberosity and is retracted slightly medially.

A full-thickness tear, in addition to pain, results in limited active movements of abduction and requires more involved surgery than that performed for a partial tear. MR is less sensitive for detecting partial thickness tears of the supraspinatus tendon than full-thickness tears. The specificity is in the range of 90%, but the sensitivity of standard MRI for detecting partial thickness tears is somewhere between 35% and 90%; these figures are significantly improved with MR arthrography.

Full-Thickness Tears. Direct evidence of a full-thickness tear by conventional MRI (not MR arthrography) consists of discontinuity of the tendon with high signal intensity fluid traversing the gap between the tendon fragments from the articular to the bursal surfaces of the tendon on T2W sequences (Fig. 10–21). MR arthrography demonstrates high signal gadolinium on T1W images in the glenohumeral joint, as well as in the subacromial/subdeltoid bursa with discontinuity of the tendon, and gadolinium filling the gap between disrupted tendon fragments (Fig. 10–22). MR also can demonstrate the size of the tear, the degree of retraction of fragments, the quality of the remaining tendon fragments, and if there is associated muscle atrophy or osseous abnormalities; these features should be commented on in the report. Muscle atrophy is seen as high signal intensity within the muscle on T1W images (Fig. 10–23).

A supraspinatus tendon tear usually is located distally in the supraspinatus tendon, either near its attachment to the greater tuberosity or in the critical zone of the tendon located about 1 cm proximal to its insertion. Tears usually start in the anterior portion of the distal supraspinatus tendon and propagate posteriorly. Complete disruption of fibers in the craniocaudal direction with communication between the joint and bursa indicate a full-thickness tear, even if it has not separated the tendons completely in the anteroposterior direction.

Disruption of the supraspinatus tendon is not always clearly evident or easy to diagnose by standard MRI. Granulation tissue or debris may obscure the tear, the tear may be very small, or it may be located far anteriorly, all of which make the diagnosis much more difficult. These difficulties can be alleviated with MR arthrography, which provides much more information (Fig. 10–22). Without benefit of MR arthrography, secondary evidence of a full-thickness tear may be helpful and may include (1) medial retraction of the musculotendinous junction that normally is located at the 12 o'clock position of the humeral head (or just lateral to the acromioclavicular joint); (2) focal thinning and irregular, indistinct margins of the tendon; (3) associated subacromial/subdeltoid bursal fluid, which also may be seen with partial tears, or represent an isolated bursitis, and is certainly not a specific finding for a completely torn tendon; and (4) atrophy of the supraspinatus muscle with fatty infiltration, which again is not specific for a tendon tear.

The sensitivity and specificity for full-thickness rotator cuff tears by MR are over 90%. MR arthrography improves these figures, as well as increases the confidence with which the diagnoses are made. The ability of MR to demonstrate complete tears of the

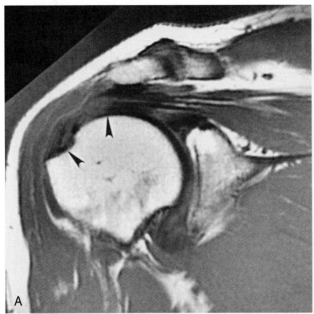

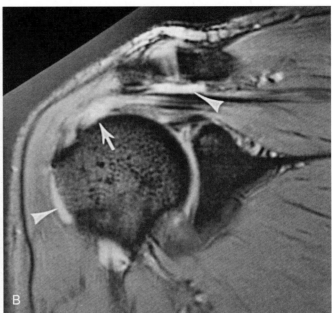

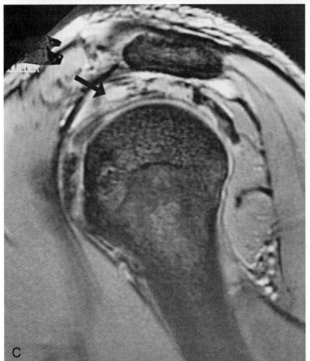

Figure 10–21. COMPLETE SUPRASPINATUS TEAR.
A, T1 coronal oblique image, shoulder. The distal 2 cm of the supraspinatus tendon (between *arrowheads*) is intermediate, rather than the normal low signal intensity, and thickened. *B,* T2* coronal oblique image, shoulder. High-signal fluid *(arrow)* fills the defect in the supraspinatus tendon. Fluid is present in the subacromial/subdeltoid bursa *(arrowheads)*. There is no retraction of the musculotendinous junction. *C,* T2* sagittal oblique image, shoulder. There is focal high signal *(arrow)* in the defect of the torn supraspinatus tendon, where normally a low-signal oval tendon should be evident.

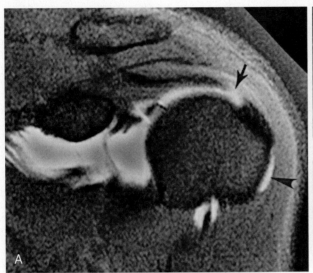

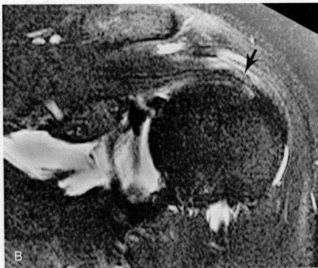

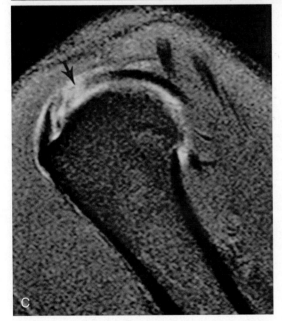

Figure 10–22. COMPLETE SUPRASPINATUS TEAR.
A, T1 fat-suppressed coronal oblique shoulder MR arthrogram. A small full-thickness tear *(arrow)* of the distal supraspinatus tendon is seen with contrast in the subacromial/subdeltoid bursa *(arrowhead).* **B,** Fast T2 fat-suppressed coronal oblique shoulder MR arthrogram. Despite the obvious tendon tear in *A* above, the defect in the tendon is not evident in this sequence *(arrow).* Fluid is evident in the bursa, but this does not prove that it is in communication with fluid from the joint. This emphasizes that making the diagnosis of a tendon tear without a dedicated MR arthrogram can be difficult and misleading, even with full-thickness tears. The diagnosis would be even more difficult if the joint had not been distended with injected fluid. **C,** T1 fat-suppressed sagittal oblique shoulder MR arthrogram. The defect in the supraspinatus tendon is easily seen *(arrow),* and contrast also is noted in the overlying bursa.

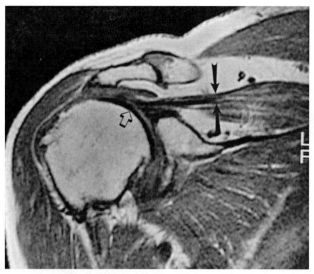

Figure 10–23. COMPLETE SUPRASPINATUS TEAR WITH SECONDARY SIGNS.
T1 coronal oblique image, shoulder. The end of the torn supraspinatus tendon is seen *(open arrow)*. There are secondary signs of a tendon tear with medial retraction of the musculotendinous junction *(solid arrows)*, atrophy of the muscle with fatty infiltration, and a decreased acromiohumeral interval. There are degenerative changes of the acromioclavicular and glenohumeral joints, as well as a subacromial spur.

rotator cuff tendons is significantly better than for partial thickness tears.

Long Head of the Biceps (Box 10–6)

Tears. The long head of the biceps tendon is completely torn in about 7% of patients with supraspi-

---

BOX 10–6: LONG HEAD OF BICEPS TENDON

Tears/Degeneration
- Attachment to superior labrum
  — Associated with SLAP lesions
- Proximal to bicipital groove
  — Associated with impingement
  — Associated with supraspinatus tears
  — Older population
- Musculotendinous junction
  — Acute, traumatic injuries
  — Younger population

Dislocation
- Associated disruptions
  — Transverse humeral ligament
  — Usually subscapularis tendon
- MRI
  — Empty bicipital groove (axial)
  — Tendon displaced medially, either anterior to or within glenohumeral joint
  — Subscapularis tendon avulsed from tuberosity (or may be intact)

---

natus tendon tears and is abnormal (degeneration or partial tears) in about one third.[21] Its proximity to the supraspinatus tendon makes it vulnerable to forces of impingement identical to those affecting the supraspinatus tendon. Long head of the biceps tendon tears associated with supraspinatus tendon tears occur in the impingement zone just proximal to the bicipital groove, and usually occur in older individuals. The distal tendon fragment and the muscle may retract distally, and an empty bicipital groove may be demonstrated on axial MR images of the shoulder (Fig. 10–24). Acute tears of the long head of the biceps tendon may occur with severe trauma in young individuals or in older "weekend" athletes. Acute tears unrelated to impingement generally occur distally in the tendon, near the musculotendinous junction.

Dislocation. Other abnormalities of the long head of the biceps tendon may occur, unassociated with impingement. Acute trauma can cause avulsion, subluxation, or dislocation of the tendon, which need to be repaired surgically. In order for subluxation or dislocation to occur, there must be disruption of the transverse humeral ligament that normally bridges the lesser and greater tuberosities and holds the long head of the biceps tendon in place. Usually, a tear of the subscapularis tendon also coexists. With dislocation, the long head of the biceps tendon may displace anteromedially, which may or may not be associated with an intact subscapularis tendon. It may dislocate medially within the shoulder joint, which is always associated with a tear of the subscapularis tendon at its attachment to the lesser tuberosity.[22, 23] Biceps tendon subluxation and dislocation are demonstrated best on axial MR images, where the bicipital groove is empty and the low-signal round tendon is seen at variable distances medial to the groove, either deep or superficial to the subscapularis tendon (Fig. 10–25).

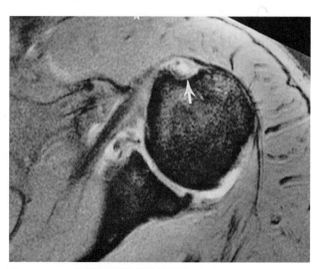

Figure 10–24. BICEPS TENDON TEAR.
T2* axial image, shoulder. The bicipital groove *(arrow)* is empty, without evidence of the oval, low-signal long head of the biceps tendon, indicating a complete rupture.

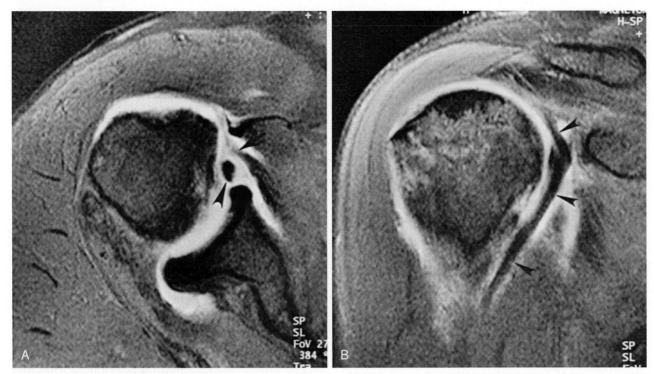

Figure 10–25. DISLOCATED BICEPS TENDON.
A, T1 fat-suppressed axial shoulder MR arthrogram. The bicipital groove is empty. The biceps tendon *(arrowhead)* is located over the anterior glenohumeral joint and posterior to the subscapularis tendon *(arrow)*, which has been avulsed from its attachment to the lesser tuberosity of the humerus. *B,* T1 fat-suppressed coronal oblique shoulder MR arthrogram. The biceps tendon *(arrowheads)* is dislocated medially overlying the shoulder joint.

Infraspinatus

Infraspinatus tendon tears can be seen in isolation after acute trauma, can occur in association with massive tears of the supraspinatus tendon, or can be associated with posterosuperior impingement of the shoulder (Fig. 10–26).

Posterosuperior Impingement (Box 10–7). This condition refers to impingement of the supraspinatus tendon, and mainly of the infraspinatus ten-

don, between the humeral head and the posterior glenoid rim during overhead movements with abduction and external rotation, such as pitching.[24] Posterosuperior impingement results in abnormali-

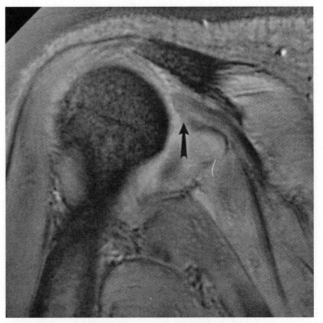

Figure 10–26. INFRASPINATUS TENDON TEAR.
T2* coronal oblique image, shoulder. The end of the torn infraspinatus tendon *(arrow)* is seen retracted inferomedially to its normal attachment to the posterolateral humerus.

BOX 10–7: POSTEROSUPERIOR IMPINGEMENT SYNDROME

Clinical
- Impingement of infra- and supraspinatus tendons between humeral head and posterosuperior labrum
- Occurs in late cocking phase of pitching
- Occurs with maximum abduction and external rotation
- Posterosuperior pain and anterior instability

MRI
- Humeral cysts adjacent to infraspinatus tendon insertion
- Infraspinatus (and supraspinatus) tendon undersurface tears
- Posterosuperior labral tear

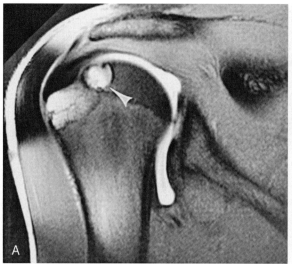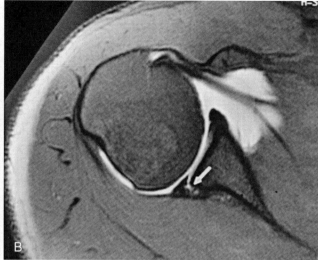

Figure 10–27. POSTERIOR IMPINGEMENT.
A, T1 fat-suppressed coronal oblique shoulder MR arthrogram. There is a large cyst in the posterolateral humeral head *(arrowhead)* that is filled with contrast at the site of impaction between the humeral head and posterior labrum during overhead movements. There is incomplete fat suppression in this image, with fat remaining high signal laterally. *B,* T1 fat-suppressed axial shoulder MR arthrogram. The posterior labrum is detached from the adjacent glenoid *(arrow).*

ties affecting the rotator cuff, most commonly the infraspinatus tendon, the posterior superior labrum, and the humeral head at the point of impaction with the posterosuperior glenoid. These patients present with posterior shoulder pain and may have associated anterior shoulder instability. MR findings include degenerative cysts on the posterior aspect of the humeral head near the insertion of the infraspinatus tendon; fraying, partial, or complete tears of the infraspinatus tendon or supraspinatus tendon; and fraying or tears of the posterior glenoid labrum (Fig. 10–27).

Subscapularis (Box 10–8)

Subscapularis tendon tears are relatively common.[25] They can result from acute trauma on an adducted arm in hyperextension or in external rota-

tion. They can result from an anterior shoulder dislocation, be associated with massive tears of the rotator cuff and with biceps tendon dislocations, or they can result from subcoracoid impingement. Subcoracoid impingement is caused by narrowing of the space between the tip of the coracoid process and the humerus, which may be congenital in origin or may result from a coracoid fracture or surgery. The narrowed space can result in impingement on, and resultant tears of, the subscapularis tendon (Fig. 10–28).[26]

Tears of the subscapularis tendon are best evaluated on axial MR images where the entire length of the tendon is evident (Fig. 10–28), or on sagittal images. The tears are seen best on T2W images or on T1W images after intraarticular gadolinium injection. Tears may be seen as tendon discontinuity, contrast media entering into the tendon substance, intrasubstance abnormal tendon signal, abnormal caliber of the tendon, and abnormal position of the tendon. Other helpful accessory signs are the leakage of intraarticular contrast under the insertion of the subscapularis tendon onto the lesser tuberosity and fatty atrophy of the subscapularis muscle, usually localized at the cranial aspect of the muscle and seen as high signal intensity streaks on T1W images. Abnormalities in the course of the long head of the biceps tendon (subluxation or dislocation) usually are associated with subscapularis tendon tears.[27] They often extend into the subscapularis muscle.

Massive Cuff Tears

Massive rotator cuff tears usually are seen in older patients with either marked tendon degeneration or with predisposing factors such as an associated

---

BOX 10–8: SUBSCAPULARIS TENDON TEARS

Associations
• Anterior shoulder dislocations
• Long head, biceps tendon dislocations
• Massive rotator cuff tears
• Subcoracoid impingement
MRI
• Evaluate on axial images
— Detachment from lesser tuberosity
— ↑ signal, thin, thick
— Contrast over the lesser tuberosity
— Associated tendon abnormalities

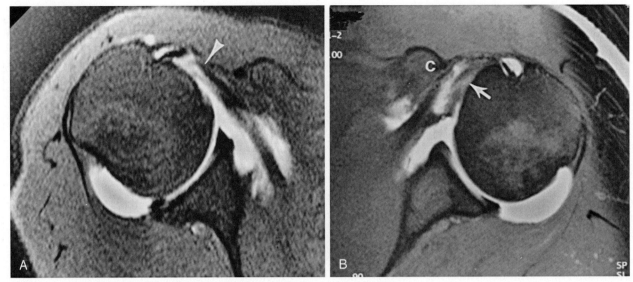

Figure 10–28. SUBSCAPULARIS TENDON TEARS; SUBCORACOID IMPINGEMENT.
A, T1 fat-suppressed axial shoulder MR arthrogram. The subscapularis has been detached from the lesser tuberosity *(arrowhead).* The biceps tendon is subluxed medially from the bicipital groove. Contrast covers the lesser tuberosity. *B,* T1 fat-suppressed axial shoulder MR arthrogram (different patient than in *A*). The coracoid process (C) was excessively long in this patient, causing narrowing of the space between it and the humerus (subcoracoid impingement). This is associated with tears of the subscapularis tendon, as was evident in this case *(arrow).* The tendon is thickened, longitudinally split, and filled with contrast.

inflammatory arthritis or diabetes, or who have been on long-term steroid therapy. These massive tears affect multiple tendons of the rotator cuff, with full-thickness tears, musculotendinous retraction, and muscle atrophy (Fig. 10–29). There is a large communication between the glenohumeral joint and the subacromial/subdeltoid bursa and, in some patients,

there will be development of a synovial cyst that extends through the acromioclavicular joint and forms a soft tissue mass on the superior aspect of the shoulder, which may be large. Associated bone changes consist of superior migration of the humeral head with associated subacromial degenerative changes and severe degenerative joint disease of the

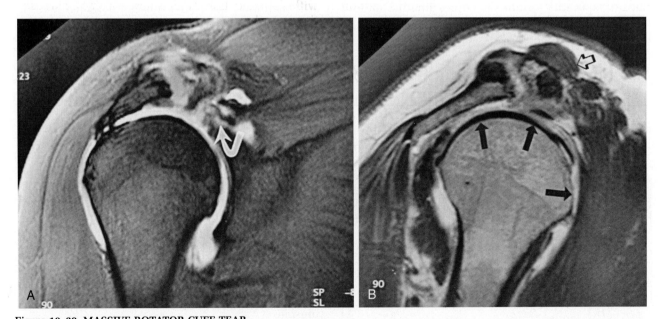

Figure 10–29. MASSIVE ROTATOR CUFF TEAR.
A, T1 fat-suppressed coronal oblique shoulder MR arthrogram. The supraspinatus tendon is torn and retracted a long distance medially *(curved arrow).* There is narrowing between the acromion and humeral head because of absence of the tendon. The acromioclavicular joint is degenerated, and high-signal contrast fills it from the glenohumeral joint injection. *B,* T1 sagittal oblique shoulder MR arthrogram. The superior mass *(open arrow)* is a small synovial cyst arising from the acromioclavicular joint. There is absence of tendons overlying the humeral head, indicating multiple tendon tears with retraction. *Solid arrows* point to the sites where the infraspinatus, supraspinatus, and subscapularis tendons (from left [posterior] to right [anterior]) should be seen, but are absent. The biceps tendon remains intact *(middle arrow),* but no supraspinatus is seen above it.

glenohumeral joint with osteophyte formation and subchondral cysts.

Rotator Interval Abnormalities
(Box 10–9)

The rotator cuff interval is a triangular space between the supraspinatus tendon and the subscapularis tendon (Fig. 10–30).[28] The base of the triangle is at the coracoid process, which separates the supraspinatus and subscapularis tendons. The apex of the triangular rotator interval is at the transverse humeral ligament, which forms the roof of the bicipital groove. The superior and inferior margins of the interval are formed by the supraspinatus and subscapularis tendons, respectively. The anterior aspect of the interval is formed by the capsule and coracohumeral ligament. The long biceps tendon courses through the rotator interval. This is the site on the anterior shoulder where arthroscopists enter the shoulder joint in order to avoid damaging tendons.

Rotator cuff interval tears may occur secondary to anterior glenohumeral dislocations or glenohumeral instability, or may represent a surgical defect from arthroscopy (Fig. 10–30). The tears are demonstrated best on T2W or postcontrast T1W sagittal oblique images. When torn, the rotator interval may become patulous, and contrast is identified extending anterosuperiorly through the coracohumeral ligament and the capsule (superior glenohumeral ligament).[4] These tears may communicate with the subacromial subdeltoid bursa, mimicking a rotator cuff tear on a shoulder MR arthrogram, without a distinct tendon tear of the rotator cuff being identified.

BOX 10–9: ROTATOR INTERVAL

Rotator interval bordered by:
- Anteriorly: coracohumeral ligament, superior glenohumeral ligament, and capsule
- Superiorly: supraspinatus tendon
- Inferiorly: supscapularis tendon
- Medially: coracoid process
- Laterally: transverse humeral ligament
- Long biceps tendon courses through the interval

Rotator interval tears from:
- Anterior shoulder dislocations
- Anterior instability
- Arthroscopy

MRI, rotator interval abnormalities
- Patulous rotator interval (sagittal oblique)
- High signal intensity through coracohumeral ligament and capsule, if torn
- May communicate with subacromial/ subdeltoid bursa, if torn

---

INSTABILITY

After impingement, instability is the major abnormality that affects the shoulder. Glenohumeral instability and impingement often coexist. Instability of the shoulder refers to subluxation or dislocation of the glenohumeral joint that may be traumatic or atraumatic in origin. It is a painful disorder that, with the exception of an acute episode of dislocation, may be difficult to diagnose.

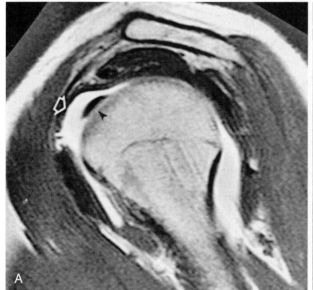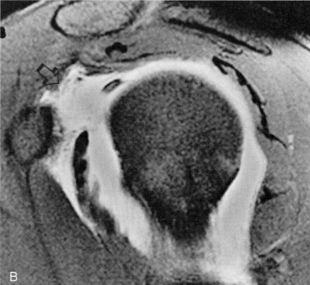

Figure 10–30. ROTATOR INTERVAL: NORMAL AND ABNORMAL.
A, T1 sagittal oblique shoulder MR arthrogram. The normal rotator interval is seen *(open arrow)* between the supraspinatus tendon superiorly and the subscapularis tendon inferiorly. The biceps tendon runs through the interval *(arrowhead)*. **B,** T1 fat-suppressed sagittal oblique shoulder MR arthrogram (different patient than in *A*). The rotator interval *(open arrow)* is patulous and irregular due to a previous anterior shoulder dislocation.

Stability of the shoulder joint is dependent on a combination of soft tissue and osseous structures surrounding and forming the glenohumeral joint. There is no isolated abnormality that accounts for instability, but rather a combination of different factors interacting with one another. Contributing factors to glenohumeral instability include labral abnormalities, a lax or torn joint capsule, deficient or torn glenohumeral ligaments, shallow or abnormal glenoid version, and Hill-Sachs and Bankart fractures from previous dislocations.

Shoulder instability can be separated clinically into two groups: functional and anatomic. With functional instability, the joint is stable on physical examination, but the patient has symptoms of clicking, pain, intermittent locking, and a subjective feeling of an unstable joint. These patients often have labral abnormalities that cause pain without clinical evidence of instability. With anatomic instability, the patient usually has recurrent episodes of subluxation or dislocation, is symptomatic, and has signs of instability on physical examination.

The different types of instabilities are (1) anterior, (2) posterior, (3) multidirectional, and (4) superior. The most common type of unstable joint subluxes or dislocates anteriorly (95%). Posterior and multidirectional instability account for most of the other 5% of all instabilities of the shoulder. Superior instability generally is associated with multidirectional instability, and superior subluxation of the humeral head may create impingement when the supraspinatus tendon is repeatedly trapped between the coracoacromial arch and the humeral head. As a consequence of any of the different types of instabilities, hypertrophy of the greater tuberosity, subacromial spur formation, and thickening of the coracoacromial ligament associated with glenohumeral osteophyte formation may develop and lead to a secondary impingement syndrome involving the rotator cuff (Box 10–10).

Many patients have instability secondary to a recognized previous traumatic dislocation. Many others have no history of a specific inciting event. It is common for athletes engaged in repetitive throwing or overhead activities such as baseball pitchers, football quarterbacks, tennis players, and swimmers (throwing oneself on the couch generally is not a risk factor) to have instability but no acute traumatic event that caused it. These athletes acquire an increased laxity of the anterior supporting structures of the shoulder in order to allow an increased range of motion, in particular in external rotation. In addition to overuse and abuse, congenital abnormalities may contribute to shoulder instability. These congenital predisposing factors include osseous abnormalities, such as congenital deficiency of the depth and radius of curvature of the glenoid fossa, and abnormal version angle of the glenoid; or soft tissue abnormalities, such as a medial (type III) capsular insertion, congenitally small or absent glenohumeral ligaments, and congenital capsular and ligamentous laxity.

BOX 10–10: GLENOHUMERAL INSTABILITY

- Subluxation or dislocation of joint
- Often coexists with impingement
  — May cause secondary impingement
- Multiple structures responsible
  — Bones, labrum, capsule, ligaments
- Clinical
  — Functional: subjective instability; clinically stable. Labral tears often are present.
  — Anatomic: subjective instability; instability on examination
- Types
  — Anterior (95%)
  — Posterior, superior, multidirectional (5%)
- Causes
  — Acute traumatic dislocation (causes disruption of several structures critical to stability that predispose to subsequent instability)
  — Chronic, repetitive overhead motions (throwing), without an acute injury
  — Congenital
    Osseous: dysplastic glenoid
    Far medial (type III) anterior capsular attachment
    Capsular/ligamentous laxity

Regardless of the type of abnormality present, or which instability pattern exists, MR arthrography is undoubtedly the best imaging study to evaluate for them.

Anatomy Relating to Instability

Capsule

The joint capsule attaches laterally on the anatomic neck of the humerus. Medially, the capsule usually attaches to the labrum or to the adjacent periosteum of the glenoid. Three types of anterior capsular insertions have been described: type I consists of a medial attachment on or very near the labrum, a type II insertion is found within one cm medial to the labrum, and a type III capsular attachment is more than one cm medial to the labrum. It is believed that a type III anterior capsular insertion may either predispose to instability or represent the sequelae of a previous dislocation with stripping of the anterior capsule and periosteum off the glenoid. The posterior capsule attaches directly on the posterior glenoid labrum.

Glenohumeral Ligaments
(Box 10–11)

The glenohumeral ligaments represent thickenings of the anterior joint capsule. The three ligaments are the superior, middle, and inferior glenohumeral ligaments. They extend from the anterior aspect of the glenoid to the lesser tuberosity of the humerus. When viewed en face, the three ligaments form a Z configuration (Fig. 10–31). Numerous variations of size and position have been described. The *superior glenohumeral ligament* originates from the region of the superior glenoid tubercle anterior to the origin of the long head of the biceps tendon and inserts on the superior aspect of the lesser tuberosity, blending with fibers of the coracohumeral ligament. The *middle glenohumeral ligament* is the most variable of the three glenohumeral ligaments and is absent in about 30% of shoulders, but its absence does not seem to increase the incidence of instability. It arises most frequently below the superior glenohumeral ligament on the anterior superior aspect of the labrum and inserts onto the medial aspect of the lesser tuberosity of the humerus. The *inferior glenohumeral ligament* is the main stabilizing ligament of the shoulder. It is composed of an anterior and a posterior band, with an intervening axillary pouch or recess. The anterior and posterior bands arise from the inferior two thirds of the anterior and posterior portions of the labrum, respectively, and they extend laterally to attach to the surgical neck of the humerus.[29–32]

The superior glenohumeral ligament is seen at the level of the body of the coracoid process on axial MR images and parallels this osseous structure (Fig. 10–32). The middle glenohumeral ligament is seen at and just inferior to the level of the tip of the coracoid process on axial cuts, and lies deep to the subscapularis tendon and adjacent to the anterior labrum, where it can mimic a torn labral fragment (Fig. 10–32). The inferior glenohumeral ligament is seen on axial images through the inferior aspect of the gle-

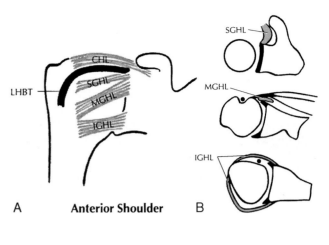

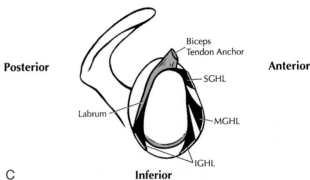

Figure 10–31. NORMAL SUPERIOR, MIDDLE, AND INFERIOR GLENOHUMERAL LIGAMENTS (SGHL, MGHL, IGHL).
A, Diagram of the GHLs en face from a coronal perspective, forming the Z configuration. The coracohumeral ligament (CHL) and long head of the biceps tendon (LHBT) are also shown. *B,* Diagram of the GHLs from an axial perspective. The SGHL parallels the coracoid process. The MGHL runs anterior to the anterior labrum at the level of the subscapularis tendon. The anterior and posterior limbs of the IGHL attach to the anterior and posterior labrum. *C,* Diagram of the GHLs from a sagittal perspective. The ligaments attach to the labrum and are a thickening of the joint capsule.

---

noid, attaching to the anterior and posterior labrum. The glenohumeral ligaments also can be identified well on sagittal oblique images (Fig. 10–32).

The glenohumeral ligaments contribute to the stability of the shoulder joint in several ways. The superior glenohumeral ligament prevents inferior displacement of the humerus when the shoulder is abducted. The middle glenohumeral ligament contributes to anterior stability in concert with the subscapularis tendon. The inferior glenohumeral ligament is the most important of the glenohumeral ligaments for anterior and posterior joint stabilization. It limits anterior translation of the humeral head with abduction and external rotation of the arm, and limits posterior translation with the shoulder in internal rotation.

The glenohumeral labroligamentous complex (the glenohumeral ligaments in combination with the labrum) to some extent passively stabilizes the glenohumeral joint. Although the labrum deepens the concavity of the glenoid fossa, its function as a

---

BOX 10–11: GLENOHUMERAL LIGAMENTS

Superior
- From supraglenoid tubercle to lesser tuberosity
- At body of coracoid on axial MR
- Limits inferior subluxation

Middle
- From supraglenoid tubercle to lesser tuberosity
- At inferior tip of coracoid, behind subscapularis tendon on axial MRI
- Variable to absent in 30%

Inferior
- From inferior glenoid labrum to anatomic neck of humerus
- Anterior and posterior bands
- Provides anterior and posterior stability
- Seen on inferior halves of labrum on sagittal oblique and axial MRI

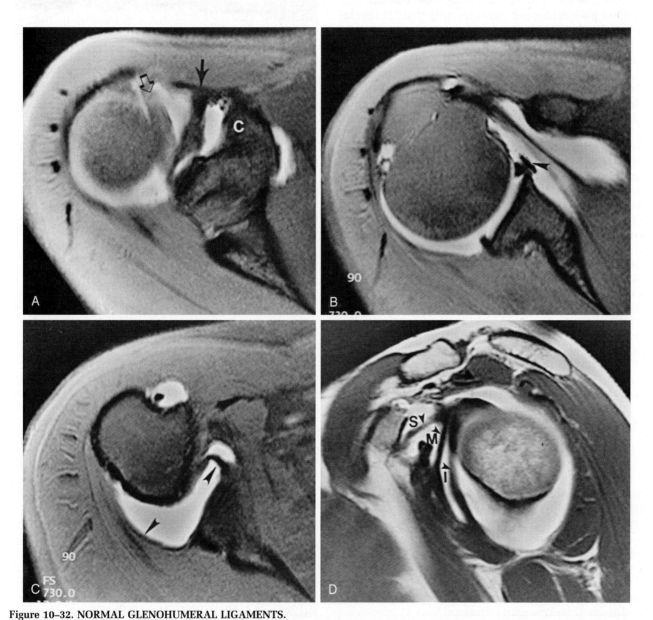

Figure 10–32. NORMAL GLENOHUMERAL LIGAMENTS.
A, T1 fat-suppressed axial shoulder MR arthrogram. The low-signal superior glenohumeral ligament *(solid arrow)* parallels the coracoid process (C) from the capsule to attach to the superior aspect of the anterior labrum. The biceps tendon *(open arrow)* also passes through the superior joint to anchor to the superior labrum. ***B,*** T1 fat-suppressed axial shoulder MR arthrogram. The linear, low-signal middle glenohumeral ligament *(arrowhead)* is located just anterior to the anterior labrum at the level of the subscapularis tendon. It may mimic a torn labrum. ***C,*** T1 fat-suppressed axial shoulder MR arthrogram. The anterior and posterior limbs of the inferior glenohumeral ligaments *(arrowheads)* extend from the humerus to the anterior and posterior glenoid labrum in the inferior shoulder joint. ***D,*** T1 sagittal oblique shoulder MR arthrogram. The glenohumeral ligaments are outlined by contrast in the anterior joint, extending from the anterior labrum to the joint capsule. S—superior, M—middle, I—inferior glenohumeral ligaments.

mechanical barrier against humeral subluxation is much less important than its function as an attachment site for the glenohumeral ligaments. Because the labrum and ligamentous collagen fibers intertwine to form a very strong histologic bond, injury is more likely to occur between the labrum and osseous glenoid (labral detachment) than at the labroligamentous junction.

The position of the shoulder and rotation of the humeral head at the time of injury determines which glenohumeral ligament develops excessive tension and, therefore, where the labral abnormality will develop. The injury most likely to lead to anterior instability of the shoulder occurs with the shoulder abducted and externally rotated, which places stress on the anterior limb of the inferior glenohumeral ligament. The ligament is taut in this position, and excessive stress leads to detachment or tear of the anterior labrum or the anterior band of the inferior glenohumeral ligament. It has been shown that imaging the shoulder in **AB**duction and **E**xternal **R**otation (ABER position) tightens the inferior glenohumeral labroligamentous complex, rendering labral tears more conspicuous.[33] This position is rarely used in our practice, however, because it considerably increases the length of time to perform an examination because of the need to reposition the patient and change surface coils.

Labrum

The labrum is a redundant fold of the joint capsule made of fibrocartilaginous tissue that attaches to the rim of the glenoid of the scapula. It serves to deepen the glenoid fossa and is the attachment site for the long head of the biceps tendon and of the glenohumeral ligaments. The glenohumeral ligaments, together with the labrum, constitute the glenohumeral labroligamentous complex. Frequently, there is a rim of hyaline cartilage interposed between the labrum and the underlying osseous glenoid, which is seen as a line of high signal intensity (the same signal as hyaline cartilage) partially separating the labrum from the glenoid (Fig. 10–33). This should not be mistaken for an avulsion or a tear of the labrum. The labrum is normally low signal intensity on all pulse sequences. It may be affected by the magic-angle phenomenon, and it also may develop myxoid degeneration with aging; in both instances, there is intrasubstance globular intermediate signal intensity on MR images. The anterior and posterior portions of the labrum are seen best on axial images (Fig. 10–34), whereas the superior labrum is depicted optimally on coronal oblique images (Fig. 10–33). The labrum may have a wide variety of shapes on MRI in asymptomatic individuals (Fig. 10–34). The most common labral shapes are triangular, followed by rounded, then cleaved, notched, flat, and absent, in decreasing order of frequency.[34, 35]

Normal Variants of the Labrum (Box 10–12). In addition to the variations in the normal shape of the

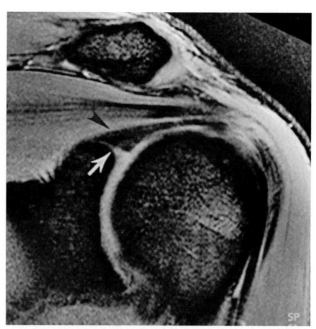

Figure 10–33. NORMAL SUPERIOR LABRUM.
T2* coronal oblique image, shoulder. The superior labrum *(arrowhead)* is seen best in this plane. The biceps tendon is seen in continuity with the labrum, where it forms its anchor. There is undercutting of hyaline cartilage on the glenoid deep to the labrum, which creates linear high signal *(arrow)* that is normal and must not be misinterpreted as a labral detachment. A portion of the labrum is clearly attached to the osseous glenoid.

labrum, there are two normal structures that may mimic tears of the superior labrum. Undercutting of articular cartilage between the labrum and the glenoid cortex or the presence of a synovial recess (sulcus) interposed between the glenoid rim and the labrum may mimic labral tears. These two normal variants follow the contour of the glenoid (go with the flow of the glenoid) (Fig. 10–35), whereas tears of the superior labrum are oriented laterally into the labrum (go against the flow or do not follow the contour of the glenoid) on coronal oblique images. Other normal variants occur at the anterosuperior aspect of the glenoid, including labral detachment from the glenoid (sublabral foramen) or congenital

---

BOX 10–12: ANTEROSUPERIOR LABRAL NORMAL VARIANTS

Sublabral foramen
• Anterior superior labrum not attached to glenoid
Buford complex
• Anterior superior labrum congenitally absent, thick middle glenohumeral ligament
Sublabral foramen versus SLAP
• Sublabral foramen does not extend posterior to the biceps attachment, whereas SLAP does

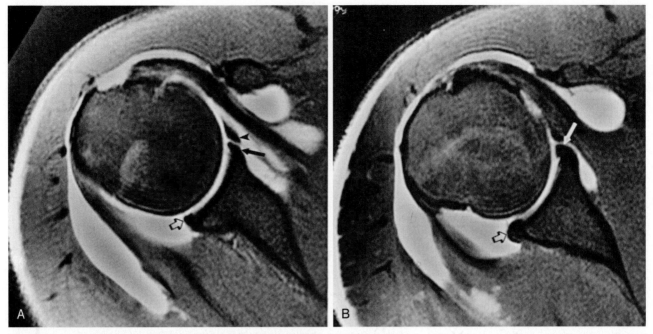

Figure 10–34. NORMAL ANTERIOR AND POSTERIOR GLENOID LABRUM.
A, T1 fat-suppressed axial shoulder MR arthrogram. The anterior labrum *(solid arrow)* and posterior labrum *(open arrow)* have a triangular, low-signal appearance. The middle glenohumeral ligament *(arrowhead)* is seen anterior to the anterior labrum. *B,* T1 fat-suppressed axial shoulder MR arthrogram (different patient than in *A*). The anterior labrum is triangular *(solid white arrow),* but the posterior labrum is rounded *(open arrow),* which is one of several normal variations in labral configuration.

absence of the labrum (Buford complex) (Fig. 10–36).[36–39]

A detached anterosuperior labrum, which is of no clinical significance, is referred to as a *sublabral foramen* or hole.[39] The anterior labrum is separated from the osseous glenoid superiorly, but reattaches to the glenoid in its mid to inferior portion (Fig. 10–37). The labrum must not be detached at any point posterior to the attachment of the long head of the biceps tendon (the biceps anchor), or else it is not a sublabral foramen, but a traumatic labral detachment instead.

Another normal labral variant is a congenitally absent anterosuperior labrum, which is associated with a markedly thickened middle glenohumeral ligament; this combination of findings is known as the *Buford complex* (Fig. 10–38).[38] Distinguishing between a sublabral foramen and a Buford complex with a thick middle glenohumeral ligament occasionally may be difficult. The thick middle glenohumeral ligament in the Buford complex can be seen to blend with the anterior joint capsule as the axial images progress inferiorly. Conversely, with a sublabral foramen, the labrum attaches to the glenoid

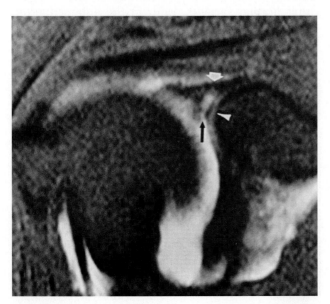

Figure 10–35. NORMAL SUPERIOR LABRUM: CARTILAGE UNDERCUTTING AND SULCUS PITFALLS.
T1 fat-suppressed coronal oblique shoulder MR arthrogram. The triangular superior labrum is attached to the glenoid *(white arrow).* The normal hyaline cartilage *(arrowhead)* that is interposed between the labrum and glenoid is lower signal than the gadolinium solution and must not be confused with a detached or torn labrum. Just lateral to the cartilage is the normal sulcus *(black arrow),* which is interposed between the labrum and the hyaline cartilage and filled with contrast. Both the sulcus and the undercutting of the cartilage are following the contour of the glenoid, pointing medially. Labral tears diverge from the glenoid (are directed laterally).

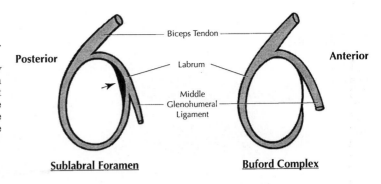

Figure 10–36. ANTEROSUPERIOR LABRAL VARIANTS.
Diagram of the sublabral foramen on the left. The *arrow* points to the gap between the anterosuperior labrum and the glenoid (the sublabral foramen), which does not extend posterior to the biceps tendon anchor. On the right is the Buford complex: congenital absence of the anterosuperior labrum with a larger-than-usual middle glenohumeral ligament.

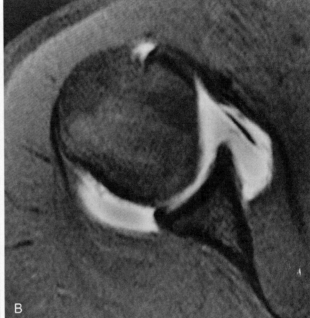

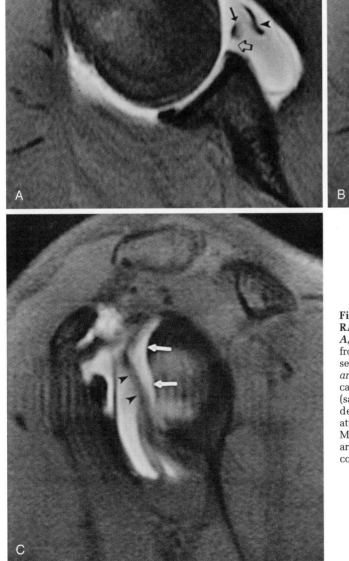

Figure 10–37. NORMAL LABRAL VARIANT: SUBLABRAL FORAMEN.
A, T1 fat-suppressed axial shoulder MR arthrogram. An image from the upper joint shows the anterior labrum *(solid arrow)* separated from the glenoid with contrast filling the space *(open arrow).* The middle glenohumeral ligament *(arrowhead)* is located anterior to the labrum. *B,* T1 fat-suppressed axial image (same sequence as in *A*). A cut obtained lower in the joint demonstrates the anterior labrum is present and solidly attached to the glenoid. *C,* T1 fat-suppressed sagittal shoulder MR arthrogram. The anterosuperior labrum *(arrowheads)* is separated from the anterior margin of the glenoid *(arrows),* with contrast between the two structures.

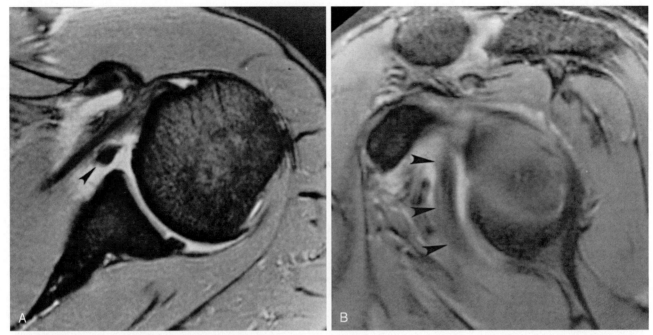

Figure 10–38. NORMAL LABRAL VARIANT: BUFORD COMPLEX.
A, T1 fat-suppressed axial shoulder MR arthrogram. No labrum is attached to the anterosuperior portion of the glenoid. The round, low-signal structure anterior to the glenoid *(arrowhead)* blended with the anterior joint capsule on lower images through the joint. Thus, this is an enlarged middle glenohumeral ligament with absence of the anterosuperior labrum. *B*, T1 fat-suppressed sagittal shoulder MR arthrogram. The large middle glenohumeral ligament *(arrowheads)* parallels the anterior glenoid, but merges with the anterior capsule distally. Contrast is interposed between the ligament and glenoid.

rather than anteriorly to the joint capsule. These variants are important to recognize on MR in order not to confuse them with significant pathology, but are of no clinical significance.

Instability Lesions

Lesions associated with instability are depicted best with shoulder MR arthrography. They may involve the labrum, the capsule, the glenohumeral ligaments, and the bones in various combinations.[40, 41] Many acronyms and eponyms have been used to name the different abnormalities, and these may **D**rive **Y**ou **N**uts (DYN) (Boxes 10–13 and 10–14).

Capsule

A type III anterior capsular attachment, patulous anterior capsule, thickening and irregularity of the capsule, and capsular shearing or stripping from the scapula can be seen on MRI and indicate anterior instability. MR arthrography with capsular distension may mimic a type III insertion. Traumatic anterior glenohumeral joint dislocation also may be associated with subscapularis tendon tears and enlargement of the subscapularis recess of the joint. The posterior capsule also may show sequelae of a posterior dislocation in the same manner as with the anterior capsule. Capsular abnormalities are best seen on MRI when fluid is present in the joint, as is usually the case with an acute injury. In other circumstances, distension of the joint with MR arthrography is the only reliable means to demonstrate the glenohumeral labroligamentous complex and the joint capsule.

A Bennett lesion is an extraarticular posterior capsular avulsive injury associated with a posterior labral injury (Box 10–15).[42] This injury is seen most commonly in pitchers, and occurs from traction of the posterior band of the inferior glenohumeral ligament during the decelerating phase of pitching. A crescent of mineralization can be identified on an axillary radiographic view or, even better, on computed tomography (CT). On MR, this mineralization appears as a low signal intensity band posterior to the posterior labrum on axial images (Fig. 10–39). If left untreated, patients progress from functional to anatomic instability.

Glenohumeral Ligaments

Torn, thickened, or absent glenohumeral ligaments are an MR manifestation of instability. The inferior glenohumeral ligament is the most important stabilizer of the glenohumeral joint and is the most frequently affected with instability. It may be affected at its labral or its humeral attachment. Avulsion of the inferior glenohumeral ligament from the humerus, called a HAGL lesion (**H**umeral **A**vulsion of the **G**lenohumeral **L**igament), may result from shoulder dislocation.[43] It often is associated with a tear of the subscapularis tendon. A **B**ony **H**umeral **A**vulsion of the **G**leno**H**umeral **L**igament (BHAGL) also can occur.

Hill-Sachs defect. This fracture may be seen in any plane of imaging, but is seen best on axial MR images on the two most superior images through the humeral head as a concave defect in the posterolateral aspect of the humeral head (Fig. 10–42). The humeral head is normally round on these superior cuts (above the coracoid process), whereas below this level a posterior flattening of the humerus is a

---

BOX 10–13: ACRONYMS AND EPONYMS OF THE SHOULDER

- **ALPSA**—**A**nterior **L**abroligamentous **P**eriosteal **S**leeve **A**vulsion. A variation of the Bankart lesion with injury to the anteroinferior labrum, but the anterior scapular periosteum is intact.
- **Bankart lesion**—Tear of the anteroinferior glenoid labrum with torn anterior scapular periosteum. May have an associated fracture of the anterior inferior glenoid rim.
- **Bennett lesion**—Mineralization of the ✓ posterior band of the inferior glenohumeral ligament and posterior capsule from chronic traction forces.
- **BHAGL lesion**—**B**ony HAGL lesion (see below).
- **Buford complex**—Congenital absence of the anterior superior glenoid labrum associated with a thickened middle glenohumeral ligament.
- **DYN**—**D**rives **Y**ou **N**uts.
- **GLAD lesion**—**G**leno**L**abral **A**rticular **D**isruption is a tear of the anterior inferior labrum with a glenoid chondral defect.
- **HAGL lesion**—**H**umeral **A**vulsion of the ✓ **G**lenohumeral **L**igament occurs from shoulder dislocation with avulsion of the inferior glenohumeral ligament from the anatomic neck of the humerus.
- **Hill-Sachs lesion**—Impaction fracture posterolateral aspect of the humeral head from anterior shoulder dislocation.
- **SLAP lesion**—**S**uperior **L**abrum tear propagating **A**nterior and **P**osterior to the biceps anchor.

HAGL lesions can be identified on axial, coronal, or sagittal MR images (Fig. 10–40). The inferior glenohumeral ligament may demonstrate high signal intensity on T2 images, may show morphologic disruption at its insertion on the anatomic neck of the humerus and wavy contours of the residual ligament, and the ligament may be displaced inferiorly. The diagnosis also can be inferred on MR arthrography when extravasation of contrast from the joint occurs in the region of the ligament insertion on the humerus.

Bones

The osseous abnormalities associated with instability can either be of developmental origin or acquired. A congenitally steep, retroverted, or shallow glenoid may predispose to instability (Fig. 10–41). An anterior dislocation may produce an acquired osseous abnormality from an impaction fracture on the posterolateral aspect of the humeral head, the

---

BOX 10–14: INSTABILITY: MR Evidence (Axial Images are Best)

Osseous
- Subluxed glenohumeral joint
- Steep, shallow glenoid
- Hill-Sachs fracture
  — Concave posterolateral defect on superior two axial cuts through humeral head (anterior dislocation)
- Bankart fracture
  — Fracture of anterior inferior glenoid rim (anterior dislocation)
- Trough sign ✓ (Reverse Hill-Sachs)
  — Impaction fracture, anteromedial humeral head (posterior dislocation)
- Reverse Bankart ✓
  — Fracture of posterior rim of glenoid (posterior dislocation)

Capsule
- Type III anterior attachment (>1 cm medial to labrum)
- Patulous capsule and stripping from scapula
- Thickened, irregular capsule
- Mineralization posteriorly (Bennett lesion)

Glenohumeral Ligaments
- Torn, thickened, absent, or avulsed
- Inferior ligament most important
  — Avulsion from humerus (HAGL lesion)
  — Avulsion from labrum

Labrum
- Tears, detachment from glenoid, crushed
  — Linear or diffuse ↑ signal in labrum (tears, crush)
  — ↑ signal between labrum and glenoid (detachment)
  — Absent or small labral remnant
- Bankart lesion
  — Detachment of anteroinferior labrum and tear of anterior scapular periosteum, ± glenoid rim fracture
- ALPSA lesion (anterior labroligamentous periosteal sleeve avulsion)
  — Same as Bankart, but scapular periosteum is not torn

Tendons
- Subscapularis
  — Tears, or detaches from tuberosity
- Biceps, long head
  — Dislocates medially

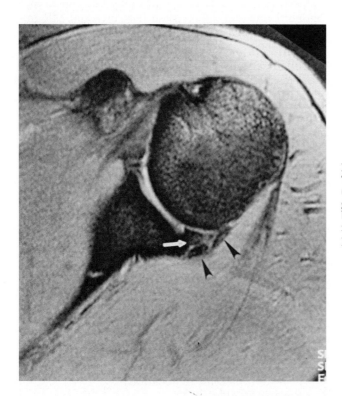

Figure 10–39. BENNETT LESION.
T2* axial image, shoulder. There is thickening and low signal (calcification) in the posterior capsule/posterior limb of the inferior glenohumeral ligament *(arrowheads)*. The adjacent posterior labrum *(arrow)* is normal. This is a traction injury to the capsule from the deceleration phase of pitching. Linear calcification was present on an axillary view radiograph.

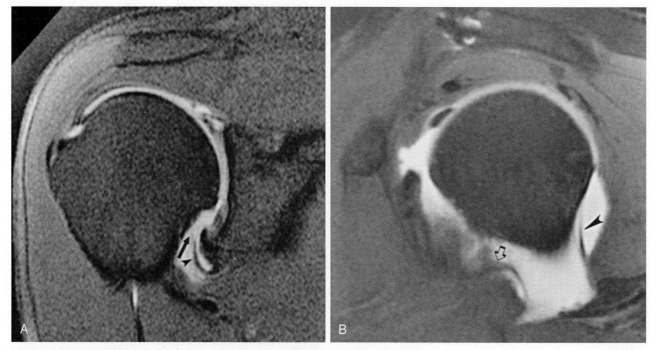

Figure 10–40. HUMERAL AVULSION OF THE GLENOHUMERAL LIGAMENT (HAGL).
A, T1 fat-suppressed coronal oblique shoulder MR arthrogram. The anterior limb of the inferior glenohumeral ligament *(arrowhead)* is detached from the humerus *(arrow)* in this patient with a previous anterior dislocation. There is also a bucket-handle superior labral anterior and posterior (SLAP) tear of the superior labrum. *B,* T1 fat-suppressed sagittal oblique shoulder MR arthrogram (different patient than in *A*). The anterior limb of the inferior glenohumeral ligament *(open arrow)* is avulsed from its humeral attachment, is thickened, and is drooping inferiorly (compare to normal posterior inferior glenohumeral ligament *[arrowhead]*). The patient had several prior dislocations.

BOX 10–15: BENNETT LESION

Clinical
- Baseball pitchers during decelerating phase of throwing
- Traction of posterior limb, inferior glenohumeral ligament on labrum
- Pain and eventually instability

MRI
- Thickened low signal posteroinferior capsule (mineralization)
- May be associated with posterior labral tear

normal appearance (Fig. 10–42).[44] Anterior dislocation of the humeral head also may create a fracture of the anterior inferior glenoid (Bankart fracture). This fracture can be demonstrated best on axial and sagittal oblique images (Fig. 10–43). A posterior shoulder dislocation may result in an impaction fracture of the anteromedial aspect of the humeral head, called a trough lesion, and the posterior aspect of the glenoid, called a reverse Bankart fracture (Fig. 10–44).

Labrum

The labrum may have partial thickness tears, full-thickness tears, be avulsed (traumatically detached) from the glenoid, or be crushed or frayed.[45, 46] There are two labral lesions definitely associated with shoulder instability: Bankart and ALPSA lesions.

The Bankart lesion is the most common injury after anterior dislocation of the glenohumeral joint. It is a detachment of the anterior inferior labrum (with or without labral tears) from the glenoid with a tear of the anterior scapular periosteum (Fig. 10–45). The Bankart lesion may or may not be associated with a fracture of the anteroinferior glenoid.

A variation of the Bankart lesion is the **A**nterior **L**abroligamentous **P**eriosteal **S**leeve **A**vulsion (AL-PSA) lesion.[45] The ALPSA lesion is an avulsion of the anterior labrum from the anteroinferior glenoid with an intact anterior scapular periosteum that has been stripped from the bone (periosteal sleeve), but which remains attached to the labrum (Fig. 10–46). The stripped periosteum allows the anterior labroligamentous complex to displace medially and rotate inferiorly on the scapular neck. If not repaired, the ALPSA lesion can heal with a resultant deformed labrum that allows for joint instability. Thus, surgical reduction of the labrum is desirable for an ALPSA lesion, because it can heal in place. This is in distinction to Bankart lesions, which have no potential for healing and are managed differently from ALPSA lesions. These differences are clinically relevant and are why we attempt to differentiate Bankart from ALPSA lesions by MRI.

A reverse Bankart lesion may occur after a posterior dislocation as the result of excessive stress on the glenohumeral joint with the arm in abduction and internal rotation. The reverse Bankart lesion consists of a detachment of the posterior inferior labrum, which may or may not be associated with a fracture of the posterior glenoid.

The MR criteria for diagnosing a labral abnormality includes linear high signal intensity (greater than hyaline cartilage) within the substance of the labrum that exists on a labral surface; diffuse high signal intensity of the labrum from a crush injury; absent or abnormally small labrum; and detachment and displacement of the labrum from the glenoid rim, with high signal intensity between the labrum and glenoid (Fig. 10–47).[46, 47] A traumatic detach-

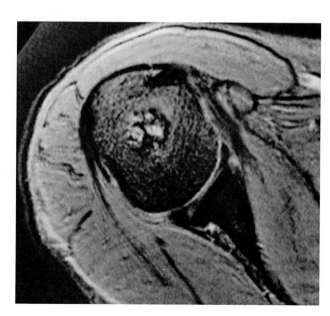

Figure 10–41. CONGENITAL OSSEOUS CAUSE OF INSTABILITY. T2* axial image, shoulder. The posterior aspect of the glenoid is retroverted, predisposing to shoulder instability. (There is an enchondroma in the humerus).

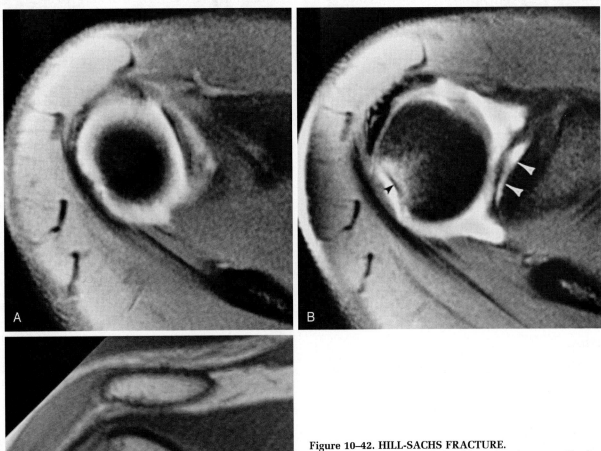

Figure 10–42. HILL-SACHS FRACTURE.
A, T1 fat-suppressed axial shoulder MR arthrogram. The first cut through the top of the humeral head is normal, with the head completely round in configuration. *B,* Same sequence as in *A,* one cut lower. The second cut through the humeral head should also show it as a round structure, but the posterolateral aspect is flattened *(black arrowhead)* from a Hill-Sachs impaction fracture as the result of an anterior dislocation. There is also a superior labral anterior and posterior (SLAP) lesion with separation of the labrum from the superior glenoid *(white arrowheads).* The posterior humerus normally becomes flattened inferior to the first two cuts through the humeral head, and must not be mistaken for a Hill-Sachs impaction fracture. *C,* T1 coronal oblique image, shoulder (different patient than in *A* and *B*). A large Hill-Sachs impaction fracture is evident *(arrow)* in the posterolateral humeral head.

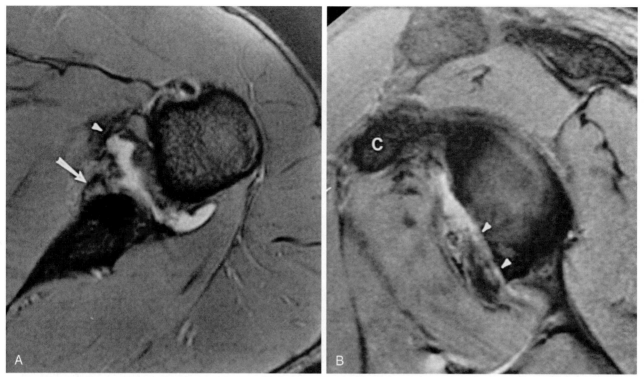

Figure 10–43. BONY BANKART LESION.
A, T1 fat-suppressed axial shoulder MR arthrogram. The anterior capsule is thickened and irregular *(arrowhead)* from injury caused by an anterior shoulder dislocation. The anterior labrum is difficult to see because of fibrillation from tears (crushed). There is also a low-signal fracture fragment *(arrow)* off of the anteroinferior glenoid (a bony Bankart lesion). *B,* T1 fat-suppressed sagittal oblique shoulder MR arthrogram. The vertical fracture line *(arrowheads)* through the anterior glenoid is obvious. C—coracoid process.

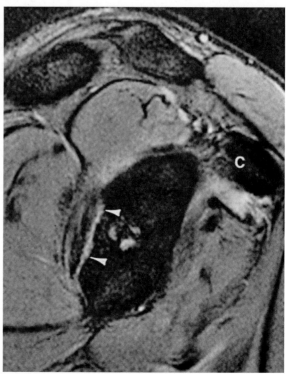

Figure 10–44. REVERSE BONY BANKART LESION.
T1 fat-suppressed sagittal oblique shoulder MR arthrogram. There is a vertical fracture through the posterior margin of the glenoid *(arrowheads)* caused by a posterior shoulder dislocation. C—coracoid process.

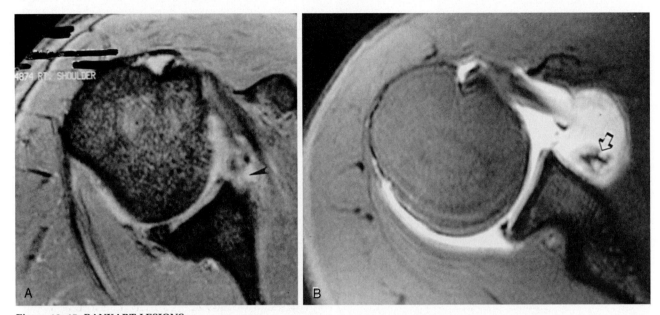

Figure 10–45. BANKART LESIONS.
A, T1 fat-suppressed axial shoulder MR arthrogram. The anteroinferior labrum is detached from the glenoid *(arrowhead)* and is irregular in shape and high signal from tears. There is no linear periosteum seen attached to the labrum because it has been torn. Incidentally, note the flat posterolateral humerus in the lower portion of the joint, which is normal and not from a Hill-Sachs impaction fracture. *B,* T1 fat-suppressed axial shoulder MR arthrogram (different patient than in *A*). The anteroinferior labrum is absent from its normal position adjacent to the glenoid; it has been completely detached and torn free of the scapular periosteum, coming to rest in the medial aspect of the joint *(open arrow).*

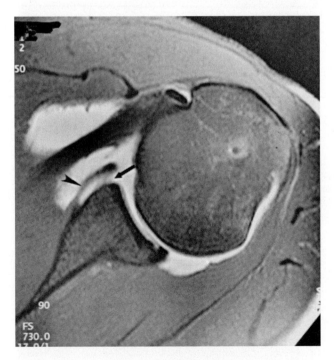

Figure 10–46. ANTERIOR LABROLIGAMENTOUS PERIOSTEAL SLEEVE AVULSION (ALPSA) LESION.
T1 fat-suppressed axial shoulder MR arthrogram. The antero-inferior labrum is detached from the bone of the glenoid *(arrow).* The detached labrum is attached to a linear, low-signal sleeve of intact periosteum *(arrowhead)* that has been stripped from the scapula. Had the periosteum been torn rather than stripped (and, therefore, not evident on MR), this would be a Bankart lesion.

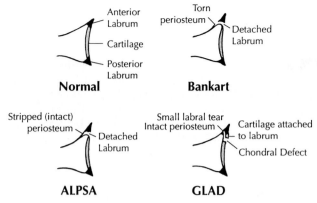

Figure 10–47. LABRAL LESIONS.
Diagram of the normal anterior labrum from an axial perspective, and the key features of Bankart, anterior labroligamentous periosteal sleeve avulsion (ALPSA), and glenolabral articular disruption (GLAD) labral lesions.

ment of the anterosuperior labrum can be distinguished from a normal variant of the labrum, the sublabral foramen, because the separation between the labrum and glenoid extends posterior to the attachment of the biceps tendon to the superior labrum. Detachment of the labrum from the glenoid at any site other than the anterosuperior glenoid is a true abnormality.

Non-Instability Labral Lesions

Lesions may affect the labrum but not be associated with anatomic glenohumeral joint instability. These include SLAP lesions, labral cysts, and glenolabral articular disruption (GLAD) lesions (Box 10–16).

SLAP Lesions

A SLAP lesion is a term applied to tears involving the **S**uperior **L**abrum that are oriented in an **A**nterior and **P**osterior direction.[4, 48] These labral tears occur at the attachment site of the long head of the biceps tendon to the superior labrum. SLAP lesions occur from compression or overhead movements that trap the labrum between the humeral head and the glenoid, or from traction on the biceps tendon that

results in avulsion of the superior labrum. Patients with a SLAP lesion have pain, catching, popping, and a sensation of instability, although the joint is stable on physical examination.

SLAP lesions initially were classified into four types: type I, fraying of the free edge of the superior glenoid labrum; type II, detachment of the superior labrum from the glenoid; type III, bucket-handle tear of the superior labrum without involvement of the long head of the biceps tendon; and type IV, bucket-handle tear of the labrum extending into the long head of the biceps tendon. Nine types of SLAP lesions have now been described. There may be many more SLAP lesions described in the future, owing to people's penchant for splitting hairs. Categorizing SLAP lesions into the different types with MR has limited practical value and may be difficult to do. There have been no large studies evaluating the accuracy of MR in staging SLAP lesions. Although the treatment may vary for certain lesions, they usually are addressed arthroscopically, and differences in treatment are based on whether or not there is involvement of the biceps anchor. Thus, it is most important to assess the integrity of the biceps tendon on the MR images and include that information in the report, rather than trying to determine which specific type of SLAP lesion exists. In general, we determine if a SLAP lesion consists of a partial or full-thickness tear of the superior labrum versus detachment from the glenoid (Fig. 10–48), and whether or not the biceps tendon is torn—that is as complex a classification system as is necessary, and all that the orthopedists expect from us (Box 10–17).

Using T2, gradient echo, or T1W images after intraarticular gadolinium injection, the various features of SLAP lesions can be diagnosed on MR images.

BOX 10–16: GLENOID LABRUM TEARS:
Stable or Unstable

Associated with instability
• Bankart lesions
• ALPSA lesions
Without associated instability
• SLAP lesions
• GLAD lesions

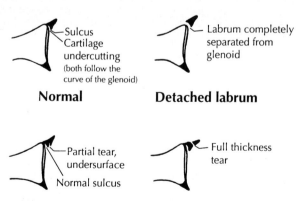

Figure 10–48. SUPERIOR LABRUM ANTERIOR AND POSTERIOR (SLAP) LESIONS.
Diagram of the normal superior labrum and SLAP lesions from a coronal perspective. The normal labrum has cartilage undercutting it, as well as a normal sulcus between cartilage and labrum. The key features of SLAP lesions demonstrated here include detachment, partial-thickness tears, and complete-thickness (bucket-handle) tears.

Fraying of the labrum is seen as irregularity of the margins and diffuse increased signal in the substance of the superior labrum.

Avulsion of the superior labrum manifests as linear high signal separating the labrum from the glenoid (Fig. 10–49). The abnormal signal extends both anterior and posterior to the attachment of the biceps tendon to the labrum, which distinguishes the SLAP lesion from a sublabral foramen, where the labrum is only separated from the glenoid anterior to the biceps tendon anchor. Superior labral detachment resembles the normal labral sulcus and undercutting of hyaline cartilage between the labrum and glenoid on coronal oblique images. However, detachment differs from normal anatomy because the labrum is completely separated from the underlying glenoid by high-signal fluid, and the separation extends posterior to the biceps anchor.

SLAP tears extend either partially through the substance of the superior labrum in a generally craniocaudal direction, extending to its inferior surface, or else extend completely through the labrum, separating it into medial and lateral labral fragments. In the latter situation, it is known as a bucket-handle tear of the labrum. In the first situation, we describe the tears as partial thickness tears of the labrum, extending to the inferior surface of the superior labrum; others call these labral detachments.

Partial thickness tears of the superior labrum may resemble the normal undercutting of hyaline carti-

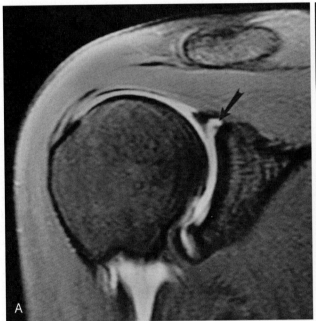

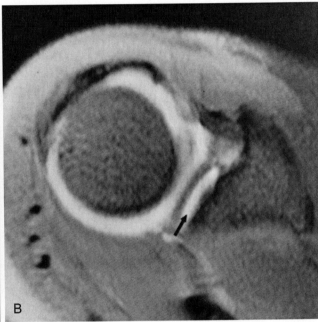

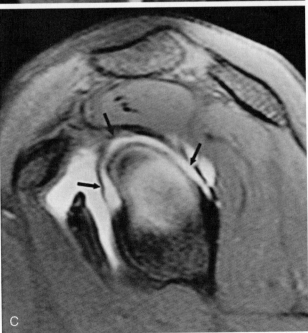

Figure 10–49. SUPERIOR LABRAL TEAR PROPAGATING ANTERIOR AND POSTERIOR (SLAP) LESION: Detachment.
A, T1 fat-suppressed coronal oblique shoulder MR arthrogram. The superior labrum is completely separated from the adjacent glenoid with no attachment identified *(arrow)*. High-signal contrast fills the space between the glenoid and the detached labrum. If the labrum had an attachment to the glenoid, this high-signal line would simply represent the normal sulcus between labrum and bone. *B,* T1 fat-suppressed axial shoulder MR arthrogram. The contrast between the detached labrum and glenoid is seen *(arrow)* all the way across the top of the labrum, extending posterior to the predicted attachment site of the biceps tendon, which is located anterior on the superior labrum. *C,* T1 fat-suppressed sagittal oblique shoulder MR arthrogram. The separation between the labrum *(arrows)* and glenoid is filled with contrast and involves the superior half of the glenoid.

- At least nine types described (at least six too many)
- Important features of SLAP lesions worth remembering:
  Labrum
  — Detached from glenoid (extends posterior to biceps-labral anchor), or
  — Partial thickness tear, or
  — Full-thickness (bucket-handle) tear
  Biceps-labral anchor
  — Torn, or
  — Not torn

lage between the labrum and adjacent glenoid. The normal sulcus between the labrum and glenoid also may create confusion with labral tears. Distinction between tears and normal anatomy is made by the fact that the linear high signal of a labral tear is oriented laterally, whereas the linear high signal from normal anatomy (sulcus or cartilage under-cutting) is oriented in the opposite (medial) direction, following the normal curve (going with the flow) of the superior glenoid on coronal oblique images (Fig. 10–50). The bucket-handle tear of the labrum results in linear high signal traversing the entire substance of the superior labrum, separating it into medial and lateral halves (Fig. 10–50). The lateral labral fragment may displace inferiorly and be evident as a low signal intensity fragment within the glenohumeral joint on both coronal oblique and axial images.

If high signal is present in the proximal biceps tendon, it indicates the tendon is abnormal and involved in the SLAP lesion. There is either diffuse high signal at the labral attachment, or linear high signal from a longitudinal split of the tendon (Fig. 10–51). Determining the integrity of the biceps tendon is critical when a SLAP lesion of the labrum is diagnosed.

Paralabral Cysts

Labral cysts occur next to the glenoid labrum, are similar to ganglion cysts, usually are associated with labral tears, and may or may not be associated with instability. The cysts may be located anywhere, but most frequently are seen posterosuperiorly in association with a posterior labral tear. These cysts form when joint fluid extravasates from the joint through the labral tear, and if a ball-valve phenomenon exists, fluid will accumulate. Water is reabsorbed from the cyst, and a thick proteinaceous material remains. MR images demonstrate a multiloculated round or oval mass of low signal intensity on T1W images and high signal intensity on T2W images (Fig. 10–52). The labral tear associated with the cyst will inconsistently be evident. These patients complain of pain more than instability. These cysts may cause symptoms of suprascapular nerve entrapment from their mass effect,[49] if located in the appropriate site where the nerve passes.

GLAD Lesions

GlenoLabral **A**rticular **D**isruption (GLAD) refers to a nondisplaced anteroinferior labral tear with an associated chondral injury (Fig. 10–47).[50] This results more from an impaction type of injury, rather than a shearing injury, as occurs with Bankart lesions. The labrum remains attached to the anterior scapular periosteum, distinguishing this from a Bankart lesion, which has torn periosteum. On MR arthrography, contrast extends into the cartilaginous defect (Fig. 10–53), but may or may not be seen in the small labral defect. The lesion results from impaction of the humeral head against the articular surface of the glenoid with the arm in abduction and external rotation. These patients complain of pain rather than instability. The lesion can be treated with arthroscopic debridment without the need for a stabilization procedure.

POSTOPERATIVE SHOULDER

MRI of the postoperative shoulder ideally is performed after intraarticular injection of gadolinium. Gradient echo sequences should be avoided because of the blooming artifact created by hemosiderin or metal deposition that is present after surgery, which may prevent proper evaluation of the joint. Knowledge of the surgical procedure performed is imperative. Postoperative MR images demonstrate metallic and hemosiderin-related round foci of very low signal intensity along the surgical path on all imaging sequences. A band of scar tissue can be seen that is low signal intensity on T1W images and may be high signal intensity on T2W images during the first postoperative year, and low signal intensity after that.

Impingement and Rotator Cuff Surgery

Acromioplasty is a common surgical treatment for mechanical impingement. This is done either through an arthroscope or with open surgery. The acromioplasty consists of removing the anteroinferior acromion, which is the insertion site of the coracoacromial ligament, and excision of the subacromial/subdeltoid bursa, if inflamed. The undersurface of the acromion is smoothed with a burr; osteophytes on the undersurface of the acromioclavicular joint are removed and, with severe degenerative joint disease of the acromioclavicular joint, the joint and the distal end of the clavicle are resected. MR depicts the surgical changes and demonstrates any

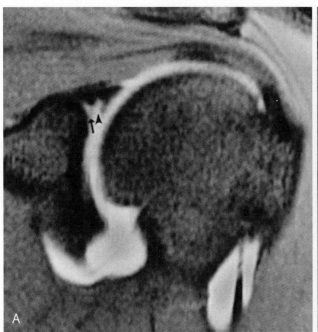

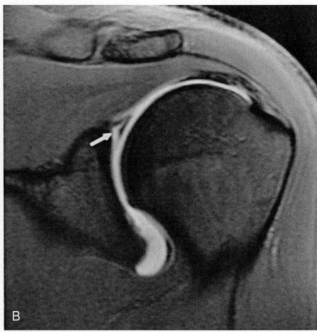

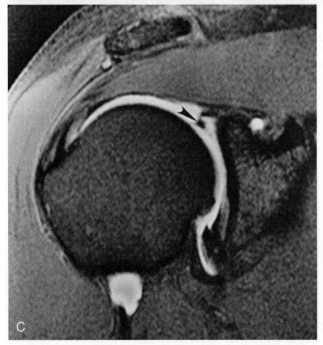

Figure 10–50. PARTIAL-THICKNESS TEAR AND BUCKET-HANDLE SUPERIOR LABRAL ANTERIOR AND POSTERIOR (SLAP) LESIONS.
A, T1 fat-suppressed coronal oblique shoulder MR arthrogram. The normal undercutting of cartilage between the superior labrum and glenoid is evident *(arrow)*, with the cartilage pointing medially and following the contour of the glenoid. Adjacent to this is another curved high-signal line *(arrowhead)* within the labrum that is directed laterally, typical of a partial-thickness tear of the labrum. *B,* T1 fat-suppressed coronal oblique shoulder MR arthrogram (different patient than in *A*). A high-signal line in the labrum does not follow the contour of the glenoid and represents a larger partial-thickness SLAP tear than in *A*. *C,* T1 fat-suppressed coronal oblique shoulder MR arthrogram (different patient than in *A* or *B*). There is high signal in the superior labrum that separates the labrum into two pieces (full-thickness or bucket-handle tear). The lateral half of the labrum *(arrowhead)* is displaced interiorly in the glenohumeral joint.

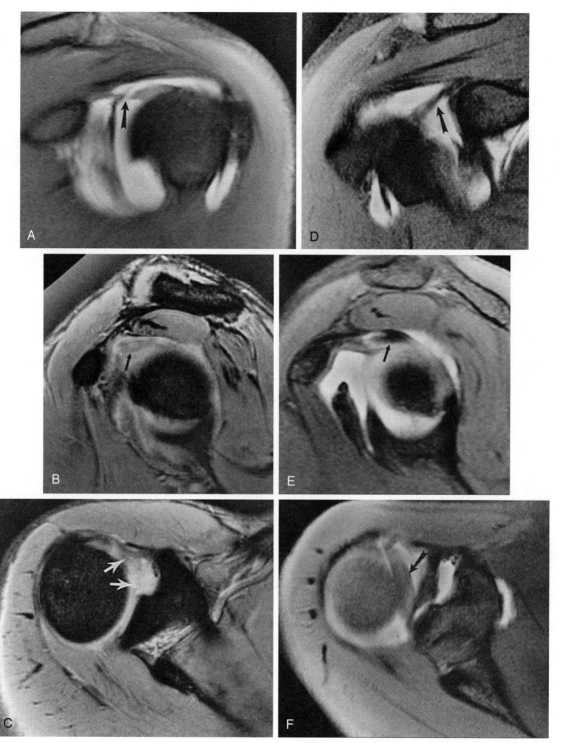

Figure 10–51. SUPERIOR LABRAL ANTERIOR AND POSTERIOR (SLAP) LESION WITH BICEPS ANCHOR TEARS; NORMAL BICEPS ANCHOR FOR COMPARISON.
BICEPS ANCHOR TEARS
A, T1 fat-suppressed coronal oblique shoulder MR arthrogram. This patient has a bucket-handle SLAP tear of the superior labrum (not shown). The biceps anchor to the superior labrum also is torn, as manifested by high signal and irregularity in the proximal tendon *(arrow).* Compare to a normal biceps anchor in *D.* *B,* T1 fat-suppressed sagittal oblique shoulder MR arthrogram. The biceps anchor to the anterosuperior labrum is abnormally high signal *(arrow)* because of partial tears. Compare to normal biceps in *E.* *C,* T1 fat-suppressed axial shoulder MR arthrogram. The biceps anchor is high signal, difficult to identify, and somewhat wavy in appearance *(arrows).* The anterosuperior labrum is not evident on this image. Compare to normal biceps anchor in *F.*
NORMAL BICEPS ANCHOR (DIFFERENT PATIENT THAN IN *A, B,* and *C*)
D, T1 fat-suppressed coronal oblique shoulder MR arthrogram. The normal biceps anchor is taut and low signal *(arrow).* *E,* T1 fat-suppressed sagittal oblique shoulder MR arthrogram. The oval biceps tendon anchor *(arrow)* on the superior labrum is low signal. *F,* T1 fat-suppressed axial shoulder MR arthrogram. The normal biceps *(arrow)* courses obliquely in the anterior aspect of the upper shoulder to anchor to the superolateral labrum. It is taut, low signal, and easy to identify.

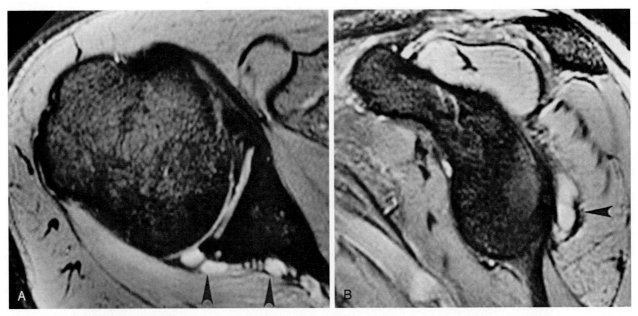

Figure 10–52. PARALABRAL CYSTS.
A, T2* axial image, shoulder. There are several high-signal round structures *(arrowheads)* posterior to the glenoid with septations between them, typical of labral cysts. *B,* T2* sagittal oblique image, shoulder. A portion of the paralabral cyst is seen posteroinferior to the glenoid *(arrowhead)* and adjacent to the labrum, which must be torn, even if the tear is not identified.

persistent causes of impingement or the development of a full-thickness tear of the rotator cuff.

After surgery that involves tendons, detection of degeneration or of partial cuff tears is not reliable by MRI.[51] Full-thickness tears of the rotator cuff usually are repaired by open surgery via a superior approach through a split made in the deltoid muscle. An anteroinferior acromioplasty is performed as

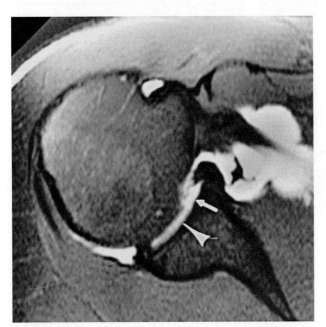

Figure 10–53. GLENOLABRAL ARTICULAR DISRUPTION (GLAD) LESION.
T1 fat-suppressed axial shoulder MR arthrogram. The anterior glenoid has a chondral defect *(arrow)*, which is filled with contrast. The slightly lower signal hyaline cartilage *(arrowhead)* is seen posterior to the chondral defect. The anterior labrum appears normal on this image.

part of the procedure; the cuff is treated with either a tendon-to-bone repair or a tendon-to-tendon anastomosis. With a tendon-to-bone repair, the surgical trough in the superolateral aspect of the greater tuberosity is seen as low signal intensity cortical irregularity. The tendon is usually of intermediate signal intensity, which may represent degeneration, postoperative granulation tissue, or partial tears. The diagnosis of a full-thickness tear is based on the presence of a high signal intensity gap in the tendon on T2W images, or on T1W images with intraarticular gadolinium, and retraction of the musculotendinous junction. The surgical repair may be incomplete and the MR arthrogram may show filling of the subacromial/subdeltoid bursa, although there is no recurrent tear.

Surgery for Instability

The role of MRI in the postoperative evaluation of patients treated for instability is still unknown. No specific abnormalities after these surgical procedures have been described. The most accurate interpretation is obtained through a thorough understanding of the surgical procedure and in direct consultation with the referring surgeon.[52]

MISCELLANEOUS CAPSULAR, BURSAL, AND TENDON ABNORMALITIES

Adhesive Capsulitis

Adhesive capsulitis, or frozen shoulder, is an inflammatory process that causes progressive capsular

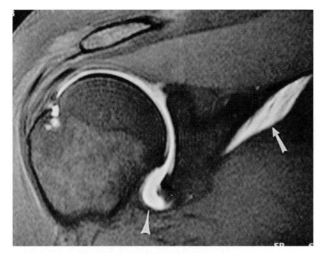

Figure 10–54. ADHESIVE CAPSULITIS.
T1 fat-suppressed coronal oblique shoulder MR arthrogram. This joint only held 5 mL of contrast, and there is extravasation of contrast from the subscapularis recess into the adjacent muscle *(arrow)*. The axillary recess is small *(arrowhead)*. At fluoroscopy, the margins of the capsule showed a serrated appearance, and the diagnosis was an easy one.

retraction. It affects women more frequently than men. Trauma, immobilization, hemiplegia, diabetes mellitus, and cervical disk disease are the most common predisposing factors. Clinically, it is characterized by shoulder pain at rest, at night, and with motion. These symptoms may mimic impingement and rotator cuff tears. Limitation of movement, mainly of abduction and external rotation, is progressive. The process is self-limited and usually lasts 12 to 18 months. Pain relief and improved range of motion can be obtained with intraarticular injection of corticosteroids followed by physical therapy. The diagnosis can be confirmed with arthrography that shows a decreased joint capacity, usually less than 7 cc, small capsular recesses, and a serrated appearance of the capsular attachments.

MR has a limited role in the diagnosis of adhesive capsulitis; it may inconsistently show thickening of the capsule greater than 4 mm as assessed on coronal oblique images at the level of the axillary recess.[53] An advantage of MR arthrography over regular MR without arthrography is the ability to make the diagnosis of adhesive capsulitis at the time of injecting the shoulder with iodinated contrast material under fluoroscopic guidance. In addition, MR arthrography demonstrates small capsular recesses and a thickened, serrated capsule (Fig. 10–54). Rupture of the capsule with extravasation of gadolinium into the extracapsular soft tissues also may be seen.

Synovial Cysts

Synovial cysts may occur at many different joints, but when they occur at the shoulder they tend to be quite large. Synovial cysts may occur as a consequence of rheumatoid arthritis, massive rotator cuff tears, or in the setting of a neuropathic arthropathy.

The shoulder is particularly predisposed to neuropathic changes in patients with a syrinx of the cervical spinal cord. Large synovial cysts may develop and dissect in the soft tissues a distance away from the shoulder joint and present a diagnostic dilemma on clinical grounds, with the masses usually being mistaken for soft tissue sarcomas. MRI is very useful to demonstrate that the masses are cystic in nature and arise from the joint.

Massive rotator cuff tears (tears of more than one of the rotator cuff tendons) result in large joint effusions, which have access to the subacromial/subdeltoid bursa. The large fluid collections can protrude through the degenerated acromioclavicular joint and create a large soft tissue mass above the shoulder joint. The MRI features allow the diagnosis to be made by showing the communication of the mass with the acromioclavicular joint, and that the mass is cystic. The mass has low signal intensity on T1W images and becomes high signal intensity on any type of T2W image (Fig. 10–55). With intravenous gadolinium, only the periphery of the mass enhances demonstrating a thin margin without irregular or thickened walls.

The origin of synovial cysts that occur as a result of rheumatoid arthritis or other inflammatory arthritides should be obvious on MRI because of the concomitant findings of thickened synovium and osseous erosions within the joint.

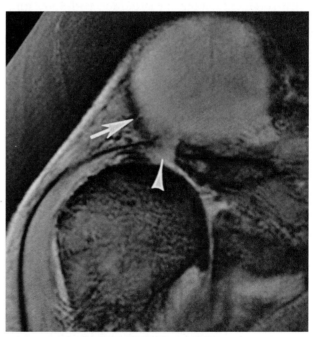

Figure 10–55. SYNOVIAL CYST SECONDARY TO A MASSIVE ROTATOR CUFF TEAR.
T2* coronal image, shoulder. This MR was done to evaluate a presumed sarcoma that was palpable above the shoulder. There is a large, round high-signal mass *(arrow)* that is in direct communication with the acromioclavicular joint *(arrowhead)*. There is absence of the supraspinatus tendon on this cut from a tear (subscapularis and infraspinatus tendons were torn on other images). There is also glenohumeral degenerative joint disease.

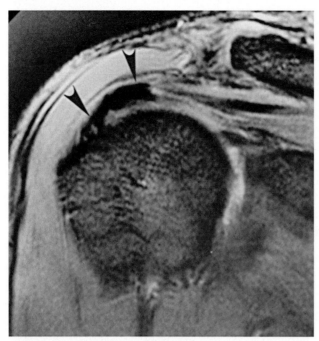

Figure 10–56. CALCIFIC TENDINITIS.
T2* coronal oblique image, shoulder. There is very low signal (lower signal than tendon) in the distal 2 to 3 cm of the supraspinatus tendon *(arrowheads)* from calcium hydroxyapatite crystal deposition.

Calcific Tendinitis and Bursitis

Calcium hydroxyapatite deposition disease occurs most commonly about the shoulder, with the supraspinatus tendon being the site most frequently involved. Many patients are asymptomatic, but those with symptoms present with pain at rest, at night, and with motion. They may have painful limitation of movement that mimicks impingement syndrome. The calcification may develop in the tendon and progressively work its way from the tendon into the adjacent glenohumeral joint or into the adjacent subacromial/subdeltoid bursa. These calcifications often are more easily recognized on radiographs than on MR images and, whenever possible, MR studies should be correlated with the radiographs (or you will make a fool of yourself more often than you can afford). The calcifications are generally low signal intensity on all pulse sequences, similar to the normal tendon. They sometimes are lower signal intensity than normal tendons, in particular on T2* sequences (Fig. 10–56). There may be associated abnormalities in the involved tendon such as thinning, thickening, and irregular margins. Calcific bursitis can be identified on MR images as a distended subacromial/subdeltoid bursa filled with low signal intensity calcifications surrounded by high signal intensity fluid and synovitis on T2W images. These findings usually are associated with an abnormal subjacent tendon.

Subcoracoid Bursitis

The subcoracoid bursa is a normal anatomic structure, located anterior to the subscapularis muscle and tendon. It may become inflamed and cause anterior shoulder pain. It does not communicate with the glenohumeral joint or the subscapularis recess of the shoulder joint. In about 20% of patients it communicates with the subacromial/subdeltoid bursa. It is positioned immediately anterior and inferior to the subscapularis recess of the shoulder joint, but is separated from it by a fibrous septum that should allow easy differentiation of the two structures should they both be distended with fluid. The subcoracoid bursa is bordered by the subscapularis tendon inferiorly and posteriorly, and the coracoid process and the attached combined tendon of the short head of the biceps and the coracobrachialis superiorly and anteriorly. On MR images, this bursa is identified only if inflamed and filled with fluid or synovitis. It appears as an oblong soft tissue mass of low signal intensity on T1W and high signal intensity on T2W images in a characteristic location inferior to the coracoid process and anterior to the subscapularis muscle (Fig. 10–57), best seen on sagittal oblique images.[54] The subcoracoid bursa may be inadvertently injected during a shoulder MR arthrogram, mistaking it for the glenohumeral joint. If the subcoracoid bursa communicates with the subacromial/subdeltoid bursa, as it normally does in 20% of people, there will be contrast in the latter bursa that may mistakenly be interpreted as evidence of a rotator cuff tear. The key to the fact that no cuff tear is present is that no contrast is evident in the glenohumeral joint, and the tendons are not disrupted.

NERVE ABNORMALITIES

Suprascapular Nerve Entrapment
(Box 10–18)

Suprascapular nerve entrapment syndrome initially was described in male weightlifters who had

---

BOX 10–18: SUPRASCAPULAR NERVE ENTRAPMENT

- Mass in suprascapular or spinoglenoid notch compressing nerve
- Mass is usually a ganglion cyst arising from a labral tear
- Causes pain, weakness, muscle atrophy in distribution of affected nerve(s)
- Suprascapular notch: nerve innervates supraspinatus and infraspinatus muscles
  Spinoglenoid notch: nerve innervates infraspinatus only
- MRI
  — Shows the mass
  — Shows supraspinatus or infraspinatus muscle atrophy (↑ signal intensity on T1 from fat infiltration of muscle)

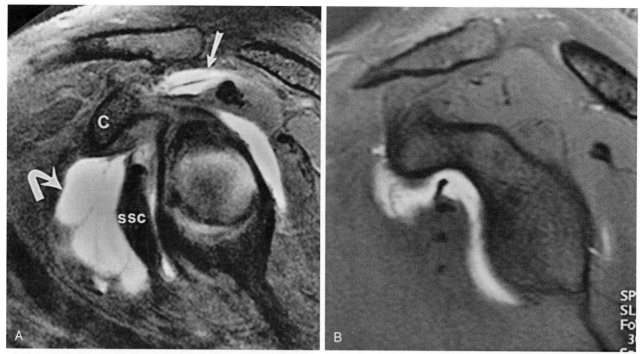

Figure 10–57. SUBCORACOID AND SUBSCAPULARIS RECESSES.
A, T1 fat-suppressed sagittal oblique shoulder MR arthrogram. The shoulder joint was injected with contrast, which filled the subacromial/subdeltoid bursa *(arrow)* due to a rotator cuff tear. The subacaromial bursa communicates with the subcoracoid bursa *(curved arrow)* in this patient, allowing filling of the bursa with contrast. The subcoracoid bursa is located inferior to the coracoid process (C) and anterior to the subscapularis tendons/muscle (SSC). *B,* T1 fat-suppressed sagittal oblique shoulder MR arthrogram (different patient than in *A*). The subscapularis recess is filled with contrast. It drapes over the top of the subscapularis tendons/ muscle beneath the coracoid process. There is no high-signal contrast anterior to the subscapularis muscle, because the subcoracoid bursa did not fill in this patient.

shoulder pain and eventually weakness and muscle atrophy. These features were the result of compression of the suprascapular nerve, which runs superior to the scapula in an anteroposterior direction in the suprascapular notch. The suprascapular nerve provides sensory innervation to the acromioclavicular and glenohumeral joints. As the nerve courses through the suprascapular notch, it provides motor innervation to the supraspinatus and infraspinatus muscles, and as it extends distally into the spinoglenoid notch, it provides motor innervation only to the infraspinatus muscle (Fig. 10–58).[49] The most common cause of suprascapular nerve compression is from a ganglion cyst, usually associated with a superior labral tear (Fig. 10–59), but other causes that affect the suprascapular notch, such as large veins (Fig. 10–60), tumor, or fracture of the scapula, have been implicated.[55] If the mass affects the suprascapular notch, both the supraspinatus and infraspinatus muscles are affected; whereas if a mass is located in the spinoglenoid notch, only the infraspinatus muscle is affected. If entrapment is caused by a ganglion cyst, MRI will show a well-defined, round or oval septated mass of low signal intensity on T1W and high signal intensity on T2W images in the region of the suprascapular or spinoglenoid notches. If intravenous gadolinium is administered, the mass remains low signal intensity, with a thin line of peripheral enhancement on T1W images. The

nerve compression is usually chronic and leads to fatty atrophy of the affected muscles, seen as high signal intensity on T1W images. Percutaneous drainage of the cyst and injection of corticosteroids in the lesion is an alternative to surgical removal, although the associated labral tear, when present, may need to be addressed surgically.

Quadrilateral Space Syndrome
(Box 10–19)

Quadrilateral space syndrome results from compression of the axillary nerve that runs through this space. The quadrilateral space is located in the posterior aspect of the axilla. It is bounded by the humerus laterally, the long head of the triceps muscle medially, the teres minor muscle superiorly, and the teres major muscle inferiorly. The axillary nerve and the posterior humeral circumflex artery travel through this space (Fig. 10–61), and compression of the nerve may occur from fibrous bands, a mass, or a fracture of the scapula or proximal humerus. Pain and paresthesias involving the lateral aspect of the shoulder and the posterosuperior region of the arm characterize the syndrome. The symptoms are exacerbated by abduction and external rotation. Eventually weakness and atrophy of the deltoid or the teres minor muscles may develop. On MR, sagittal

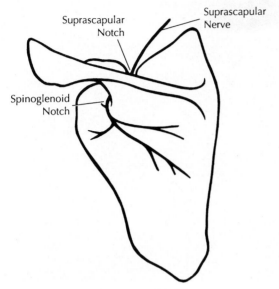

Figure 10–58. SUPRASCAPULAR NERVE.
Diagram of the normal anatomy of the suprascapular nerve from a posterior perspective (innervates both supraspinatus and infraspinatus) in the suprascapular notch on top of the scapula. Inferior to the suprascapular notch is the spinoglenoid notch, which contains only the nerve to the infraspinatus muscle.

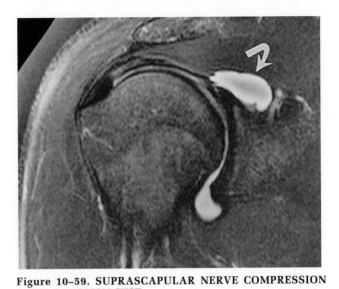

Figure 10–59. SUPRASCAPULAR NERVE COMPRESSION FROM GANGLION CYST.
Fast T2 with fat suppression coronal oblique image, shoulder. There is a high-signal mass *(curved arrow)* in the suprascapular notch that compresses the suprascapular nerve.

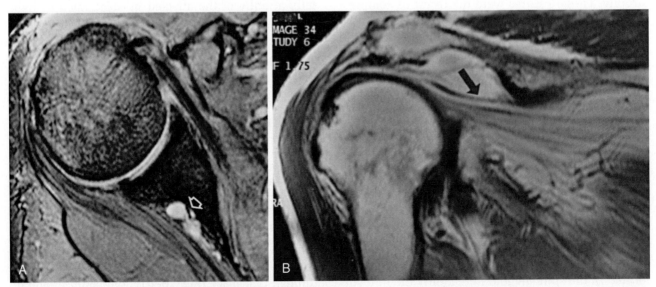

Figure 10–60. SPINOGLENOID NOTCH NERVE COMPRESSION.
A, T2* axial image, shoulder. There are high-signal varices *(open arrow)* in the spinoglenoid notch. The infraspinatus muscle posterior to the shoulder joint has a striated appearance caused by atrophy. *B,* T1 coronal oblique image, shoulder. The infraspinatus muscle *(arrow)* is nearly totally replaced by fat because of atrophy from compression of the nerve by the varices in the spinoglenoid notch.

BOX 10–19: QUADRILATERAL SPACE SYNDROME

Anatomic boundaries of the space
  Lateral—Humerus
  Medial—Long head, triceps
  Superior—Teres minor
  Inferior—Teres major
Clinical
  Compression of axillary nerve in quadrilateral space
  — Fibrous bands, mass, fracture fragments
  Pain, paresthesia, muscle atrophy
MRI
  Fatty atrophy of deltoid or teres minor

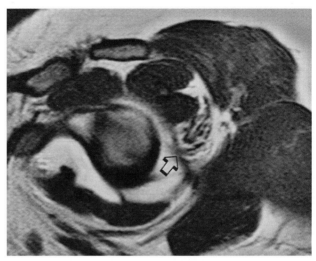

Figure 10–62. QUADRILATERAL SPACE SYNDROME: Atrophy of teres minor.
T1 sagittal oblique shoulder MR arthrogram. The teres minor muscle *(open arrow)* is atrophied and has fat infiltrating it, which creates a speckled appearance compared to the normal adjacent muscles. No mass was identified in the quadrilateral space and this was presumed to be due to fibrous bands compressing the axillary nerve.

oblique images demonstrate best the fatty atrophy of these muscles, seen as high signal intensity on T1W images (Fig. 10–62).[56]

Parsonage-Turner Syndrome

Shoulder pain and weakness may be caused by acute brachial neuritis (Parsonage-Turner syndrome), which is probably the consequence of a viral inflammation of the nerves. The MRI findings of this acute neuromuscular disorder are initially those of muscle edema with high signal in muscle on T2W images; later muscle atrophy occurs with fatty infiltration that is high signal intensity within muscle on T1W images (Fig. 10–63). The muscles that have been shown to be affected with this syndrome are the supraspinatus, infraspinatus, or deltoid.[57] (Box 10–20).

BONE ABNORMALITIES

Posttraumatic Osteolysis of the Clavicle

Posttraumatic osteolysis of the clavicle relates to bone resorption of the distal end of the clavicle after a single episode of severe trauma, or it may occur from repetitive trauma. People who play contact sports, weightlifters, and swimmers are particularly

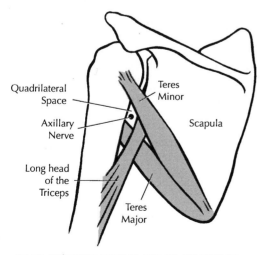

Figure 10–61. QUADRILATERAL SPACE ANATOMY.
Diagram of the quadrilateral space from a posterior perspective. The axillary nerve passes through the space formed by the humerus, teres major, triceps, and teres minor tendons.

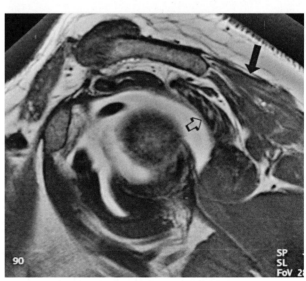

Figure 10–63. PARSONAGE-TURNER SYNDROME: Atrophy of deltoid and infraspinatus muscles.
T1 sagittal oblique shoulder MR arthrogram. There is fat streaking in the deltoid *(solid arrow)* and the infraspinatus *(open arrow)* muscles. The patient had pain and weakness. The tendons were not torn. This was presumably from a viral brachial neuritis.

BOX 10–20: MUSCLE ATROPHY FROM NERVE ABNORMALITIES

Suprascapular notch
— Supraspinatus
— Infraspinatus
Spinoglenoid notch
— Infraspinatus
Quadrilateral space
— Teres minor
— Deltoid
Parsonage-Turner syndrome
— Supraspinatus
— Infraspinatus
— Deltoid

prone to this problem. Clinically, they present with localized pain increased by movement, with or without impingement, and swelling of the acromioclavicular joint.

MR demonstrates joint effusion or synovitis involving the acromioclavicular joint; loss of the black cortical line with resorption of the distal clavicle and, occasionally, of the medial end of the acromion; and bone marrow edema involving the distal end of the clavicle and acromion (Fig. 10–64).[58] In addition, signs of impingement may be present, such as loss or interruption of the fat plane separating the inferior aspect of the clavicle from the supraspinatus muscle, and swelling and synovial hypertrophy of the acromioclavicular joint indenting the supraspinatus muscle.

Occult Fractures

Fractures involving the proximal humerus or the glenoid may result from direct trauma or dislocation. These fractures may not be apparent on radiographs, but show on MRI as either bone contusions or fractures. The characteristic sites of involvement after a shoulder dislocation have been described in the instability portion of this chapter. Another common site of occult fracture involves the greater tuberosity. Bone contusions are seen as poorly defined, heterogeneous, reticulated areas of intermediate to low signal intensity on T1W and high signal intensity on T2W images, that involves the cancellous bone. An acute, radiographically occult fracture is depicted by a linear or curvilinear line of low signal intensity, usually on both T1W and T2W images, surrounded by poorly defined bone marrow edema of intermediate signal intensity on T1W and high signal intensity on T2W images (Fig. 10–65).

Avascular Necrosis

The humeral head is the second most common site of osteonecrosis after the femoral head. Osteonecrosis usually occurs secondary to a predisposing risk factor such as corticosteroids, marrow infiltrative disorders, or after a fracture of the anatomic neck of the humerus. MR permits early detection of osteonecrosis in the shoulder, just as elsewhere in the skeleton. On T1W images, the area of necrosis is delineated by a well-defined, low signal intensity,

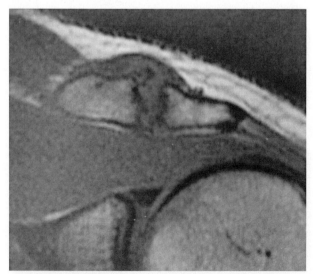

Figure 10–64. OSTEOLYSIS OF THE DISTAL CLAVICLE.
T1 coronal oblique image, shoulder. The distal end of the clavicle and, to a lesser extent, the medial acromion are irregular from bone resorption. There is synovitis of the acromioclavicular joint, with a soft tissue mass centered at the joint. The synovitis impinges on the underlying supraspinatus muscle and obliterates the fat plane between the joint and muscle. This patient was a weightlifter.

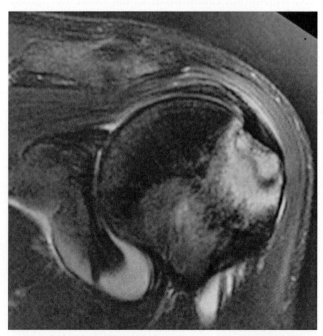

Figure 10–65. RADIOGRAPHICALLY OCCULT FRACTURE.
Fast T2 with fat suppression coronal oblique image, shoulder. There is a nondisplaced fracture of the greater tuberosity with surrounding marrow edema. This was not evident radiographically.

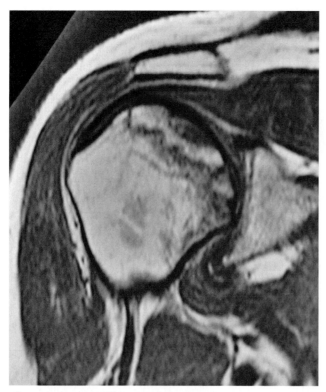

Figure 10–66. AVASCULAR NECROSIS.
T1 coronal oblique image, shoulder. There is a serpiginous line in the humeral epiphysis, typical of avascular necrosis. A fracture could have a very similar appearance, but is rare in this location and should have lots of surrounding edema in the acute phase.

serpiginous line or arc (Fig. 10–66). The center of the lesion is of variable signal intensity, depending on the pathologic alterations of the fragment, but most frequently the signal intensity is that of fat.

Tumors (Box 10–21)

The shoulder girdle is not a site specific for any particular bone tumor. The most common primary bone tumor found incidentally on shoulder MR is a

---

BOX 10–21: TUMORS OF THE SHOULDER

Bone tumors
• Enchondroma, chondrosarcoma
Soft tissue tumors
• Benign
— Lipoma
— Benign fibrous histiocytoma
— Synovial cysts
— Elastofibroma
• Malignant
— Malignant fibrous histiocytoma
— Liposarcoma

---

benign enchondroma. It is a well-defined, lobular lesion of low signal intensity on T1W images and high signal intensity on T2W images, which may have stippled calcifications of low signal intensity (Fig. 10–67). Its malignant counterpart, chondrosarcoma, is the most common focal primary malignant tumor in the shoulder; the distinction from a benign enchondroma may be difficult to make unless there is endosteal scalloping that affects more than two thirds of the cortical thickness, destruction of the adjacent cortex, or a soft tissue mass.[59] Metastases and myeloma remain the most common malignant processes that affect the shoulder.

SOFT TISSUE ABNORMALITIES

Benign and Malignant Tumors

MR is particularly helpful in detecting a soft tissue mass, defining its extent, and planning a biopsy. Lipoma and benign fibrous histiocytoma are the most common benign tumors that affect the shoulder girdle, whereas malignant fibrous histiocytoma and liposarcoma are the most common malignant soft tissue tumors in the shoulder. Elastofibromas are soft tissue masses that occur almost exclusively in the shoulder region, and their specific location may allow the diagnosis to be made by MRI.

Elastofibroma dorsi is a benign fibroelastic lesion that usually occurs in older women in a periscapu-

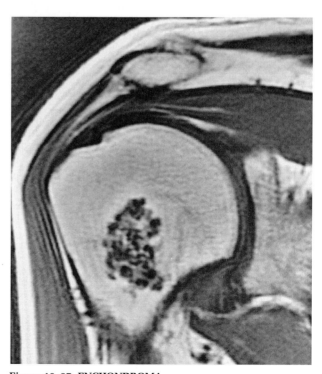

Figure 10–67. ENCHONDROMA.
T1 coronal oblique image, shoulder. There are stippled, low-signal calcifications in the humeral metaphysis from a benign enchondroma. There is no soft tissue mass, erosion of cortex, or other signs of an aggressive lesion to suggest a chondrosarcoma.

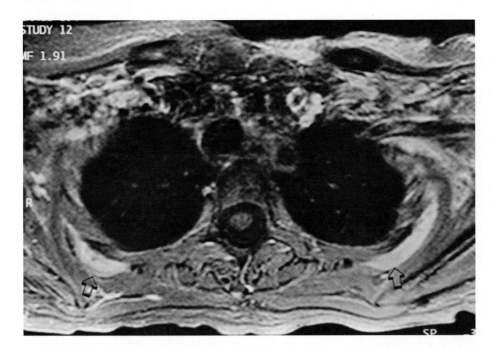

Figure 10–68. ELASTOFIBROMAS. T1 axial fat-suppressed, contrast-enhanced image, chest. There is diffuse contrast enhancement of bilateral periscapular masses *(open arrows)* in this elderly woman.

lar location. These lesions often are asymptomatic and bilateral. Elastofibromas are located deep to the scapula or inferior to the tip of the scapula, usually involving the medial border. The MR characteristics are of a mass with signal intensity similar to muscle on T1W and T2W images, with interspersed streaks of fat that are high signal on T1 (Fig. 10–68).[60]

MR characteristics of soft tissue lesions usually are not sufficiently specific to permit a histologic diagnosis, or to differentiate between benign and malignant lesions, with the possible exceptions of lipomas, hemangiomas, paralabral ganglion cysts, and possibly elastofibromas.

Pectoralis Muscle Injuries

Tears of the pectoralis major muscle or tendon occasionally occur in athletes, especially in weight-lifters as a result of bench-pressing. These tears result in pain and some loss of abduction strength. Treatment is either conservative or surgical, depending on precisely where the tear occurred. Thus, MRI can be valuable in making the diagnosis and in determining what type of therapy is optimal.[61]

The pectoralis major muscle is composed of two major heads, the clavicular and sternal, which converge laterally as they approach the humerus. The pectoralis major tendon attaches to the proximal shaft of the humerus at the bicipital groove.

Pectoralis major tears are usually partial, but also may be complete. They may occur at different sites: the muscle belly, musculotendinous junction, or the attachment of the tendon to the humerus. Surgery generally is the treatment for avulsions of the tendon from the humerus, whereas conservative treatment usually is warranted for injuries to the muscle or musculotendinous junction.

MRI in the axial and coronal oblique planes can show the muscle and tendon well. Tears have the same appearance as in all other muscles and are dependent on the age of the injury. Hemorrhage and edema (high signal on T2W images) can be seen in the lateral aspect of the muscle and surrounding the tendon (Fig. 10–69). High signal on T2W images around the humeral cortex is an important sign that the humeral periosteum has been stripped from the bone during an avulsion injury of the tendinous attachment to the bone.

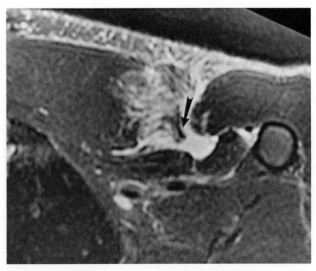

Figure 10–69. PECTORALIS MAJOR MUSCLE TEAR. Fast T2 with fat suppression axial image, shoulder. There is edema on the medial side of the humerus, indicating avulsion of the pectoralis tendon attachment from the bone. The retracted tendon *(arrow)* is seen surrounded by high-signal edema and hemorrhage in the muscle and fat planes. This patient was a weightlifter.

References

1. Kwak SM, Brown RR, Trudell D, et al. Glenohumeral joint: comparison of shoulder positions at MR arthrography. *Radiology* 1998; 208:375–380.
2. Davis SJ, Teresi LM, Bradley WG, et al. Effect of arm rotation on MR imaging of the rotator cuff. *Radiology* 1991; 181:265–268.
3. Siebold CJ, Mallisee TA, Erickson SJ, et al. Rotator cuff: evaluation with US and MR imaging. *Radiographics* 1999; 19:685–705.
4. Stoller DW, Wolf EM. The shoulder. In Stoller DW (ed): *Magnetic Resonance Imaging in Orthopaedics and Sports Medicine*. Philadelphia: JB Lippincott; 1997:597–742.
5. Vangsness CT Jr, Jorgenson SS, Watson T, et al. The origin of the long head of the biceps from the scapula and glenoid labrum: an anatomical study of 100 shoulders. *J Bone Joint Surg [Br]* 1994; 76:951–954.
6. Kaplan PA, Bryans KC, Davick JP, et al. MR imaging of the normal shoulder: variants and pitfalls. *Radiology* 1992; 184:519–524.
7. Timins ME, Erickson SJ, Estkowski LD, et al. Increased signal in the normal supraspinatus tendon on MR imaging: diagnostic pitfall caused by the magic-angle effect. *AJR* 1995; 165:109–114.
8. Erickson SJ, Cox IH, Hyde JS, et al. Effect of tendon orientation on MR imaging signal intensity: a manifestation of the "magic angle" phenomenon. *Radiology* 1991; 181:389–392.
9. Farley TE, Neumann CH, Steinbach LS, et al. The coracoacromial arch: MR evaluation and correlation with rotator cuff pathology. *Skeletal Radiol* 1994; 23:641–645.
10. Rockwood CA Jr, Lyons FR. Shoulder impingement syndrome: diagnosis, radiographic evaluation and treatment with a modified Neer acromioplasty. *J Bone Joint Surg [Am]* 1993; 75:409–424.
11. Kieft GJ, Bloem JL, Rozing PM, et al. Rotator cuff impingement syndrome: MR imaging. *Radiology* 1988; 166:211–214.
12. Seeger LL, Gold RH, Bassett LW, et al. Shoulder impingement syndrome: MR findings in 53 shoulders. *AJR* 1988; 150:343–347.
13. Bigliani LU, Ticker JB, Flatlow EL, et al. The relationship of the acromial architecture to rotator cuff disease. *Clin Sports Med* 1991; 10:823–838.
14. Edelson JG. The "hooked" acromion revisited. *J Bone Joint Surg [Br]* 1995; 77:284–287.
15. Peh WCG, Farmer THR, Totty WG: Acromial arch shape: assessment with MR imaging. *Radiology* 1995; 195:501–505.
16. Park JG, Lee JK, Phelps CT. Os acromiale associated with rotator cuff impingement: MR imaging of the shoulder. *Radiology* 1994; 193:255–257.
17. Hijioka A, Suzuki K, Nakamura T, et al. Degenerative change and rotator cuff tears: an anatomical study in 160 shoulders of 80 cadavers. *Arch Orthop Trauma Surg* 1993; 112:61–64.
18. Getz JD, Recht MP, Piraino DW, et al. Acromial morphology: relation to sex, age, symmetry, and subacromial enthesophytes. *Radiology* 1996; 199:737–742.
19. Feller JF, Tirman PFJ, Steinbach LS, et al. Magnetic resonance imaging of the shoulder: review. *Semin Roentgenol* 1995; 30:224–239.
20. Rafii M, Hossein F, Sherman O, et al. Rotator cuff lesions: signal patterns at MR imaging. *Radiology* 1990; 177:817–823.
21. Tuckman GA. Abnormalities of the long head of the biceps tendon of the shoulder: MR imaging findings. *AJR* 1994; 163:1183–1188.
22. Cervilla V, Schweitzer ME, Ho C, et al. Medial dislocation of the biceps brachii tendon: appearance at MR imaging. *Radiology* 1991; 180:523–526.
23. Chan TW, Dalinka MK, Kneeland JB, et al. Biceps tendon dislocation: evaluation with MR imaging. *Radiology* 1991; 179:649–652.
24. Tirman PFJ, Bost FW, Garvin GJ, et al. Posterosuperior glenoid impingement of the shoulder: findings at MR imaging and MR arthrography with arthroscopic correlation. *Radiology* 1994; 193:431–436.
25. Gerber C, Krushell RJ. Isolated rupture of the tendon of the subscapularis muscle: clinical features in 16 cases. *J Bone Joint Surg [Br]* 1991; 73:389–394.
26. Patte D. The subcoracoid impingement. *Clin Orthop* 1990; 254:55–59.
27. Patten RM. Tears of the anterior portion of the rotator cuff (the subscapularis tendon): MR imaging findings. *AJR* 1994; 162:351–354.
28. Harryman DT, Sidles JA, Harris SL, et al. The role of the rotator interval capsule in passive motion and stability of the shoulder. *J Bone Joint Surg [Am]* 1992; 74:53–66.
29. Massengill AD, Seeger LL, Yao L, et al. Labrocapsular ligamentous complex of the shoulder: normal anatomy, anatomic variation, and pitfalls of MR imaging and MR arthrography. *Radiographics* 1994; 14:1211–1223.
30. Palmer WE, Caslowitz PL, Chew FS. MR arthrography of the shoulder: normal intraarticular structures and common abnormalities. *AJR* 1995; 164:141–146.
31. Chandnani VP, Gagliardi JA, Murnane TG, et al. Glenohumeral ligaments and shoulder capsular mechanism: evaluation with MR arthrography. *Radiology* 1995; 196:27–32.
32. Yeh LR, Kwak S, Kim Y-S, et al. Anterior labroligamentous structures of the glenohumeral joint: correlation of MR arthrography and anatomic dissection in cadavers. *AJR* 1998; 171:1229–1236.
33. Cvitanic O, Tirman PF, Feller JF, et al. Using abduction and external rotation of the shoulder to increase the sensitivity of MR arthrography in revealing tears of the anterior glenoid labrum. *AJR* 1997; 169:837–844.
34. McCauley TR, Pope CF, Jokl P. Normal and abnormal glenoid labrum: assessment with multiplanar gradient-echo MR imaging. *Radiology* 1992; 183:35–37.
35. Loredo R, Longo C, Salonen D, et al. Glenoid labrum: MR imaging with histologic correlation. *Radiology* 1995; 196:33–41.
36. Kwak SM, Brown RR, Resnick D, et al. Anatomy, anatomic variations, and pathology of the 11-to 3-o'clock position of the glenoid labrum: findings on MR arthrography and anatomic sections. *AJR* 1998; 171:235–238.
37. Tuite MJ, Orwin JF. Anterosuperior labral variants of the shoulder: appearance on gradient-recalled echo and fast spin-echo MR images. *Radiology* 1996; 199:537–540.
38. Tirman PFJ, Feller JF, Palmer WE, et al. The Buford complex—a variation of normal shoulder anatomy: MR arthrographic imaging features. *AJR* 1996; 166:869–873.
39. Smith DK, Chopp TM, Aufdemorte TB, et al. Sublabral recess of the superior glenoid labrum: study of cadavers with conventional nonenhanced MR imaging, MR arthrography, anatomic dissection, and limited histologic examination. *Radiology* 1996; 201:251–156.
40. Resnick D, Kang HS. Shoulder. In *Internal Derangements of Joints; Emphasis on MR Imaging*. Philadelphia: W. B. Saunders; 1997:163–333.
41. Beltran J, Rosenberg ZS, Chandnani VP, et al. Glenohumeral instability: evaluation with MR arthrography. *Radiographics* 1997; 17:657–673.
42. Ferrari JD, Ferrari DA, Coumas J, et al. Posterior ossification of the shoulder: the Bennett lesion. *Am J Sports Med* 1994; 22:171–175.
43. Tirman PFJ, Steinbach LS, Feller JF, et al. Humeral avulsion of the anterior shoulder stabilizing structures after anterior shoulder dislocation: demonstration by MRI and MR arthrography. *Skeletal Radiol* 1996; 25:743–748.
44. Richards RD, Sartoris DJ, Pathria MN, et al. Hill-Sachs lesion and normal humeral groove: MR imaging features allowing their differentiation. *Radiology* 1994; 190:665–668.
45. Neviaser TJ. The anterior labroligamentous periosteal sleeve avulsion lesion: a cause of anterior instability of the shoulder. *Arthroscopy* 1993; 9:17–21.
46. Chandnani VP, Yeager TD, DeBeradino T, et al. Glenoid labral tears: prospective evaluation with MR imaging, MR arthrography, and CT arthrography. *AJR* 1993; 161:1229–1235.
47. Palmer WE, Caslowitz PL. Anterior shoulder instability: diagnostic criteria determined from prospective analysis of 121 MR arthrograms. *Radiology* 1995; 197:819–825.
48. Shankman S, Bencardino J, Beltran J. Glenohumeral instabil-

ity: evaluation using MR arthrography of the shoulder. *Skeletal Radiol* 1999; 28:365–382.

49. Fritz RC, Helms CA, Steinbach LS, et al. Suprascapular nerve entrapment: evaluation with MR imaging. *Radiology* 1992; 182:437–444.

50. Saunders TG, Tirman PFJ, Linares R, et al. The glenolabral articular disruption lesion: MR arthrography with arthroscopic correlation. *AJR* 1999; 172:171–175.

51. Gaenslen ES, Satterlee CC, Hinson GW. Magnetic resonance imaging for evaluation of failed repairs of the rotator cuff: relationship to operative findings. *J Bone Joint Surg [Am]* 1996; 78:1391–1396.

52. Haygood TM, Oxner KG, Kneeland JB, et al. Magnetic resonance imaging of the postoperative shoulder. *Magn Reson Imaging Clin North Am* 1993; 1:143–156.

53. Emig EW, Schweiter ME, Karasick D, et al. Adhesive capsulitis of the shoulder: MR diagnosis. *AJR* 1995; 164:1457–1459.

54. Schraner AB, Major NM. MR imaging of the subcoracoid bursa. *AJR* 1999; 172:1567–1571.

55. Tirman PFJ, Feller JF, Janzen DL, et al. Association of glenoid labral cysts with labral tears and glenohumeral instability: radiologic findings and clinical significance. *Radiology* 1994; 190:653–658.

56. Linker CS, Helms CA, Fritz RC. Quadrilateral space syndrome: findings at MR imaging. *Radiology* 1993; 188:675–676.

57. Helms CA, Martinez S, Speer KP. Acute brachial neuritis (Parsonage-Turner syndrome): MR imaging appearance—report of three cases. *Radiology* 1998; 207:255–259.

58. De la Puente R, Boutin RD, Theodorou DJ, et al. Post-traumatic and stress-induced osteolysis of the distal clavicle: MR imaging findings in 17 patients. *Skeletal Radiol* 1999; 28:202–208.

59. Murphey MD, Flemming DJ, Boyea SR, et al. Enchondroma versus chondrosarcoma in the appendicular skeleton: differentiating features. *Radiographics* 1998; 18:1213–1237.

60. Naylor MF, Nascimento AG, Sherrick AD, McLeod RA. Elastofibroma dorsi: radiologic findings in 12 patients. *AJR* 1996; 167:683–687.

61. Connell DA, Potter HG, Sherman MF, Wickiewicz TL. Injuries of the pectoralis major muscle: evaluation with MR imaging. *Radiology* 1999; 210:785–791.

SHOULDER PROTOCOLS

This is one set of suggested protocols; there are many variations that would work equally well.

SHOULDER MR ARTHROGRAM				
Sequence #	1	2	3	4
Sequence Type	T1 fat saturation	T2 fat saturation	T1	T1
Orientation	Coronal oblique	Coronal oblique	Axial	Sagittal oblique
Field of View (cm)	14	14	14	14
Slice Thickness (mm)	4	4	4	4
Contrast	Intraarticular			
Recipe for MR arthrography				

A. In a 20-mL syringe, draw up
  - 3 mL iodinated contrast material
  - 10 mL sterile saline
B. In a tuberculin syringe, draw up
  - 0.1 mL gadolinium—DTPA
C. Inject the gadolinium into the needle end of the 20-mL syringe in *A*. Mix the concoction (shaken, not stirred) and inject 10 to 12 mL.

SHOULDER: WITHOUT ARTHROGRPHY					
Sequence #	1	2	3	4	5
Sequence Type	T1	T2*	Fast T2 fat saturation	T2*	T2*
Orientation	Coronal oblique	Coronal oblique	Coronal oblique	Axial	Sagittal oblique
Field of View (cm)	14	14	14	14	14
Slice Thickness (mm)	4	4	4	4	4
Contrast	No	No	No	No	No

Scout		Final Image
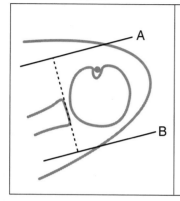	• Axial scout • Obtain coronal oblique images perpendicular to glenoid articular surface (dashed line) • Cover from line A to B • Film from posterior to anterior • Obtain coronal plane first (most valuable)	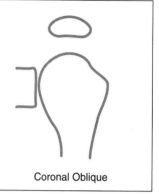 Coronal Oblique

Scout		Final Image
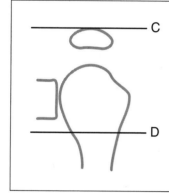	• Coronal scout • Obtain axial images • Cover from line C at acromion to line D at inferior glenoid	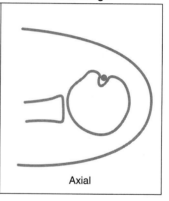 Axial

Scout		Final Image
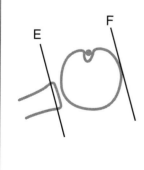	• Axial scout • Obtain sagittal images parallel to glenoid articular surface • Cover from line E at glenohumeral joint to line F at edge of humeral head	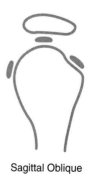 Sagittal Oblique

HOW TO IMAGE THE ELBOW
NORMAL AND ABNORMAL
Bones
  Normal Relationships
  Osseous Disorders
    Osteochondritis dissecans/
      Panner's disease
    Fractures
Ligaments
  Radial Collateral Ligament
    Complex
  Normal radial collateral ligaments
  Abnormal radial collateral
    ligaments
  Ulnar Collateral Ligament Complex
  Normal ulnar collateral ligaments
  Abnormal ulnar collateral
    ligaments

Muscles/Tendons
  Anterior Compartment
    Normal anatomy
    Abnormal anatomy
  Posterior Compartment
    Normal anatomy
    Abnormal anatomy
  Medial Compartment
    Normal anatomy
    Abnormal anatomy
  Lateral Compartment
    Normal anatomy
    Abnormal anatomy

Nerves
  Ulnar Nerve
  Median Nerve
  Radial Nerve
Articular Disorders
  Masses
  Epitrochlear Adenopathy
  Bursae

HOW TO IMAGE THE ELBOW

Coils/Patient Position. The elbow typically is scanned with the patient in a supine position with the arm at the side. A surface coil is imperative for obtaining high-quality images. Occasionally, the size of the patient precludes supine imaging, because the surface coil will be too close to the magnet. These patients can be scanned prone with the arm overhead and the elbow as completely extended as possible. This position has been referred to as the "Superman" position, but to be technically correct, this should be referred to as the "Mighty Mouse" position, because Superman flies with both hands overhead. Nevertheless, patient comfort is most important. Positioning the patient comfortably results in a higher yield of images not degraded by motion artifact. Using a vitamin E capsule to mark the area of the patient's pain or palpable mass is useful for assessing whether the area of concern has been imaged; this is especially important if the examination is normal.

Image Orientation (Box 11–1). The elbow should be scanned beginning about 10 cm above the elbow joint through the bicipital tuberosity distally. For convenience, the image should be oriented in the same way as in conventional radiography. That is, the humerus at the top of the image, and the distal structures hung distally. The axial images should be oriented with volar surface superiorly.

Pulse Sequence/Regions of Interest. Axial imaging enables evaluation of tendons, ligaments, bone pathology, and neurovascular bundles. Coronal imaging is ideal for assessing the integrity of the collateral ligaments. Sagittal images are useful for evaluation of the biceps and triceps tendons.

In general, as with most joint imaging, a slice thickness of 4 mm is reasonable, with a 10% interslice gap (translation: 0.4 mm). T2W images show pathologic processes by taking advantage of the long relaxation time for "water," and thus edema is shown to greater advantage. T2W sequences include spin echo T2, fast spin echo T2, (fast) short TI inversion recovery (STIR), and gradient echo (T2*) imaging. It is useful to apply fat suppression to the fast spin echo imaging. This makes the appearance of pathologic fluid more conspicuous. Because of the unique magnetic susceptibility properties of T2* imaging, this technique can be used when searching for loose bodies. It is not a technique that should be used in a post-surgical elbow because of the amount of artifact created by micrometallic debris. The degree of artifact surrounding orthopedic hardware is most prominent on T2* sequences because of the lack of a 180 degree refocusing pulse, and is least prominent on fast spin echo sequences because of the presence of multiple 180 degree pulses.

Contrast. Intravenous gadolinium may provide useful information in the assessment of synovial-based processes or to distinguish cystic from solid masses about the elbow. Intraarticular gadolinium

Axial	Tendons
	Annular ligament
	Bones
	Neurovascular
	Muscles
Sagittal	Biceps, triceps tendons
	(longitudinally)
	Anterior/posterior muscle masses
Coronal	Ligaments (medial and lateral)
	Medial/lateral muscle masses
	Bones (especially medial/lateral
	epicondyles)
	Extensor-supinator and flexor-
	pronator conjoined tendons
	longitudinally

is useful in patients without a joint effusion to detect loose bodies, capsular disruption, and partial tears of the ulnar collateral ligament or to assess the stability of an osteochondral fracture fragment. The dilution is the same for shoulder arthrography (1/200–250) of gadolinium in normal saline. The solution is injected to maximal distention of the joint as indicated by resistance to further injection. This usually occurs at about 10 mL of fluid injected.

NORMAL AND ABNORMAL

Elbow abnormalities are increasing as the number of people participating in weight lifting and throwing and racquet sports continues to rise. Even couch potatoes are at risk from overuse of the elbow in consuming 12-oz. beverages. The understanding of elbow pathology is becoming more sophisticated with the advent of improved imaging techniques and the evolution of surface coils. MRI offers superior depiction of muscles, ligaments, and tendons, as well as the ability to directly visualize bone marrow, articular cartilage, and neurovascular structures.

Bones

Normal Relationships

The osseous anatomy of the elbow allows for two complex motions: flexion-extension and pronation-supination. The elbow is composed of three articulations contained within a common joint cavity. The radius articulates with the capitellum and the ulna articulates with the trochlea of the humerus in a hinge fashion. The proximal radioulnar joint is composed of the radial head, which rotates within the radial (sigmoid) notch of the ulna, allowing supina-

tion and pronation distally. The ulnohumeral articulation of the elbow is almost a true hinge joint. The radius articulates with the proximal ulna and rounded capitellum of the distal humerus. This radiocapitellar joint allows for pronation-supination.

Osseous Disorders

Osteochondritis Dissecans/Panner's Disease (Box 11–2). Although osteochondritis dissecans can occur in throwers and nonthrowers, in dominant and nondominant elbows, in both the capitellum and the radial head, it tends to occur in the capitellum of the dominant arm in throwers.[1–6] The exact cause is uncertain, but the leading hypothesis is that the lesion results from a combination of tenuous blood supply to the capitellum and repetitive trauma at the radiocapitellar joint, resulting in bone death.[7]

MRI can determine the stability of the osteochondral injury. Unstable lesions are characterized by high-signal fluid that encircles the osteochondral fragment on T2W images. Round, cystic lesions may be seen beneath the osteochondral fragment, and abnormal high signal may be seen on the T2W images within the fragment of bone (Fig. 11–1). The overlying cartilage is not necessarily damaged and therefore should be closely inspected. The overlying cartilage is intact in stable lesions and, therefore, usually is treated with rest and splinting. Unstable lesions are either pinned or excised.

Osteochondritis dissecans should be distinguished from Panner's disease (an osteochondrosis of the capitellum), which coincidentally also occurs in throwers from trauma. The MR appearance, patient's age, and prognosis differ. Osteochondritis dissecans is seen in slightly older patients (12 to 16 years), whereas Panner's disease is in the 5- to 10-year age range. Loose body formation usually is not seen with Panner's disease, and the entire capitellum generally is abnormal in signal (low in signal on T1W images and high in signal on T2W images) and may demonstrate irregular contour to the capitellum. Subsequent follow-up imaging in Panner's disease reveals normalization of these changes with little to no residual deformity at the articular surface. Osteochondritis dissecans can lead to intraar-

OSTEOCHONDRITIS DISSECANS
12–16 yrs of age
Part or whole capitellum
May lead to loose bodies
PANNER'S DISEASE
5–10 yrs of age
Whole capitellum
No long-term deformity or loose bodies

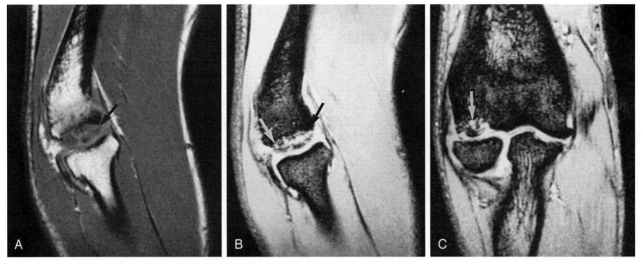

Figure 11–1. OSTEOCHONDRITIS DISSECANS (UNSTABLE).
A, Sagittal T1-weighted image demonstrating irregularity to the capitellum with low-signal bone marrow edema *(arrow).* *B,* Sagittal T2* revealing high signal around the bone fragment *(arrows).* Bone marrow edema is not appreciated in the gradient echo image. *C,* Coronal T2* showing the unstable fragment. High signal is identified around the bone fragment *(arrow).*

ticular loose bodies and significant residual deformity of the capitellum (Fig. 11–2).

A pitfall in diagnosing osteochondritis dissecans is the pseudodefect of the capitellum. This occurs because the most posterior portion of the capitellum has an abrupt slope. A coronal image through the posterior capitellum mimics a defect. Examination of this area in another plane and the lack of edema support the pseudodefect as the cause of the irregularity of the capitellum (Fig. 11–3). Additionally, osteochondritis dissecans occurs on the anterior convex margin of the capitellum, rather than posteriorly.

Unstable osteochondral lesions may fragment and migrate throughout the joint as loose bodies. Loose bodies also can occur from purely cartilaginous fragments breaking off in the joint from acute trauma or degenerative joint disease. Loose bodies can become large and cause mechanical symptoms, limiting mo-

bility of the joint, or produce a synovitis that results in an effusion and stiff elbow (Fig. 11–4). Loose bodies may be identified in the posterior compartment in the throwing athlete and are easier to detect on MRI when joint fluid is present. Occasionally, a loose body can have marrow within it. The signal characteristics follow that of fatty marrow, high in signal on the T1W images. The loose bodies are identified on MR as low-signal structures within the high signal of the joint fluid. Instilling intraarticular dilute gadolinium can increase identification of loose bodies when joint fluid is not present. Axial and sagittal images aid in the diagnosis and location of the loose bodies. Small fragments of cortical bone result in blooming on T2* sequences, which may make them more conspicuous than on other imaging sequences.

Fractures. MRI is useful in evaluating radiographically occult fractures when there is radiographic

Figure 11–2. OSTEOCHONDRITIS DISSECANS.
In a male little league baseball pitcher with elbow pain. *A,* Sagittal T1W image shows low signal in the convex portion of the capitellum *(arrow).* *B,* Fast spin echo fat-suppressed T2-weighted image shows the bone marrow edema *(arrow).* No loose body was identified.

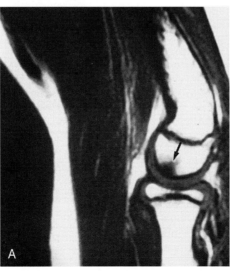
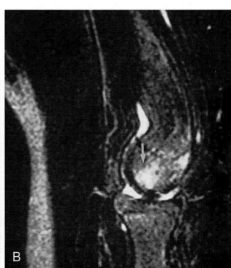

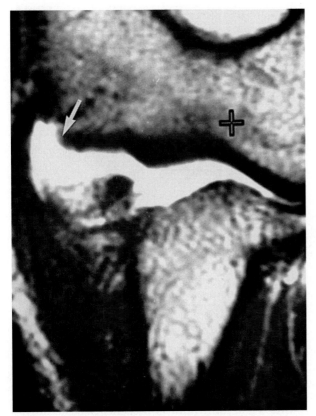

Figure 11–3. PSEUDODEFECT OF CAPITELLUM.
Coronal T1W image located posteriorly shows irregularity of the capitellum without surrounding edema *(arrow)*. Knowledge of this appearance will prevent overdiagnosing osteochondritis dissecans of the capitellum.

evidence of a joint effusion but a fracture is not visualized. Marrow-sensitive sequences (T1W imaging, [fast] STIR, and fat-suppressed fast spin echo) are the most sensitive for assessing the fracture and edema associated with it (Fig. 11–5). Gradient echo is the least sensitive technique for evaluating the marrow. MRI is outstanding for evaluating stress fractures. One type of stress fracture diagnosis that is important in the elbow involves the middle third of the olecranon. This type of fracture is seen in throwing athletes as a result of overload by the triceps mechanism. These fractures can displace and require surgical fixation. Similarly, non-union of an injury through the olecranon physeal plate can be detected and also may require surgical intervention. MRI can adequately assess fractures extending through the cartilage of the physis.

Ligaments

The anterior and posterior portions of the joint capsule are relatively thin. The medial and lateral portions are thickened to form the collateral ligaments. The ligaments of the elbow are divided into the lateral (radial) and medial (ulnar) collateral ligament complexes.

Radial Collateral Ligament Complex
(Box 11–3)

Normal Radial Collateral Ligaments. The lateral or radial collateral ligament complex provides varus stability. This complex consists of the radial collateral ligament (RCL), the annular ligament, the accessory collateral ligament, and the posterolateral (lateral ulnar) collateral ligament (LUCL) (Fig. 11–6). The annular ligament surrounds the radial head and originates and inserts onto the anterior and posterior margins of the lesser sigmoid notch of the ulna. It is the primary stabilizer of the proximal radioulnar joint and is best seen on axial images. The radial collateral ligament proper arises from the anterior margin of the lateral epicondyle and inserts onto the annular ligament and fascia of the supinator muscle. The LUCL is more posterior and is absent in 10% of anatomic specimens; it is thought to provide the primary restraint to varus. It is a more superficial and posterior continuation of the RCL, arising from the lateral epicondyle and extending along the lateral and posterior aspect of the proximal radius to insert on the ulna at the crista supina-

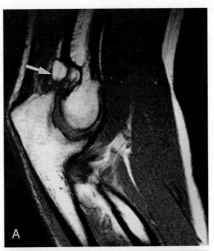

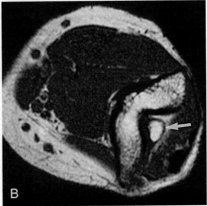

Figure 11–4. LOOSE BODY.
A, Sagittal T1-weighted image shows marrow in the posteriorly located loose body *(arrow)*. *B,* Axial T1-weighted image shows the posteriorly located loose body *(arrow)* that has marrow within it.

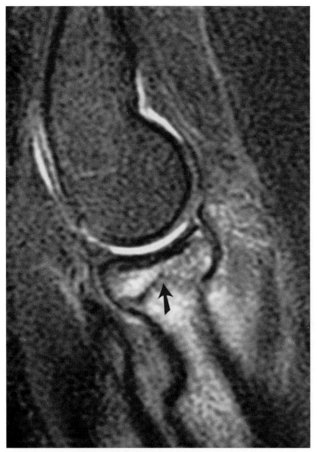

Figure 11–5. OCCULT RADIAL HEAD FRACTURE.
Female had a clinical diagnosis of biceps tendon tear. Sagittal fast spin echo T2-weighted, fat-suppressed image shows a linear low-signal fracture line along radial head *(arrow)*, with surrounding edema. There was no biceps tendon tear.

toris (Fig. 11–7). Both ligaments provide lateral stability to the elbow and constraint to varus stress. Functionally, the LUCL is more important, because it is the primary posterolateral elbow stabilizer. Both the RCL proper and the LUCL are well seen on coronal images and both should be evaluated as

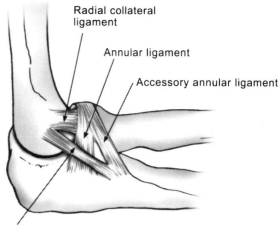

Radial collateral ligament

Annular ligament

Accessory annular ligament

Lateral ulnar collateral ligament

Figure 11–6. Diagram of the lateral side of elbow showing components of the radial collateral ligament complex.

discrete structures because of their difference in functional significance.

Abnormal Radial Collateral Ligaments. Disruption of the lateral collateral ligament complex is more unusual than that of the ulnar collateral ligament complex. Job-or sports-related injuries usually are caused by chronic, repetitive microtrauma that produces varus stress. Injury to the radial collateral ligament complex commonly is associated with lateral epicondylar soft tissue degeneration and tearing

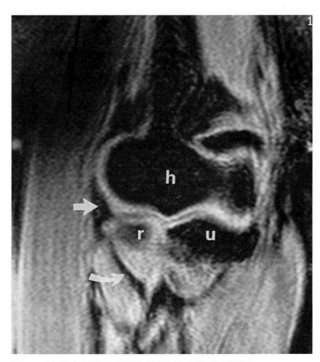

Figure 11–7. RADIAL COLLATERAL LIGAMENTS.
Coronal T2* image showing normal triangular-appearing radial collateral ligament *(straight arrow)* and obliquely oriented lateral ulnar collateral ligament (LUCL) *(curved arrow)* running posterior to the radius. h—humerus; r—radial head; u—ulna.

BOX 11–3: RADIAL COLLATERAL LIGAMENT COMPLEX

- Restrains varus stress
- Lateral ulnar collateral ligament (LUCL)—the most important
- Radial collateral ligament (RCL)—less important
- Radial collateral ligament complex injury:
  MR: ↑ T2 or complete disruption
  LUCL insufficiency → posterolateral rotatory instability
  Associated with lateral epicondylitis ("tennis elbow")

of the common extensor tendon (lateral epicondylitis or "tennis elbow"). Acute varus injury or elbow dislocation also can be associated with radial collateral ligament complex injury. Insufficiency of the LUCL may result in posterolateral rotatory instability, which allows transient rotatory subluxation of the ulnohumeral joint and secondary subluxation or dislocation of the radiohumeral joint. Rupture of this ligament occurs most commonly as a result of a posterior dislocation or varus stress. Insufficiency of the LUCL also may occur after a lateral extensor release for tennis elbow or resection of the radial head.[8] This injury most often is seen in patients who sustain a fall on an outstretched hand with resulting hyperextension and varus stress. Laxity of the LUCL after surgical lateral extensor release for tennis elbow also has been described as a result of extensive subperiosteal elevation of the common extensor tendon and radial collateral ligament complex during surgery, and also from unrecognized LUCL insufficiency preoperatively.[8, 9] Patients frequently complain of locking or snapping of the elbow. The physical examination may reveal pain over the lateral aspect of the elbow, a subjective complaint of laxity or instability with varus stress, and a positive lateral pivot shift maneuver. At surgery, laxity or disruption of the LUCL and the posterolateral portion of the capsule can be identified, as well as possible RCL laxity. Reconstruction or reattachment of the LUCL on the lateral epicondyle is performed.

A sprain of the radial collateral ligament complex appears as a thickened or thinned ligament with high signal in and around it. A complete tear demonstrates discontinuous fibers along the RCL or LUCL. Proximal detachment or avulsion of their common origin on the lateral epicondyle shows edema and hemorrhage extending into the defect and absence of the fibers of the radial collateral ligament complex (Figs. 11–8 and 11–9).[10–12] When seen in association with lateral epicondylitis, bone marrow edema in the lateral epicondyle as well as high signal in the extensor tendon group can be identified. If surgical release of the common extensor tendon is being considered, the integrity of the LUCL must be assessed.

Ulnar Collateral Ligament Complex
(Box 11–4)

Normal Ulnar Collateral Ligaments. The ulnar or medial collateral ligament complex consists of three ligaments: the anterior, posterior, and transverse ligaments (Fig. 11–10). The anterior ligament is a thick, discrete ligament with parallel fibers arising from the medial epicondyle and inserting onto the medial coronoid process; it is the most important of the ligaments and is well seen on coronal images. The MR appearance is that of a low-signal linear structure that is flared proximally and tapers distally on all imaging sequences. It is normal to see slight high signal in the proximally flared portion of the

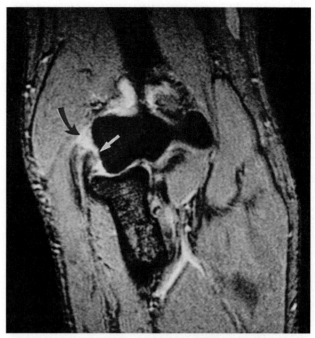

Figure 11–8. RADIAL COLLATERAL LIGAMENT TEAR. Coronal T2* image demonstrating high signal at the proximal aspect of the ulnar collateral ligament *(arrow)*. This appearance is compatible with a tear of the radial collateral ligament. Note also a partial tear of the extensor tendon *(curved arrow)*.

anterior bundle (Fig. 11–11). The anterior bundle of the ulnar collateral ligament (UCL) provides the primary restraint to valgus stress and commonly is damaged secondary to overuse in throwers.

The fan-shaped posterior bundle of the UCL is a thickening of the capsule that is best defined with the elbow flexed at 90 degrees. The transverse bundle of the UCL is formed from horizontally oriented capsule fibers joining the inferior margins of the anterior and posterior bundles. It stretches between the tip of the olecranon and the coronoid, and contributes little to elbow stability. The transverse and posterior bundles are located deep to the ulnar

---

BOX 11–4: ULNAR COLLATERAL LIGAMENT (UCL)

Restrains valgus stress
  Bundles
    Anterior (the important one)
    Posterior
    Transverse
    Best seen on coronal images
  UCL injury
    MR: ↑ T2, thickening (partial tear) or
      complete disruption
  Partial UCL tear
    Fluid between distal ligament and to ulna
      (deep fibers disrupted)

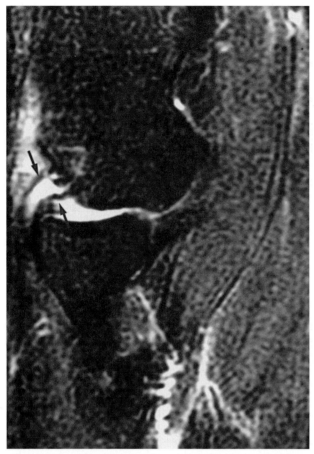

Figure 11–9. RADIAL COLLATERAL LIGAMENT RCL TEAR. Symptoms of tennis elbow. Oblique coronal (fast) STIR image shows abnormal high signal surrounding the torn RCL *(arrows)*.

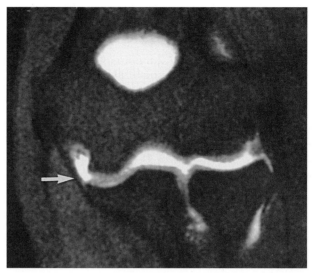

Figure 11–11. NORMAL ULNAR COLLATERAL LIGAMENT. Coronal T2-weighted image with intraarticular contrast demonstrating a normal ulnar collateral ligament (anterior bundle). The ulnar collateral ligament adheres tightly to the olecranon *(arrow)*.

nerve and, in conjunction with the capsule, form the floor of the cubital tunnel. The posterior and transverse bundles are not well depicted on MRI, but their integrity is inferred based on the floor of the cubital tunnel; regardless, they are of limited importance, inconsistently present, and are not further considered here.

Abnormal Ulnar Collateral Ligaments. UCL in-

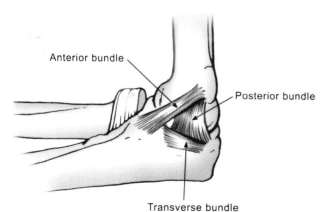

Figure 11–10. Diagram of the medial aspect of elbow, showing components of the medial collateral ligament.

Anterior bundle

Posterior bundle

Transverse bundle

jury commonly occurs in throwing athletes and may accompany an injury to the common flexor tendon group. Injury to these medial stabilizing structures is caused by chronic microtrauma from repetitive valgus stress during the acceleration phase of throwing.[13–15]

Complete rupture of the anterior bundle of the UCL usually occurs as a sudden event. Patients with acute UCL ruptures report sudden pain with or without a popping sensation that occurred with throwing, and they are unable to throw after the injury. These injuries are well seen on coronal MR images. Abnormal signal is identified in the expected location of the linear, low-signal structure of the UCL (Fig. 11–12). The torn fragments also can be identified.

In a large series of throwing athletes, midsubstance ruptures of the anterior bundle of the UCL accounted for 87% of UCL tears, whereas distal and proximal avulsions were found in 10% and 3%, respectively.[16] Chronic degeneration of the UCL is characterized by thickening of the ligament secondary to scarring, often accompanied by foci of calcification or heterotopic bone.[16] Treatment for acute UCL tears is changing. Conservative treatment is recommended for the nonelite athlete (mere mortals), because the flexor-pronator mass will keep the elbow functionally stable, although throwing will be limited. Surgical reconstruction for the competitive athlete has been recommended for many years.

Partial detachment of the deep undersurface fibers of the anterior bundle of the UCL also may occur. These patients present with medial elbow pain. The diagnosis with routine MRI is difficult. This type of tear of the UCL spares the superficial fibers of the anterior bundle and is not visible from an open surgical approach unless the undersurface of the ligament is inspected.[17, 18] Identification of these

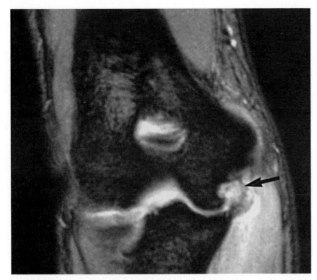

Figure 11–12. COMPLETE ULNAR COLLATERAL LIGAMENT (UCL) TEAR.
Patient with medial elbow pain. Coronal spin echo T2-weighted image shows abnormal high signal through the disrupted (UCL) *(arrow)*.

BOX 11–5: ANATOMY OF MUSCLES AROUND THE ELBOW

Anterior
Biceps superficial to brachialis
Bicipital aponeurosis
Biceps tendon; extrasynovial paratenon
Posterior
Triceps, anconeus
Medial
Pronator teres, flexors of hand and wrist
Common flexor tendon
Lateral
Supinator, brachioradialis, extensors of hand and wrist

tears is more easily made after the injection of intraarticular contrast (MR arthrography). The capsular fibers of the anterior bundle, which normally insert on the medial margin of the coronoid process, will demonstrate fluid beneath the distal extension of the anterior bundle (Fig. 11–13).[18, 19] This is often a very subtle finding, but can cause functional debilitation in a throwing athlete. Partial tears are treated with repair or reconstruction in athletes.

Muscles/Tendons (Box 11–5)

The muscles around the elbow can be divided into anterior, posterior, medial, and lateral compartments.

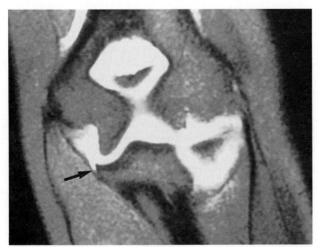

Figure 11–13. PARTIAL ULNAR COLLATERAL LIGAMENT (UCL) TEAR.
Female field hockey player with medial elbow pain. T1-weighted, fat-suppressed coronal image after intraarticular contrast administration demonstrates high signal (gadolinium) deep to the fibers of the UCL, separating bone from ligament *(arrow)*. This has been referred to as the T-sign. The ligament normally is tightly adherent to the ulna.

Anterior Compartment

Normal Anatomy. The biceps and brachialis muscles are located anteriorly. These muscles and tendons are best evaluated on axial and sagittal images. The brachialis extends along the anterior joint capsule and inserts on the ulnar tuberosity. The tendon is surrounded by its muscle, and the brachialis tendon is much smaller than the adjacent biceps tendon. The biceps muscle lies superficial to the brachialis and has a long segment of tendon that is not surrounded by muscle, making it more susceptible to injury than the brachialis. The biceps tendon inserts on the radial tuberosity. The bicipital aponeurosis (or lacertus fibrosus) helps keep the biceps tendon located in proper position. The distal aspect of the biceps tendon is covered by an extrasynovial paratenon and is separated from the radial tuberosity by the bicipital-radial bursa (normally not visualized unless distended with fluid) (Fig. 11–14).

Abnormal Anatomy (Box 11–6). Injuries to the brachialis muscle are less common than to the biceps tendon. The brachialis can be injured in association with repetitive pull-ups, hyperextension, repeated forceful supination or, occasionally, from violent extension against a forceful contraction extrinsic overload (such as an arm-wrestling match that went bad).[20] Climber's elbow is defined as a

BOX 11–6: ANTERIOR TENDON PATHOLOGY

Brachialis
• Repetitive pull-ups/climbing
Biceps
• Distal rupture rare (3%)
• Majority complete tears
• Sudden forceful load near midflexion
• Sagittal and axial images show gap/retraction

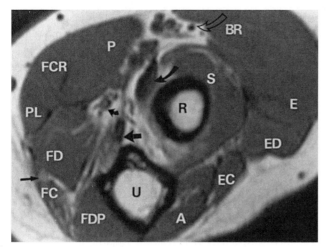

Figure 11–14. NORMAL MUSCLE, NERVE, ANATOMY.
T1-weighted axial image just distal to the elbow joint. Long *curved arrow* indicates biceps tendon. *Straight arrow* indicates brachialis tendon. *Short black arrow* indicates ulnar nerve. *Short curved arrow* indicates ulnar artery and median nerve. *Open arrow* indicates radial artery and superficial radial nerve. U—ulna; R—radius; S—supinator muscle; E—extensor carpi radialis longus/brevis muscle; BR—brachioradialis muscle; P—pronator teres muscle; FCR—flexor carpi radialis muscle; PL—palmaris longus muscle; FD—flexor digitorum superficialis muscle; FC—flexor carpi ulnaris muscle; FDP—flexor digitorum profundus muscle; A—anconeus muscle; EC—extensor carpi ulnaris muscle; ED—extensor digitorum muscle.

strain of the brachialis tendon.[21] This musculotendinous unit is believed to be involved because climbing (when done correctly) involves the use of the forearms in a pronated and semiflexed position[21] (Fig. 11–15).

Distal biceps tendon rupture is an uncommon injury, representing only 3% of all biceps ruptures.[22] Conversely, it is the most commonly (completely) torn tendon of the elbow. The majority of distal biceps tendon ruptures are complete, although partial tears have been reported.[23, 24] Partial tears often are associated with bicipitoradial bursitis; patients present with a painful mass. The mechanism of injury is a sudden, forceful overload with the elbow near midflexion. The tendon typically tears from its attachment on the radial tuberosity as a result of resisted elbow flexion[25] (Fig. 11–16); however, tears may be found anywhere along the length of the tendon. MRI is useful in evaluating these injuries because tendinopathy, partial tears, and complete ruptures may be distinguished, and tearing of the aponeurosis can be identified.

Clinical diagnosis can be difficult because the bicipital aponeurosis (lacertus fibrosus) may remain intact, with minimal retraction of the muscle. The flexion strength at the elbow may be preserved if the aponeurosis remains intact, but supination of the forearm usually is weakened.

T2W axial images are most useful for determining the degree of tearing. Partial tears can be seen as either thickening or relative thinning of the tendon with or without abnormal high signal within the tendon. These changes may be seen focally or more diffusely in the tendon. A full-thickness tear is identified as a gap that exists with the two ends of the tendon retracted from each other. The axial images must extend from the musculotendinous junction to the insertion of the tendon on the radial tuberosity. Using sagittal and axial images, the size of the gap and the location of the tear can be assessed accurately for preoperative planning.

Current treatment is primary repair that allows for reinsertion of the biceps tendon to restore power while also reducing the risk of radial nerve injury. Nonoperative treatment can be expected to yield strength deficits of 30% to 40% in flexion and supination, whereas immediate repairs result in near-normal strength.[26]

Posterior Compartment

Normal Anatomy. Within the posterior compartment are the triceps and anconeus muscles. These are best evaluated on axial and sagittal images. The triceps inserts on the proximal portion of the olecranon. At the insertion site, striated high signal can be identified on both T1W and T2W images because of the fibrofatty slips between the tendon fibers (Fig. 11–17). This should be noted so that an erroneous diagnosis of a partial tear of the triceps can be avoided. The anconeus arises from the posterior aspect of the lateral epicondyle and inserts more distally on the olecranon. The anconeus provides dynamic support to the lateral collateral ligament in resisting varus stress. A real use of the anconeus is that identification of this structure helps the radiologist become oriented as to radial and ulnar aspects of the elbow on axial imaging—the anconeus is lateral (radial).

Abnormal Anatomy. Triceps tendon rupture is the least common of all tendon ruptures in the body and

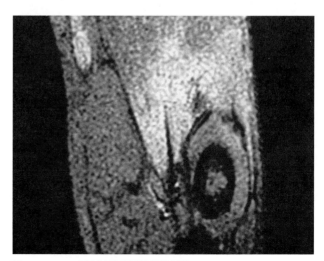

Figure 11–15. BRACHIALIS STRAIN.
Football player injured while tackling an opponent. The clinical concern was a biceps tendon injury. Coronal (fast) STIR image shows high signal in the brachialis muscle.

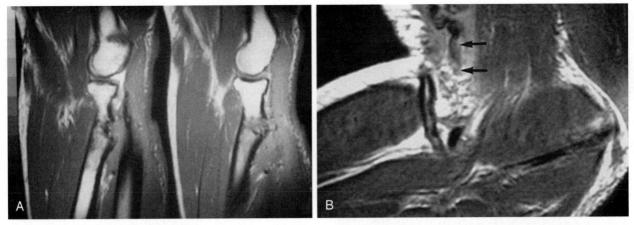

Figure 11–16. BICEPS TENDON TEAR.
Weight-lifter. Sagittal T1-weighted image shows *(A)*, avulsion of bicipital tuberosity, and *(B)* torn, retracted tendon *(arrows)*.

is an uncommon cause of posterior elbow pain.[26] Similarly, triceps tendinopathy is an uncommon cause of posterior elbow pain. The usual mechanisms of injury include a direct blow to the tendon or a decelerating counterforce during active extension.[27] The tendon also may undergo degeneration or erosion in association with olecranon bursitis.

Axial and sagittal imaging are necessary to evaluate the degree of tendinopathy, partial versus complete tear, and the size of the gap associated with the tear. This aids in preoperative planning. Abnormal signal may be seen in the tendon in a partial tear or tendinopathy, and discontinuous fibers are noted with a complete tear. Most tears occur at the insertion onto the olecranon (Fig. 11–18). However, there

have been reports of tears at the musculotendinous junction.[26–30] Often, there is associated distention of the olecranon bursa with injury to the triceps tendon. If there is distention of the olecranon bursa, a well-defined fluid collection will be noted on the T2W image posterior to the triceps tendon (Fig. 11–19).

These injuries should be treated as soon as possible with primary repair. The results are universally good.[26, 31]

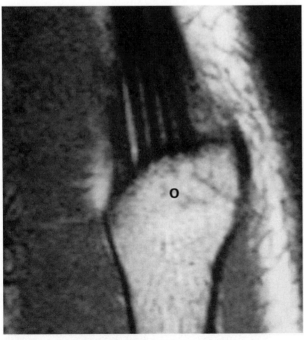

Figure 11–17. TRICEPS TENDON STRIATIONS.
Coronal T1-weighted image showing a striated appearance to the triceps tendon due to fibrofatty tissue insinuating between the tendon slips. o—olecranon.

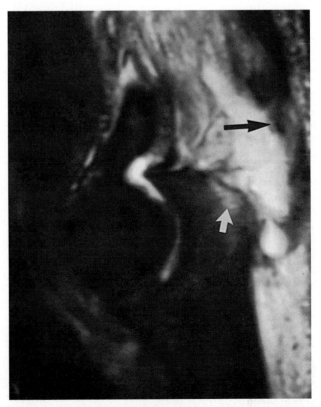

Figure 11–18. TRICEPS TENDON TEAR.
Football player. Sagittal fast spin echo, T2-weighted, fat-suppressed image shows a completely torn and retracted triceps tendon *(black arrow)*. Note abnormal high signal on olecranon from avulsion *(white arrow)*.

ELBOW ■ 235

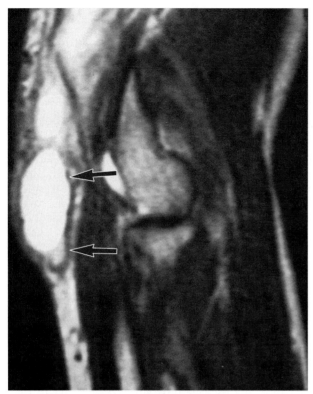

Figure 11–19. OLECRANON BURSITIS.
Sagittal T2-weighted image shows a focal fluid collection posteriorly *(arrows)* in a patient with triceps tendon tear (not shown on this image).

Medial Compartment (Box 11–7)

Normal Anatomy. The medial compartment includes the pronator tears and the flexors of the hand and wrist that arise from the medial epicondyle as the common flexor tendon. The common flexor tendon provides dynamic support to the underlying UCL in resisting valgus stress. These structures are

---

BOX 11–7: MEDIAL TENDON PATHOLOGY ("MEDIAL EPICONDYLITIS")

- Repetitive valgus stress
- Tendon degeneration, partial tear, disruption
- MR: ↑ T1 and T2 signal or disruption, thickening or thinning of tendon, +/− marrow edema in adjacent epicondyle
- Best identified in axial and coronal planes

---

best evaluated on axial and coronal images and are seen as uniformly low signal, round to oval structures inserting onto the medial epicondyle on T1W and T2W axial images (Fig. 11–20).

Abnormal Anatomy. Repetitive valgus stress injuries of the elbow are common overuse injuries seen in baseball pitchers ("Little Leaguer elbow") and other sports that use a throwing motion. Medial epicondylitis also is known as "golfer's elbow" (associated with both good and bad golf swings) or "medial tennis elbow." The term "epicondylitis" is a misnomer, because no inflammatory cells are necessarily found histologically. Nevertheless, because the term is used commonly in the literature, we are not going to attempt to change it here. It is caused by overload of the flexor-pronator muscle group, which has its origin at the medial epicondyle. Disruption of the flexor-pronator muscle group medially is more common than of the extensor muscle group laterally, even though epicondylitis is more common on the lateral side.

The findings at MRI in medial epicondylitis include tendon degeneration, partial tear, tendon disruption, and muscle strain. Coronal and axial imaging is most useful for evaluating the flexor-

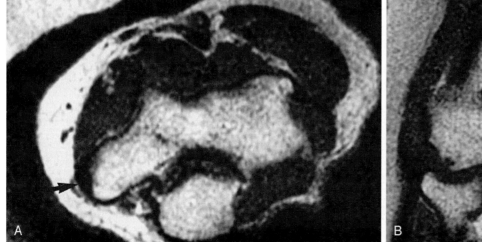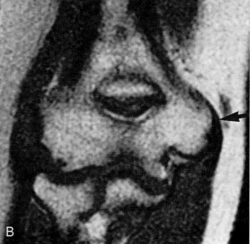

Figure 11–20. NORMAL MEDIAL TENDON.
A, Axial T1-weighted image shows normal low-signal structure inserting on medial epicondyle *(arrow).* *B,* Coronal T1-weighted image demonstrating low signal of flexor-pronator conjoined tendon as it inserts on medial epicondyle *(arrow).*

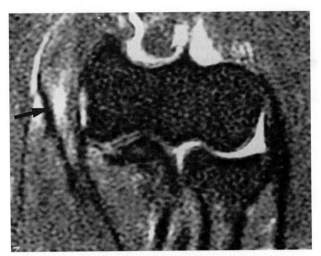

Figure 11–21. MEDIAL EPICONDYLITIS.
Male golfer with medial elbow pain. Coronal fast spin echo, T2-weighted, fat-suppressed image shows abnormal high signal at the insertion site of the flexor tendon group *(arrow).*

pronator group. MRI shows abnormal signal with possible alteration in tendon thickness on T2W images in tendon degeneration and partial tear. Discontinuity of the fibers is seen with complete rupture (Fig. 11–21). MRI facilitates surgical planning by differentiating complete from partial tears, as well as evaluating the underlying UCL complex. The increased preoperative information may lessen the need for extensive surgical exploration.

Avulsion of the medial epicondylar apophysis may occur in the skeletally immature throwing athlete as a result of failure of the flexor muscle group. MRI may detect this injury prior to complete avulsion by showing abnormal high signal on the T2W image in the adjacent soft tissues and medial apophysis. Additionally, the ulnar collateral ligament must be inspected for its integrity.

Lateral Compartment

Normal Anatomy. The lateral compartment structures consist of the supinator, the brachioradialis, and the extensors of the hand and wrist that arise from the lateral epicondyle as the common extensor tendon. As in the medial compartment, these structures are best evaluated on axial and coronal images (Fig. 11–22).

Abnormal Anatomy. Lateral tendons (Box 11–8). The lateral aspect of the elbow is the most common location of elbow pain in the general population. It occurs 7 to 20 times more frequently than medial epicondylitis.[25] Lateral epicondylitis is a chronic tendinopathy of the extensor muscles, primarily the extensor carpi radialis brevis, caused by overuse (either increased intensity or duration). Degeneration and tearing of the common extensor tendon causes the symptoms of lateral epicondylitis or "tennis elbow." Typically, the extensor carpi radialis brevis tendon is partially avulsed from the lateral epicondyle (Fig. 11–23). Scar tissue forms in response to this partial avulsion, which is then susceptible to further tearing with repeated trauma.

Lateral epicondylitis presents as lateral elbow pain that has an insidious onset, beginning gradually after vigorous activity and progressing to pain with activity.

Radiographs frequently are normal, although some patients will have evidence of a spur at the lateral epicondyle or calcification of the common extensor tendon.

In patients refractory to conservative therapy, MRI is useful in assessing the degree of tendon damage and associated ligament abnormality. The axial and coronal planes are necessary for assessing the lateral tendons. Partial tears or tendinopathy are characterized by thickening or thinning of the tendon with high signal on T2W images in or around the tendon.

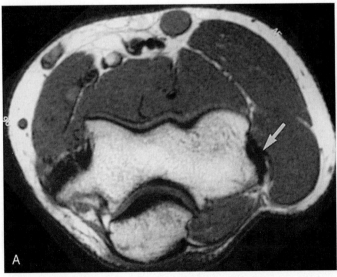

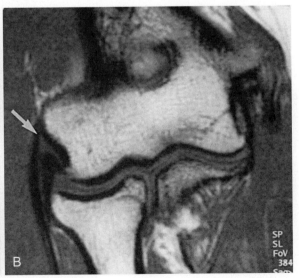

Figure 11–22. NORMAL LATERAL TENDON.
A, Axial T1-weighted image shows low signal around tendon inserting onto lateral epicondyle *(arrow).* *B,* Coronal T1-weighted image shows extensor-supinator conjoined tendon as it inserts onto lateral epicondyle *(arrow).*

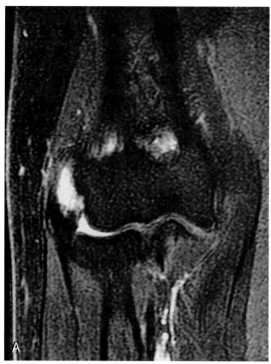

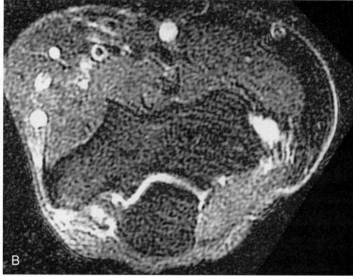

Figure 11–23. LATERAL EPICONDYLITIS.
Male with symptoms of tennis elbow. *A,* Coronal fast spin echo, T2W image shows high signal replacing extensor tendon. *B,* Axial fast spin echo T2W image shows high signal in the expected location of extensor carpi radialis brevis tendon. The tendon was completely torn.

Complete tears may be diagnosed on MRI by identifying a fluid-filled gap separating the tendon from its adjacent bony attachment site (Fig. 11–24). MRI is useful in identifying high-grade partial tears and complete tears that are unlikely to respond to nonsurgical therapies. Additionally, MRI is useful in providing assessment of additional structures that may explain the lack of response to therapy. For example, rupture or injury to the radial collateral ligament may occur in association with tears of the common extensor tendon. Moreover, the lack of significant abnormality involving the common extensor tendon on MRI may prompt consideration of an alternate diagnosis, such as radial nerve entrapment, which may occur with or mimic lateral epicondylitis.

Nerves (Box 11–9)

The nerves about the elbow are the ulnar, median, and radial nerves. They travel through numerous compartments and are subject to a variety of entrapment syndromes. The nerves are relatively small and are surrounded by fat.

MRI findings of neuropathies include increased signal of the nerve on T2W images, indistinct fascicles, enlargement of the nerve, and fluid (edema) surrounding the nerve.[32] Homogeneous high signal resembling a fluid collection on T2W images also can be seen. Nerve thickening can be focal or fusiform. The nerves are best evaluated on axial images. The amount of fat around a nerve increases the ability to identify it, particularly the radial and median nerves. MRI may be complementary to electromyography and nerve conduction studies in cases of nerve entrapment about the elbow.[32] Affected muscles in subacute denervation have prolongation of T1 and T2 relaxation times secondary to muscle

---

BOX 11–8: LATERAL TENDON PATHOLOGY ("LATERAL EPICONDYLITIS")

- More common than medial
- Repetitive varus stress
- Extensor carpi radialis brevis partially avulsed from lateral epicondyle
- MR: ↑ T1 and T2 signal or disruption, thickening or thinning of tendon, +/− marrow edema
- Radial collateral ligament also may be disrupted
- Best identified in axial and coronal planes

BOX 11–9: MRI OF NEUROPATHY

- ↑ T2 signal
- Indistinct fascicles
- Focal or diffuse thickening
- Best seen on axial images
- Neurogenic edema in muscles show ↑ signal on T2, late findings show atrophy of muscle

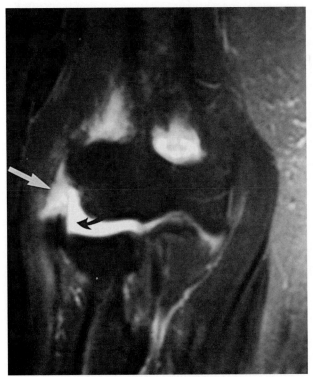

Figure 11–24. LATERAL EPICONDYLITIS.
Female with clinically suspected chronic lateral epicondylitis. Coronal fast spin echo, T2-weighted, fat-suppressed image shows abnormal high signal in the expected location of the extensor tendon group *(straight arrow)*. Note also disruption of the radial collateral ligament *(curved arrow)*.

fiber shrinkage and associated increase in extracellular water[33] (Fig. 11–25). Entrapment of a nerve about the elbow may therefore cause increased signal within the muscles innervated by the nerve on T2W images. These changes may be followed to

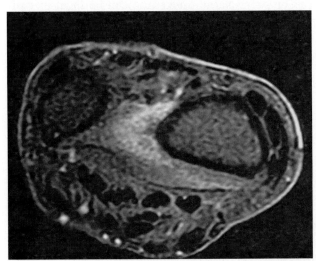

Figure 11–25. NEUROGENIC EDEMA FROM ANTERIOR INTEROSSEOUS NERVE SYNDROME.
Axial fast spin echo, T2-weighted, fat-suppressed image shows high signal in the pronator quadratus muscle that is innervated by the anterior interosseous nerve.

resolution or progress to atrophy and fatty infiltration with high signal in the muscle on T1W images.

Ulnar Nerve (Box 11–10)

Normal Ulnar Nerve. The ulnar nerve is most superficial, especially in the cubital tunnel. It is seen best on axial images. The roof of the cubital tunnel is formed by the flexor carpi ulnaris aponeurosis distally and the cubital tunnel retinaculum proximally (Fig. 11–26). The cubital tunnel retinaculum is normally a thin fibrous structure that extends from the olecranon to the medial epicondyle; this structure may be complete, partial, or absent. This structure also may be referred to as the arcuate ligament. The capsule of the elbow and the posterior and transverse portions of the medial collateral ligament form the floor of the cubital tunnel.

Abnormal Ulnar Nerve. The ulnar nerve is the most frequently injured nerve in the elbow. Anatomic as well as physiologic factors can result in abnormal nerve function and traction. The most common neuropathy is cubital tunnel syndrome (Fig. 11–27).

The ulnar nerve is well seen on axial MR images because it is surrounded by fat, especially as it passes through the superficially located cubital tunnel. Anatomic variations of the cubital tunnel retinaculum may contribute to ulnar neuropathy. These variations in the retinaculum and the appearance of the ulnar nerve are well seen with MRI. The retinaculum may be thickened, resulting in dynamic compression of the ulnar nerve during flexion. Thickening of the ulnar collateral ligament and medial bone spurring from the ulna may undermine the floor of the cubital tunnel, resulting in ulnar neuropathy.[34, 35] In 11% of the population an anomalous muscle, the anconeus epitrochlearis, replaces the retinaculum, resulting in static compression of the ulnar nerve.[35] The cubital tunnel retinaculum may be absent in 10% of the population, allowing anterior subluxation of the nerve over the medial epicondyle with flexion, leading to a friction neuritis.

A common cause of external compression on the ulnar nerve is due to prolonged hospitalization, after surgery caused by pressure from the operating room table, and in bedridden or wheelchair-bound

---

BOX 11–10: ULNAR NEUROPATHY

- Most frequent neuropathy
- Cubital tunnel most common (superficial)
- Thickened retinaculum, ulnar collateral ligament
- Bone spur
- Anconeus epitrochlearis
- Friction (absent retinaculum)
- Pressure (OR table, wheelchair)
- Masses

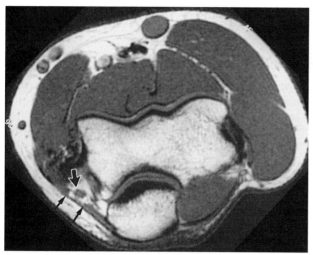

Figure 11–26. NORMAL CUBITAL TUNNEL.
Axial T1-weighted image demonstrating the normal ulnar nerve *(arrow)* surrounded by fat. The retinaculum (a portion of the flexor carpi ulnaris) is seen as the thin, linear, low-signal structure containing the ulnar nerve *(small arrows)*.

patients. Pressure from space-occupying lesions also can result in cubital tunnel syndrome. Such masses include ganglions, bursae, hematoma, tumors, osteophytes and loose bodies.

Early symptoms of cubital tunnel syndrome are paresthesias in the ring and little fingers, as well as varying degrees of sensory and motor loss in the muscles of the hand along the ulnar nerve distribution.

Cubital tunnel syndrome should be differentiated clinically from other sites of ulnar nerve compression, such as the distal humerus (eg, supracondylar process syndrome), Guyon's canal in the wrist, and the palm of the hand.

Treatment of ulnar neuropathy is conservative initially, with rest, removal of the causative agent, and steroid injection. Surgery should be performed if symptoms are not relieved after a few weeks of

conservative management. Surgical procedures include arcuate ligament (cubital tunnel retinaculum) release, medial epicondylectomy, and anterior transposition of the nerve with or without the vascular bundle. Postsurgical ulnar nerve compression is avoided by releasing the arcade of Struthers (when present), the common aponeurosis for the humeral head, origin of the flexor carpi ulnaris, the origin of the flexor digitorum superficialis, and the common intermuscular septum.

Median Nerve (Box 11–11)

Normal Median Nerve. The median nerve—as with the other nerves—is best evaluated on axial imaging, but is best seen with prone positioning of the forearm. This position allows more fat to be present around the nerve, enabling easier identification of this tiny structure. The median nerve at the elbow is located superficially, behind the lacertus fibrosus (bicipital aponeurosis) and anterior to the brachialis muscle. As it leaves the cubital fossa (this fossa, not to be confused with the cubital tunnel, is ventral to the elbow joint), the median nerve passes between the ulnar and humeral heads of the pronator teres. The anterior interosseus nerve branches off the median nerve in close proximity to the bifurcation of the brachial artery, then courses over the interosseous membrane toward the wrist.

Abnormal Median Nerve. The most common cause of median nerve entrapment is the pronator syndrome, which can present as anterior elbow pain, with or without numbness and tingling in the distribution of the median nerve, and is a result of median nerve compression between the two heads of the pronator teres muscle with pronation, or the fibrous arch of the flexor digitorum superficialis muscle, the lacertus fibrosus, or a supracondylar process (mass effect from bone spur or ligament). The most frequent cause is dynamic compression by the pronator teres muscle. The nerve gets trapped

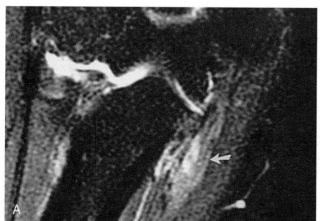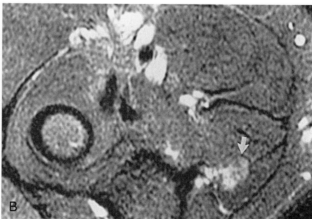

Figure 11–27. ULNAR NEUROPATHY.
Female with symptoms of ulnar neuritis. *A,* Sagittal fast spin echo, T2-weighted image shows high signal with fusiform swelling in the ulnar nerve *(arrow)*. *B,* Fast spin echo, T2-weighted axial image demonstrates fusiform swelling and abnormal high signal in the ulnar nerve *(arrow)*.

BOX 11–11: MEDIAN NEUROPATHY

Pronator syndrome occurs from compression by
- Two heads of pronator teres (most common)
- Fibrous arch of flexor digitorum superficialis
- Lacertus fibrosus
- Supracondylar process
- Irritation secondary to bicipitoradial bursitis, biceps injury
- MR: ↑ T2 signal in anterior compartment of forearm, sparing flexor carpi ulnaris and ulnar half of flexor digitorum profundus

Anterior interosseous syndrome (Kiloh-Nevin)
- Motor branch of medial nerve
- Inability to flex distal joints of thumb and index finger
- MR: ↑ T2 in flexor pollicis longus, pronator quadratus, and a part of flexor digitorum profundus

between the superficial humeral head and the deep, ulnar head.

The lacertus fibrosus (bicipital aponeurosis) arises from the biceps tendon and courses obliquely over the flexor-pronator group of muscles to insert on the antebrachial fascia. An unusually thick lacertus fibrosus can produce compression of the pronator muscle and median nerve. Bicipital-radial bursitis and partial tendon tears of the biceps may cause irritation of the adjacent median nerve, complicating the clinical findings.

The initial course of treatment is conservative and includes rest, immobilization and avoidance of exacerbating activities (pronation and finger flexion). If symptoms are severe, surgery is indicated. The region of the two heads of the pronator teres, lacertus fibrosus, and the fibrous arch of the flexor digitorum superficialis should be explored. A supracondylar spur can be identified on conventional radiographs.

The anterior interosseous syndrome (Kiloh-Nevin syndrome) is a rare compression neuropathy confined to the anterior interosseous nerve, which is purely a motor branch of the median nerve. The nerve courses along the interosseous membrane and ends in the pronator quadratus. Common causes of compression include masses, fibrous bands, accessory muscles, or an enlarged bicipital-radial bursa. Abnormal high signal can be seen in the pronator quadratus, flexor pollicis longus, and a part of flexor digitorum profundus.

Patients have pure motor loss and a characteristic pinch caused by the inability to flex the distal joints of the thumb and index fingers (such patients cannot pick dog or cat hair off clothing). Conservative treatment is warranted initially, because the condition may be reversible (Fig. 11–25). Surgery should be

performed if no improvement is seen within 6 to 8 weeks.

Radial Nerve (Box 11–12)

Normal Radial Nerve. The radial nerve is located between the brachialis and brachioradialis muscles anterior to the lateral epicondyle. At the elbow it divides into a deep motor branch (posterior interosseous nerve) and a superficial branch (sensory). The posterior interosseous nerve gains access to the posterior compartment via the superficial and deep heads of the supinator muscle. Up to 35% of individuals have a fibrous arch, called the arcade of Frohse. The superficial branch of the radial nerve passes between the supinator and the brachioradialis muscles.

Abnormal Radial Nerve. Radial nerve injury above the elbow frequently is associated with trauma such as displaced fracture of the humeral shaft, inappropriate use of crutches, prolonged tourniquet application, and lateral or posterior intramuscular injection. Pressure from a cast also may result in radial nerve injury. Nontraumatic radial neuropathy is much less common. Thickening of the arcade of Frohse (fibrous arch) along the proximal edge of the supinator muscle can lead to posterior interosseous nerve syndrome or supinator syndrome. The posterior interosseous nerve branches from the radial nerve at the capitellum and proceeds to the supinator muscle; it is a purely motor nerve. The fibrous arch limits the space for the posterior interosseous nerve. Mass effect from fracture or dislocation of the proximal radius, neoplasms, or proliferative synovitis can further compromise the tunnel. Occupations that require frequent pronation-supination or forceful extension, such as violinists, conductors, swimmers, basketball players who illegally "palm" the ball, and housewives who vigorously clean and make bread from scratch, are susceptible to this neuropathy. Abnormal high signal can be identified in the muscles of the posterior compartment of the forearm with a prolonged abnormality of the posterior interosseous nerve.

Because posterior interosseous syndrome can coexist or mimic lateral epicondylitis, MRI becomes extremely valuable in making the diagnosis in refractory cases of tennis elbow.

BOX 11–12: RADIAL NEUROPATHY

- Above elbow, secondary to trauma, fractures, cast, tourniquet, intramuscular injections
- Below elbow, less common, thickening of arcade of Frohse
- Posterior interosseous nerve, purely motor
- MR: ↑ T2 in muscles of posterior compartment of forearm

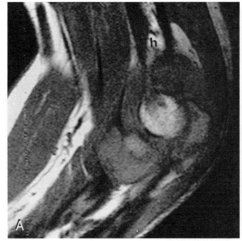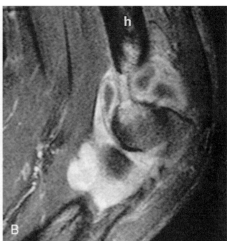

Figure 11–28. RHEUMATOID AR-THRITIS.
A, Sagittal T1-weighted image shows a distended joint as indicated by the low signal surrounding the distal humerus (h) in a patient with rheumatoid arthritis. **B,** Sagittal T1-weighted, fat-suppressed image after intravenous contrast administration. Diffuse enhancement of the pannus is easily identified.

Treatment of radial nerve compression includes conservative treatment consisting of rest, paraneural steroid injections, and physical therapy. Surgical decompression is recommended within four months of symptoms in order to avoid permanent nerve damage.

Articular Disorders

Because the distribution of articular findings is important in evaluating an arthropathy, plain films should be evaluated at the time of reviewing the MRI. Some arthropathies have a propensity to affect the elbow, such as rheumatoid arthritis, osteoarthritis, crystal deposition diseases (gout and calcium pyrophosphate deposition disease), septic arthritis, and synovial osteochondromatosis.

Rheumatoid arthritis, a pancompartmental process, has involvement of the wrist and hands if the elbow is involved (Fig. 11–28). Also, it is a bilateral process, but can be asymmetric in symptoms and appearance. Synovial proliferation occurs in this arthropathy, as well as in a number of arthritides. To assess for synovial proliferation, MRI can be used to monitor therapy by performing contrast-enhanced imaging. Subchondral cysts or erosions with bone marrow edema can occur with any of the arthritides.

Osteoarthritis typically affects a portion of the joint and, when present, has a predisposing factor such as trauma, underlying rheumatoid arthritis, calcium pyrophosphate deposition, neuropathy, or infection. Usually, osteophytes can be identified.

A joint effusion can be diagnosed by MRI if the fluid in the synovial recesses of the elbow has convex margins in the synovial recesses. An effusion is not specific for any type of arthropathy.

Gradient echo imaging can be valuable in identifying loose bodies (Fig. 11–29). The magnetic susceptibility properties of gradient echo imaging cause blooming of the cortical portions of the loose bodies, which can be seen in primary (same-sized bodies) or secondary (different-sized bodies) osteochondromatosis (Fig. 11–30). The loose bodies image as low signal structures within the high-signal joint fluid. Often, the loose bodies are multiple. Degenerative joint changes also can be seen with secondary (post traumatic) osteochondromatosis. In addition to evaluating for loose bodies, gradient echo imaging also can identify the blooming property of hemosiderin, which is seen in pigmented villonodular synovitis and hemophilia (Fig. 11–31).

Masses

Masses described for other areas of the body also can occur around the elbow. However, a few deserve special mention, because they can occur with increased frequency around the elbow.

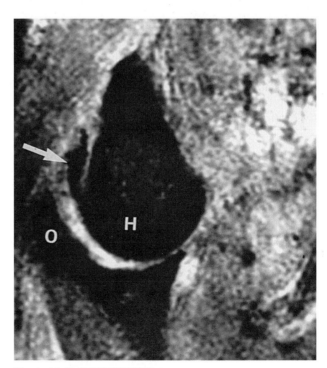

Figure 11–29. LOOSE BODY.
Sagittal T2* image demonstrating curvilinear, low-signal loose body (arrow) in a patient who suffered posterior elbow dislocation. H—humerus; O—olecranon.

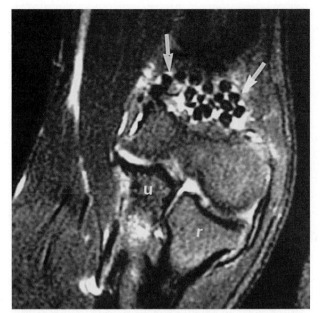

Figure 11–30. SYNOVIAL OSTEOCHONDROMATOSIS.
Coronal T2-weighted image at the anterior aspect of the joint demonstrates multiple low-signal loose bodies that are relatively similar in size *(arrow)*. This is consistent with primary synovial osteochondromatosis. r—radius; u—ulna.

Epitrochlear Adenopathy

Cat-scratch disease is characterized by local lymphadenitis within 1 or 2 weeks after being scratched by a cat. A soft tissue mass, representing swollen epitrochlear nodes, can easily be identified on MRI. The history is important to help distinguish this entity from a worrisome soft tissue mass such as a sarcoma. The distribution of the mass along the nodal chain in the epitrochlear region also is helpful. The nodes image as high signal on the T2W images, but their appearance is nonspecific. Hematogenous dissemination and spread from a contiguous contaminated source, such as a lymph node, represent potential mechanisms of osseous involvement. The responsible organism is reported to be *Afipia felis.*

Bursae

Two bursae can be identified at the biceps tendon insertion on the radial tuberosity. These are the bicipitoradial and the interosseous bursae. These bursae are located anterior to the biceps tendon. These bursae should be considered if a well-defined, isointense mass is identified on T1W images that becomes high signal on T2W images and is located anterior to the biceps tendon. Bursitis in either of these locations may impair flexion and extension. Posterior interosseous nerve compression can result from distention of the bicipitoradial bursa (Fig. 11–32). The median nerve can be affected by enlargement of the interosseous bursa. These bursae may communicate with each other, and both bursae may affect both nerves. Enlargement of either of these bursae occasionally may present as a nonspecific antecubital fossa mass. Intravenous administration of gadolinium may aid in recognition of this enlarged bursa and differentiates this benign entity from a solid neoplasm by demonstrating peripheral enhancement for the bursa, whereas a solid neoplasm demonstrates diffuse enhancement.

Gout typically is extraarticular and affects the olecranon bursa. Fluid in this bursa is considered an olecranon bursitis, and any fluid in this bursa is considered abnormal. The most common causes for fluid in the olecranon bursa are gout, trauma (hemorrhage), and infection.

Septic olecranon bursitis usually is clinically apparent, and MRI has limited application in evaluating the uncomplicated cases. MRI is useful to exclude osteomyelitis in patients refractory to therapy and has limited application in septic arthritis. Possible uses include evaluation to exclude osteomyelitis and to assess cartilage. Many of the arthritides can mimic infection by MRI appearance. Superimposed infection also can exist with arthritis. Aspiration of

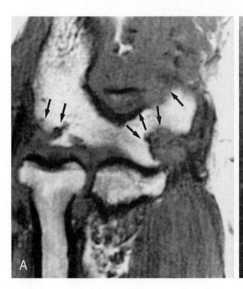
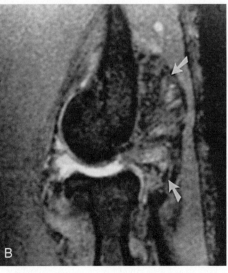

Figure 11–31. PIGMENTED VILLONODULAR SYNOVITIS.
Male with elbow pain and fullness. *A,* Coronal T1-weighted image shows erosions involving lateral and medial epicondyles, as well as the trochlea *(black arrows). B,* Sagittal gradient echo image shows low signal in the posterior aspect of the joint, representing hemosiderin *(white arrows).*

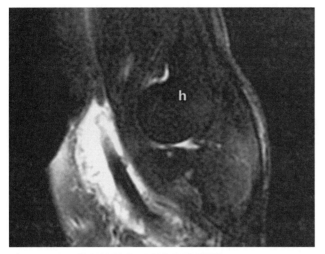

Figure 11–32. BICIPITO-RADIAL BURSITIS.
Female with mass in antecubital fossa and median nerve symptoms. Sagittal (fast) STIR image shows abnormal signal around the biceps tendon in this patient with rheumatoid arthritis. The median nerve had mass effect from the distended bicipito-radial bursa. h—humerus.

the joint remains the most efficacious diagnostic study.

References

1. Aronen J. Problems of the upper extremity in gymnastics. *Clin Sports Med* 1985; 4:61–71.
2. Ellman H. Unusual affections of the preadolescent elbow. *J Bone Joint Surg [Am]* 1967; 49:203.
3. Fixsen J, Maffulli N. Bilateral intra-articular loose bodies of the elbow in an adolescent BMX rider. *Injury* 1989; 20:363–364.
4. Gugenheim J, Stanley R, Woods G, Tullos H. Little League survey: the Houston study. *Am J Sports Med* 1976; 4:189.
5. Hang V, Lippert F, Spolek G, et al. Biomechanical study of the pitching elbow. *Int Orthop* 1979; 3:217.
6. Pintore E, Maffulli N. Osteochondritis dissecans of the lateral humeral condyle in a table tennis player. *Med Sci Sports Exerc* 1991; 23:889–891.
7. Bennett J, Tullos H. Ligamentous and articular injuries in the athlete. In Morrey BF (ed): *The Elbow and Its Disorders.* Philadelphia: W.B. Saunders; 1985; 502–522.
8. Nestor B, O'Driscoll S, Morrey B. Ligamentous reconstruction for posterolateral rotatory instability of the elbow. *J Bone Joint Surg [Am]* 1992; 74:1235–1241.
9. O'Driscoll S, Bell D, Morrey B. Posterolateral rotatory instability of the elbow. *J Bone Joint Surg [Am]* 1991; 73:440–446.
10. Fritz R, Steinbach L. Magnetic resonance imaging of the musculoskeletal system. Part 3: the elbow. *Clin Orthop* 1996; 324:321–339.
11. Herzog R. Efficacy of magnetic resonance imaging of the elbow. *Med Sci Sports Exerc* 1994; 26:1193–1202.
12. Ho C. Sports and occupational injuries of the elbow: MR imaging findings. *AJR* 1995; 164:1465–1471.
13. Kvitne R, Jobe F. Ligamentous and posterior compartment injuries. In Jobe FW (ed). *Operative Techniques in Upper Extremity Sports Injuries.* St. Louis: Mosby–Year Book; 1996:411–430.
14. Fleisig G, Andrews J, Dillman C, Escamilla R. Kinetics of baseball pitching with implications about injury mechanisms. *Am J Sports Med* 1995; 23:233–239.
15. Joyce M, Jelsma R, Andrews J. Throwing injuries to the elbow. *Sports Med Arthroscop Rev* 1995; 3:224–236.
16. Conway J, Jobe F, Glousman R, Pink M. Medial instability of the elbow in throwing athletes: treatment by repair of reconstruction of the ulnar collateral ligament. *J Bone Joint Surg [Am]* 1992; 74:67–83.
17. Timmerman LA, Schwartz ML, Andrews JR. Preoperative evaluation of the ulnar collateral ligament by magnetic resonance imaging and computed tomography arthrography: evaluation in 25 baseball players with surgical confirmation. *Am J Sports Med* 1994; 22:26–32.
18. Timmerman LA, Andrews JR. Undersurface tear of the ulnar collateral ligament in baseball players: a newly recognized lesion. *Am J Sports Med* 1994; 22:33–36.
19. Schwartz ML, al-Zahrani S, Morwessel RM, Andrews JR. Ulnar collateral ligament injury in the throwing athlete: evaluation with saline-enhanced MR arthrography. *Radiology* 1995; 197:297–299.
20. Safran M. Elbow injuries in athletes. *Clin Orthop* 1995; 310:257–277.
21. Bollen S. Soft tissue injury in extreme rock climbers. *Br J Sports Med* 1988; 22:145–147.
22. Seiler J, Parker L, Chamberland P, et al. The distal biceps tendon. Two potential mechanisms involved in its rupture: arterial supply and mechanical impingement. *J Shoulder Elbow Surg* 1995; 4:149.
23. Bourne M, Morrey B. Partial rupture of the distal biceps tendon. *Clin Orthop* 1991; 271:143–148.
24. Nielsen K. Partial rupture of the distal biceps brachii tendon. *Acta Orthop Scand* 1987; 58:287.
25. Coonrad R. Tendinopathies at the elbow. AAOS *Instructional Course Lecture* 1991; 40:25–42.
26. Morrey B. Tendon injuries about the elbow. In Morrey BF (ed): *The Elbow and Its Disorders* Philadelphia: W.B. Saunders, 1985; 452–463.
27. Tarsney F. Rupture and avulsion of the triceps. *Clin Orthop* 1972; 83:177–183.
28. Farrar E III, Lippert F. III. Avulsion of the triceps tendon. *Clin Orthop* 1981; 161:242.
29. Gilcreest E. Rupture of muscles and tendons. *JAMA* 1925; 84:1819.
30. Montgomery A. Two cases of muscle injury. *Surgical Clinics of Chirurgia* 1920; 4:871.
31. Bennett B. Triceps tendon rupture: case report and method of repair. *J Bone Joint Surg [Am]* 1962; 44:741–744.
32. Rosenberg ZS, Beltran J, Cheung YY, et al. The elbow: MR features of nerve disorders. *Radiology* 1993; 188:235–240.
33. Polak J, Jolesz F, Adams D. Magnetic resonance imaging examination of skeletal muscle prolongation of T1 and T2 subsequent to denervation. *Invest Radiol* 1991; 23:365–369.
34. McPherson S, Meals R. Cubital tunnel syndrome. *Orthop Clin North Am* 1992; 23:111–123.
35. O'Driscoll S, Horii E, Carmichael S, Morrey B. The cubital tunnel and ulnar neuropathy. *J Bone Joint Surg [Br]* 1991; 73:613–617.

ELBOW PROTOCOLS

	ELBOW MRI: NON-ARTHROGRAM					
Sequence #	1	2	3	4	5	6
Sequence Type	T1	Fast spin echo with fat suppression	T1	Fast spin echo with fat suppression	T2* 20° Flip angle	
Orientation	Axial	Axial	Coronal	Coronal	Sagittal	
Field of View (cm)	12–14	12–14	12–14	12–14	12–14	
Slice Thickness (mm)	4	4	4	4	4	
Contrast	No	No	No	No	No	

	ELBOW MRI: ARTHROGRAM					
Sequence #	1	2	3	4	5	6
Sequence Type	T1 with fat suppression	Fast spin echo with fat suppression	T1 with fat suppression	Fast spin echo with fat suppression	Gradient echo	
Orientation	Axial	Axial	Coronal	Coronal	Sagittal	
Field of View (cm)	12–14	12–14	12–14	12–14	12–14	
Slice Thickness (mm)	4	4	4	4	4	
Contrast	Intrarticular done in fluoroscopy					

Same dilution as shoulder arthrogram.

Elbow MRI

Scout		Final Image
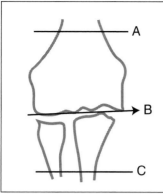	• Coronal scout • Obtain axial images parallel to line B, tangent to humeral condyle surface • Cover from line A (distal humeral metaphysis) to C (proximal radial metaphysis) • Axials should be obtained as first (most valuable) plane • Final image should fill entire frame	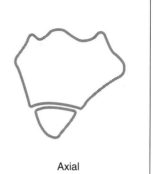 Axial
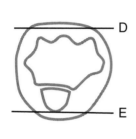	• Axial scout • Obtain coronal images parallel to line connecting humeral condyles anteriorly • Cover from line D to E • Coronals should be obtained as second plane	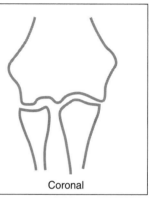 Coronal
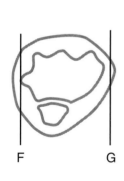	• Axial scout • Obtain sagittal images perpendicular to coronal plane • Cover from line F to G • First and last images should include epicondyle tips • Sagittals should be obtained as last plane (least valuable)	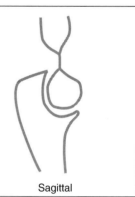 Sagittal

WRIST AND HAND

HOW TO IMAGE THE WRIST AND
  HAND
NORMAL AND ABNORMAL
Ligaments
  Intrinsic Ligaments
    Normal scapholunate and
      lunotriquetal ligaments
  Extrinsic Ligaments
    Volar and dorsal ligaments
Triangular Fibrocartilage Complex
  Triangular Fibrocartilage
  Radioulnar Ligaments
  Meniscus Homologue
  Extensor Carpi Ulnaris Sheath
  Ulnar Collateral Ligament (Wrist)
**Ulnar Collateral Ligament of the
  Thumb (Gamekeeper's Thumb)**
Tendons
  Normal Anatomy

Tendon Pathology
  De Quervain syndrome
  Extensor carpi ulnaris
  Bowstringing
  Other tendons
Carpal Tunnel
Nerves
  Median Nerve
    Carpal tunnel syndrome
  Ulnar Nerve
    Ulnar tunnel syndrome
  Fibrolipomatous Hamartoma
Osseous Structures
  Normal Relationships
  Osseous Abnormalities
    Os styloideum
    Carpal instability
    Ulnolunate impaction

Occult fractures
Physeal injuries
Osteonecrosis
Other congenital osseous lesions
Tumors
  Osseous Lesions
    Enchondromas
    Intraosseous ganglion cysts
  Soft Tissue Lesions
    Ganglion cysts
    Giant cell tumors of the tendon
      sheath
    Glomus tumors
    Anomalous muscles
Arthritis
  Synovial Cysts
Infection
Wrist/Hand Protocols

HOW TO IMAGE THE WRIST AND HAND

See the wrist protocols at the end of the chapter.

Coils/Patient Position. Some type of surface coil is an absolute requirement for proper wrist imaging. There are many different coils that may be used, including dedicated wrist coils. In general, the smaller the coil, the better the images of the wrist.

If the patient is not too large, the wrist may be imaged with the patient supine and the arm alongside their body. Many of our patients are too large to be imaged in this position; thus, we usually have them prone with the arm over the head and the elbow flexed. This position can become rapidly tiring and painful. The technologist must be aware of how to position and properly pad the patient at pressure points in order to ensure the patient's comfort and prevent motion during the study. Padding under the shoulder and elbow are particularly useful. The best way to understand what is uncomfortable about an examination is to have it done to yourself.

Image Orientation (Box 12–1). We image the wrist in three anatomic orthogonal planes, based on an axial scout view obtained through the proximal carpal row. This allows for acquiring true anatomic coronal, axial, and sagittal images. Many radiologists do not obtain sagittal images in the wrist, and this may be considered an optional sequence. We prefer to have sagittal images because they give an additional look at the osseous structures and their alignment, which may not be evaluated as well in the other imaging planes.

Pulse Sequences/Regions of Interest. Pulse sequences are a combination of T1 and some type of T2 images. T2* (gradient echo) images are particularly excellent for ligament evaluation. Three-dimensional (3D) volume acquisition using gradient echo images allows for very thin (1- to 2-mm) slices, which are necessary for identifying the ligaments well. Two-dimensional (2D) gradient echo images that have a section thickness less than 3 mm also work well. The specific protocols are selected based on pulse sequences needed for the following clinical indications: "routine" (pain), mass/infection, gamekeeper's thumb, and trauma (screening for fractures only).

We do dedicated imaging of only the wrist, unless there is a clinical reason given for imaging any portion of the hand as well. The field of view for a wrist examination is approximately 10 cm (plus or minus, depending on patient size), and this allows the distal radius and ulna, carpal bones, and bases of the metacarpal bones to be included. An MRI examination of the hand includes the wrist, metacarpals, and most (or all) of the fingers, using the same pulse sequences and planes of imaging as for the wrist, but the field of view is enlarged to 14 cm (plus or minus) in order to include the additional

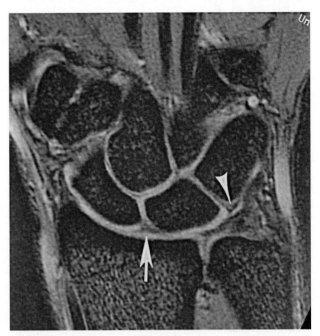

Figure 12–1. NORMAL INTRINSIC CARPAL LIGAMENTS. T2* coronal image, wrist. The scapholunate *(arrow)* and lunotriquetral *(arrowhead)* ligaments are located on the proximal aspects of the carpal bones to which they attach, best depicted on coronal images.

anatomy. We also perform dedicated examinations of the fingers, in which case a 6- to 8-cm field of view is used.

The coronal plane of imaging is where the small ligaments of the wrist are best demonstrated, and it is essential to have thin slices in this plane. For evaluation of ligaments, the slice thickness should be 1 to 2 mm. A slice thickness of 3 mm can be used in the other imaging planes and for evaluation of masses, fractures, and other abnormalities aside from ligaments.

Contrast. Intravenous contrast administration is used for evaluation of a mass in order to differentiate a cystic from a solid lesion, and for infection in order to better appreciate abscess formation. We do not perform MR arthrography in the wrist.

NORMAL AND ABNORMAL

Ligaments

The ligaments of the wrist are divided into intrinsic and extrinsic ligaments. The intrinsic carpal ligaments connect carpal bones to one another and limit their motion. The extrinsic ligaments connect the bones of the forearm to those of the wrist, allowing stability of the wrist with the distal forearm.

Intrinsic Ligaments (Box 12–2)

Normal Scapholunate and Lunotriquetral Ligaments. The scapholunate ligament and the lunotriquetral ligament are the two intrinsic carpal ligaments of greatest clinical significance; disruption of these ligaments may cause instability and pain. Both of these ligaments can be evaluated best on gradient echo T2* coronal images using thin sections. These ligaments are horseshoe-shaped, band-like, or triangular-shaped structures on the proximal aspects of the carpal bones to which they attach (Fig. 12–1).[1, 2]

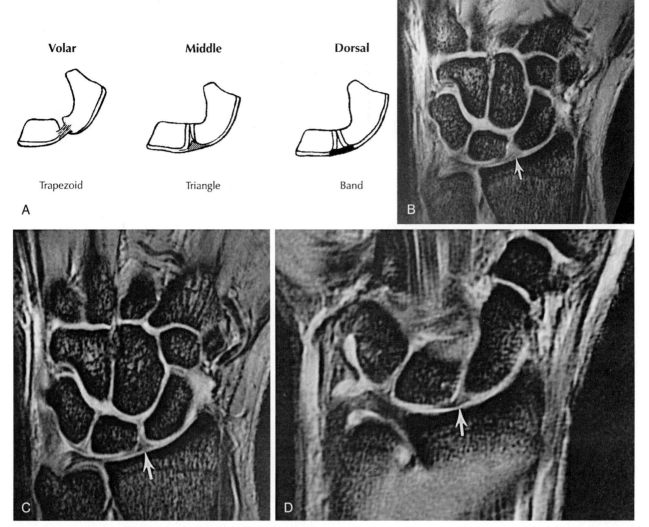

Figure 12–2. NORMAL SCAPHOLUNATE LIGAMENT: Three Portions.
A, Diagram showing the different appearances of the volar, middle, and dorsal portions of the scapholunate ligament, which correspond to the MRI appearances. *B,* T2* coronal image, wrist. The volar portion of the ligament *(arrow)* is trapezoidal and intermediate signal. *C,* T2* coronal image, wrist. The middle portion of the scapholunate ligament *(arrow)* is lower signal than the volar portion and triangular in configuration. *D,* T2* coronal image, wrist. The dorsal portion *(arrow)* is a band of even lower signal, and the strongest portion of the ligament.

The scapholunate ligament has volar, middle, and dorsal portions (Fig. 12–2). Studies have shown that only the volar and, especially, the dorsal portions are important for wrist stability. Perforations (or communicating defects) in the middle portion are common and do not seem to relate to symptoms when they are an isolated finding.[3]

The volar portion of the scapholunate ligament is trapezoidal in configuration, with intermediate signal intensity on gradient echo images. The middle portion of the scapholunate ligament is triangular in shape, with somewhat lower signal intensity than the volar component, and both portions are routinely heterogeneous. The dorsal portion is a low signal intensity homogenous band. In general, the volar portion of the scapholunate ligament attaches to cortical bone, whereas the middle and dorsal portions attach to hyaline cartilage or a combination of cartilage and cortical bone. The reason for the relatively higher signal intensity of the volar and middle portions of the scapholunate ligament, as compared to the dorsal portion, is related to the lower density of collagen fibers and the higher proportion of loose connective tissue and vascular tissue in these regions.[4]

The lunotriquetral ligament is smaller than the scapholunate ligament but has a similar shape and frequently displays a heterogeneous low signal intensity on coronal gradient echo images. The lunotriquetral ligament may attach to hyaline articular cartilage or cortical bone.

Intermediate signal intensity may partially or completely traverse the substance of the lunotriquetral ligament and scapholunate ligament in asymptomatic individuals (Fig. 12–3). Only if this signal intensity becomes as high a signal as that of fluid on whatever type of T2 sequence is being used should it be considered an abnormal finding (torn

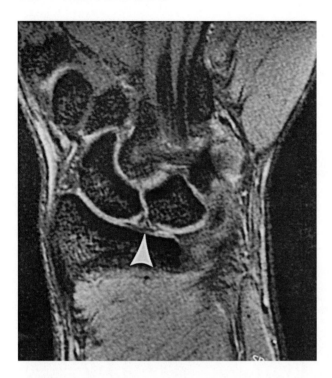

Figure 12–3. SCAPHOLUNATE LIGAMENT: Normal Variation.
T2* coronal image, wrist. High signal traversing the intercarpal ligaments is a normal finding *(arrowhead)* because it does not become as high signal as fluid.

ligament). Similarly, high signal intensity between articular cartilage and the ligament should indicate an avulsed ligament only if the signal intensity becomes as bright as fluid.

Abnormal Scapholunate and Lunotriquetral Ligaments. The abnormalities on MRI that indicate a scapholunate ligament abnormality are (1) discontinuity of the ligament, with or without an increased space between the scaphoid and lunate bones; (2) complete absence of the scapholunate ligament; (3) distorted morphology with fraying, thinning, and irregularity, and (4) elongated ligament with an increased intercarpal space (Fig. 12–4). The accuracy of MRI has been reported as 90% when compared with arthrography and 95% when compared to surgery (arthroscopy and arthrotomy).[5]

Scapholunate instability occurs when the scapholunate ligament is completely torn or stretched, allowing the scaphoid and lunate bones to dissociate. The scaphoid tilts in a volar direction (rotatory subluxation), whereas the lunate tilts in a dorsal direction (dorsal intercalated segmental instability, or DISI). The relationship of the osseous structures can be detected on sagittal MR images (Fig. 12–5). Rotatory subluxation is the most common instability pattern in the wrist. The DISI pattern of carpal instability also can occur with an unstable fracture of the scaphoid, even though the scapholunate ligament is intact.[6, 7]

Scapholunate ligament disruption and chronic rotatory instability of the scaphoid also may lead to the capitate migrating proximally and may cause

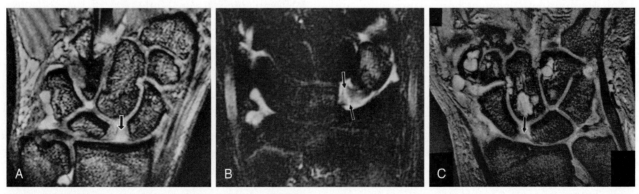

Figure 12–4. SCAPHOLUNATE LIGAMENT ABNORMALITIES.
A, Three-dimensional T2* coronal image, wrist. *Arrow* points to the widened space between the scaphoid and lunate. The torn ligament is absent. *B,* Fast T2 with fat saturation coronal image, wrist (different patient than in *A*). Distortion of the morphology of the scapholunate ligament, which is frayed and with a vertical high–signal tear through it *(arrows)*. *C,* T2* coronal image, wrist (different patient than in *A* and *B*). The space between the scaphoid and lunate bones is increased and the ligament *(arrow)* is stretched, although it remains intact. This was the result of inflammation associated with rheumatoid arthritis. Multiple bone erosions, subchondral cysts, and a triangular fibrocartilage tear are also present.

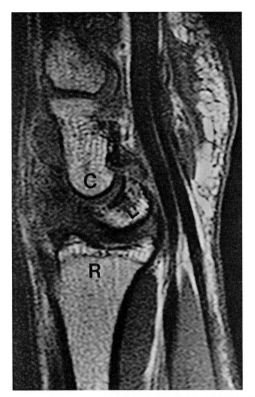

Figure 12–5. DORSAL INTERCALATED SEGMENTAL INSTABILITY (DISI).
T1 sagittal image, wrist (same patient as Figure 12–4B). The lunate (L) is tipped in a dorsal direction relative to the capitate (C) and radius (R) as the result of rotatory subluxation of the scaphoid that occurred from disruption of the scapholunate ligament.

be evaluated to see an entire ligament. The volar ligaments are stronger and thicker than the dorsal ligaments. Extrinsic ligaments are located between the wrist joint capsule and the synovial lining of the joint (intracapsular, extrasynovial). Extrinsic ligaments appear as striated fascicular structures with alternating bands of low and intermediate signal intensity on coronal MR images.

The most important volar ligaments are the radioscaphocapitate and radiolunotriquetral ligaments. The radioscophocapitate ligament originates on the volar surface of the radial styloid process and courses obliquely across the waist of the scaphoid without attaching to it (it acts as a seatbelt to maintain the position of the scaphoid), to insert on the center of the capitate. The radiolunotriquetral ligament is the largest ligament of the wrist. It arises adjacent to (on the ulnar side of) the radioscaphocapitate ligament on the radial styloid. It runs obliquely to attach to the volar surfaces of the lunate and triquetrum.

The dorsal extrinsic ligaments of the wrist run obliquely between the distal radius and to each of the carpal bones of the proximal carpal row (radioscaphoid, radiolunate, and radiotriquetral ligaments).[8–10] There are other small extrinsic carpal ligaments that are not discussed here.

The good news about all of these extrinsic ligaments is that no one knows with certainty what importance they have clinically. The MRI appearance of normal extrinsic ligaments has been exten-

the SLAC (**S**capho **L**unate **A**dvanced **C**ollapse) wrist. The SLAC wrist consists of scapholunate ligament disruption, degenerative changes between the scaphoid and distal radius, and proximal migration of the capitate between the scaphoid and lunate bones (Fig. 12–6).

Disruption of the lunotriquetral ligament is not as easy to diagnose as that of the scapholunate ligament, because of its relatively smaller size. Similar abnormalities to those seen in an abnormal scapholunate ligament are present in an abnormal lunotriquetral ligament (Fig. 12–7). Tears of the lunotriquetral ligament are the second most common cause of carpal instability and result in the lunate tilting in a volar direction (volar intercalated segmental instability, or VISI). There is a strong association between tears of the triangular fibrocartilage and lunotriquetral ligament tears.

Extrinsic Ligaments

Volar and Dorsal Ligaments. The extrinsic carpal ligaments can be seen best on gradient echo coronal images; they are seen in cross section on sagittal images (Fig. 12–8). These course between the carpal bones and the radius on both the volar and dorsal sides of the wrist. The extrinsic ligaments run obliquely and, usually, several adjacent images must

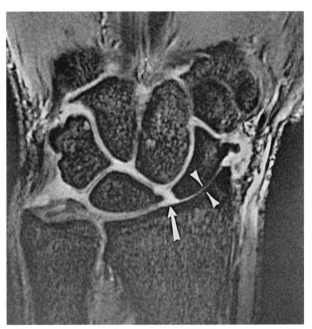

Figure 12–6. SCAPHOLUNATE ADVANCED COLLAPSE (SLAC) WRIST.
T2* coronal image, wrist. The scapholunate ligament is absent (arrow) and the space between the bones is increased. The capitate is migrating proximally between the two bones. There is loss of cartilage and a decreased space between the scaphoid and radius from degenerative joint disease (arrowheads). Incidentally, there is also a triangular fibrocartilage tear.

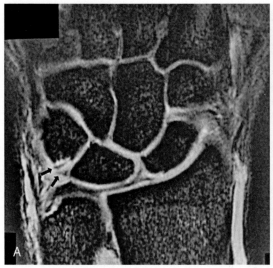
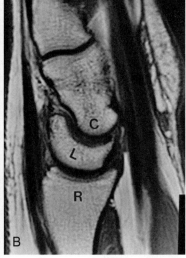

Figure 12–7. LUNOTRIQUETRAL TEAR AND CONSEQUENT VOLAR INTERCALATED SEGMENTAL INSTABILITY (VISI).
A, T2* coronal image, wrist. There is high signal through a disruption of the lunotriquetral ligament with fragments of the ligament *(arrow)* seen on either side of the tear. *B,* T1 sagittal image, wrist. The lunate (L) is tipped in a volar direction relative to the capitate (C) and radius (R) as the result of the lunotriquetral ligament tear, causing carpal instability (VISI).

sively described, but the ability of MRI to detect abnormalities is unknown. The only value in radiologists knowing about them is so that they do not cause confusion during interpretation of MR images of the wrist. We spend little to no time analyzing these ligaments.

Triangular Fibrocartilage Complex
(Box 12–3)

The triangular fibrocartilage complex (TFCC) is made up of several soft tissue structures on the ulnar side of the wrist: the triangular fibrocartilage, volar and dorsal radioulnar ligaments, meniscus homologue, ulnar collateral ligament, and the sheath of the extensor carpi ulnaris (ECU) tendon (Fig. 12–9).

The functions of the structures that compose the TFCC include cushioning forces across the ulnar side of the wrist during axial loading and stabilizing the ulnar side of the wrist and the distal radioulnar

joint. With neutral ulnar variance, about 80% of axial loading forces pass through the radial side of the wrist. The ulna absorbs about 20% of the axial loading forces through the TFCC.[6, 11]

Triangular Fibrocartilage

Normal Triangular Fibrocartilage. The triangular fibrocartilage (TFC) is a fibrocartilagenous biconcave disk with an asymmetric bow-tie shape, similar to the temporomandibular joint disk (Fig. 12–10). The TFC is positioned in the ulnocarpal space with attachments on the medial side to the ulnar styloid process by two thin bands of TFC tissue, and laterally to the side of the radius. At its radial attachment, there is hyaline cartilage interposed between the TFC and the radius that must not be confused with a detached or torn TFC. The TFC attaches directly to the cartilage, which is the articular surface of the distal radioulnar joint. The thickness of the TFC is inversely proportional to the degree of ulnar variance. In other words, the TFC is thinner

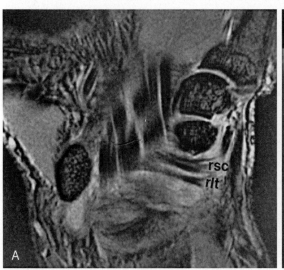
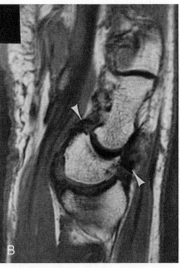

Figure 12–8. EXTRINSIC LIGAMENTS.
A, T2* coronal image, wrist. Portions of the two major volar carpal extrinsic ligaments are shown coursing obliquely as striated low-signal structures. rsc—radioscaphocapitate; rlt—radiolunotriquetral ligaments. *B,* T1 sagittal image, wrist. Both volar and dorsal extrinsic ligaments are seen as round, low-signal structures *(arrowheads)* in cross section in this plane of imaging.

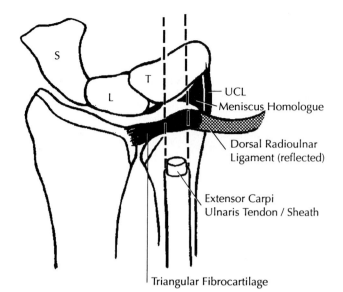

Figure 12–9. TRIANGULAR FIBROCARTILAGE COMPLEX (TFCC).
Diagram of the anatomic components of the TFCC from a dorsal perspective. S—scaphoid; L—lunate; T—triquetrum; UCL—ulnar collateral ligament.

BOX 12–3: TRIANGULAR FIBROCARTILAGE COMPLEX (TFCC)

Components:
  Triangular fibrocartilage (TFC)
  Radioulnar ligaments (dorsal and volar)
  Extensor carpi ulnaris (ECU) tendon sheath
  Ulnar collateral ligament
  Meniscus homologue
Function:
  Absorbs axial loading forces (20% pass through ulnar side of wrist)
  Stabilizes ulnar side of wrist and distal radioulnar joint
Abnormalities:
  • TFC
    —Partial or full thickness tears, detachment, degeneration
    —High signal through surface on T2 = tear
  • Radioulnar ligaments
    —High signal through these structures indicates a tear
    —Tear leads to instability of the distal radioulnar joint
  • ECU sheath
    —Tenosynovitis commonly affects this tendon
      High signal surrounding the tendon on axial T2 images
    —Disruption of the sheath leads to medial subluxation of the ECU from its groove in ulna

in patients with positive ulnar variance, and thicker in those with negative ulnar variance.

The TFC is depicted best on coronal MR images. It may be diffusely low signal intensity regardless of pulse sequence, or have intermediate signal intensity in its substance from asymptomatic myxoid degeneration.

Abnormal Triangular Fibrocartilage. Any structure of the TFCC can be abnormal, but the TFC is the main component to show abnormalities. The TFC can be evaluated similarly to the meniscus in the knee. High signal intensity within the substance of the TFC has no clinical significance, whereas high signal intensity extending through either the proximal or distal surface of the TFC indicates a tear (Fig. 12–11).[5, 12–15] TFC tears may be partial or full thickness, extending partially or completely through the substance of the TFC. Fluid in the distal

radioulnar joint was once believed to be a secondary sign of a TFC tear, but fluid is normally present in this joint in most individuals.

The location of a tear has therapeutic implications because of the vascular supply of the TFC.[16] The peripheral 20% of the TFC on the ulnar margin is

Figure 12–10. NORMAL TRIANGULAR FIBROCARTILAGE.
A, T2* coronal image, wrist. The triangular fibrocartilage *(small black arrowhead;* TFC) is a biconcave structure attaching to the high-signal cartilage on the radius *(white arrowhead).* This image also shows the ulnar collateral ligament well *(large black arrowheads).* *B,* T2* coronal image, wrist. The ulnar attachment of the TFC consists of two thin bands of tissue *(arrowheads).*

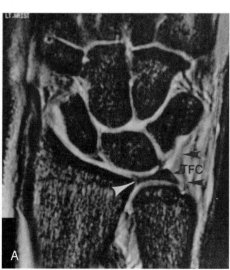

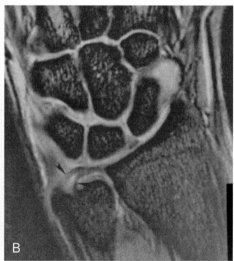

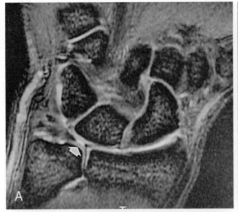
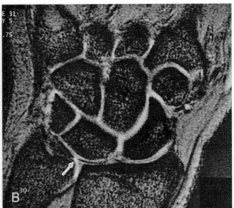
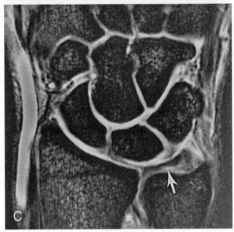

Figure 12–11. TRIANGULAR FIBROCARTI-LAGE (TFC) TEARS. *A,* T2* coronal image, wrist. There is a large gap in the midsubstance of the TFC *(arrow)* from a tear. *B,* T2* coronal image, wrist (different patient than in *A*). A tiny perforation at the radial attachment of the TFC is evident as a high-signal line *(arrow)* traversing the TFC. *C,* T2* coronal image, wrist (different patient than *A* and *B*). There is a high-signal irregularity *(arrow)* on the proximal surface of the TFC from a partial tear.

well vascularized, and tears may heal with nonoperative therapy. The remainder of the TFC is essentially avascular, and perforations or tears in the central and radial portions of the TFC usually are debrided. Many people have high signal intensity within the substance of the TFC, as well as perforations, but have no symptoms. The intrasubstance signal is probably from myxoid degeneration. The asymptomatic perforations are probably degenerative in nature, because most traumatic tears are symptomatic. As with all imaging, the presence of abnormal findings does not ensure that symptoms are a consequence of the abnormalities, and correla-

tion of the MRI and clinical findings is mandatory in planning proper management of patients. The TFC may be traumatically detached from its ulnar attachment and may even become interposed between the radius and ulna, preventing proper reduction of the distal radioulnar joint (Fig. 12–12).

Traumatic tears of the TFC often are associated with injuries of adjacent structures, which MRI can demonstrate well. Disruption of the ECU tendon sheath and partial or complete tears of the lunotriquetral ligament are associated.

MRI is very accurate for diagnosing TFC tears; compared with arthrography and surgery, it has an

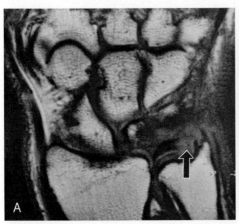
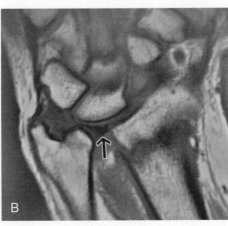

Figure 12–12. TRIANGULAR FIBROCARTILAGE (TFC) DETACHMENT.
A, T1 coronal image, wrist. The ulnar attachment of the TFC has been traumatically detached with discontinuity and a gap of the TFC *(arrow)* through the two thin bands that attach it to the ulnar styloid process. *B,* T1 coronal image, wrist (different patient than in *A*). The TFC has been detached from the ulnar styloid and is displaced and trapped in the distal radioulnar joint *(arrow),* preventing reduction of the joint. The distal radius also is fractured.

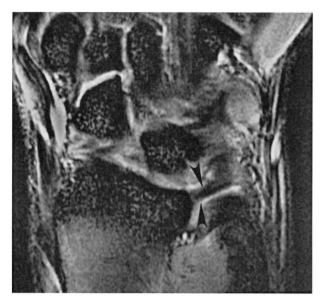

Figure 12–13. NORMAL RADIOULNAR LIGAMENT.
T2* coronal image, wrist. The volar radioulnar ligament is seen as a low-signal structure *(arrowheads)* attaching to the bones of the radius and ulna, with straight proximal and distal margins. These are all features distinguishing it from the adjacent triangular fibrocartilage proper. The dorsal radioulnar ligament has an identical appearance to the volar ligament.

accuracy rate of 95%. Tears in the central and radial portions are best demonstrated, whereas tears near the ulnar attachment are less accurately diagnosed because synovitis or synovial proliferation in the prestyloid recess may mimic a tear.

Radioulnar Ligaments

Normal Radioulnar Ligaments. The volar and dorsal radioulnar ligaments are broad, striated bands that originate on the volar and dorsal cortex of the sigmoid notch of the distal radius. The ligaments pass on the volar and dorsal surfaces of the TFC and blend with it. The radioulnar ligaments attach to the ulnar styloid process medially, and to the distal radius laterally. The dorsal and volar radioulnar ligaments can be distinguished from the TFC proper because they tend to have flat superior and inferior margins, rather than being biconcave, and they attach directly to bone, rather than to cartilage on the radius (Fig. 12–13). These structures are low signal intensity on all pulse sequences and are best depicted on coronal images.[6]

Abnormal Radioulnar Ligaments. Disruption of the volar or dorsal radioulnar ligaments is associated with instability of the distal radioulnar joint (DRUJ).[17] Disrupted ligaments can be seen on MRI, and subluxation or dislocation of the DRUJ can be easily demonstrated on axial MR images (Fig. 12–14). DRUJ instability is diagnosed when the ulna does not articulate properly with the sigmoid notch of the distal radius, and is displaced in either a dorsal or volar direction from this notch.

Meniscus Homologue

The meniscus homologue can be thought of as a thickening of the ulnar side of the joint capsule that is inconsistently present. It is located just distal to the prestyloid recess and attaches to the triquetrum. If present, it is demonstrated on coronal MR images as a low signal intensity, triangular-shaped structure (Fig. 12–15).[11] The prestyloid recess is a triangular-shaped space bordered by the meniscus homologue distally, the TFCC attachments to the ulnar styloid process proximally, and the central TFC disk radially. The prestyloid recess normally contains fluid.

Extensor Carpi Ulnaris Sheath

Normal Extensor Carpi Ulnaris. The ECU tendon and its sheath, which is a component of the TFCC, can be seen on coronal MR images, but is best depicted in the axial plane, as is the case with many

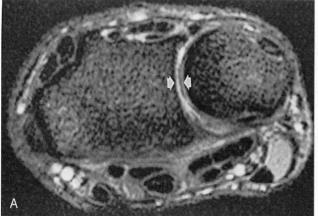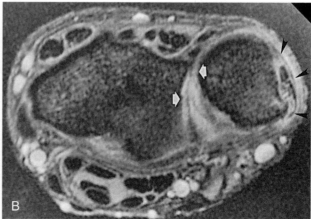

Figure 12–14. DISTAL RADIOULNAR JOINT (DRUJ): NORMAL AND ABNORMAL.
A, T2* axial image, wrist. The normal concentric relationship of the radius and ulna is demonstrated *(arrows)* in the DRUJ of this patient with intact radioulnar ligaments. *B,* T2* axial image, wrist (different patient than in *A*). Disruption of the dorsal radioulnar ligament resulted in dorsal subluxation of the ulna relative to the radius with loss of the concentric relationship of the two bones in the DRUJ *(arrows)*. There is also extensor carpi ulnaris tenosynovitis *(arrowheads)*.

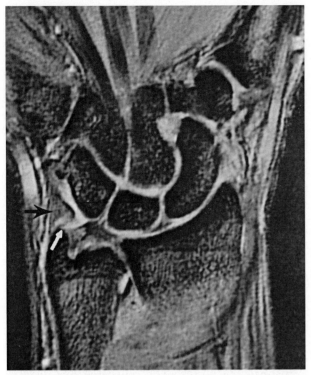

Figure 12–15. MENISCUS HOMOLOGUE AND PRESTYLOID RECESS.
T2* coronal image, wrist. The meniscus homologue is a triangular, low-signal structure *(black arrow)* on the ulnar side of the wrist. It is the distal boundary of the prestyloid recess *(white arrow),* which is a space also bounded by the triangular fibrocartilage proximally and radially.

other tendons (Fig. 12–16). The tendon sheath is not evident on MRI unless there is fluid in it. The ECU tendon is located in the groove on the dorsum of the ulna.

Abnormal Extensor Carpi Ulnaris Sheath. Trau-

matic disruption of the ECU tendon sheath can result in subluxation or dislocation of the ECU tendon at the level of the distal ulna, out of its normal groove, in a medial direction. Associated tenosynovitis is common. Subluxation and tenosynovitis are best demonstrated on axial images (Fig. 12–17).[18]

Ulnar Collateral Ligament (Wrist)

The ulnar collateral ligament (UCL) of the wrist is an additional support structure comprising the TFCC that may be seen on coronal MR images (Fig. 12–10A). It represents a thickening of the wrist joint capsule and provides little mechanical strength. The UCL extends from the ulnar styloid process to the triquetrum. A similar structure exists on the lateral side, the radial collateral ligament, which extends from the radial styloid process to the scaphoid.

Ulnar Collateral Ligament of the Thumb (Gamekeeper's Thumb)

Normal Ulnar Collateral Ligament of the Thumb. The normal ligament is a taut structure that attaches to the base of the proximal phalanx of the thumb and to the distal end of the first metacarpal. It stabilizes the ulnar aspect of the first metacarpophalangeal joint. On MRI, the ligament is a low signal intensity band that spans the first metacarpophalangeal joint, located deep to a similar, vertically oriented low signal intensity band, which is the adductor aponeurosis (Fig. 12–18).[19]

Gamekeeper's Thumb. An abduction injury to the first metacarpophalangeal joint may cause an avulsion fracture at the site of attachment of the UCL, to the base of the proximal phalanx of the thumb (one third of cases), or it may injure only the UCL with-

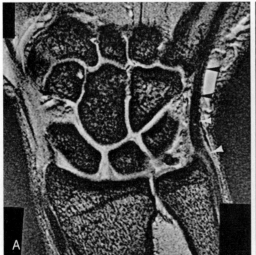
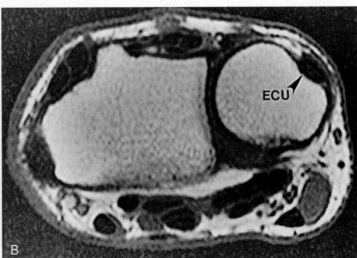

Figure 12–16. NORMAL EXTENSOR CARPI ULNARIS (ECU) TENDON.
A, T2* coronal image, wrist. The ECU tendon is seen on the ulnar and dorsal side of the wrist *(arrowheads).* There is also a triangular fibrocartilage tear present. *B,* T1 axial image, wrist. The normal position of the ECU is evident in the groove on the dorsum of the ulna *(arrowhead).*

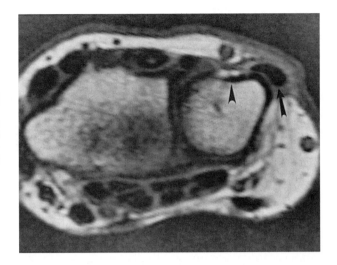

Figure 12–17. DISLOCATED EXTENSOR CARPI ULNARIS (ECU) TENDON.
T1 axial image, wrist. The extensor carpi ulnaris tendon *(arrow)* is dislocated in an ulnar direction from its normal position in the groove *(arrowhead)* on the dorsum of the ulna, indicating disruption of the ECU tendon sheath, which is a component of the triangular fibrocartilage complex.

out radiographic evidence of an osseous abnormality (two thirds of cases). When the UCL is retracted proximally and displaced superficial to the adductor aponeurosis, it is referred to as a Stener lesion. Stener lesions occur in about one third of all gamekeeper's thumbs. The interposition of the adductor aponeurosis between the torn ligament and the bone prevents healing, which may lead to chronic laxity,

loss of grip, and degenerative joint disease. Treatment of the Stener lesion in the first 3 weeks after injury has a better outcome than more delayed treatment and may warrant an MRI for diagnosis, because physical examination is not accurate for this lesion.

MRI of a tear of the UCL *without* a Stener lesion simply demonstrates the thin, low signal intensity

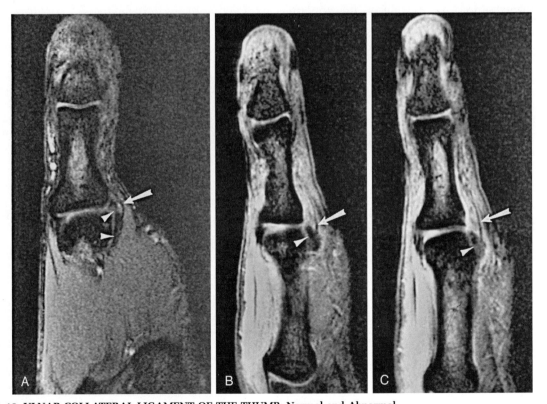

Figure 12–18. ULNAR COLLATERAL LIGAMENT OF THE THUMB: Normal and Abnormal.
A, T2* coronal image, thumb. Normal ulnar collateral ligament *(arrowheads)* is spanning the first metacarpophalangeal joint as a continuous, low-signal band. The adductor aponeurosis *(arrow)* is a thin, low-signal band superficial to the collateral ligament. *B,* T2* coronal image, thumb (different patient than in *A*). The ulnar collateral ligament *(arrowhead)* has been avulsed from its attachment to the base of the proximal phalanx of the thumb (gamekeeper's or skier's thumb), but remains deep to the adductor aponeurosis *(arrow).* *C,* T2* coronal image, thumb (different patient than in *A* and *B*) with a Stener lesion. The ulnar collateral ligament *(arrowhead)* is detached from the base of the thumb, thickened, intermediate signal, and retracted proximally so that it gives the "yoyo on a string" appearance. The string of the yoyo is the adductor aponeurosis *(arrow).*

ligament avulsed from the base of the thumb or discontinuity of the ligament with hemorrhage and edema surrounding the torn end(s) of the ligament (Fig. 12–18). The ligament remains deep to the linear adductor aponeurosis. The edema and hemorrhage are high signal intensity on T2W images. Gradient echo images are excellent for showing the ligament well.

The Stener lesion has been described as having the appearance of a yoyo on a string on MRI.[20] The yoyo is created by the balled-up and retracted UCL, whereas the string of the yoyo is the adductor aponeurosis (Fig. 12–18). An image with high resolution and small field of view that is oriented like an anteroposterior view of the thumb is necessary to see these structures properly. The ligament must be seen throughout its length, rather than in cross section, to make the diagnosis.

Tendons

Normal Anatomy

Tendons in the wrist are best depicted in the axial plane. Most of the flexor tendons (nine of them) pass through the carpal tunnel on the volar aspect of the wrist. It is not necessary to know the names of individual flexor tendons.

The extensor tendons are located on the dorsum of the wrist and are important to know. The extensor tendons are stabilized on the dorsum of the wrist by an extensor retinaculum. Fascial septations form six dorsal compartments that contain the extensor tendons (Fig. 12–19).

The first dorsal compartment, on the radial side of the wrist, contains the abductor pollicis longus and extensor pollicis brevis tendons. The second dorsal compartment contains the extensor carpi radialis longus and brevis tendons and is separated from the extensor pollicis longus tendon in the third dorsal compartment by Lister's tubercle, a bony protuberance on the dorsum of the radius. The fourth compartment holds the extensor digitorum and extensor indicis tendons. The extensor digiti minimi tendon lies in the fifth dorsal compartment. The extensor carpi ulnaris tendon is located in the sixth compartment in the notch of the ulna. It is hard enough to remember the names of these tendons, much less whether they are a longus or a brevis. A trick that helps us to remember if a tendon is a longus or a brevis is to recall that the tendon on the ulnar aspect of Lister's tubercle is the extensor pollicis longus (and it has a very longus way to go to get to the thumb). As one progresses from the extensor pollicis longus in a radial direction, the tendons alternate as to longus and brevis: extensor pollicis *longus*, extensor carpi radialis *brevis*, extensor carpi radialis *longus*, extensor pollicis *brevis*, and abductor pollicis *longus*. So, longus and brevis become easy as you get into the rhythm, and it

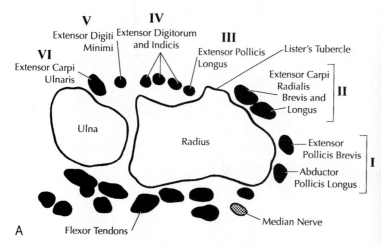

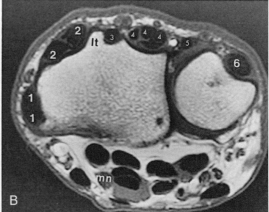

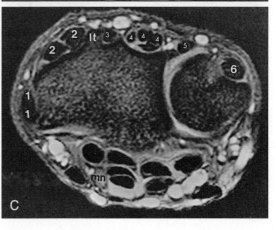

Figure 12–19. NORMAL TENDONS OF THE WRIST.
A, Diagram of the wrist in the axial plane at the level of the distal radioulnar joint (DRUJ). This shows the six dorsal compartments that contain the tendons, which are labeled. The flexor tendons and median nerve are present volarly. *B*, T1 axial image, wrist through the DRUJ. The dorsal tendons are labeled with numbers that correlate with the dorsal compartments shown in the diagram in *A*. mn—median nerve; lt—Lister's tubercle. *C*, T2* axial image, wrist through DRUJ. The dorsal tendons are labeled as in *B* to correspond to the six dorsal compartments in the diagram in *A*. mn—median nerve; lt = Lister's tubercle.

is only the names of the tendons you are left to struggle with.

The tendons of the wrist are oval to round, low signal intensity structures. The extensor carpi ulnaris tendon, in particular, normally may have some high signal intensity within it for reasons that are not understood.[21] The magic-angle phenomenon is a likely culprit, but it is not entirely clear why high signal in this tendon is common in patients without symptoms. Unless the tendon has fluid around it (tenosynovitis) or is abnormally enlarged or thinned, we do not call it abnormal based on small amounts of intrasubstance high signal intensity. Small amounts of fluid in tendon sheaths are considered normal, and only if it completely surrounds the tendon is fluid considered abnormal.

Tendon Pathology

Abnormalities of the tendons in the wrist and hand are common and range from tenosynovitis to degeneration and tears. Chronic repetitive trauma from overuse and inflammatory arthritis are common causes for tendon problems in the wrist.

De Quervain Syndrome (Box 12–4). Entrapment and tenosynovitis of the abductor pollicis longus and extensor pollicis brevis tendons in the first dorsal compartment is known as De Quervain syn-

---

BOX 12–4: DE QUERVAIN SYNDROME

Entrapment/irritation of tendons, first dorsal compartment
—Abductor pollicis longus
—Extensor pollicis brevis
Associated with overuse (manual laborers) and pregnancy
MRI appearance
—Tendons may have normal size and signal, be thickened, or have intratendinous signal
—Abnormal signal around tendons is common: low signal on T1; either low or high (fibrosis or tenosynovitis) on T2.

---

drome.[6, 18, 22] The diagnosis usually is made clinically, but sometimes the findings are not obvious and cannot be distinguished from those of a scaphoid fracture, flexor carpi radialis tenosynovitis, or degenerative arthritis of the first carpometacarpal joint. De Quervain syndrome may be idiopathic, but also is associated with pregnancy or repetitive trauma in manual laborers.

MRI findings in De Quervain syndrome may have a varied appearance (Fig. 12–20). There may be

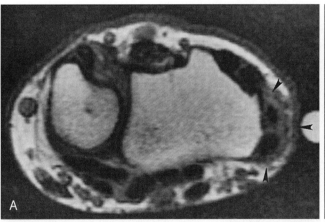

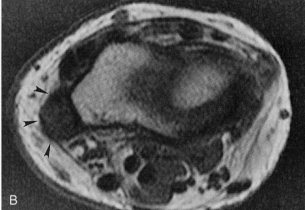

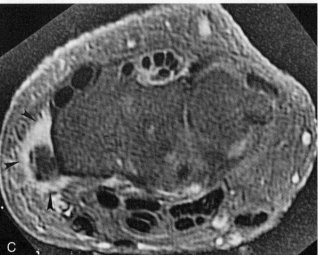

Figure 12–20. DE QUERVAIN TENOSYNOVITIS.
A, T1 axial image, wrist. Painful mass over the radial styoid process in this postpartum woman proved to be fibrosis surrounding the extensor pollicis brevis and abductor pollicis longus tendons *(arrowheads),* causing obliteration of the subcutaneous fat that normally surrounds these tendons. *B,* T1 axial image, wrist (different patient than in *A*). The tendons of the first dorsal compartment are not discrete, low-signal structures like the other wrist tendons, and appear enlarged *(arrowheads).* The subcutaneous fat surrounding the tendons remains normal in this patient. *C,* T1 fat-saturation image, with contrast, axial wrist (different patient than in *A* and *B*). There is increased signal and size of the tendons of the first dorsal compartment and contrast enhancement surrounding the tendons *(arrowheads)* from extensive tenosynovitis.

obliteration of subcutaneous fat surrounding the tendons, with the tendons surrounded by intermediate signal intensity tissue on all pulse sequences, or there may be tenosynovitis with high-signal fluid surrounding them on T2W images. The tendons may be normal in caliber or thickened, or there may be high signal within the tendons from partial tears or degeneration.

Injection of steroids into the tendon sheath cures this disease in most patients, but surgical decompression occasionally is required.

Extensor Carpi Ulnaris. The ECU tendon commonly is involved with tenosynovitis or partial tears.[6, 18] This may occur secondary to repetitive subluxation or dislocation, which occurs when the ECU tendon sheath has been disrupted from an injury to the TFCC. We only diagnose tenosynovitis or partial tendon tears of the ECU tendon when there is fluid surrounding the entire tendon or the tendon is abnormally thick or thin (Fig. 12–21). High signal intensity within this particular tendon is not enough to call an abnormality, because it is present in many asymptomatic individuals.

Bowstringing. The flexor digitorum tendons in the fingers normally are closely apposed to the adjacent osseous structures because they are held in position by a system of pulley ligaments. When there is rupture of the pulley system ligaments, the tendons are free to displace from the bones of the digit, creating a "bowstring" appearance. This diagnosis, along with the quality of the displaced tendon, can easily be made by MRI when the tendons are separated from the bone to a greater extent than normal or when compared to the adjacent normal digits (Fig. 12–22).

Other Tendons. Tenosynovitis and partial and complete tears also may affect other tendons of the wrist. Tenosynovitis of the flexor digitorum tendons in the carpal tunnel is a common cause of the carpal tunnel syndrome.

Carpal Tunnel

The carpal tunnel is a fibro-osseous space formed by the concave volar aspects of the carpal bones on the dorsal surface, and by the flexor retinaculum on the volar surface. The tunnel contains the flexor tendons and the median nerve. The flexor retinaculum is a dense, fibrous band that attaches to the scaphoid and tubercle of the trapezium on the radial aspect of the tunnel and to the pisiform and hook of the hamate on the ulnar side of the tunnel. The retinaculum normally shows some slight palmar bowing.[23] There is normally very little fat within the carpal tunnel, but when present, it should be found only in the dorsal aspect. The median nerve lies within the volar and lateral aspect of the carpal tunnel and can be easily differentiated from the lower signal intensity tendons that surround it.

It is helpful to evaluate the structures passing through the carpal tunnel at three standard locations on axial MR images (Fig. 12–23): (1) the level of the distal radioulnar joint just before the median nerve enters the tunnel, (2) at the level of the pisiform bone in the proximal tunnel, and (3) at the level of the hook of the hamate in the distal tunnel, where it is most constricted.

Nerves

Median Nerve

The median nerve lies in the volar and radial aspect of the carpal tunnel, just deep to the retinaculum, although the position may vary somewhat with wrist position. The nerve has higher signal intensity and is more oval in shape than the adjacent flexor tendons in the carpal tunnel (Fig. 12–23). The size of the median nerve is maintained or slightly decreases as it progresses distally through the tunnel.

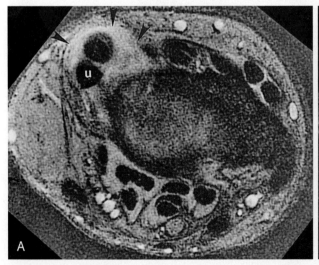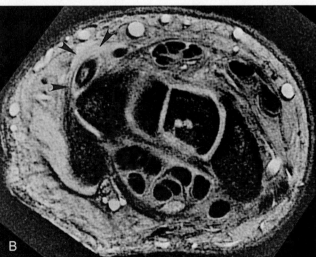

Figure 12–21. EXTENSOR CARPI ULNARIS (ECU) TENOSYNOVITIS/PARTIAL TEARS.
A, T2* axial image, wrist. There is extensive high signal from tenosynovitis in the soft tissues *(arrowheads)* surrounding the ECU. The ECU is slightly enlarged. u—ulnar styloid process. *B*, T2* axial image, wrist (different patient than in *A*). The ECU tendon is enlarged with more than the usual high signal within it, indicating partial tears. There is also surrounding high signal *(arrowheads)* from tenosynovitis.

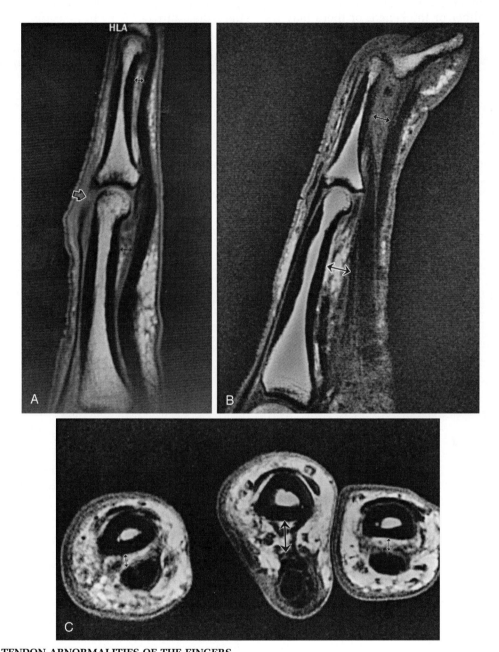

Figure 12–22. TENDON ABNORMALITIES OF THE FINGERS.
A, T1 sagittal image, finger. Tear of the extensor tendon *(open arrow),* which is discontinuous, intermediate signal, and thickened. This also shows the relationship of the normal flexor tendons to the phalanges *(double-headed arrows).* *B,* T1 sagittal image, finger (different patient than in *A*). Bowstringing of the flexor tendons is manifest as significant displacement (compare to *A*) of the tendons in a volar direction from the osseous phalanges *(double-headed arrows).* Scarring surrounds the tendons with partial obliteration of the volar subcutaneous fat. In addition, there is a mallet finger (flexion of the distal interphalangeal joint) from rupture of the distal extensor tendon. *C,* T1 axial image, finger (same patient as in *B*). The large distance between the bone and the flexor tendons is demonstrated *(double-headed arrow)* in the middle finger from a bowstringing injury. The normal distance between bone and flexor tendons *(small double-headed arrows)* can be seen in the normal digits on either side of the injured finger.

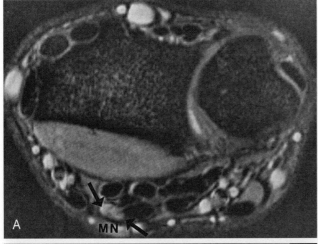

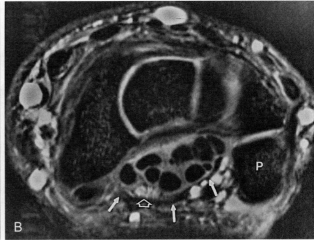

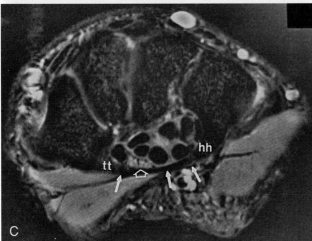

Figure 12–23. CARPAL TUNNEL, NORMAL ANATOMY.
A, T2* axial image, wrist at the distal radioulnar joint (DRUJ) shows the oval and relatively high signal median nerve (MN; *arrows*) immediately before it enters the carpal tunnel. *B,* T2* axial image, wrist at the pisiform (P). The median nerve *(open arrow)* maintains the same size as at the level of the DRUJ. The normal flexor retinaculum *(white solid arrows)* is slightly bowed volarly. *C,* T2* axial image, wrist at the distal carpal tunnel at the level of the hook of the hamate (hh) and tubercle of the trapezium (tt). The median nerve *(open arrow)* is slightly smaller than at the more proximal levels, with a fasciculated intermediate- to high-signal appearance.

The tunnel becomes progressively smaller from proximal to distal, and the nerve may have a somewhat flattened appearance at the level of the hook of the hamate, where the tunnel is most constricted and the nerve is in close apposition to adjacent flexor tendons.[24]

Carpal Tunnel Syndrome (Box 12–5). Carpal tunnel syndrome is a common compressive neuropathy that affects the wrist and which results from the median nerve being compressed in the carpal tunnel. Symptoms generally make this an easy clinical diagnosis, so imaging is not necessary. Patients have pain and paresthesias in the thumb, index finger, third finger, and radial half of the fourth finger, which are usually worse at night.

There are many causes of carpal tunnel syndrome. Anything that increases the volume of the tunnel or narrows the tunnel can create nerve entrapment. The most common cause of this syndrome is tenosynovitis of the flexor tendons from overuse of the hands (typists).

MR generally is not used to diagnose carpal tunnel syndrome, because nerve conduction studies and clinical history suffice in most cases. MR may be useful to define the underlying cause of carpal tunnel syndrome if it is evident, when nerve conduction studies are equivocal, or after surgery if patients have recurrent or persistent symptoms.

MR findings of carpal tunnel syndrome are seen best on axial images. There are four major signs of carpal tunnel syndrome (Figs. 12–24 and 12–25).[23, 24]

1. Focal or segmental swelling (pseudoneuroma) of the median nerve, best determined by subjectively comparing the size of the nerve at the level of the distal radius with its size at the pisiform. Normally, the nerve should stay the same size or

---

BOX 12–5: CARPAL TUNNEL SYNDROME

MRI Features
- Swollen median nerve (larger at level of pisiform than at distal radioulnar joint
- Flattened median nerve (evaluate at level of hamate hook)
- Increased signal of nerve on T2
- Flexor retinaculum (bowing ratio >15%)

Postop Appearance, Carpal Tunnel Release
- Flexor retinaculum
  —Absent, or
  —Incised free ends displaced volarly
- Flexor tendons volarly displaced

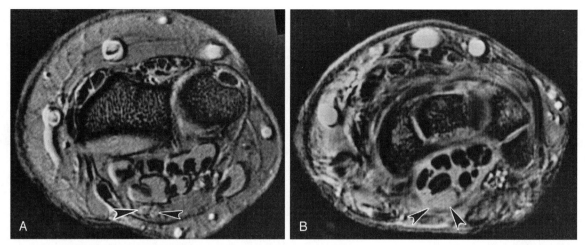

Figure 12–24. CARPAL TUNNEL SYNDROME.
A, T2* axial image, wrist at the distal radioulnar joint (DRUJ). The median nerve *(arrowheads)* has a normal size and signal prior to entering the carpal tunnel. *B,* T2* axial image, wrist at the pisiform. The median nerve *(arrowheads)* is enlarged and high signal. The flexor retinaculum is bowed volarly, and there is increased signal and space between the flexor tendons from tenosynovitis.

decrease distally. If the nerve is larger on progressively more distal images, it is swollen.

2. Flattening or angulation of the nerve. This is best evaluated at the distal carpal tunnel at the level of the hook of the hamate. If the nerve is compressed against adjacent tendons and bones, the surface becomes faceted or angled.

3. Bowing of the flexor retinaculum caused by increased volume of the carpal tunnel contents. This is called the bowing ratio. The bowing ratio is calculated by drawing a line from the triquetrum to the hook of the hamate on an axial image

(length = TH). The distance from this line to the flexor retinaculum (palmar displacement = PD) is divided by the length TH. The ratio is up to 15% in normal subjects and ranges from 14% to 26% in patients with carpal tunnel syndrome.

4. Increased signal intensity of the median nerve on T2 images may occur from obstruction of venous return from the nerve with resultant edema.

Perhaps more important than diagnosing carpal tunnel syndrome is evaluating the cause of persistent or recurrent carpal tunnel syndrome in patients

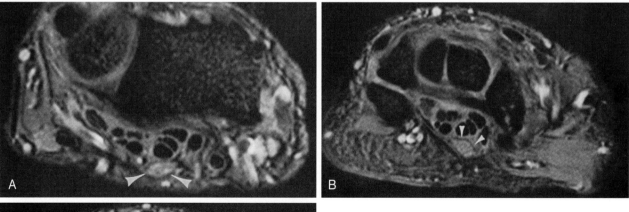

Figure 12–25. CARPAL TUNNEL SYNDROME.
A, T2* axial image, wrist at the distal radioulnar joint (DRUJ). The median nerve *(arrowheads)* has a normal appearance at this level. *B,* T2* axial image, wrist at the pisiform. The median nerve *(arrowheads)* is somewhat enlarged and has an angled or faceted appearance from pressure where it abuts the adjacent flexor tendons. *C,* T2* axial image, wrist at the distal carpal tunnel (h—hook of hamate; t—tubercle of trapezium). The median nerve *(arrowhead)* is significantly larger than on more proximal images. There is an abnormal bowing ratio. The bowing ratio is calculated by drawing a line from the hook of the hamate to the tubercle of the trapezium (line th) and dividing that distance by the amount of palmar displacement (pd), which is the distance from line th to the flexor retinaculum.

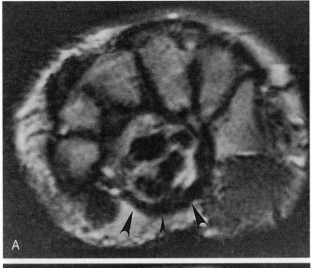

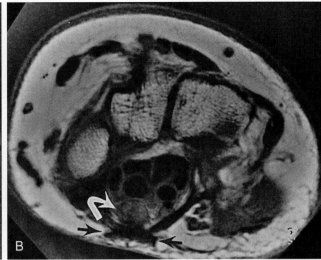

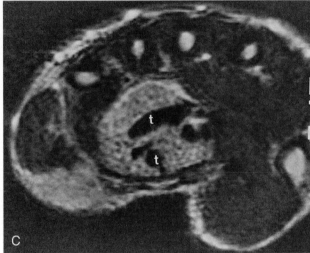

Figure 12–26. CAUSES OF FAILED CARPAL TUNNEL RELEASE. *A,* Proton density axial image, wrist. Incomplete release of the flexor retinaculum, which is thickened and bowed *(arrowheads).* *B,* T1 axial image, wrist (different patient than in *A*). The median nerve *(curved white arrow)* is huge and its volar surface is surrounded by scar *(black arrows)* from previous surgery. *C,* Proton density axial image, wrist (different patient than *A* and *B*). Recurrent carpal tunnel syndrome occurred, caused by the development of rice bodies in the tendon sheaths surrounding the flexor tendons (t). The rice bodies give the stippled appearance in the carpal tunnel surrounding the tendons and create a mass effect on the nerve.

who have been treated for it surgically without success. Postoperative failures may be from several causes, the most common of which is incomplete release of the flexor retinaculum.[25] MRI findings suggestive of an anatomic basis for recurrent symptoms include identification of an intact portion of the flexor retinaculum, the development of low signal intensity fibrotic scarring around the median nerve, and proximal swelling of the nerve (Fig. 12–26). MRI also may demonstrate a persistent or recurrent mass lesion within the carpal tunnel or the development of a median nerve neuroma. The normal postoperative appearances of the carpal tunnel after complete incision of the retinaculum are the retinaculum is not visible, the free ends of the retinaculum are displaced in a volar direction, and the contents of the carpal tunnel are displaced in a volar direction relative to the tunnel (Fig. 12–27).

Ulnar Nerve

The ulnar nerve, artery, and vein pass through Guyon's canal on the ulnar side of the wrist (Fig. 12–28). The canal is formed by the flexor retinacu-

lum and hypothenar musculature, the volar aspect is formed by a layer of fascia, and the pisiform and hook of the hamate form the osseous margins of the canal.

Ulnar Tunnel Syndrome. The ulnar nerve may become compressed along Guyon's canal. Causes for this include ganglion cysts (Fig. 12–29) or other masses, fracture of the hamate, or repetitive occupational trauma to this region. The course, size, and signal intensity of the nerve, as well as any adjacent masses, can be assessed on axial MR images.[26]

Fibrolipomatous Hamartoma

Fibrolipomatous hamartoma of a nerve is a benign lesion that arises in and causes profound enlargement of a nerve.[27] The median nerve in the wrist is by far the most common nerve in the body to be affected. The lesion may be asymptomatic, but nerve compression may develop. Two thirds of patients with macrodactyly (macrodystrophia lipomatosa) have fibrolipomatous hamartoma. There is infiltration of the nerve by fibrous and fatty tissue.

There is a distinctive MR appearance for this le-

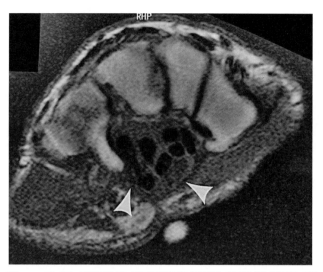

Figure 12–27. NORMAL POSTOPERATIVE APPEARANCE OF THE CARPAL TUNNEL.
T1 axial image, wrist. The flexor retinaculum is partially missing, the free ends of the retinaculum are displaced volarly *(arrowheads)*, and the contents of the tunnel are displaced volarly.

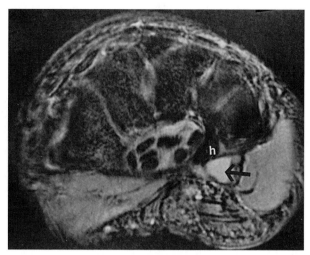

Figure 12–29. ULNAR TUNNEL SYNDROME.
T2* axial image, wrist. There is a ganglion cyst *(arrow)* in the ulnar tunnel adjacent to the hook of the hamate (h), causing a compressive neuropathy of the ulnar nerve.

sion (Fig. 12–30). It is seen as a mass along the course of the median nerve, composed of tubular low signal intensity structures, probably corresponding to nerve fascicles surrounded by epineural and perineural fibrosis, within a background of high signal intensity fat.

Osseous Structures

Normal Relationships

Certain osseous anatomy of the wrist needs to be emphasized, so that abnormalities will be easier to understand. The relationship of the distal articular

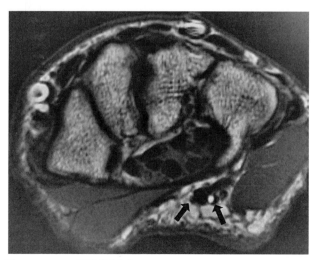

Figure 12–28. GUYON'S CANAL.
T1 axial image, wrist. The ulnar tunnel (Guyon's canal) is formed by the flexor retinaculum, hypothenar musculature, and pisiform and hook of the hamate bones. The ulnar nerve, artery, and vein pass through the tunnel *(arrows)*.

surface of the radius with the convex head of the ulna is important (Fig. 12–31). These structures are normally at the same level on coronal MR images, and this is referred to as neutral ulnar variance. If the ulna is more than two mm proximal to the radial articular surface, it is called negative ulnar variance (or ulnar minus variance). If the ulna is situated distal to the radius, it is positive ulnar (or ulnar plus) variance. Any alteration from the normal neutral ulnar variance changes the stresses on the wrist and can result in pathology. Specifically, ulnar plus variance is associated with the ulnolunate impaction syndrome and triangular fibrocartilage tears, whereas ulnar minus variance is associated with osteonecrosis of the lunate (Box 12–6).

The alignment of the carpal bones on sagittal images depends on wrist position. The lunate tends to volarflex and dorsiflex relative to the radius when the wrist is placed in radial and ulnar deviation, respectively.[6] Proper positioning of the hand and wrist in the magnet is important in order to prevent this pitfall. Normally the distal radius, lunate, and

---

BOX 12–6: ASSOCIATIONS WITH ULNAR VARIANCE

Positive ulnar variance
- Triangular fibrocartilage (TFC) tears
- Ulnolunate impaction syndrome
  —Cartilage degeneration of lunate and ulna
  —TFC tears
  —Proximal lunate marrow edema or subchondral cyst

Negative ulnar variance
- Osteonecrosis of the lunate (Kienböck disease)

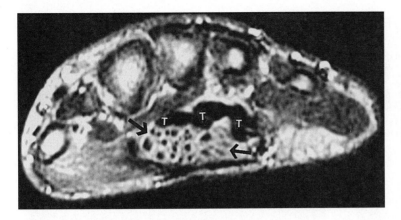

Figure 12–30. FIBROLIPOMATOUS HAMARTOMA.
Spin echo-T2 axial image, wrist. The stippled area *(arrows)* volar to the flexor tendons (T) represents a gigantic median nerve. The low-signal stippled appearance is from enlarged nerve fascicles and fatty tissue infiltrates around the fascicles.

capitate all align colinearly, or nearly so, just as they do on a lateral wrist radiograph.

Osseous Abnormalities

Os Styloideum. There are many accessory ossicles in the wrist, but the os styloideum is one that may be associated with pain and be confused with tumor or fracture. It is a common bony protuberance on the dorsal aspect of the wrist that is located at the base of the second and third metacarpals. This variant occasionally can cause pain because of degenerative changes that develop between it and the underlying bones (Fig. 12–32), because of an overlying bursitis or ganglion cyst, or because of trauma, because it projects from the surface of the wrist and is predisposed to injury. This usually is easily seen with conventional radiographs, and MRI generally is not required to make this specific diagnosis.

MRI shows a small piece of bone that articulates with the underlying capitate and trapezoid on axial or sagittal images. Bursitis and degenerative changes can be demonstrated.

Carpal Instability (Box 12–7). This also was discussed under the sections on scapholunate and lu-

notriquetral ligament ruptures (Fig. 12–5 through 12–7). Scapholunate ligament disruption may lead to scapholunate dissociation, which is the most common carpal instability syndrome. This results in rotatory subluxation of the scaphoid and dorsal tipping of the lunate (DISI). The ruptured scapholunate ligament can be diagnosed on coronal MR images, and DISI can be diagnosed on sagittal images. This also may cause SLAC wrist.

A tear of the lunotriquetral ligament can be diagnosed on coronal MR images, and any associated instability between the lunate and triquetrum can be detected on sagittal MR images with volar tipping of the lunate (VISI).

Ulnolunate Impaction. The ulnolunate impaction syndrome is a pain syndrome that occurs because of chronic abutment of the distal ulna against the proximal lunate. There is a strong association between ulnar plus variance and ulnolunate impaction syndrome. Ulnar plus variance leads to altered and increased forces transmitted across the ulnar side of the wrist. Ulnar plus variance may be a congenital variant or may develop as the result of an impacted distal radial fracture. The chronic repetitive impaction of the two bones against one another ini-

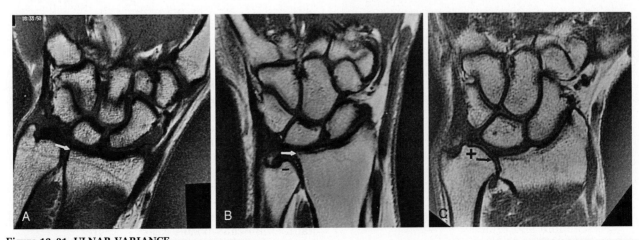

Figure 12–31. ULNAR VARIANCE.
A, T1 coronal image, wrist. Neutral ulnar variance exists when the distal radius and head of the ulna are at the same level *(arrow)* or the ulna is within 2 mm proximal to the radius. *B,* T1 coronal image, wrist. Ulnar minus variance occurs when the head of the ulna is located more than 2 mm proximal to the distal radius *(arrow).* *C,* T1 coronal image, wrist. Ulnar plus variance results if the head of the ulna projects distal to the radius *(arrow).*

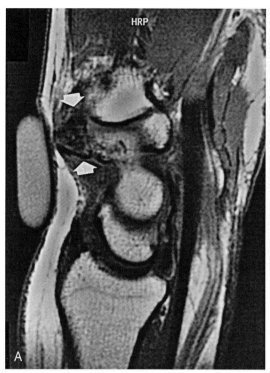

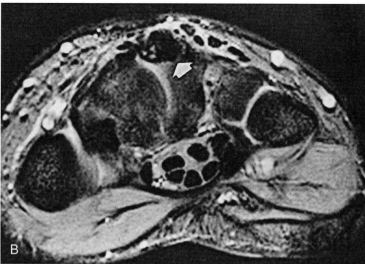

Figure 12–32. OS STYLOIDEUM.
A, T1 sagittal image, wrist. An os styloideum *(arrows)* is present on the dorsum of the wrist. It is low signal because of sclerosis from degenerative changes that developed with the underlying carpal bones. *B,* T2* axial image, wrist (same patient as *A*). There are small high-signal foci in the os styloideum *(arrow)* from degenerative changes.

tially results in degenerative changes of the cartilage covering both bones. The intervening triangular fibrocartilage often is torn. Ultimately, degenerative changes affect the bones, especially the proximal surface of the lunate.[28]

MRI can show the bone changes in the lunate when radiographs are normal. The triangular fibrocartilage tears also are easily identified. MRI shows cartilage destruction, and underlying bone marrow edema, subchondral cyst formation, or sclerosis in the proximal lunate or head of the ulna (Fig. 12–33).

Occult Fractures. Persistent pain in the wrist after trauma may be the result of bone or soft tissue injuries. MR is the best imaging technique for identifying abnormalities affecting both the osseous and soft tissue structures. If a radiographically occult fracture is the only clinical concern, a limited trauma screening MR examination can be done. MRI offers an exquisitely sensitive and specific method of diagnosing radiographically occult traumatic bone lesions.

The scaphoid is the most commonly fractured carpal bone. Delayed fracture union and osteonecrosis of the proximal fracture fragment are complications that may be prevented by early detection of the fracture and appropriate treatment. About 16% of scaphoid fractures are not evident on the initial radiographs, and MRI is an excellent method for detecting these lesions (Fig. 12–34).[29–31] Many other bones in the carpus also may fracture and not be evident on radiographs. These radiographically occult fractures can be seen as marrow edema from bone contusions (Fig. 12–35) or true linear fracture lines. The appearance of contusions with marrow edema but no fracture line does not necessarily indicate a less significant injury, because at follow-up a true fracture line may be evident on radiographs.[29]

Physeal Injuries. Trauma to the physis (growthplate) of the distal radius and ulna may occur in young competitive gymnasts. This may result in the formation of a fibrous or osseous bridge across the physis, or slowing of growth in a portion of the physis, which can cause a growth disturbance. The metaphysis may have associated contusions and radiographically occult stress fractures.

MRI can demonstrate the fractures, contusions, physeal injury, or focal bridge formation. The osseous lesions are identical to those described above. The cartilage of the physis is thickened initially,

---

BOX 12–7: CARPAL INSTABILITY

Scapholunate ligament disruption may lead to
- Increased scapholunate interval
- Rotary subluxation of scaphoid
- Dorsal tipping of lunate (DISI)
- Scapholunate advanced collaspe (SLAC) wrist
  —Increased scapholunate interval
  —Degenerative changes between scaphoid and radius
  —Proximal migration of capitate between scaphoid and lunate

Lunotriquetral ligament disruption may lead to
- Volar tipping of lunate (VISI)

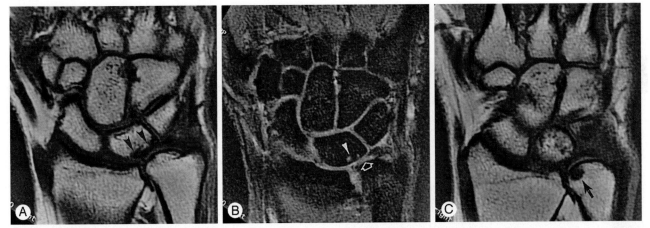

Figure 12–33. ULNOLUNATE IMPACTION.
A, T1 coronal image, wrist. Subchondral sclerosis in the lunate *(arrowheads)* is a response to the ulnar plus variance. *B,* T2* coronal image, wrist (different patient than *A*). There is ulnar plus variance, a triangular fibrocartilage tear *(open arrow),* and subchondral cyst/marrow edema in the lunate *(arrowhead). C,* T1 coronal image, wrist (different patient than *A* and *B*). A cyst *(arrow)* in the head of the ulna is a manifestation of ulnolunate impaction from the ulnar plus variance.

with persistent cartilagenous foci found later within the metaphysis. Physeal bridges are focal areas of either bone or low signal intensity fibrous material that extend vertically from the metaphysis to the epiphysis, traversing the cartilaginous physis. Gradient echo or STIR sequences are excellent for showing these abnormalities.[32, 33]

Osteonecrosis (Box 12–8). The two most common sites for osteonecrosis in the wrist are the proximal pole of the scaphoid after a scaphoid fracture and the lunate bone. Rarely, the proximal portion of the capitate may undergo osteonecrosis after being fractured.

The *proximal pole of the scaphoid* is at high risk for osteonecrosis because of its tenuous blood supply. This also can lead to delayed or nonunion of the fracture. Assessment of the viability of the proximal fragment is important for management and for surgical planning in patients who do not heal properly.

Normal fatty marrow signal intensity on T1W images indicates viability of the fragment. Low signal intensity on T1W and T2W images indicates necrosis (Fig. 12–36). If there is low signal intensity on T1W images and high signal intensity on T2W images, the significance is less clear and could be the result of either bone marrow edema, changes of healing, or ischemic changes.[34, 35]

Kienböck's osteonecrosis of the lunate may occur as the result of repetitive trauma, acute fracture, or ulnar minus variance. Men usually are affected and describe wrist pain that worsens with activity. Most patients with this disease are involved in manual labor.

The blood supply to the lunate is tenuous with much of it being supplied by end arteries. It is subjected to strong compressive forces because of its central position in the wrist. The forces on the lunate are even greater in patients with negative ulnar variance.

MRI can show several patterns of abnormality based on the stage of the disease at the time of imaging. If there is low signal intensity on T1W

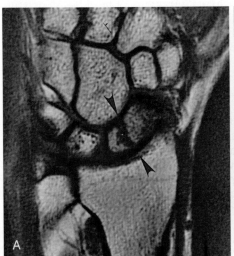

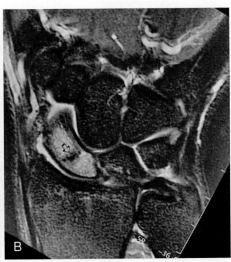

Figure 12–34. OCCULT CARPAL FRACTURES.
A, T1 coronal image, wrist. A radiographically occult fracture of the proximal pole of the scaphoid *(arrowheads)* is obvious on MRI, without evidence of ischemic changes. *B,* STIR coronal image, wrist. A radiographically occult scaphoid fracture is seen in this patient 3 months after the injury. The fracture line is linear low signal *(open arrow)* and there is diffuse, surrounding edema throughout the bone.

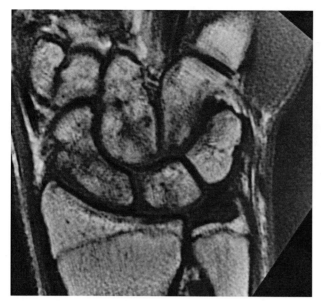

Figure 12–35. BONE CONTUSIONS.
T1 coronal image, wrist. Patchy abnormal intermediate signal is present in the scaphoid, capitate, hamate, triquetrum, and lunate from multiple bone contusions without discrete fracture lines seen.

and T2W images that involve the entire lunate, the findings are diagnostic for osteonecrosis (Fig. 12–37). If only a portion of the lunate is involved or if there is increased signal intensity on T2W images, the diagnosis is less definite because other pathologies may cause a similar appearance (Fig. 12–38). High signal intensity on T2W images from os-

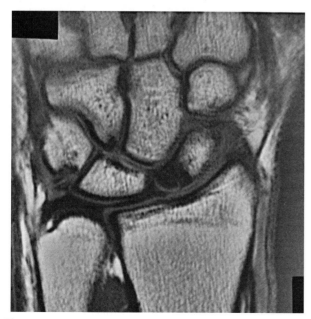

Figure 12–36. OSTEONECROSIS, SCAPHOID.
T1 coronal image, wrist. Osteonecrosis manifests as diffuse low signal in the proximal pole of the scaphoid without collapse. Incidentally, there is a type II lunate with marrow edema in the proximal hamate (see text).

BOX 12–8: OSTEONECROSIS (AVN) IN THE WRIST

Scaphoid
• Proximal pole at risk after fracture
• MRI
  —Low signal on T1 and T2 = AVN
  —Low signal on T1, high on T2 = questionable significance:
    —possible ischemia, marrow edema, or healing
  —High signal on T1, intermediate on T2 (fat) = normal
Lunate (Keinböck disease)
• Associated with repetitive trauma, fracture, ulnar minus
• MRI
  —Low signal on T1 and T2 of entire bone = AVN
  —If only a portion of the lunate is involved with low signal on T1 and T2, or there is low signal on T1 and high signal on T2, consider:
    Early stage of AVN
    Intraosseous ganglion
    Marrow edema/subchondral cyst from ulnolunate impaction (look for ulnar plus)

AVN, avascular necrosis.

teonecrosis indicates an earlier stage of the disease process and a better outcome.[6, 36, 37]

Other lesions in the lunate that may simulate Kienböck's disease include intraosseous ganglion cyst and marrow edema or subchondral cyst formation that can occur from ulnolunate impaction. Both of these entities are focal and have high signal intensity on T2W images. The diagnosis of Kienböck's disease is certainly more definite when the entire bone is involved or when there is low signal intensity on both T1W and T2W images, but must be considered in the differential for focal lesions that are high signal intensity on T2W images as well. Obviously, ulnolunate impaction syndrome should not be difficult to distinguish because ulnar plus variance is necessary for this entity to occur, whereas osteonecrosis of the lunate tends to occur with ulnar minus variance.

Other Congenital Osseous Lesions. The most common *carpal coalition* is between the lunate and triquetrum. Lunotriquetral coalition may be osseous, fibrous, or cartilaginous. Fibrocartilagenous coalitions often have associated marrow edema or cystic changes adjacent to the coalition, which mimic degenerative joint disease (Fig. 12–39).

A *type II lunate* has an extra facet that articulates with the proximal hamate. A type I lunate articulates only with the capitate. The articulation between the hamate and lunate that occurs with a type

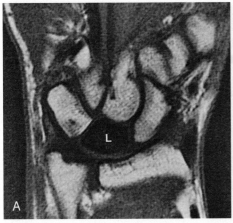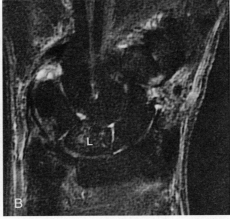

Figure 12–37. OSTEONECROSIS, LUNATE.
A, T1 coronal image, wrist. The lunate (L) is diffusely low signal from Kienböck's osteonecrosis. **B,** Fast T2 image with fat saturation (same patient as *A*). Signal in the lunate (L) remains nearly completely low signal.

II lunate may lead to chondromalacia of the hamate, and MR may demonstrate these changes as marrow edema or subchondral cysts in the proximal pole of the hamate (Fig. 12–39). These changes are seen as a focal area of signal abnormality in the proximal hamate that is low signal on T1W and high signal on T2W images. Chondromalacia is found at surgery much more commonly than MR abnormalities are seen in the hamate.

Tumors

Bone and soft tissue tumors and tumor-like lesions of the hand and wrist are common and of varying causes. Only those lesions that are very common or occur almost exclusively in the wrist and hand are discussed here.

Osseous Lesions

Benign lesions of bone are far more common in the hand and wrist than malignant lesions. The most common of these lesions are enchondromas, intraosseous ganglion cysts, and epidermoid inclusion cysts.

Enchondromas. Enchondromas are cartilagenous rests within bone that have lobulated margins and often erode the endosteal surface of the cortical bone. They are located in the proximal and middle phalanges of the fingers and in the metacarpal bones. They often have calcifications seen by conventional radiography, but these may be difficult to identify by MRI. Enchondromas are low signal intensity on T1W images and become high signal intensity on T2W images. The characteristic location and lobulated configuration should allow the diagnosis to be made by MRI, where they usually are detected as incidental findings.

Intraosseous Ganglion Cysts. These lesions are common in the carpal bones, particularly in the radial aspect of the lunate. They consist of a dense fibrous wall and a mucoid fluid inside the wall. They generally are located in the subchondral region of bone and may be confined to the bone or

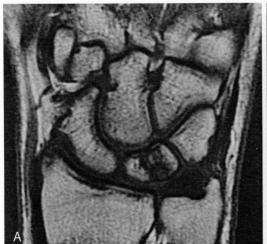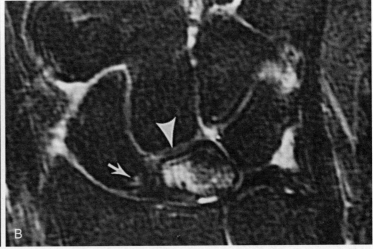

Figure 12–38. OSTEONECROSIS, LUNATE PARTIAL INVOLVEMENT.
A, T1 coronal image, wrist. There is focal low signal in the lunate with normal fatty marrow on either side of the abnormality. This makes osteonecrosis less certain than if the entire lunate were involved. **B,** Fast T2 with fat saturation coronal image, wrist (different patient than *A*). There is focal high signal in the radial side of the lunate *(arrowhead)*, as well as a small area of high signal in the proximal pole of the scaphoid *(arrow)*. Partial involvement of the lunate makes osteonecrosis a less definite diagnosis. This was proven osteonecrosis from steroid use in both the scaphoid and lunate.

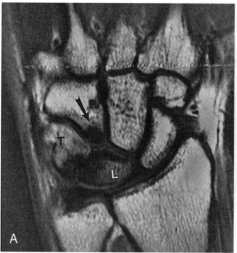 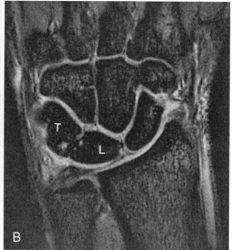

Figure 12–39. CARPAL COALITION AND TYPE II LUNATE. *A,* T1 coronal image, wrist. The space between the lunate (L) and the triquetrum (T) is narrowed and there is low signal from degenerative sclerosis in the bones on either side of the lunotriquetral joint, which has congenital coalition. There also happens to be abnormal signal in the proximal hamate *(arrow)* because of the type II lunate, which has a facet that articulates with the hamate. *B,* T2* coronal image, wrist (same patient as in *A*). Subchondral cysts from the congenital coalition between the lunate (L) and triquetrum (T) are evident and the joint is narrowed.

result from extension of a soft tissue ganglion cyst into the adjacent bone. These may be painful lesions. A small ganglion cyst arising in the scapholunate ligament commonly erodes the radial aspect of the lunate bone, resulting in a very common site for an intraosseous ganglion (Fig. 12–40).[38, 39]

MRI can demonstrate intraosseous ganglion cysts when radiographs are normal and radionuclide bone scans are nonspecific. MRI can demonstrate whether the lesion is confined to bone or the result of erosion from an adjacent soft tissue ganglion cyst. These lesions are small, rounded, well-circumscribed foci with low signal intensity on T1W images and high signal intensity on T2W images.

Soft Tissue Lesions

The most common soft tissue masses in the hand and wrist are ganglion cysts, giant cell tumors of

the tendon sheath, nerve sheath tumors, soft tissue chondromas, glomus tumors, and anomalous muscles.

Ganglion Cysts. The most common cause of a mass involving the wrist is a ganglion cyst.[40] These are fibrous-walled masses that contain thick mucoid fluid that resembles petroleum jelly. Ganglion cysts arise from synovial tissue, so they may be found attached by a pedicle to a tendon sheath, joint capsule, ligament, or within a fascial plane. These lesions may or may not be symptomatic. They usually occur in women during their thirties. Their cause is uncertain, but probably relates to chronic irritation at the site of formation. Ganglion cysts may erode the adjacent osseous structures. It is important to examine the scapholunate ligament carefully for small, occult ganglion cysts that are clinically not palpable but are a common source of dorsal wrist pain (Fig. 12–41).

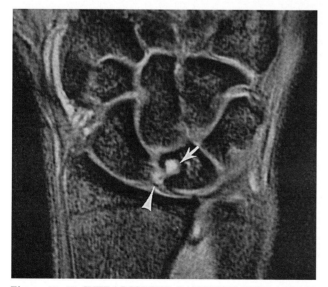

Figure 12–40. INTRAOSSEOUS GANGLION CYST ASSOCIATED WITH SCAPHOLUNATE LIGAMENT DEGENERATION. T2* coronal image, wrist. An intraosseous ganglion cyst in the radial aspect of the lunate *(arrow)* is in continuity with a ganglion cyst in the scapholunate ligament *(arrowhead).*

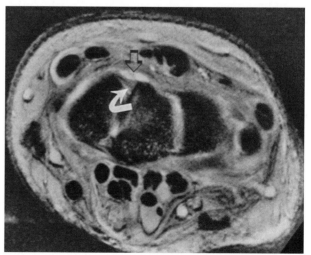

Figure 12–41. OCCULT GANGLION CYST OF THE SCAPHOLUNATE LIGAMENT. T2* axial image, wrist. There is a small, high-signal mass with a septation in it representing a ganglion cyst *(open arrow)* dorsal to the low-signal band of scapholunate ligament *(curved white arrow).*

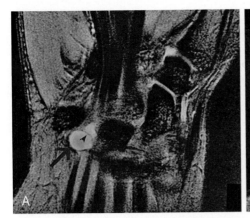
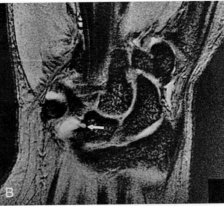

Figure 12–42. GANGLION CYST. *A*, T2* coronal image, wrist. The ganglion cyst arising from the flexor tendons is a high-signal mass *(arrow)* with a thin septation *(arrowhead)* within it. *B*, T2* coronal image, wrist (same patient as *A*). The high-signal ganglion cyst is eroding into the ulnar aspect of the lunate *(white arrow)*.

MRI shows ganglion cysts as low signal intensity masses on T1W images, although occasionally they are higher signal intensity because of a high protein concentration. On T2W images, the lesions generally are diffusely high signal intensity. A common feature that is somewhat characteristic for ganglion cysts is the presence of thin septations within the mass that are seen as low signal intensity lines on T2W images (Fig. 12–42).[41, 42]

Gadolinium may be given to differentiate a ganglion cyst from a solid mass. Enhancement is evident in the very thin fibrous wall, as well as in the thin septations. The remainder of the lesion should show no enhancement.

Giant Cell Tumors of the Tendon Sheath. This represents the second most common soft tissue mass of the hand and wrist. It is an extraarticular, localized form of pigmented villonodular synovitis, a hyperplastic synovial process of unknown cause. The mass shows low signal intensity on both T1W and T2W images, which significantly limits the differential diagnostic possibilities (Fig. 12–43). Amyloid deposits and gouty tophi also may present as soft tissue masses with the same signal characteristics, but there are generally other features on the MR images or clinical history that help to differentiate these entities. For example, gout usually has multiple lesions and joint involvement, and amyloid is generally a systemic process from an underlying known disease.

Glomus Tumors. These are benign tumors that arise from a neuromyoarterial glomus, which are present in the deepest layer of the dermis throughout the body. Glomus bodies are highly concentrated in the fingertips, especially beneath the fingernails. Thus, the lesions usually are found dorsal to the distal phalanges of the digits, but occasionally can be present on the volar surface. The glomus functions to regulate body temperature. These lesions can cause severe aching pain, point tenderness, and sensitivity to cold. Pressure erosion of the adjacent bone may occur from a glomus tumor.

MRI is valuable for evaluation of glomus tumors in order to establish the diagnosis, demonstrate if multiple lesions are present, and to direct surgery to the proper location because the lesions are generally extremely small and may be difficult to find.[43] Glomus tumors are small, well-defined soft tissue masses that demonstrate low signal intensity on T1W images and are hyperintense on T2W images (Fig. 12–44). Intravenous contrast administration demonstrates these lesions to have strong enhancement. A thin capsule may be seen as low signal intensity surrounding the lesion on all pulse sequences and after contrast is given. Axial and sagittal images are the best for demonstrating glomus tumors, and bone erosion often is evident when none is seen by conventional radiography.

Anomalous Muscles. These are relatively common in the hand and wrist. They may present as a soft tissue mass, or may cause compression of the median or ulnar nerve, depending on the location of the anomalous muscle. A common anomalous

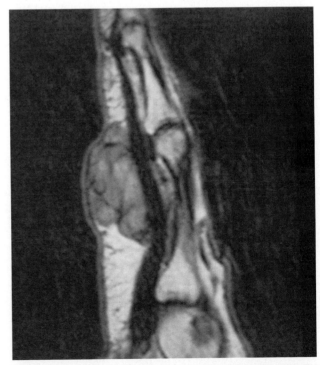

Figure 12–43. GIANT CELL TUMOR OF THE TENDON SHEATH. T1 sagittal image, finger. There is a lobulated, intermediate signal mass volar to the flexor tendon of the index finger.

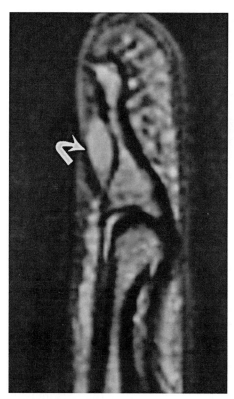

Figure 12–44. GLOMUS TUMOR.
Fast T2 sagittal image, finger. There is a small, high-signal mass *(curved arrow)* on the dorsum of the distal phalanx, causing bone erosion.

muscle is the extensor digitorum manus brevis, found on the dorsum of the wrist and hand along the ulnar side of the extensor indicis tendon.[44] Clinically, this anomalous muscle easily may be confused with a ganglion cyst.

MRI serves to document the presence of muscle in predictable locations (Fig. 12–45). The signal intensity follows that of other skeletal muscle on all pulse sequences, which serves to differentiate it from a mass of other origin.

Arthritis

Inflammatory, degenerative, and metabolic arthritides commonly affect the hand and wrist. The tomographic nature and superb contrast resolution of MRI allows erosions, subchondral cysts, synovitis, tenosynovitis, and other manifestations of arthritis to be exquisitely demonstrated when other imaging techniques show no or minimal abnormalities. A separate chapter is devoted to the findings in arthritis and the role of MRI in these diseases.

Synovial Cysts

Synovial cysts may occur in the wrist. These may be a manifestation of rheumatoid arthritis, but a synovial cyst arising from the pisotriquetral joint is so common and unrelated to an inflammatory arthri-

tis that it deserves attention here. Small amounts of fluid in the pisotriquetral synovial recess normally may be seen, but when it becomes large in amount, it may be a possible source of pain. These probably occur in patients who have pisotriquetral degenerative joint disease. A ball-valve mechanism may exist that allows synovial fluid to enter the cyst, but not exit it. The fluid is absorbed, and what remains behind in the synovial cyst is very thick, mucoid material similar to that found in ganglion cysts. The enlarged pisotriquetral synovial cyst is anatomically a similar situation to the popliteal (Baker) cyst in the knee, and may become symptomatic and usually enlarges as a response to abnormalities in the adjacent joint. We have aspirated and injected several enlarged pisotriquetral cysts with anesthetic and steroid and patients received pain relief. If the injections do not relieve symptoms, surgical removal of the pisiform bone may be performed for pain relief.

The MR appearance of the pisotriquetral synovial cyst is that of a rounded or elongated mass on the volar aspect of the wrist, just proximal to the pisiform, that is low signal intensity on T1W images and high signal intensity on T2W images (Fig. 12–46). When it measures one cm or more in diameter, we mention it as a synovial cyst that may be a pain source.

Infection

Septic arthritis, abscesses, cellulitis, and osteomyelitis may occur in the hand and wrist. These

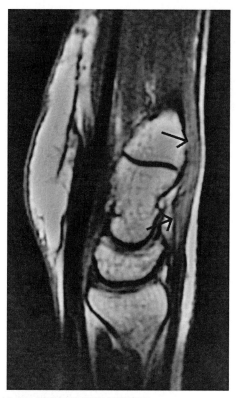

Figure 12–45. ANOMALOUS MUSCLE.
T1 sagittal image, wrist. A dorsal soft tissue mass *(arrows)* with signal typical of muscle is the extensor digitorum manus brevis.

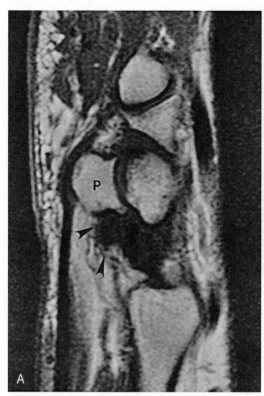

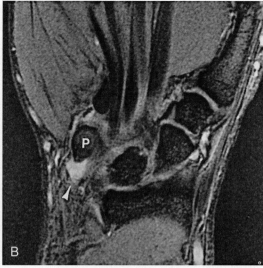

Figure 12–46. PISOTRIQUETRAL SYNOVIAL CYST.
A, T1 sagittal image, wrist. A low-signal mass *(arrowheads)* just proximal to the pisiform (P) is a synovial cyst from the pisotriquetral joint. Note the mild degenerative changes in the joint with osteophytes. *B,* T2* coronal image, wrist (same patient as *A*). The synovial cyst becomes high signal *(arrowhead)* and is located just proximal to the pisiform (P).

processes are more common in other anatomic locations and are discussed in detail elsewhere. The MR findings of infection in the hand and wrist are no different than in other anatomic sites. One feature of this anatomic region to keep in mind is that infection spreads rapidly along compartments and tendon sheaths (Fig. 12–47). Any suspicion of infection needs to be aggressively worked up and treated because of the devastating consequences in the hand. Fluid in a tendon sheath (tenosynovitis) may be sterile or infected, and one should always remember to consider a purulent tenosynovitis in the differential diagnosis for tenosynovitis.

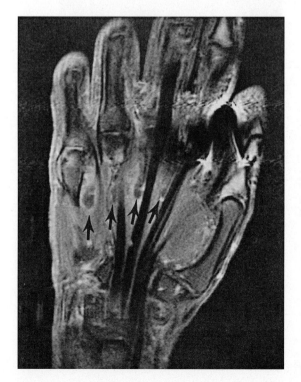

Figure 12–47. INFECTION.
T1 fat saturation coronal image, with contrast, hand. High-signal contrast outlines four low-signal linear abscesses *(arrows)* in different compartments in the hand.

References

1. Smith DK. Scapholunate interosseous ligament of the wrist: MR appearances in asymptomatic volunteers and arthrographically normal wrists. *Radiology* 1994; 192:217–221.

2. Smith DK, Snearly WN. Lunotriquetral interosseous ligament of the wrist: MR appearances in asymptomatic volunteers and arthrographically normal wrists. *Radiology* 1994; 191:199–202.

3. Wright TW, Del Charco M, Wheeler D. Incidence of ligament lesions and associated degenerative changes in the elderly wrist. *J Hand Surg [Am]* 1994; 19:313.

4. Totterman SMS, Miller RJ. Scapholunate ligament: normal MR appearance on three-dimensional gradient-recalled-echo images. *Radiology* 1996; 200:237–241.

5. Zlatkin MB, Chao PC, Osterman AL, et al. Chronic wrist pain: evaluation with high-resolution MR imaging. *Radiology* 1989; 173:723–729.

6. Anderson MW, Kaplan PA, Dussault RG, Degnan GG. Magnetic resonance imaging of the wrist. *Curr Probl Diagn Radiol* 1998; 27:191–226.

7. Timins ME, Jahnke JP, Krah SF, et al. MR imaging of the major carpal stabilizing ligaments: normal anatomy and clinical examples. *Radiographics* 1995; 25:575–587.

8. Smith DK. Dorsal carpal ligaments of the wrist: normal appearance on multiplanar reconstructions of three-dimensional fourier transform MR imaging. *AJR* 1993; 161:119–125.

9. Smith DK. Volar carpal ligaments of the wrist: normal appearance on multiplanar reconstructions of three-dimensional fourier transform MR imaging. *AJR* 1993; 353–357.

10. Brown RR, Fliszar E, Cotten A, et al. Extrinsic and intrinsic ligaments of the wrist: normal and pathologic anatomy at MR arthrography with three-compartment enhancement. *Radiographics* 1998; 18:667–674.

11. Totterman SMS, Miller RJ. Triangular fibrocartilage complex: normal appearance on coronal three-dimensional gradient-recalled-echo MR images. *Radiology* 1995; 195:521–527.

12. Schweitzer ME, Brahme SK, Hodler J, et al. Chronic wrist pain: spin echo and short tau inversion recovery MR imaging and conventional and MR arthrography. *Radiology* 1992; 182:205–211.

13. Oneson SR, Timins ME, Scales LM, et al. MR imaging diagnosis of triangular fibrocartilage pathology with arthroscopic correlation. *AJR* 1997; 168:1513–1518.

14. Golimbu CN, Firooznia H, Melone CP Jr, et al. Tears of the triangular fibrocartilage of the wrist: MR imaging. *Radiology* 1989; 173:731–733.

15. Totterman SMS, Miller RJ, McCance SE, Meyers SP. Lesions of the triangular fibrocartilage complex: MR findings with a three-dimensional gradient-recalled-echo sequence. *Radiology* 1996; 199:227–232.

16. Palmer AK. Triangular fibrocartilage complex lesions: a classification. *J Hand Surg [Am]* 1989; 14:594–606.

17. Staron RB, Feldman F, Haramati N, et al. Abnormal geometry of the distal radioulnar joint: MR findings. *Skeletal Radiol* 1994; 23:369–372.

18. Klug JD. MR diagnosis of tenosynovitis about the wrist. *Magn Reson Imaging Clin N Am* 1995; 3:305–312.

19. Spaeth HJ, Abrams RA, Bock GW, et al. Gamekeeper thumb: differentiation of nondisplaced and displaced tears of the ulnar collateral ligament with MR imaging—work in progress. *Radiology* 1993; 188:553–556.

20. Hinke DH, Erickson SJ, Chamoy L, Timins ME. Ulnar collateral ligament of the thumb: MR findings in cadavers, volunteers, and patients with ligamentous injury (gamekeeper's thumb). *AJR* 1994; 163:1431–1434.

21. Rubens DJ, Blebea JS, Totterman SMS, Hooper MM. Rheumatoid arthritis: evaluation of wrist extensor tendons with clinical examination versus MR imaging—a preliminary report. *Radiology* 1993; 187:831–838.

22. Glajchen N, Schweitzer M. MRI features in de Quervain's tenosynovitis of the wrist. *Skeletal Radiol* 1996; 25:63–65.

23. Mesgarzadeh M, Schneck CE, Bonakdarpour A. Carpal tunnel: MR imaging I: Normal anatomy. *Radiology* 1989; 171:743–748.

24. Ikeda K, Haughton VM, Ho K-C, et al. Correlative MR-anatomic study of the median nerve. *AJR* 1996; 167:1233–1236.

25. Murphy RX, Chernofsky MA, Osborne MA, Wolson AH. Magnetic resonance imaging in the evaluation of persistent carpal tunnel syndrome. *J Hand Surg [Am]* 1993; 18:113–120.

26. Binkovitz LA, Berquist TH, McLeod RA. Masses of the hand and wrist: detection and characterization with MR imaging. *AJR* 1990; 154:323–326.

27. Cavallaro MC, Taylor JAM, Gorman JD, et al. Imaging findings in a patient with fibrolipomatous hamartoma of the median nerve. *AJR* 1993; 161:837–838.

28. Escobedo EM, Bergman AG, Hunter JC. MR imaging of ulnar impaction. *Skeletal Radiol* 1995; 24:85–90.

29. Breitenseher MJ, Metz VM, Gilula LA, et al. Radiographically occult scaphoid fractures: value of MR imaging in detection. *Radiology* 1997; 203:245–250.

30. Hunter JC, Escobedo EM, Wilson AH, et al. MR imaging of clinically suspected scaphoid fractures. *AJR* 1997; 168:1287–1293.

31. Gaebler C, Kukla C, Breitenseher M, et al. Magnetic resonance imaging of occult scaphoid fractures. *J Trauma* 1996; 41:73–76.

32. Shih C, Chang C-Y, Penn I-W, et al. Chronically stressed wrists in adolescent gymnasts: MR imaging appearance. *Radiology* 1995; 195:855–859.

33. Chang C-Y, Shih C, Penn I-W, et al. Wrist injuries in adolescent gymnasts of a Chinese opera school: radiographic survey. *Radiology* 1995; 195:861–864.

34. Trumble TE. Avascular necrosis after scaphoid fracture: a correlation of magnetic resonance imaging and histology. *J Hand Surg [Am]* 1990; 15:557–564.

35. Desser TS, McCarthy S, Trumble T. Scaphoid fractures and Kienböck's disease of the lunate: MR imaging with histopathologic correlation. *Magn Reson Imaging* 1990; 8:357–361.

36. Golimbu CN, Firooznia H, Rafii M. Avascular necrosis of carpal bones. *Magn Reson Imaging Clin N Am* 1995; 3:281–303.

37. Trumble TE, Irving J. Histologic and magnetic resonance imaging correlations in Kienböck's disease. *J Hand Surg [Am]* 1990; 15:879–884.

38. Pope TL, Fechner RE, Keats TE. Intra-osseous ganglion. *Skeletal Radiol* 1989; 18:185–187.

39. Magee TH, Rowedder AM, Degnan GG. Intraosseous ganglia of the wrist. *Radiology* 1995; 195:517–520.

40. Bogumill GP, Sullivan EJ, Baker GI. Tumors of the hand. *Clin Orthop* 1975; 108:214–222.

41. Vo P, Wright T, Hayden F, et al. Evaluating dorsal wrist pain: MRI diagnosis of occult dorsal wrist ganglion. *J Hand Surg [Am]* 1995; 10:667–670.

42. Kransdorf MJ, Murphey MD. MR imaging of musculoskeletal tumors of the hand and wrist. *Magn Reson Imaging Clin N Am* 1995; 3:327–344.

43. Drape J, Idy-Peretti J, Goettmann S, et al. Subungual glomus tumors: evaluation with MR imaging. *Radiology* 1995; 195:507–515.

44. Anderson MW, Benedetti P, Walter J, Steinberg DR. MR appearance of the extensor digitorum manus brevis muscle: a pseudotumor of the hand. *AJR* 1995; 164:1477–1479.

WRIST/HAND PROTOCOLS
This is one set of suggested protocols; there are many variations that would work equally well.

WRIST: ROUTINE						
Sequence #	1	2	3	4	5	6
Sequence Type	T1	T2*	Turbo T2	T2*	T1	T1
Orientation	Coronal	Coronal	Coronal	Axial	Axial	Sagittal
Field of View (cm)	8–10	8–10	8–10	8–10	8–10	8–10
Slice Thickness (mm)	3	1 or 2	3	3	3	3
Contrast	No	No	No	No	No	No

WRIST: MASS OR INFECTION						
Sequence #	1	2	3	4	5	6
Sequence Type	T1	STIR	T1	STIR	T1 fat saturation	T1 fat saturation
Orientation	Coronal	Coronal	Axial	Sagittal	Coronal	Axial
Field of View (cm)	8–10	8–10	8–10	8–10	8–10	8–10
Slice Thickness (mm)	3	3	3	3	3	3
Contrast	No	No	No	No	Yes	Yes

WRIST: TRAUMA SCREENING						
Sequence #	1	2	3	4	5	6
Sequence Type	T1	Turbo T2				
Orientation	Cor	Cor				
Field of View (cm)	8–10	8–10				
Slice Thickness (mm)	3	3				
Contrast	No	No				

THUMB: GAMEKEEPER'S THUMB SCREENING PROTOCOL						
Sequence #	1	2	3	4	5	6
Sequence Type	T1	T2*				
Orientation	Coronal	Coronal				
Field of View (cm)	6–8	6–8				
Slice Thickness (mm)	3	2				
Contrast	No	No				

Scout		Final Image
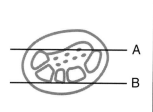	• Axial scout • Obtain coronal images tangent to line A • Cover from line A to B • Coronals should be first sequence in study (most valuable plane) • Final image should include bases of metacarpals and distal radioulnar joint	Coronal 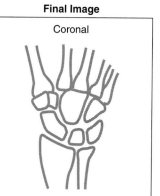

Scout		Final Image
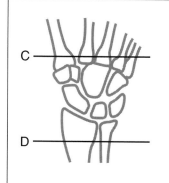	• Coronal scout • Obtain axial images between lines C and D • Final image should fill the entire frame	Axial 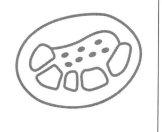

Scout		Final Image
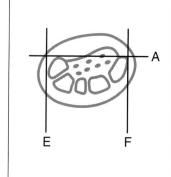	• Axial scout • Obtain sagittal images perpendicular to line A • Cover from line E to F • Sagittal should be last sequence in study (least valuable plane)	Sagittal 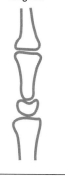

- Patient prone with wrist in coil above head, elbow in flexion
- Coil centered on point 1 cm distal to palpated ulnar styloid
- Comfort, padding, relaxed fingers are crucial

Scout		Final Image
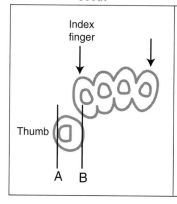	• 3 plane scout, use axial • Obtain coronal images of thumb parallel to flat volar surface of thumb bones • Cover between lines A & B • Final coronal image should appear as AP thumb x-ray	Coronal 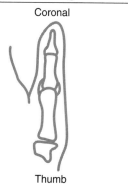 Thumb

- Small coil, patient prone, elbow in flexion
- Center coil over MCP joint of thumb.

277

13 SPINE

HOW TO IMAGE THE SPINE
NORMAL AND ABNORMAL
Degenerative Changes
  Disk Aging/Degeneration
    Normal disk
    Abnormal nucleus
    Abnormal annulus
    Abnormalities in disk
      morphology
    Disk bulge
    Disk protrusion
    Disk extrusion
    Sequestered disk
    Location of focal disk
      abnormalities
    Significance of disk contour
      abnormalities
    Disk-related compressive
      myelopathy/epidural hematoma
    Disk mimickers
    Vacuum disks and vertebral bodies
    Calcified disks
  Osseous Degenerative Changes
    Vertebral bodies
    Facet joints
    Posterior spinous processes
Spinal Stenosis
  Central Canal Stenosis

  Lateral Recess Stenosis
  Neural Foramen Stenosis
Postoperative Changes
  Uncomplicated Postoperative
    MRI
  Failed Back Surgery
Inflammatory Changes
  Spondylodiskitis
  Epidural Abscess
  Arachnoiditis
  Ankylosing Spondylitis
Traumatic Changes
  Spondylolysis and
    Spondylolisthesis
  Intraosseous Disk Herniations
  Major Trauma
    Osseous
    Ligaments
    Traumatic disks
    Epidural fluid collections
    Vascular abnormalities
    Cord injuries
    Other soft tissues
Osseous Spine Tumors
  Benign Bone Tumors
    Intraosseous hemangiomas

  Malignant Bone Tumors
    Metastases and multiple myeloma
    Chordomas
    Primary bone tumors
Spinal Canal Contents
  Epidural Space
    Epidural abscess
    Epidural hematoma
    Epidural lipomatosis
    Epidural cysts
    Miscellaneous
  Intradural Space
    Nerve sheath tumors
    Meningioma
    Other tumors
    Lipomas
    Intradural cystic lesions
    Metastases
  Spinal Cord Lesions
    Demyelination abnormalities
    Cysts
    Infarction
    Tumors
  Tethered Cord
SPINE PROTOCOLS

HOW TO IMAGE THE SPINE

See spine protocols at the end of the chapter.

Coils/Patient Position. Phased array spine coils should be used for all spine imaging. Patients are supine in the magnet.

Image Orientation (Box 13–1). Both sagittal and axial images are acquired in the cervical, thoracic, and lumbar regions. In the axial imaging plane, we obtain stacked cuts that cover an entire block of the spine, as well as images angled with the disks when the indications are for pain, degenerative changes, or to rule out disk or radiculopathy. Some people obtain stacked images only and do not bother angling with the disks on any sequence; this is a matter of personal preference. Conversely, acquiring images angled only through the disks (without obtaining stacked images) is considered inadequate, because portions of the spinal canal will not be imaged in the axial plane and sequestered disk frag-

ments could be missed. Sagittal images alone are sometimes not adequate to detect a disk fragment that has migrated from the parent disk. Because sequestered disks are a cause of failed back surgery and persistent symptoms, it is important to identify them on MRI by obtaining stacked axial images in addition to sagittal images through the canal. In the unoperated lumbar spine, we obtain stacked axial images from the middle of the L3 vertebral body to the middle of the S1 vertebral body. In the postoperative spine, stacked axial images (matched images pre- and post-contrast) are obtained by centering at the level of the previous surgery. Axial images are often better than sagittal for detecting lesions in the neural foramina. In general, we consider axial and sagittal planes of imaging to be complementary, and do not recommend doing without either. Coronal images may be useful to better define the anatomy in patients with scoliosis.

Pulse Sequences/Regions of Interest. The pulse

BOX 13–1: SPINAL STRUCTURES TO EVALUATE IN DIFFERENT PLANES

Sagittal
  Cord
  Disk signal, height
  Disk contour ($\pm$)
  Vertebral bodies
  Spinous processes
  Nerve roots
  Neural foramen
  Central canal
  Ligaments (anterior and posterior
    longitudinal, interspinous, supraspinous)
  Epidural space
Axial
  Nerve roots
  Cord
  Disk contour
  Vertebral bodies
  Neural foramen
  Central canal
  Lateral recesses
  Ligaments (ligamentum flavum)
  Epidural space
  Facet joints

sequences are determined by the clinical indications for the examination, based on the following major categories: (1) degenerative disease (including radicular symptoms), (2) trauma, (3) cord compression/bone metastases, and (4) infection (disk or epidural)/intradural lesion.

TlW and fast T2W images are the standard for sagittal imaging in any segment of the spine. Gradient echo sagittal sequences are used when looking for blood in the cord after trauma to take advantage of the blooming effect. A fast STIR sagittal sequence also is useful in trauma patients when looking for ligamentous injury with changes of hemorrhage and edema. Gradient echo axials are used to detect disk disease in the cervical spine, whereas fast T2W axial images are used in the thoracic and lumbar spine for the same indications. Both TlW and some type of T2W images are selected in both the sagittal and axial planes for most indications. Details are given in the tables of spine protocols.

Slice thickness in general is 3 or 4 mm. Axial gradient echo images through the cervical disks are 2 mm thick. The fields of view are as small as possible; larger ones are required for sagittal than for the axial imaging planes. In the cervical, thoracic, and lumbar spine, the sagittal fields of view are usually 14 cm, 16 cm, and 16 cm, respectively; recommended fields of view for the axial images are 11 cm, 12 cm, and 14 cm, respectively.

Phase and frequency encoding gradients should be reversed for imaging the spine in the sagittal plane, so that chemical shift artifacts at the discovertebral interfaces do not obscure pathology in the vertebral body endplates or disks.

Contrast. Contrast is always used for postoperative spine imaging, suspected infection, or intradural or nontraumatic cord lesions. If any abnormality is identified in the epidural space when evaluating for osseous metastases or cord compression, gadolinium is given to better demonstrate these lesions.

NORMAL AND ABNORMAL

Degenerative Changes

Without a doubt, the most prevalent abnormalities of the spine are degenerative changes of the joints and osseous structures. Remember that, in the spine, the major joints consist of the paired, freely movable (diarthrodial) synovial facet joints running along the dorsal aspect of the spine and the minimally movable (amphiarthrodial) cartilagenous articulations formed by the intervertebral disks. Primary stability of the spine below C2 is provided by this three-joint complex, composed of the intervertebral disk and paired facet joints at each vertebral level. Anatomic and biochemical changes occur in these joints as the result of aging, but such changes may or may not cause symptoms.

The major focus of spine imaging over the years has been on the mechanical effect that osseous, disk, and joint structures have on adjacent nerves. Although it is important to detect this mechanical effect with imaging, it must be remembered that most symptoms of back pain are not related to compression or stretching of an exiting or descending nerve. Pain may arise from the facet joints or disks, regardless of what these structures do to an adjacent spinal nerve root. It has been well established that asymptomatic individuals of all ages have disk abnormalities on imaging studies.[1] Defining the source of a patient's neck or back pain must be done very carefully by integrating the findings of clinical examination and MRI, often with the aid of diagnostic injections of anesthetic to different spinal structures for confirmation.

Disk Aging/Degeneration (Box 13–2)

Features of normal and abnormal disks discussed here apply to disks at any level in the spine, because they appear the same whether in the cervical, thoracic, or lumbar regions.

Normal Disk. Intervertebral disks consist of a central gelatinous nucleus pulposus composed of water and proteoglycans. The nucleus pulposus is surrounded by the annulus fibrosus. The inner portion of the annulus is composed of fibrocartilage, whereas the outer fibers are made of concentrically oriented lamellae of collagen fibers. The annulus is anchored to the adjacent vertebral bodies by Sharpey's fibers.

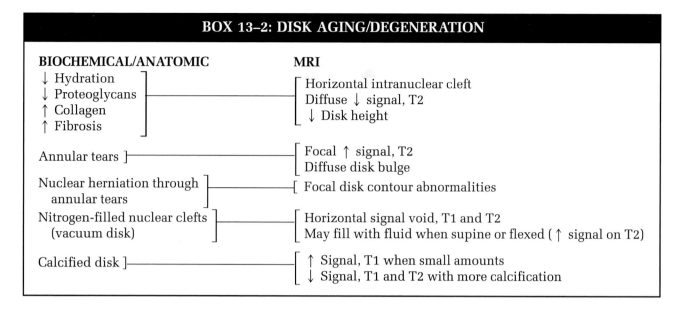

BOX 13–2: DISK AGING/DEGENERATION

BIOCHEMICAL/ANATOMIC	MRI
↓ Hydration ↓ Proteoglycans ↑ Collagen ↑ Fibrosis	Horizontal intranuclear cleft Diffuse ↓ signal, T2 ↓ Disk height
Annular tears	Focal ↑ signal, T2 Diffuse disk bulge
Nuclear herniation through annular tears	Focal disk contour abnormalities
Nitrogen-filled nuclear clefts (vacuum disk)	Horizontal signal void, T1 and T2 May fill with fluid when supine or flexed (↑ signal on T2)
Calcified disk	↑ Signal, T1 when small amounts ↓ Signal, T1 and T2 with more calcification

On MRI, the ideal normal disk is low signal intensity on T1W images, being slightly lower signal than adjacent normal red marrow, and very similar to muscle (Fig. 13–1). T2W images show diffuse high signal intensity throughout the disk, except for the outer fibers of the annulus, which are homogeneously low signal intensity (Fig. 13–1). Distinction between the nucleus pulposus and the inner annulus fibrosus is not possible by MRI.

Normal disks typically do not extend beyond the margins of the adjacent vertebral bodies; however, diffuse extension beyond the margins by 1 to 2 mm may certainly occur in some histologically normal disks.[2] The posterior margins of disks tend to be mildly concave in the upper lumbar spine, straight at the L4–5 level, and slightly convex at the lumbosacral junction.

Abnormal Nucleus. With aging and degeneration, the intervertebral disks lose hydration, lose proteoglycans, and gain collagen as they become more fibrous. A horizontally oriented fibrous intranuclear cleft develops in the nucleus.

MRI demonstrates the intranuclear cleft as a horizontal, low signal intensity line that divides the disk into upper and lower halves on T2W sagittal images (Fig. 13–2). Eventually, there is diffuse decreased signal intensity on T2W images from the increased collagen content in the nucleus (Fig. 13–2). The disk progressively loses height with increasing degrees of degeneration.

Abnormal Annulus (Box 13–3). Aging and biochemical changes in the disks as described above are associated with the development of multiple, focal annular tears. Three types of annular tears have been described, but only one type is of practical interest, and that is the radial type of tear.[3]

Radial tears (or fissures) involve either part or the entire thickness of the annulus from the nucleus to the outer annular fibers. Radial tears run perpendicular to the long axis of the annulus and occur more commonly in the posterior half of the disk, usually at L4–5 and L5–S1. The radial annular tear is considered by many to be responsible for pain. It may be a pain source because vascularized granulation tissue grows into the tear and causes painful stimulation of nerve endings that also extend into the defect from the surface of the disk; this would result in diskogenic pain.[4] It also may be a pain source because of the instability of the disk that accompanies these fissures, and the chemical as well as mechanical irritation to the nociceptive fibers that normally exist in the annulus. Radial fissures that cause diskogenic pain can be treated by minimally invasive intradiskal therapy (thermal or chemical) or by spinal fusion.

MRI of annular tears shows focal areas of high signal intensity on T2W images or on contrast-enhanced T1W images.[5] Radial tears (Fig. 13–3) may be seen on T2W sagittal images within the posterior annulus as globular or horizontal lines of high signal intensity. On axial images, radial tears may be seen as focal areas of high signal intensity that parallel

BOX 13–3: RADIAL TEARS OF THE ANNULUS

—Also called high intensity zones (HIZ)
—Often painful
—Linear fissures through all or part of thickness of annulus
—Run perpendicular to long axis
—Usually in posterior annulus of lower lumbar disks
—Nerve ingrowth from surface of disk causes pain
—Globular or horizontal lines of ↑ signal in disk substance, T2 and postcontrast T1

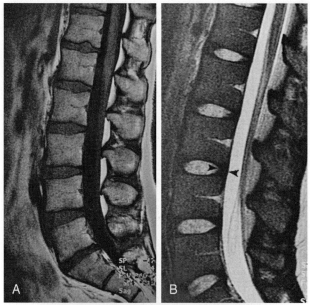

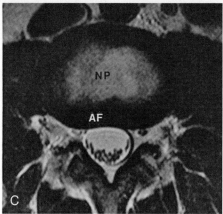

Figure 13–1. NORMAL DISKS.
A, T1 sagittal image, lumbar spine. Disks are intermediate signal intensity, lower signal than bone marrow, on T1W images. *B,* Fast T2 sagittal image, lumbar spine. The nucleus is diffusely high signal, whereas the annulus fibrosus is low signal (between *arrowheads,* at L3–4). *C,* Fast T2 axial image, L3–4 disk. The nucleus pulposus (NP) is high signal, whereas the annulus fibrosus (AF) around the periphery of the disk is low signal.

the outer disk margin for a short distance. Radial tears or fissures on MRI also are referred to as high-intensity zones (HIZ).[5]

Abnormalities in Disk Morphology (Box 13–4). The terminology for disk abnormalities is very confusing and inconsistent in the literature. Many physicians have referred to any and all disk abnormalities that extend beyond the margin of the vertebral body or disk as a herniated disk or herniated nucleus pulposus (HNP). The problem with this approach is that most of the abnormalities are of no consequence to the patient and are not associated with symptoms. This explains the high incidence of disk "herniations" reported in an asymptomatic population.[1] Analogies to this situation would be to call benign bone islands "sclerotic foci of undetermined etiology" or calcified granulomas in the lungs

on a chest x-ray as "changes of infection." These latter statements are true, but of absolutely no help to the referring clinician or patient. They do not put the abnormality seen on the imaging study in proper perspective and indeed may be very misleading.

Most surgeons dealing with spine disorders are starting to use a more standardized nomenclature that helps to distinguish what are likely to be clinically relevant lesions from those that probably are not. We use the same terminology as our surgeons to describe abnormalities in disk morphology: diffuse disk bulge, broad-based protrusion, focal disk protrusion, disk extrusion, and sequestered disk (Fig. 13–4). Focal disk abnormalities occur when material from the nucleus extends either partially or completely through radial tears in the annulus. Thus, focal disk abnormalities generally occur in a degenerated disk. The term "herniated disk" can be used as a general term to encompass all of the other more specific terms outlined here, but in our opinion it should never be the diagnosis in a report of a spine MRI examination.

Once it has been determined that there is a diffuse or focal abnormality in disk contour, we generally try to quantify the abnormality as mild, moderate, or severe in extent. Unfortunately, there are no agreed-upon definitions for what constitutes these different categories. Our method of quantifying the severity of disk disease is *mild* if the anterior epidural fat is not obliterated, *moderate* if the epidural fat is obliterated and the thecal sac is being displaced, or *severe* if the cord is being effaced or nerve root(s) displaced.

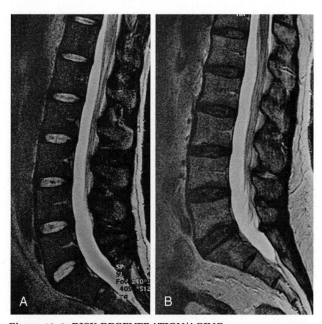

Figure 13–2. DISK DEGENERATION/AGING.
A, Fast T2 sagittal image, lumbar spine. Horizontal low-signal fibrous intranuclear clefts at each level divide the disks into upper and lower halves as an early manifestation of degeneration. *B,* Fast T2 sagittal image, lumbar spine (different patient than in *A*). Diffuse low signal intensity throughout the disks is a more advanced change of degeneration and aging.

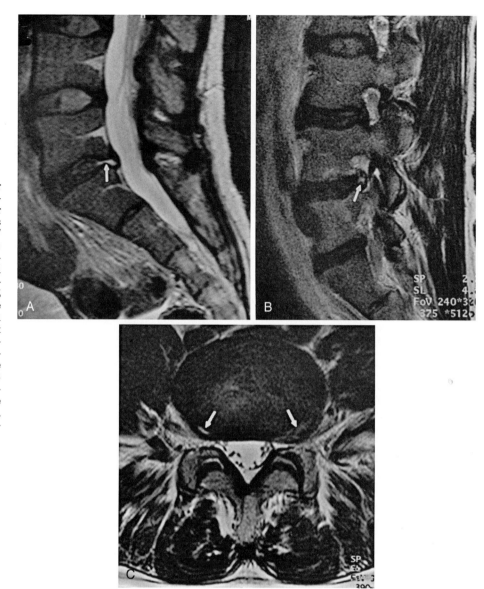

Figure 13–3. ANNULAR TEARS. *A,* Fast T2 sagittal image, lumbar spine. There is a focal line of increased signal in the posterior midline of the L5–S1 annulus *(arrow),* representing a radial tear/fissure or high-intensity zone (HIZ). The disk is protruding posteriorly slightly. *B,* Fast T2 sagittal image, lumbar spine (different patient than in *A*). A focal HIZ *(arrow)* from a radial tear of the L4–5 annulus is seen in the region of the left neural foramen. *C,* Fast T2 axial image, L4–5 (same patient as in *B*). Short, linear segments of high signal *(arrows)* are present in the posterolateral L4–5 disk from annular tears in the foraminal regions. The disks are protruding at the sites of the tears, resulting in mild bilateral foraminal narrowing.

This is not rocket science. The greatest difficulty is consistency and agreeing to the terms. All we are really evaluating when it comes to abnormalities in disk morphology is whether or not something is sticking out from the normal margin of a disk (like a wart from the skin surface), and by how far (how big the wart is).

Disk Bulge. A diffusely bulging disk extends symmetrically and circumferentially by more than 2 mm beyond the margins of the adjacent vertebral bodies. This diagnosis is based on axial and sagittal images by comparing the size of the disk with the size of the adjacent vertebral bodies and determining if the central canal and neural foramina are narrowed by the disk (Fig. 13–5). Identifying disk material protruding beyond the vertebral body margins on sagittal images does not clearly define if it is a diffuse or focal disk abnormality. The annulus can be considered as lax, and a decrease in disk height and disk signal usually is present on MRI. There are tears in

the annulus when there is disk bulging, although they may not be evident on MRI. A long segment of disk tissue that projects beyond the margin of the vertebral body but that does not involve the entire circumference of the disk can be called either a focal bulge or a broad-based protrusion (Fig. 13–6).

Disk Protrusion. This is a focal, asymmetric extension of disk tissue beyond the vertebral body margin, usually into the spinal canal or neural foramen, that often does not cause symptoms. The base (the mediolateral dimension along the posterior margin of the disk) is broader than any other dimension (Fig. 13–7).[6] Some of the outer annular fibers remain intact, and some people refer to this as a contained disk. The protruded disk does not extend in a cranial or caudal direction from the parent disk. MRI shows most disk protrusions and their parent disks to have low signal intensity on both T1W and T2W images.

Disk Extrusion. An extruded disk is a more pro-

BOX 13–4: DISK CONTOUR ABNORMALITIES: "Talk the Talk"

Herniated Disk
—All-encompassing, nonspecific term to indicate disk extends in some abnormal manner beyond margin of vertebral body

Disk Bulge
—Diffuse extension of disk by >2 mm beyond vertebral margin

Disk Protrusion
—Focal, small extension of disk beyond vertebral margin
—Anteroposterior < mediolateral diameter
—No cranial or caudal extension
—Usually asymptomatic
—Low signal T1 and T2

Disk Extrusion
—Greater extension of focal disk material than a protrusion
—Frequently symptomatic
—Anteroposterior ≥ mediolateral diameter
—May migrate craniocaudally, but maintains attachment to parent disk
— ↓ Signal on T1, ↓ (or ↑) on T2

Sequestered Disk
—Loss of continuity between extruded disk material and parent disk
—Usually symptomatic
—Fragment migrates
 • Cranial or caudal (equally)
 • Anterior or posterior to posterior longitudinal ligament
 • Epidural, intrathecal, paraspinous
—Contraindication to limited disk procedures
—Common cause of failed back surgery, if unrecognized
— ↓ Signal on T1, ↓ or ↑ on T2 or contrast T1

ous reduction in size of disk extrusions and protrusions that were managed conservatively has been well documented with imaging (Fig. 13–9).[8–12] The larger the disk extrusion, the greater the amount of regression in size of the extruded fragment with time.[11] The regression in disk size may not be the reason for reduction in pain. Again, much of the pain from extruded disks is probably from the inflammatory response to them, rather than from compression of neural elements from the mass effect.

Sequestered Disk. When extruded disk material loses its attachment to the parent disk, it is called a sequestered fragment (Fig. 13–10). These may migrate in a cranial or caudal direction with equal frequency and generally remain within about 5 mm of the parent disk. They may be located between the posterior longitudinal ligament and the osseous spine or extend through the posterior ligament into the epidural space. They almost always remain in the anterior epidural space, but occasionally the fragment may migrate into the posterior epidural space. Rarely, sequestered fragments may enter the dural sac or migrate into the paraspinous soft tissues. It is extremely important to recognize these fragments, because they may be overlooked at surgery and are a contraindication to chymopapain, percutaneous discectomy, and other limited disk procedures. The fragment of disk material that mi-

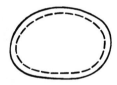

A. **Diffuse Disk Bulge**

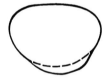

B. **Broad-based Protrusion**
(or focal disk bulge)

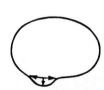

C. **Focal Disk Protrusion**
AP< Mediolateral dimension

D. **Disk Extrusion**
AP≥Mediolateral dimension

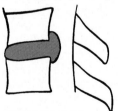

E. **Disk Extrusion**
Disk migrates above and/or below parent disk, maintaining continuity with it

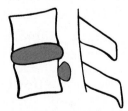

F. **Sequestered Disk**
Separate from parent disk

Figure 13–4. DISK MORPHOLOGY.
Diagram demonstrating abnormalities in morphology of the disks. The dashed lines in *A* and *B* indicate the vertebral bodies, whereas the solid lines represent the disks.

nounced version of a protrusion and often is responsible for symptoms (Fig. 13–8). There is disruption of the outer fibers of the annulus, and the disk abnormality usually is greater in its anteroposterior dimension than it is at its base (mediolateral dimension). The extruded disk may migrate up or down behind the adjacent vertebral bodies, but maintains continuity with the parent disk. These also may be referred to as noncontained disks. MRI shows the described contour abnormalities and, because of a significant inflammatory reaction that may occur in response to the extruded disk material, there may be high signal intensity on T2W and contrast-enhanced T1W images in or surrounding the disk. The typical appearance, however, is the same signal intensity as the parent disk on all pulse sequences.

Lumbar disk extrusions that cause radiculopathy but that are managed nonoperatively have been shown to do well about 90% of the time.[7] Spontane-

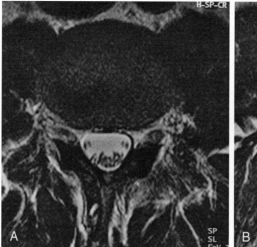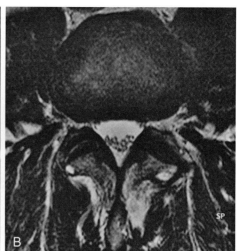

Figure 13–5. DIFFUSE DISK BULGE.
A, Fast T2 axial image through vertebral body. This demonstrates the size of the vertebral body, which must be compared to the size of the adjacent disk (in *B*). *B*, Fast T2 axial image through the adjacent disk. The oval configuration of the disk is slightly larger than the vertebral body in *A*, indicating mild diffuse disk bulging. Also, the neural foramina and the thecal sac are slightly narrowed compared to *A*, due to the bulging disk.

grates from the parent disk often shows peripheral or diffuse high signal intensity on T2W and contrast-enhanced T1W images, caused by the inflammatory reaction within or surrounding it. Otherwise, a low signal intensity mass resembling the signal of the parent disk is seen.

Location of Focal Disk Abnormalities (Box 13–5). A focal disk abnormality should be defined as to size, contour, location, and relationship to nerves or other important structures. The location of a focal disk abnormality needs to be conveyed accurately so the surgical approach can be properly planned, or so that it can be determined whether symptoms

correlate to the anatomic abnormality seen on MRI. Focal disk abnormalities that remain at the level of the parent disk should be described as being central, left or right paracentral, left or right foraminal, or left or right extraforaminal (also called lateral or far lateral) (Fig. 13–11).

Over 90% of focal lumbar disk abnormalities affect the spinal canal (central and paracentral regions), whereas approximately 4% occur in the neural foramen, and another 4% in the extraforaminal regions. Thus, individuals with symptoms of an L5 nerve abnormality almost always have a disk abnormality in the canal at the L4–5 level in the central

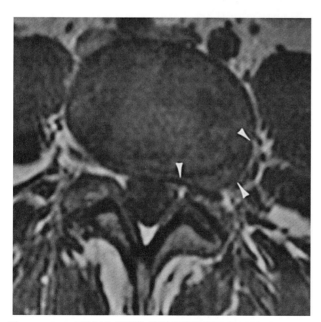

Figure 13–6. FOCAL DISK BULGE/BROAD-BASED PROTRUSION.
T1 axial image, L4–5. There is extension of disk beyond the margin of the vertebral body (between *arrowheads*) that is relatively long, referred to as either a broad-based protrusion or a focal disk bulge.

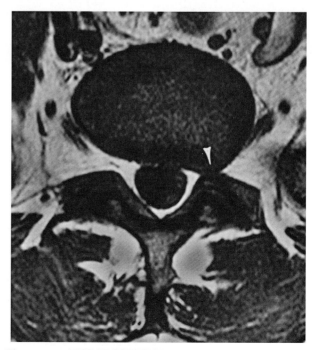

Figure 13–7. DISK PROTRUSION.
T1 axial image, L4–5. There is a short segment of disk protruding into the left neural foramen *(arrowhead)* and narrowing it. The base of the disk abnormality is greater than its anteroposterior dimension, typical of a focal disk protrusion.

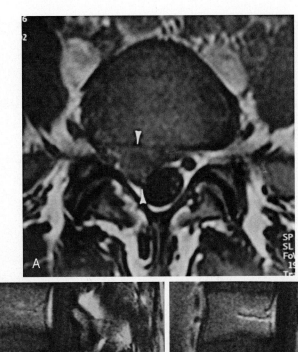

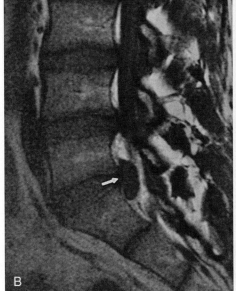

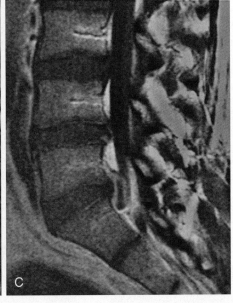

Figure 13–8. DISK EXTRUSION.
A, T1 axial image, L5–S1. There is a large piece of disk extending into the spinal canal in the right paracentral region. Its base is shorter than its anteroposterior dimension (between *arrowheads*), making this a disk extrusion. The descending S1 nerve is not identified because of displacement by the disk. **B,** T1 sagittal image, L5–S1. The disk extends both superior and inferior to the level of the parent disk *(arrow),* which is an additional criterion for calling this a disk extrusion **C,** T1 sagittal image with contrast enhancement, L5–S1. There is a peripheral rim of high signal surrounding the disk extrusion from enhancement of inflammatory reactive tissue.

Figure 13–9. SPONTANEOUS REGRESSION OF DISK EXTRUSION.
A, T1 sagittal image, L5–S1. There is a large disk extrusion extending behind the S1 vertebral body *(arrow).* **B,** T1 sagittal image, L5–S1. This image was obtained almost 1 year after the one in *A.* The patient had no surgery or other interventional therapy for the extruded disk. The disk extrusion is markedly reduced in size and now has the appearance of a disk protrusion.

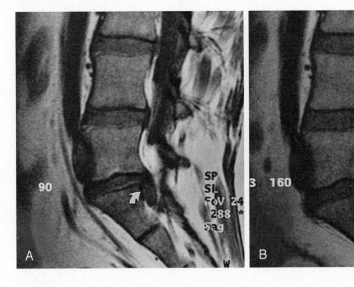

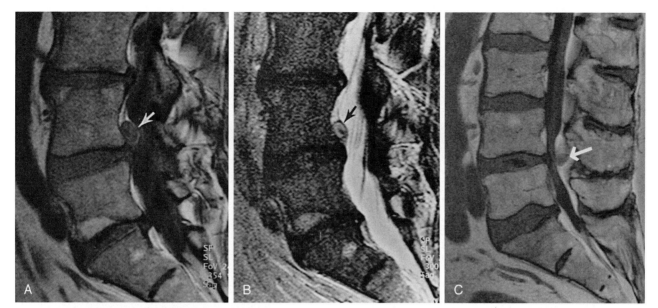

Figure 13–10. SEQUESTERED DISK.
A, T1 sagittal image, lumbar spine. There is a fragment of disk *(arrow)* posterior to the L4 vertebral body. There is a discrete line separating it from the L4–5 disk. Because this fragment has no attachment to a disk, it is a sequestered disk fragment. It may have originated from the L3–4 disk, which is narrowed and degenerated. *B,* Fast T2 sagittal image, lumbar spine. The sequestered fragment *(arrow)* is much higher signal than are any of the lumbar disks, because of inflammatory reaction in and around the fragment. *C,* T1 sagittal image, lumbar spine (different patient than in *A* and *B*). There is a large fragment of disk *(arrow)* in the posterior epidural space at the L4–5 level that is compressing the thecal sac. This was a sequestered fragment at surgery. An MRI done 2 weeks earlier showed a disk extrusion at L4–5, but no abnormality posteriorly. The MRI was repeated because of acute onset of severe back pain and radicular symptoms. Incidentally noted is Baastrup's disease involving the spinous processes (see text).

or paracentral regions. However, an extraforaminal (lateral) disk at L5–S1 could cause the same symptoms as a posterior L4–5 disk, because it would be impinging on the L5 nerve that already exited.

About 90% of all focal disk abnormalities in the lumbar spine occur at L4–5 or L5–S1. Most focal degenerative disk abnormalities occur at C5–6 and C6–7 in the cervical spine, and very few focal disk abnormalities occur scattered throughout the thoracic spine. It is helpful to describe which nerve(s) is affected by a disk abnormality. Therefore, it is important to remember that cervical nerves exit above the level of their respective disk level until C8, and then the nerves exit below. For example, a

right paracentral C4–5 disk extrusion will impinge upon the descending C6 nerve; similarly positioned right paracentral disk extrusions at T4–5 and L4–5 will nail the right descending T5 and L5 nerves. Intraforaminal extrusions at C4–5 will affect the exiting C5 nerve, whereas at T4–5 and L4–5 the exiting T4 and L4 nerves, respectively, will be impinged upon.

Significance of Disk Contour Abnormalities (Box

BOX 13–5: DISKS AT RISK

- Approximately one third of asymptomatic people have focal lumbar disk contour abnormalities on MRI.
- Only 1% of asymptomatic patients have a disk *extrusion* by MRI.
- About 90% of focal disk contour abnormalities occur at L4–5 and L5–S1 in the lumbar region, and at C5–6 and C6–7 in the cervical spine.
- Over 90% of focal disk contour abnormalities in the lumbar spine affect the central and paracentral regions.

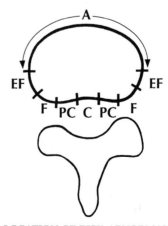

Figure 13–11. LOCATION OF DISK ABNORMALITIES.
Diagram depicting how to describe the location of disk abnormalities. Focal disk contour abnormalities may be central (C); left or right paracentral (PC); left or right foraminal (F); left or right extraforaminal (EF), which also may be called far lateral disk abnormalities; or anterior (A). Ninety percent of focal disk contour abnormalities affect the central and paracentral regions.

13–6). MRI is extremely sensitive in detecting abnormalities in the configuration of disks.[13–16] The problem is that many of these abnormalities do not cause symptoms, or at least not on the basis of nerve compression at that site.

Disk abnormalities are frequent in asymptomatic patients. Twenty percent of subjects younger than 60 years old and 36% of patients over 60 years old have one or more focal disk abnormalities of the lumbar spine, but no symptoms.[1] However, if the distinction is made between disk protrusions and extrusions, the findings are much more encouraging. Only 1% of asymptomatic patients have evidence of a disk extrusion by MRI.[6] Thus, extrusions are much more likely to be significant and cause symptoms.

Mechanical compression of a nerve by a focal disk abnormality certainly can cause symptoms of dysesthesias and muscle weakness, but not necessarily pain symptoms. One theory for back pain is that the body reacts to displaced nucleus pulposus material with a foreign body-type inflammatory reaction. High levels of phospholipase A2 enzyme have been found in degenerated disk material; this is also the active enzyme in snake venom and in the pannus of rheumatoid arthritis that generates inflammatory mediators such as prostaglandins, leukotrienes, and platelet activating factor. It is believed that a severe inflammatory reaction to displaced nuclear material may irritate surrounding nerves and produce pain and radicular symptoms, even in the absence of extension of disk into the spinal canal.[4, 17–19]

Disk-related Compressive Myelopathy/Epidural Hematoma. High signal intensity areas on T2W images can be seen within the spinal cord at the point of spinal stenosis secondary to a disk bulge or extrusion (Fig. 13–12). This may be from focal myelomalacia as the result of ischemia to the cord. These cord lesions may or may not disappear after decompressive surgery.[20]

Small spontaneous epidural hematomas may sometimes occur in association with disk herniations from tearing of the fragile epidural vessels. This may be impossible to distinguish from a sequestered or extruded disk located posterior to the vertebral body (Fig. 13–13).

Disk Mimickers (Box 13–7). Abnormalities and normal variants may mimic an extruded or seques-

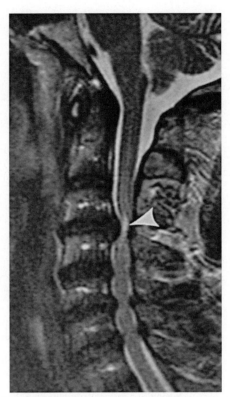

Figure 13–12. DISK-RELATED MYELOPATHY.
Fast T2 sagittal image, cervical spine. The C3–4 disk is protruding into the spinal canal and there is compression of the cord with high signal within it *(arrowhead)*. The cord abnormality is the result of cord ischemia with myelomalacia. The disks are protruding to a lesser extent at lower levels, causing multilevel canal stenosis.

tered disk on MRI: synovial cysts from the facet joints, conjoined nerve roots, arachnoid diverticulae, perineural cysts, and nerve sheath tumors arising from the nerve roots may cause confusion. We also have seen bullet fragments and cement from vertebroplasties (Fig. 13–14) within the spinal canal resembling the appearance of a sequestered disk, so keep your mind open to the possibilities.

The signal intensity of dilated nerve root sleeves (arachnoid diverticulae), which is identical to cerebral spinal fluid, should allow differentiation from a disk fragment. A conjoined nerve is two nerve roots exiting the thecal sac at the same location; the roots can be seen within the mass on T2W images, and the lateral recess on the side of the conjoined nerve root is enlarged, indicating that this is a long-standing process.[21]

Vacuum Disks and Vertebral Bodies. Aside from abnormalities in disk contour, another manifestation of disk degeneration occurs from dessication of the disk with the formation of cracks or clefts in the nuclear material, which may fill with nitrogen that comes out of solution from adjacent extracellular fluid. When this finding is present, it essentially excludes the possibility of superimposed infection or tumor involving the disk.[22] MRI shows the vacuum disk as a horizontally oriented linear-signal void on all pulse sequences (Fig. 13–15).

BOX 13–6: DISK AGING/ DEGENERATION: Possible Consequences

Neural compression
Chemical irritation of nerves
Osseous abnormalities
Segmental instability
Spinal stenosis
Pain

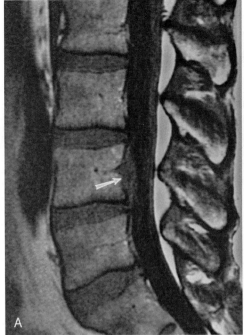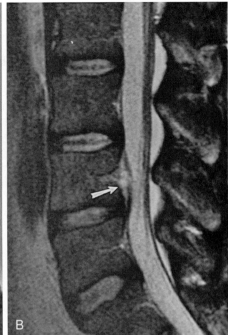

Figure 13–13. SPONTANEOUS EPIDURAL HEMATOMA.
A, T1 sagittal image, lumbar spine. There is an intermediate-signal mass with a convex posterior margin posterior to L3 *(arrow)* that causes narrowing of the thecal sac. *B,* Fast T2 sagittal image, lumbar spine. The mass becomes high signal *(arrow).* This is compatible with a spontaneous epidural hematoma. It also could be an extruded disk, but the symptoms resolved rapidly and there is no narrowing of the disks to indicate that a large amount of disk material has been extruded.

Cracks in the vertebral body endplates can allow nitrogen from the adjacent vacuum disk to seep into the vertebral body, forming an intraosseous vacuum cleft. This appearance has long been thought to be the result of osteonecrosis; in fact, in many cases it is simply a manifestation of degenerative disk disease and osteoporotic fractures combining to create this appearance.[23–25] The intraosseous vacuum has an appearance similar to the vacuum disk, with linear-signal void on all MRI pulse sequences if it is filled with gas, or intermediate signal on T1 and high signal on T2W images if it is filled with fluid (see below).

The presence of a vacuum cleft within a disk or vertebral body tends to occur with extension of the spine. The contents of the clefts may change when the patient is in a supine or flexed position. Within 1 hour of being placed supine in an MR unit, the nitrogen-filled clefts may be replaced with fluid that will be high signal intensity on T2W images (Figs. 13–15 and 13–16). These must not be confused with infection or other pathology.

Calcified Disks. Intervertebral disks are nourished by way of a vascular supply to the outermost fibers of the annulus fibrosus, but the bulk of the disk receives nourishment by diffusion through the adjacent endplates, which requires motion and stresses in order to occur.

Calcification of the disks may occur from degenerative changes and aging, limited motion of the spine (ankylosing spondylitis, diffuse idiopathic skeletal

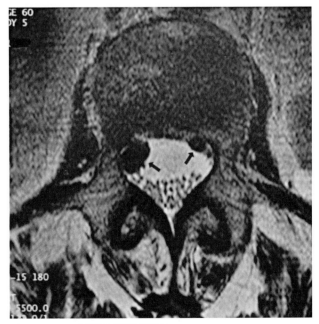

Figure 13–14. DISK MIMICKERS.
Fast T2 axial image, lumbar spine. There are rounded low-signal masses in both lateral recesses *(arrows)* in this patient with worsening radiculopathy. The signal is much lower than would be expected from sequestered disk fragments. This condition is caused by extruded cement from a vertebroplasty and is one of several entities that can mimic disk herniations.

BOX 13–7: MIMICKERS OF EXTRUDED/SEQUESTERED DISKS

—Synovial cyst
—Conjoined nerve root
—Arachnoid diverticulum
—Perineural (Tarlov) cyst
—Nerve sheath tumors
—Small epidural hematoma

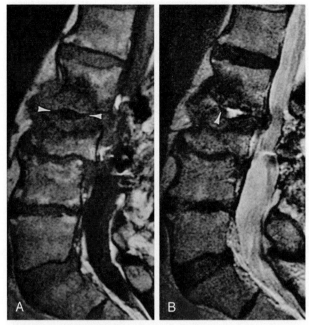

Figure 13–15. VACUUM DISK.
A, T1 sagittal image, lumbar spine. There is horizontal, very low signal in the L2–3 disk *(arrowheads)* compatible with nitrogen in a vacuum disk from degeneration. The adjacent vertebral bodies have large areas of low-signal marrow adjacent to the degenerated disk. *B,* Fast T2 sagittal image, lumbar spine. This sequence was obtained later than the T1 sequence. High-signal fluid is now filling most of the cleft in the disk. Low-signal nitrogen is still present anteriorly *(arrowhead)* in the nondependent portion of the disk. The marrow changes remain low signal, indicating discogenic sclerosis (type 3 marrow signal changes). This appearance could be confused with disk infection if careful analysis of the signal is not made.

hyperostosis, surgical fusion, old trauma, or infection), calcium pyrophosphate dihydrate crystal deposition disease, ochronosis, or hemochromatosis, among others.

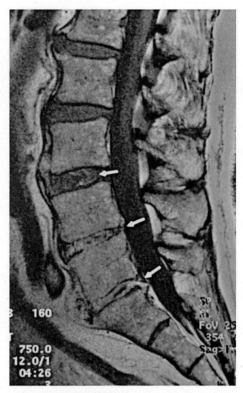

Figure 13–17. CALCIFIED DISKS.
T1 sagittal image, lumbar spine. The lower three lumbar disks have large areas of heterogeneous high signal *(arrows)*. This occurs when calcium is present in certain quantities.

MRI may show small amounts of calcium in the disks that are not evident by plain film or computed tomography (CT), which are high signal intensity on T1W images (Fig. 13–17).[26] The appearance on T2W images is variable. As more calcium is deposited in the disks, they show low signal intensity on T1W and T2W images (Fig. 13–16).

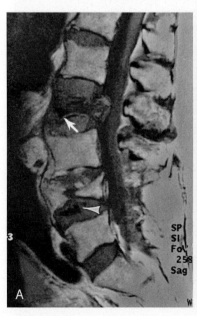
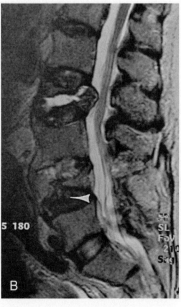

Figure 13–16. VACUUM VERTEBRAL BODY AND CALCIFIED DISK.
A, T1 sagittal image, lumbar spine. The L2 vertebral body is fractured with retropulsion into the spinal canal. The center of the vertebral body has intermediate signal, except anteriorly, where very low signal *(arrow)* caused by nitrogen in a vacuum vertebra is seen. There is also linear low signal in the L4–5 disk *(arrowhead)* from a calcified disk. The low signal is too thick and irregular to be from vacuum disk. *B,* Fast T2 sagittal image, lumbar spine. Most of the defect in the L2 vertebra has become high signal. Only a small area of low signal is present anteriorly from the small amount of nitrogen that remains. The low signal at L4–5 *(arrowhead)* persists from disk calcification.

Osseous Degenerative Changes
(Box 13–8)

Vertebral Bodies. The vertebral bodies respond to degenerative changes in the adjacent interverbral disks in two major ways: (1) formation of osteophytes, and (2) marrow changes paralleling the endplates.

Osteophytes are the all too familiar excrescences of bone that occur on the upper or lower margins of vertebral bodies. They occur as disks degenerate and bulge, placing traction stresses on Sharpey's fibers, which attach the disks to the vertebral bodies. Osteophytes usually are located anteriorly in the lumbar and thoracic spine, but are commonly anterior or posterior in the cervical spine.

In the cervical spine, disk abnormalities so commonly are accompanied by osteophytes that we refer to the combination of osteophytes and disk as diskoosteophytic material. Thus, diffuse disko-osteophytic bulging or focal disko-osteophytic protrusions are common in the cervical spine. MRI of most osteophytes shows low signal intensity cortical margins with fatty marrow centers that follow the signal of fat on all pulse sequences. In the cervical spine, osteophytes may be more diffusely sclerotic (mainly cortical rather than medullary bone) and sometimes difficult to distinguish from disk material. Cervical disks are relatively high signal intensity on gradient echo axial images, but the low signal outer fibers of the annulus and of the posterior longitudinal ligament may be difficult to distinguish from the cortical bone of osteophytes. This sometimes makes it difficult to determine if there is only a disk protruding into the canal, or if there is an osteophyte as well. On gradient echo axial sequences through the cervical spine, osteophytes are very low signal intensity. There may be blooming artifact from the sclerotic portions of the osteophytes that results in inaccurate overestimation of the size of osteophytes and their effect on the neural foramina or central canal. T1W images may be helpful in more accurately estimating stenosis and in determining what is osteophyte versus disk.

The *marrow* in vertebral bodies adjacent to degenerated disks may change in response to the disk disease. Parallel bands of abnormal signal in the end plates have been divided into two types by Modic et al.,[27] and a third type by others; these typically are called Modic type 1, 2, or 3 changes. These marrow changes may be focal or diffuse along the endplate, but tend to be linear and always parallel to the endplates.

Type 1 changes are the earliest marrow changes encountered. These consist of inflammatory and granulomatous tissue in the marrow that is low signal intensity on T1W images and becomes high signal intensity on T2W sequences (Fig. 13–18). This appearance may raise the question of spondylodiskitis, but disk infection demonstrates intradiskal high signal intensity on T2W images, whereas it would be unusual to have high signal intensity in

an uninfected, degenerated disk adjacent to these osseous changes, making the distinction relatively straightforward. Intact cortical endplates, lack of paraspinous inflammatory change, as well as preservation of the intranuclear cleft also allow the diagnosis of infection to be excluded with confidence.

Type 2 changes consist of signal intensity typical of fat on all pulse sequences, caused by focal fatty marrow conversion (Fig. 13–18). These findings are very common on spine MRI.

Type 3 endplate changes are the result of sclerosis and demonstrate low signal intensity on all pulse sequences (Fig. 13–15).

Facet Joints. The facet joints are formed by the inferior articular process of the vertebra above articulating with the superior articular process of the lower vertebra. The articular surfaces are covered with hyaline cartilage. The osseous structures are enveloped in a joint capsule lined by synovium; thus, these are true synovial joints. The anterior aspects of the facet joints and the laminae are covered by the ligamentum flavum.

These joints frequently undergo degenerative

BOX 13–8: OSSEOUS CHANGES RELATED TO DISK DEGENERATION

Vertebral Bodies
- Osteophytes
- Marrow changes (Modic)
  —Focal or diffuse bands parallel to endplates

  Type 1: ↓ signal T1, ↑ signal T2 (inflammatory tissue)

  Type 2: ↑ signal T1, follows fat on T2 (focal conversion to fat)

  Type 3: ↓ signal T1 and T2 (sclerosis)

Facet Joints
- Degenerative joint disease (DJD)
  —Cartilage loss, subchondral sclerosis, or cysts
  —Osteophytes with overgrowth of articular processes
  —Synovial cysts
  —Buckling of ligamentum flavum into canal
  —Marrow changes in adjacent pedicles

Posterior Spinous Processes (Baastrup disease)
- Associated with lordosis, facet DJD, disk degeneration
- Breakdown of interspinous ligaments
  —Bursae form between spinous processes (high signal on T2)
  — ↓ Space between spinous processes
- Spinous processes in contact
  —Subcortical sclerosis, cysts
  —Faceted appearance
  —Osteophytes, enthesophytes

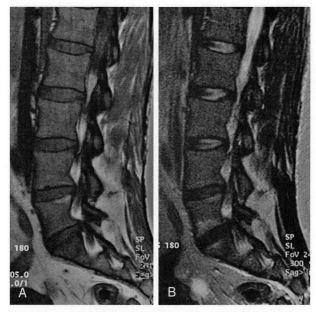

Figure 13–18. OSSEOUS DEGENERATIVE CHANGES (TYPE 1 AND 2 CHANGES).
A, T1 sagittal image, lumbar spine. Linear high-signal fat parallels the inferior endplate of L4 and superior endplate of L5 from type 2 marrow signal changes associated with adjacent degenerative disk disease. *B,* Fast T2 sagittal image, lumbar spine. High-signal fat in the L4 and L5 endplates is still evident because fat is not suppressed on fast T2 sequences. There is also linear high-signal paralleling the inferior endplate of L5 and superior endplate of S1 that was not evident on the T1 sequence, compatible with type 1 marrow signal changes from the degenerative disk disease.

changes, especially in the middle and lower cervical spine and the lower lumbar spine and lumbosacral junction. Degenerative changes of the facet joints manifest as cartilage fibrillation with joint space narrowing, subchondral sclerosis, subchondral cysts, and osteophyte formation that result in overgrowth or hypertrophy of the osseous portions of the joints. Changes in the marrow of pedicles adjacent to facet degenerative joint disease may occur, similar to that seen in vertebral body endplates adjacent to degenerative disk disease, as a result of increased stresses. Synovial cysts may develop from degenerated spinal facet joints and project either anteriorly (through the ligamentum flavum) or posteriorly from the joints. Loss of cartilage from degenerative changes in the facet joints in concert with loss of disk height from degenerative disk disease leads to inward buckling of the ligamentum flavum, which in turn causes narrowing of the neural foramen or central canal.

Symptoms from degenerative changes of the facet joints may be the result of compression of adjacent neural structures (spinal stenosis) by overgrowth of the bone, inward buckling of the ligamentum flavum, protrusion of synovial cysts into the spinal canal, or from the joints themselves being painful. Degenerated facet joints can cause local pain at the facet joints, but also frequently are responsible for referred pain patterns to the shoulders or interscap-

ular regions from cervical disease, or to the buttocks, thighs, and hips from lumbar facet syndromes.[28, 29] As always, the presence of abnormalities on MRI examination does not indicate which, if any, of these joints is responsible for pain in a given patient. Additional work-up with injection of anesthetic into facet joints is the only way to document if a facet joint is responsible for some or all of the symptoms.

MRI of degenerative facet joint disease (Fig. 13–19) is typical of degenerative changes in any joint (subchondral sclerosis is low signal intensity on all pulse sequences, cysts are low signal intensity on T1W and high signal on T2W images). There often are increased amounts of fluid in the joints, seen as high signal on T2W images. The osteophytes and hypertrophic osseous changes create a rounded and enlarged (portobello mushroom) appearance of the articular processes of the facets on axial images that may affect the appearance of the adjacent spinal canal, lateral recesses, or neural foramina. Signal intensity changes (Modic changes) in the pedicles adjacent to facet joint degeneration may be seen (Fig. 13–19), and sometimes are easier to identify than the degenerative changes themselves. These can be Modic type 1, 2, or 3 signal changes, but are most commonly type 2 (fat signal).

Synovial cysts are rounded masses of varying size and sometimes variable signal intensity (Fig. 13–20). They are generally low signal intensity on T1W images, but because of hemorrhage into the cyst or high protein content, they occasionally may be relatively high signal intensity on T1W images. T2W images generally demonstrate high signal intensity, or mixed signal intensity relating to the presence of calcifications (in up to 30%) and vacuum phenomenon. Contrast-enhanced images show peripheral enhancement with an appearance similar to a sequestered disk. Most sequestered disk fragments are not located posteriorly in the spinal canal or are not diffusely high signal intensity on T2W images, whereas a synovial cyst is. A synovial cyst always lies immediately adjacent to the facet joint, but a communication is not demonstrated on MRI. Differentiation of a synovial cyst from a sequestered disk fragment can be made with certainty by injecting contrast material into the facet joint and demonstrating filling of the cyst under fluoroscopy.

Posterior Spinous Processes. Degenerative changes of the spinous processes and intervening interspinous soft tissues (kissing spine or Baastrup disease) may occur as the result of hyperlordosis in the cervical or lumbar spine or from associated degenerative disk or facet joint disease, which places increased stresses on these posterior structures.[30]

Close apposition of adjacent spinous processes causes laxity of the overlying supraspinous ligament and damage to the intervening interspinous ligaments. The interspinous ligament becomes fibrillated and torn, producing spaces in the ligament that may lead to formation of bursae or, eventually, true synovial joints between spinous processes.

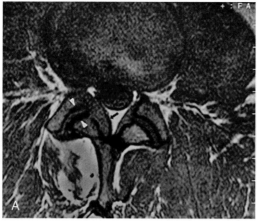

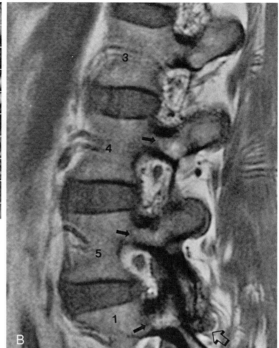

Figure 13–19. DEGENERATIVE FACET JOINT DISEASE.

A, T1 axial image, lumbar spine. The right facet joint shows mild hypertrophic changes of the bones from osteophyte formation, subchondral sclerosis *(arrowheads),* and ligamentum flavum thickening *(arrow),* all of which are very different in appearance than on the normal left side. *B,* T1 sagittal image, lumbar spine. Severe degenerative disease of the L5–S1 facet is seen *(open arrow)* with hypertrophic changes, a large inferior recess, and inward buckling of the ligamentum flavum into the neural foramen. Marrow signal intensity changes are evident in the pedicles, which are associated with adjacent degenerative facet joint disease. High-signal fat (type 2 changes) is seen in the pedicles of L4, L5, and S1 *(arrows).* The L3 pedicle has normal signal that matches the signal in the adjacent vertebral body.

Breakdown of the interspinous ligaments causes excessive motion and leads to instability with direct contact between spinous processes that may result in eburnation of the bone, a faceted appearance, osteophytes, or degenerative enthesophytes. These changes sometimes cause symptoms of pain.

The main appearance to be aware of on MRI is the high signal intensity bursal fluid collections between spinous processes on T2W images (Fig. 13–21). Also, the lack of space between adjacent spinous processes, flattening of the superior or inferior surfaces (faceted appearance), and low signal intensity eburnation (sclerosis) on all pulse sequences are identified. There are sometimes degenerative cysts noted in the spinous processes where they chronically abut, which have low signal intensity on T1W images that becomes hyperintense on T2W images.

Spinal Stenosis (Box 13–9)

Spinal stenosis is narrowing of the central spinal canal, neural foramen, lateral recess, or any combination of these anatomic regions, by soft tissue or osseous structures that impinge on neural elements and may result in symptoms.

The standard classification for spinal stenosis is based on cause and includes congenital (eg, short pedicle syndrome, achondroplasia) or acquired (usually degenerative) causes. Even if there are congenital abnormalities of the spine that narrow the canal, patients rarely have symptoms of spinal ste-

nosis unless they have superimposed degenerative changes (acquired stenosis). Among some miscellaneous causes of spinal stenosis are spondylolysis (pars defect) with spondylolisthesis (anterior or posterior subluxation), ossification of the posterior longitudinal ligament, epidural lipomatosis, or osseous abnormalities such as fracture or Paget's disease, among many others.

Symptoms from multilevel spinal stenosis are often nonspecific and include back pain, intermittent neurogenic claudication, extremity radiculopathy, pain with hyperextension relieved by flexion, and pain on standing relieved by lying down. The presence of imaging findings of spinal stenosis does not indicate that a patient necessarily has symptoms from the stenosis. Just as arteriosclerotic calcification of the coronary arteries on a chest CT does not confirm that the patient's chest pain is from angina, abnormalities of the spine by imaging do not indicate the patient must have symptoms relating to the abnormalities. Clinical examination and other tests must be correlated with MRI studies in the spine (and elsewhere) in order to avoid errors in managing patients.

Spinal stenosis may occur at one or more levels in the spine and almost always is the result of several degenerative processes occurring in concert. When disks degenerate and lose height, and the articular cartilage in the facet joints is lost, there may be motion of one vertebral segment relative to the adjacent one; this motion causes degenerative spondylolisthesis, which results in spinal stenosis. As the

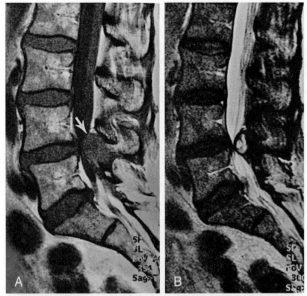

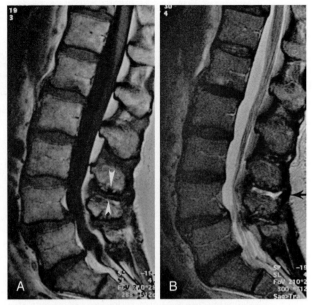

Figure 13–21. BAASTRUP DISEASE (KISSING SPINE).
A, T1 sagittal image, lumbar spine. The spinous processes of L3 and L4 are closer together than at the other levels. There is sclerosis in the bones *(arrowheads)* where they abut one another, and the bones are angled and faceted from chronic wear against each other. *B,* Fast T2 sagittal image, lumbar spine. There is high signal between the L3 and L4 spinous processes from breakdown of the interspinous ligament and formation of a bursa *(arrow).*

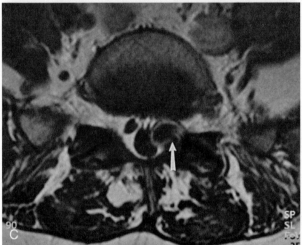

Figure 13–20. SYNOVIAL CYST FROM DEGENERATIVE FACET JOINT DISEASE.
A, T1 sagittal image, lumbar spine. There is an intermediate-signal mass *(arrow)* in the posterior epidural space compressing the thecal sac at the L4–5 level. *B,* Fast T2 sagittal image, lumbar spine. The mass becomes mainly high signal with a low-signal rim. *C,* T1 contrast-enhanced axial image, lumbar spine. There is peripheral rim enhancement of the left-sided mass *(arrow).* It is immediately adjacent to the degenerated left facet joint, but a communication cannot be seen. The thecal sac and nerve are displaced.

spine loses height from these same degenerative changes, the ligamentum flavum buckles inward toward the canal and neural foramina, also resulting in spinal stenosis. Other degenerative changes that lead to spinal stenosis include diffuse or focal abnormalities in disk contour, vertebral body osteophytes, facet joint osteophytes (hypertrophy), and facet joint synovial cysts.

Central Canal Stenosis. This usually is the result of facet joint osteophytes and inward buckling of the ligamentum flavum posteriorly, with disk bulging anteriorly in the canal. Vertebral body osteophytes (especially in the cervical spine) also may contribute to central canal stenosis, as can postoperative

---

BOX 13–9: SPINAL STENOSIS

Sites of Involvement
• Central canal
• Neural foramina
• Lateral recesses
Causes
• Degenerative
—Disk contour abnormalities (bulges, herniations)
—Vertebral body osteophytes
—Degenerative spondylolisthesis
—Facet joint degeneration, osteophytes, synovial cysts
—Ligamentum flavum buckling
• Congenital short pedicles
—Usually requires superimposed degeneration to be symptomatic
• Any mass arising from bone, disk, or within canal
—Osseous tumor, fracture fragments
—Spondylolysis, spondylolisthesis
—Ossification of posterior longitudinal ligament
—Epidural lipomatosis, hematoma, abscess, tumor, scarring
Complications
• Pain symptoms
• Cord myelomalacia from ischemia
• Nerve root edema

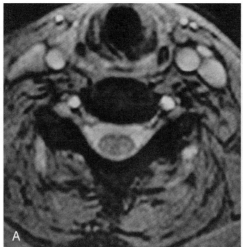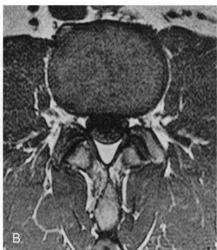

Figure 13–22. NORMAL CENTRAL SPINAL CANAL.
A, T2* axial image, cervical spine. The central canal is normal, with the high-signal thecal sac having a rounded, plump oval configuration. *B,* T1 axial image, lumbar spine. The central canal is normal at this level, with the low-signal thecal sac again having the appearance of a rounded, plump oval.

scarring. We do not use measurements to determine if there is central stenosis, but use the shape of the canal and thecal sac instead. Normally, the central canal and thecal sac are round or nearly round (a plump oval) structures on axial images (Fig. 13–22); if they become flattened ovals or triangular in shape, it indicates central stenosis (Fig. 13–23 through 13–25). Quantitating the degree of stenosis as to mild, moderate, or severe is part of our dictated report, but there is no universally agreed-upon objective definitions for these terms.

Severe central stenosis can cause edema in the

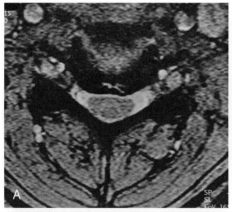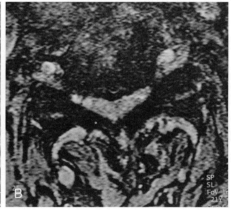

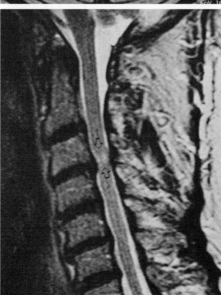

Figure 13–23. CENTRAL CANAL STENOSIS: Cervical (Acquired).
A, T2* axial image, cervical spine. There is diffuse disko-osteophytic bulging into the central canal, causing the thecal sac to lose its rounded appearance. This is mild in extent because there is still cerebrospinal fluid (CSF) present between the osteophyte and the cord. The neural foramina are normal and unaffected by the degenerative process. *B,* T2* axial image, cervical spine (same patient as in *A* but different level). The central canal is markedly narrowed with essentially no CSF seen, and the cord is flattened by the diffuse disko-osteophytic bulge. Both neural foramina are narrowed from osteophytes, worse on the right than on the left side. **C,** Fast T2 sagittal image, cervical spine (different patient than in *A* and *B).* There is focal high signal in the cord *(open arrows)* at the level of the bulging disk/osteophytes from myelomalacia.

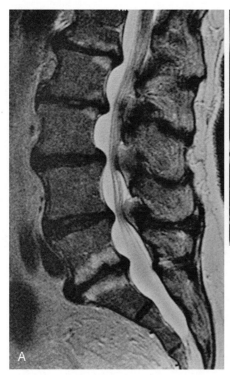

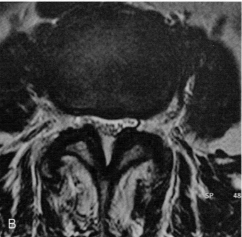

Figure 13–24. CENTRAL CANAL STENOSIS: Lumbar (Acquired). *A,* Fast T2 sagittal image, lumbar spine. Disks and ligamentum flavum protrude into the spinal canal, causing multilevel canal stenosis with narrowing of the thecal sac at the disk levels. *B,* Fast T2 axial image, lumbar spine. The central canal is markedly narrowed and has a triangular shape, rather than the normal plump oval. The central stenosis is from a diffusely bulging disk in concert with bilateral facet degenerative joint disease.

affected nerve roots or, in the cervical spine, there may be abnormalities of the cord, probably myelomalacia from ischemia at the site of stenosis which is high signal intensity on T2W images (Fig. 13–23).

Lateral Recess Stenosis. This usually is caused by hypertrophic degenerative changes of the facet joints, or less commonly by a disk fragment postoperative fibrosis. Remember that lateral recesses are located on the medial aspects of pedicles. Nerve roots lie in these recesses after leaving the thecal sac, but before entering the exiting neural foramina. There is a neural foramen bordering both the upper and lower margins of a lateral recess. Measurements are not used to determine if this recess is stenotic. If there is deformity in the shape of the recess and the descending nerve is displaced or compressed, there is lateral recess stenosis (Fig. 13–26). This space is best evaluated in the axial plane of imaging.

Neural Foramen Stenosis. This occurs from degenerative osteophytes of the facet joints or of the unconvertebral joints in the cervical spine; inward buckling of the ligamentum flavum (which forms the posterior aspect of the foramina); a foraminal disk protrusion, extrusion, or sequestered fragment;

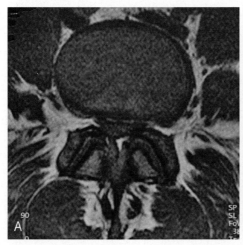

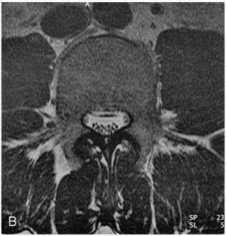

Figure 13–25. CENTRAL CANAL STENOSIS: Lumbar (Congenital With Superimposed Acquired).
A, T1 axial image, lumbar spine. There are mild hypertrophic changes of the left facet joint from degenerative disease, and a very mild diffuse disk bulge. The central canal is severely narrowed, with a flattened thecal sac and triangular shape of the canal. *B,* Fast T2 axial image, lumbar spine (same patient as in *A).* An image obtained through the pedicles shows that the pedicles are congenitally short and the central canal is small at this level (a flattened oval rather than a plump oval), even without the presence of superimposed degenerative changes.

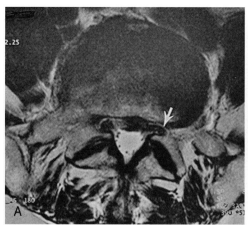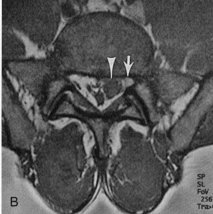

Figure 13–26. LATERAL RECESS STENOSIS.
A, Fast T2 axial image, lumbar spine. Both lateral recesses are narrowed as the result of osteophytes from facet degenerative joint disease. The left side is more severe than the right *(arrow),* and the nerve that runs in the lateral recess is compressed between osteophyte and the vertebral body. *B,* T1 axial image, lumbar spine (different patient than in *A*). There is a large, extruded disk fragment *(arrowhead)* narrowing the left lateral recess *(arrow)* and compressing the nerve in it.

a diffuse disk bulge; or postoperative fibrosis. Narrowing of the neural foramina can be evaluated on both sagittal and axial images. On sagittal images, the normal neural foramen has the appearance of a vertical oval. If disk material extends into the foramen, the oval narrows inferiorly, creating a keyhole shape (Fig. 13–27). Axial images may be more accurate for diagnosis, because they show more of the extent of each foramen (Figs. 13–28 and 13–29).

Something that really impinges on our nerves is the concept we repeatedly hear from our residents that the nerve must be unaffected by a disk abnormality if they see the nerve surrounded by fat in the superior aspect of the neural foramen on sagittal images. They see a big disk abnormality in the lower neural foramen and say, "but the nerve got out." This thinking is inaccurate and certainly not based on anatomic fact. What we see in the superior portion of the neural foramen is the large dorsal root ganglion and ventral root cut in cross section. As the nerve progresses laterally and inferiorly in the neural foramen, it divides into approximately 15 fascicles, which compose the short segment spinal nerve. The fascicles, which cannot be seen well on MRI, regroup to form the dorsal and ventral rami. The dorsal and ventral nerve roots, the spinal nerve, and the dorsal and ventral rami run obliquely through the neural foramen in a superior to inferior and medial to lateral direction; this can be appreciated on coronal MR images through the neural foramen (Fig. 13–30). Disk or other material that narrows the mid or inferior portion of the neural foramen may compress or irritate the spinal nerve or dorsal and ventral rami, whereas the dorsal root ganglion looks pristine and unaffected, surrounded by fat in the superior portion of the foramen. In addition, any mass projecting lateral to the foramen may impinge on the nerve that exited through the foramen at one level above and cause nerve symp-

toms. The point is that anything narrowing *any* portion of the neural foramen may affect a nerve, because there is nerve passing through all levels of the foramen and just outside the foramen—we just happen to see the nerve best in the superior and medial aspect of the foramen because we are looking at the large dorsal root ganglion.

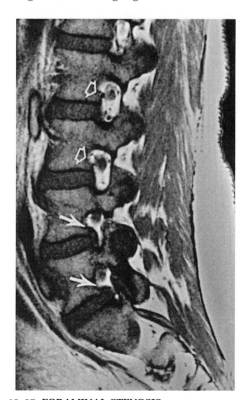

Figure 13–27. FORAMINAL STENOSIS.
Normal neural foramina on sagittal images should have a vertical oval appearance *(open arrows).* Stenosis from disk abnormalities creates narrowing of the lower portion of the foramen so that it has a keyhole appearance *(solid arrows).* The dorsal root ganglion is evident in the superior portion of the lumbar foramina.

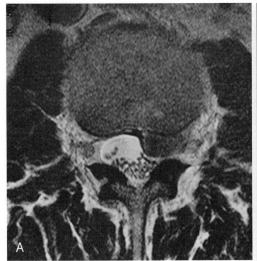

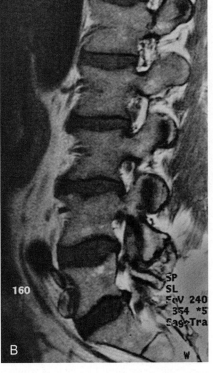

Figure 13–28. FORAMINAL STENOSIS: Lumbar.
A, Fast T2 axial image, lumbar spine. There is a large L3–4 intraforaminal disk extrusion that essentially obliterates the left neural foramen. *B,* T1 sagittal image, lumbar spine. The disk extrusion seen on axial images was not evident on any of the sagittal images. It is essential to use both axial and sagittal images to evaluate the neural foramina and extraforaminal regions because they are sometimes complementary to one another.

Postoperative Changes

Uncomplicated Postoperative MRI
(Box 13–10)

Many changes occur in both the osseous and soft tissues of the spine after surgery. It is important to know their MRI appearance, in order not to confuse normal postoperative changes with pathology that requires treatment.

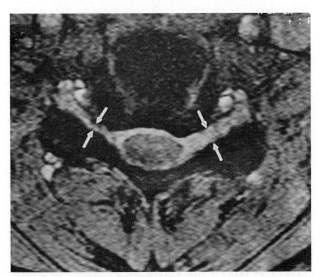

Figure 13–29. FORAMINAL STENOSIS: Cervical.
T2* axial image, cervical spine. There is moderate narrowing of the right neural foramen as compared to the normal left foramen *(arrows)*. The stenosis of the right foramen is from osteophytes arising from the uncovertebral joint.

Osseous abnormalities include removal of portions of the spine (lamina, facets) or additions of bone graft or hardware to the spine. Dura and cerebrospinal fluid sometimes may protrude through a laminar defect and result in a postoperative meningocele (Fig. 13–31). Distinguishing a meningocele from a pseudomeningocele (a defect in the dura with leak of spinal fluid) is not generally possible on MRI.

Marrow in the vertebral bodies adjacent to an operated disk generally remains normal after surgery (or maintains the same disk-related Modic marrow abnormalities that were present before surgery) and does not enhance with contrast (although Modic 1 changes will enhance).

Epidural scarring after osseous decompression or disk surgery is extremely common and occurs to varying extent in different individuals. Fibrosis is shown to best advantage after injection of intravenous gadolinium. The degree of contrast enhancement is greatest during the first year after surgery, but contrast enhancement may persist for years. The fibrosis or scarring in the anterior epidural space where surgery was performed is often an irregular epidural mass that mimics a persistent or recurrent disk (Fig. 13–32).[31–33] The mass effect from scarring at the operated disk level may take months to resolve and may never resolve completely. During the first 6 months after surgery, there may be peripheral contrast enhancement of the mass of granulation tissue and fibrosis, making it impossible to distinguish scarring from extruded disk in the early postoperative period.

Enhancement of intrathecal *nerve roots* after con-

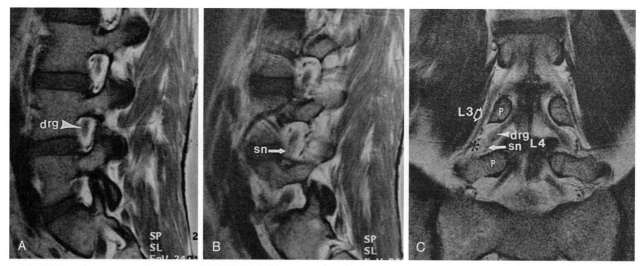

Figure 13–30. NEURAL FORAMEN ANATOMY: How the Nerve Really Gets Out.
A, T1 sagittal image, lumbar spine. The oval neural foramina are seen with the dorsal root ganglia (drg; *arrowhead*) cut in cross section in the superior foramina. *B,* T1 sagittal image, lumbar spine. This is one cut more lateral than that in *A*. The lateral aspect of the neural foramen is imaged and the striated fascicles of the spinal nerve (sn; *arrow*) are evident in the inferior aspect of the foramen at the level of the disk. Thus, if the dorsal root ganglion is surrounded by fat, but there is a disk protruding into the inferior foramen, the nerve did not "get out"—the dorsal root ganglion got out, but the spinal nerve or dorsal and ventral rami did not. There *is* nerve traversing the lower foramen at the level of the disk. *C,* T1 coronal image, lumbar spine. The neural foramen is shown between the pedicles (p). The nerve runs through it obliquely from superomedial to inferolateral. The dorsal root ganglion (drg; *arrowhead*) is located in the superomedial foramen, whereas the spinal nerve (sn; *arrow*) is located in the inferior and lateral portion of the foramen. The L3 nerve *(open arrow)* is seen coming from above, and it is obvious why a far lateral disk in the location marked by the asterisk (*) could affect the L3 or L4 nerves.

trast administration is common during the first 6 months after surgery, but should not persist after that (Fig. 13–33).[31–33]

Postoperative changes in *disks* often are seen after intravenous gadolinium is given and may persist for years (Fig. 13–34). Most patients have enhancement of the posterior annulus at the operative site from curettage, whereas only a few have enhancement within the center of the disk. This has the appearance of high signal intensity on T2W and contrast-enhanced T1W images. This should not be confused with a disk infection, because the adjacent vertebral bodies should maintain a normal appearance postoperatively.

Failed Back Surgery

Patients may have persistent, recurrent, or new and different symptoms after surgery of the spine.

BOX 13–10: POSTOPERATIVE CHANGES: Uncomplicated

Vertebral Marrow
• Unchanged from before surgery; no enhancement (unless Modic 1 changes are present)
Nerve roots
• May enhance for 6 months
Disks
• Contrast enhancement of posterior annulus, and ↑ signal on T2 for years
Epidural
• Scarring/fibrosis common
• Contrast enhancement of fibrosis for years
• Fibrosis is often nodular, resembling persistent or recurrent disk extrusion
 —Peripheral enhancement may mimic disk extrusion in first 6 months
 —Diffuse enhancement is typical after 6 months, allowing differentiation from disk (peripheral enhancement only)

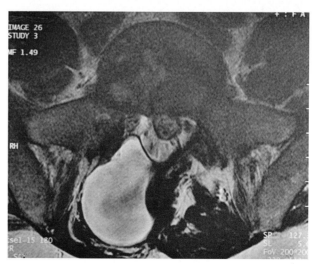

Figure 13–31. POSTOPERATIVE CHANGES: Meningocele.
Fast T2 axial image, L5. There are postoperative changes of a right laminectomy, through which a large, high-signal mass protrudes into the posterior soft tissues.

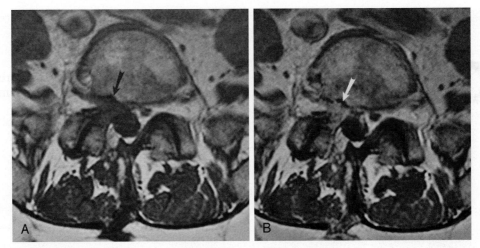

Figure 13–32. POSTOPERATIVE CHANGES: Scarring/Fibrosis (Versus Disk).
A, T1 axial image, L5. There is an intermediate signal mass *(arrow)* in the right paracentral region of this patient with a right laminectomy. The descending right L5 nerve is not seen. This could be a disk fragment or scarring. *B,* T1 contrast-enhanced axial image (same level as in *A*). There is diffuse enhancement of the right paracentral mass, indicating this is from scarring/fibrosis, rather than from a disk fragment.

The reasons for these problems are many and varied. The most common reasons are recurrent or persistent disk extrusions, postoperative scarring, nerve root damage (neuritis), and inadequate surgery (missed free fragments, inadequate decompression of spinal stenosis, wrong level treated, or what was treated was not the pain source). Spondylodiskitis and epidural abscess, epidural hematoma (Fig. 13–35), failure of fusion of bone graft material, arachnoiditis, and a defect in the dural sac that creates a pseudomeningocele all may occur as complications of spinal surgery.

Distinguishing postoperative scarring (epidural fibrosis) from extruded disk material is one of the most important tasks for radiologists in evaluating postoperative MRIs. All postoperative spine MRIs are done with contrast enhancement in order to distinguish between these two common causes of symptoms in postoperative patients.[34] Scar tissue that is over 6 months old enhances diffusely and early after the intravenous administration of gadolinium (high signal intensity on T1W images) (Fig. 13–32). Disk material does not enhance until late, if at all, and usually only enhances peripherally (Fig. 13–36). These rules are great, except they do not work as well during the first 6 months after surgery,

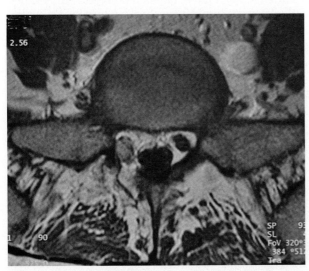

Figure 13–33. POSTOPERATIVE CHANGES: Nerve Root Enhancement.
T1 contrast-enhanced axial image, L5. The right lamina is surgically absent. The right descending L5 nerve is enlarged and high signal compared to the normal left nerve. This is expected during the first 6 months after surgery.

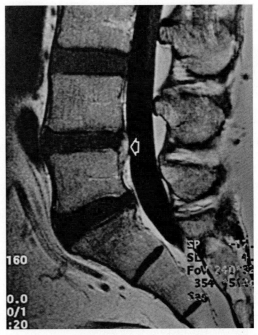

Figure 13–34. POSTOPERATIVE CHANGES: Disk Enhancement.
T1 contrast-enhanced sagittal image, lumbar spine. The posterior annulus of the L4–5 disk shows focal enhancement *(open arrow)* from previous surgery with curettage. This finding may last indefinitely after surgery.

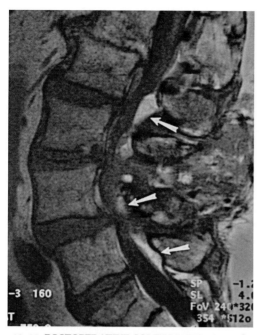

Figure 13–35. POSTOPERATIVE COMPLICATIONS: Epidural Hematoma.
T1 sagittal image, lumbar spine. There was posterior decompression surgery at the L4 level. While still hospitalized, the patient developed pain and weakness. The MRI shows a heterogeneous hematoma posteriorly at the level of the L4 spinous process. In addition, there are irregular high- and intermediate-signal masses in the posterior epidural space *(arrows),* representing a subacute hematoma that is compressing the dural sac and cauda equina.

when asymptomatic fibrosis may show peripheral rather than diffuse contrast enhancement that is indistinguishable from an extruded disk. MRI has more value in differentiating scar from disk material after the first 6 months postoperatively. Extruded disk material may be an indication for another operation, whereas there is no benefit from reoperating on a patient with epidural fibrosis.

> ### BOX 13–11: SPONDYLODISKITIS
>
> Classic MRI Triad
> • T1: low signal vertebral body marrow
> • T1, postcontrast: marrow enhancement (and possibly disk)
> • T2: high signal in disk (and possibly marrow)
> Associated Abnormalities
> • ↓ Disk height
> • Destruction of endplate
> • Phlegmon or abscess
>   —Epidural, subligamentous, paraspinous

Other signs that may help distinguish epidural fibrosis from a disk abnormality are that epidural fibrosis often has irregular margins, may not be contiguous with the adjacent disk and, instead of producing a mass effect on the dural sac, it may cause retraction. Recurrent disk herniations, conversely, usually are contiguous with the disk, have sharp margins, and cause mass effect on the dural sac.

Inflammatory Changes

Spondylodiskitis (Box 13–11)

Infection of the spine generally occurs from hematogenous spread of *Staphylococcus aureus* from a distant site. In adults, the marrow in the region of a vertebral body endplate usually is affected first (osteomyelitis or spondylitis), and the infection rapidly spreads to the adjacent disk (diskitis) and to the closest adjacent vertebral body. When both the bone and disk are infected, it is referred to as spondylodiskitis. Unlike adults, children have disks with

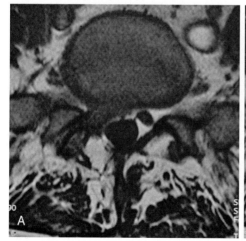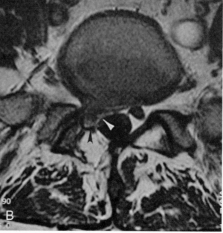

Figure 13–36. POSTOPERATIVE COMPLICATIONS: Recurrent Disk (Versus Scarring).
A, T1 axial image, L5–S1 disk. A right laminectomy has been performed. The patient has recurrent symptoms, and the MR shows intermediate signal in the right paracentral region that could be either scarring or a recurrent disk extrusion. The descending S1 nerve root is not identified. *B,* T1 contrast-enhanced axial image, L5–S1. There is a thin peripheral rim of enhancement *(arrowheads)* around the mass, typical of a disk, rather than scarring, which would have diffuse enhancement.

significant vascularity, so the initial infection may occur in the disk and then spread secondarily to the adjacent bone.

The MRI appearance depends on the extent of disease and the body's response to it at the time of imaging. Patients usually do not present for imaging until the infection has spread across a disk and involves at least two adjacent vertebral bodies. The MRI findings consist of a triad of (1) low signal intensity on T1W images in vertebral body marrow; (2) contrast enhancement of marrow on T1W images, and possibly of the disk if an abscess has not formed; and (3) high signal intensity of the disk on T2W images (Fig. 13–37).[35] High signal intensity in marrow on T2W images is sometimes present, but if reactive changes or sclerosis in the bone exist, the marrow may be low signal intensity on T2W images. Associated abnormalities that may be detected with spondylodiskitis include decreased disk height; destruction of the low signal intensity cortical endplate; and subligamentous, epidural, or paraspinous inflammatory phlegmon or abscess. MRI of soft tissue inflammatory/hyperemic phlegmonous response shows soft tissue swelling or a mass in the epidural or paraspinous regions that is high signal on T2W images or enhances diffusely with contrast on T1W images. If an abscess has formed, the soft tissue mass is low signal intensity on T1W images,

high signal intensity on T2W images, and shows peripheral rim enhancement on contrast-enhanced T1W images. Contrast administration is mandatory for complete evaluation of a spine with a suspected infection.

Granulomatous infections such as tuberculosis or fungal infections may be more clinically indolent than pyogenic infections. There is almost always bone destruction evident at the time of imaging, rather than just marrow edema. The disks may be spared, or nearly so, as the infection spreads beneath the anterior or posterior longitudinal ligaments of the spine to adjacent vertebrae.[36] The posterior elements often are involved, and epidural and paraspinous abscesses are common and large at the time of presentation.

Epidural Abscess

Direct extension of infection from spondylodiskitis can cause an epidural abscess, as described earlier. Other times, there is hematogenous seeding of the epidural space from infection at a remote site, or direct implantation of bacteria from instrumentation may occur (Fig. 13–38). Spondylodiskitis is present in 80% of patients with an epidural abscess at the time of imaging.[37] Two stages may be evident: the phlegmon (diffuse soft tissue inflammation),

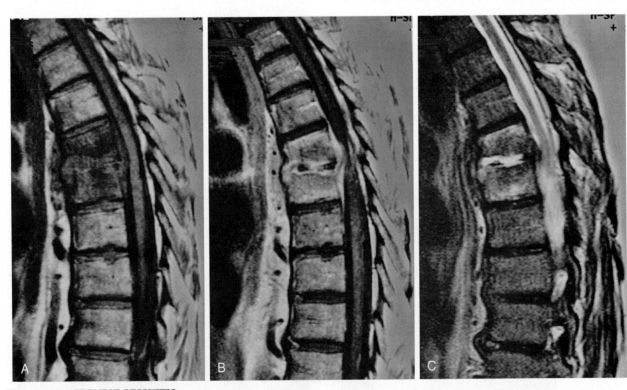

Figure 13–37. SPONDYLODISKITIS.
A, T1 sagittal image, thoracic spine. There is abnormal low signal in two adjacent vertebral bodies. The endplates show destruction. There are soft tissue masses extending both anterior and posterior to the vertebral bodies. The posterior mass is displacing the cord. *B*, T1 contrast-enhanced sagittal image, thoracic spine. The marrow shows contrast enhancement, as does the mass in the anterior epidural space and the mass anterior to the spine. The diffuse enhancement of the soft tissue masses indicates that these are phlegmonous masses rather than abscesses. The disk demonstrates rim enhancement only, which means there is an abscess in the disk. *C*, T2 sagittal image, thoracic spine. The vertebral bodies show heterogeneous high signal. The soft tissue phlegmon is difficult to see compared to the contrast-enhanced images. The pus in the disk is diffusely high signal.

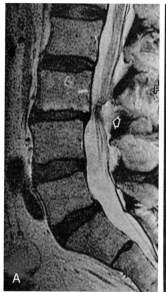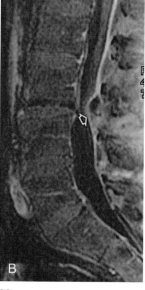

Figure 13–38. EPIDURAL ABSCESS.
A, Fast T2 sagittal image, lumbar spine. Fever and neurologic symptoms occurred in this person after instrumentation for placement of an epidural catheter. There is a high-signal mass *(open arrow)* displacing the dura and cauda equina anteriorly. **B,** T1 sagittal image with fat suppression and contrast-enhancement, lumbar spine. There is peripheral rim enhancement *(open arrow)* of the mass, which indicates it is cystic (abscess).

which progresses to an abscess (focal fluid collection), with MRI features as described above.

Arachnoiditis

This is an inflammatory process that may occur after surgery from agents being injected into the subarachnoid space (anesthetics, contrast material, steroids), from infection, or from intrathecal hemorrhage. An inflammatory response occurs and adhesions form; fibrous inflammatory masses also may occasionally be evident. On MRI, the findings are best demonstrated on T2W images (Figs. 13–39 through 13–41). The nerve roots may be clumped instead of evenly distributed through the thecal sac. Nerves may adhere to the dura so that there is the appearance of an empty thecal sac without nerve roots present. On sagittal images, the nerves of the cauda equina may have an irregular, angled, or wavy appearance, rather than the normal gentle curve as they descend. Contrast administration serves no useful purpose for making this diagnosis.[38]

Ankylosing Spondylitis

Many different arthritides may affect the spine, but ankylosing spondylitis involves the spine by definition. Occasionally, young patients with back pain are sent for MRI and we are able to make the first diagnosis of their ankylosing spondylitis by MRI. Although we do not believe MRI is routinely necessary to diagnose early ankylosing spondylitis, there are certainly occasions where the sequence of events creates such a situation, and it is necessary to know the MRI changes in the spine.

The classic changes of ankylosing spondylitis involve the sacroiliac joints and spine, usually becoming clinically manifest in the late teens or early 20s. The earliest changes are sacroiliitis with microerosions of the cartilage and subchondral bone and associated marrow edema. The changes in the sacroiliac joints on a spine MRI consist of high signal intensity on T2W images that parallel the joints,

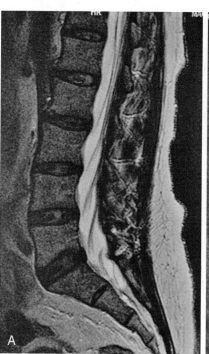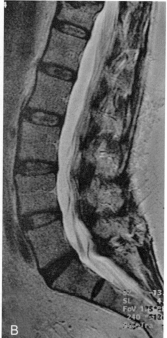

Figure 13–39. ARACHNOIDITIS: Normal and Abnormal Nerves, Sagittal Plane.
A, Fast T2 sagittal image, lumbar spine. This is an example of the normal appearance of the cauda equina nerves descending in the dural sac with a gentle curve. Compare with arachnoiditis in *B*. **B,** Fast T2 sagittal image, lumbar spine (different patient than in *A*). The nerves of the cauda equina have a wavy, angled, and irregular appearance typical of arachnoiditis in the sagittal plane.

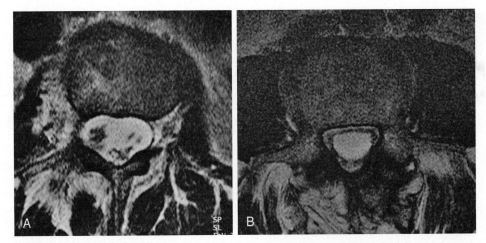

Figure 13–40. ARACHNOIDITIS: Axial Plane.
A, Fast T2 axial image, lumbar spine. The nerve roots are clumped and demonstrate an uneven distribution in the thecal sac from arachnoiditis. *B,* Fast T2 axial image, lumbar spine (different patient than in *A*). The nerves adhere to the dura, creating the empty thecal sac appearance of arachnoiditis.

involving the iliac side of the joint to a greater extent than the sacral side. This can have an appearance very similar to insufficiency fractures, but these diseases usually affect patients of different ages and gender, and usually no osteoporosis is seen in young people with ankylosing spondylitis. Infection of the sacroiliac joint could have an identical appearance, but this is usually a unilateral process, whereas ankylosing spondylitis affects the sacroiliac joints bilaterally.

The earliest changes of ankylosing spondylitis in the spine occur from marrow edema at the anterior corners of the vertebral bodies at the thoracolumbar junction. This is caused by inflammatory changes beneath the attachments of the anterior longitudinal ligament to the spine and where Sharpey's fibers

from the disk annulus attach to the vertebral body. This appears on MRI as low signal intensity on T1W images (or no abnormality evident at all) and high signal intensity on T2W images (Fig. 13–42). The sequence of events would then lead to squaring of the vertebral bodies from the erosion of bone and sclerosis of the corners of the vertebral bodies ("shiny corner" sign on conventional radiographs) as the bone attempts to heal from the inflammatory process. The sclerotic bone would be low signal intensity on both T1W and T2W MR images.

Because of the stiffness and rigidity of the spine in patients with more advanced ankylosing spondylitis, fractures may occur, often through the disks. These may be difficult to identify on conventional radiographs, but MRI may be useful in showing the

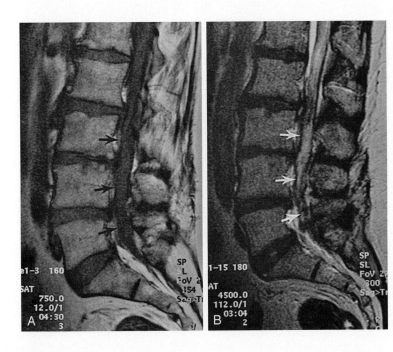

Figure 13–41. ARACHNOIDITIS: Fibrous Mass.
A, T1 sagittal image, lumbar spine. The thecal sac has heterogeneous intermediate signal, rather than the normal low signal of cerebrospinal fluid *(arrows). B,* Fast T2 sagittal image, lumbar spine. There is persistent heterogeneous intermediate signal in the dural sac *(arrows).* These are changes of a fibrous inflammatory mass from arachnoiditis.

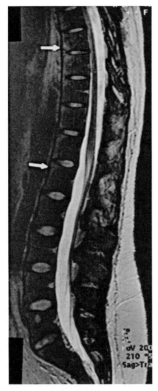

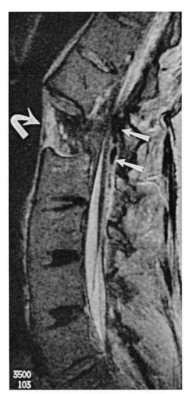

Figure 13–42. ANKYLOSING SPONDYLITIS: Early Changes.
Fast T2 sagittal image, thoracolumbar spine. MRI shows abnormal high signal in the anterior vertebral bodies of several lower thoracic and upper lumbar vertebral bodies (between *arrows*) from marrow edema. The vertebrae also are squared.

Figure 13–43. ANKYLOSING-SPONDYLITIS: Fracture.
Fast T2 sagittal image, thoracolumbar junction. There is a fracture through the disk *(curved arrow)* with marked displacement of fragments. Low signal in the posterior spinal canal from an epidural hematoma *(arrows)* is present. Changes of ankylosing spondylitis are evident in the vertebral bodies inferior to the fracture: the squared bodies are fused anteriorly with high signal evident in the disks from ossification and calcification.

fracture and any associated epidural hematomas, which are particularly common in patients with this disease (Fig. 13–43).

Traumatic Changes

Spondylolysis and Spondylolisthesis
(Box 13–12)

Spondylolysis is an osseous defect (fracture) of the pars interarticularis of the spine. These usually occur in the lower lumbar spine and may cause back pain, instability, or be asymptomatic. These osseous abnormalities probably are the result of chronic repetitive trauma, causing stress fractures of a congenitally weakened pars. Large amounts of osseous, fibrous, and cartilagenous material may build up around the defect, resulting in spinal stenosis, and a pseudoarthrosis may occur. The vertebral body above may slip forward on the vertebral body below (spondylolisthesis) to variable extents and may lead to spinal stenosis.

Findings of spondylolysis may be difficult to detect on MRI (Fig. 13–44). Direct visualization of the defect in the pars is possible, but it is not as easily seen as it is on radiographs or CT. On sagittal MR images, the break in the pars may be seen as a focus of low signal intensity. An intact pars sometimes has sclerosis with low signal intensity on all pulse

sequences, which appears to be a spondylolytic defect on MRI when none is present. It is helpful to directly identify a pars defect on axial images, where a cut through the mid-vertebral body (at the inferior aspect of the pedicles) shows disruption of the pars where normally there is an intact bony ring made of the pedicles and laminae (Fig. 13–45). This

---

BOX 13–12: SPONDYLOLYSIS

Direct Evidence
• Defect in pars interarticularis
  —Difficult diagnosis by MRI
  —Sclerotic (low signal) intact pars may mimic lysis
Indirect Evidence
• Neural foramen
  —Obliquely oriented figure-of-eight configuration
• Modic marrow changes in adjacent pedicles
• ↓ Posterior vertebral body height
• Widened canal compared to L1 level by >25% (even when no spondylolisthesis is present)

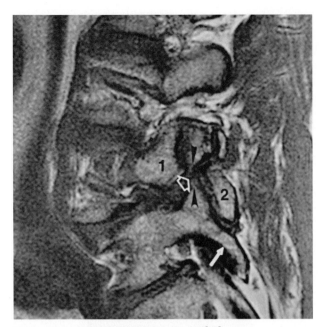

Figure 13–44. SPONDYLOLYSIS: Sagittal Plane.
T1 sagittal image, lumbar spine. The normal pars interarticularis at L5 is shown for reference *(solid white arrow)*. The pars at L4 is in two separate fragments (1,2), and a large spondylolytic defect in the pars is shown *(open arrow)*. The gap created by the L4 pars defect is filled by inferior and superior articular processes that are resting on each other *(arrowheads)*, so that the foot of the "Scottie dog" above is resting on the ear of the one below.

has an appearance similar to a cut through the facet joints (with the pars defects mimicking the facet joints), but the facet joints should not be present at this location.

Because of the difficulty in making the diagnosis of spondylolysis on MRI, especially when no spondylolisthesis is present, several secondary signs have been described that may help (Fig. 13–46).[39] The neural foramen at the affected level becomes somewhat horizontal in orientation and may have a lobulated, oblique, figure-of-eight appearance. The pedicles and articular processes adjacent to the pars defect may have reactive marrow changes (Modic changes) from abnormal stresses, usually with fatty marrow that has signal intensity that follows fat on all pulse sequences. Wedging, with a decreased height of the posterior vertebral body at the level of the spondylolysis, can be seen as a secondary finding. Widening of the anteroposterior diameter of the canal at the affected level can occur even when there is no anterior spondylolisthesis, because the posterior elements displace slightly posteriorly. This widened spinal canal can be shown as abnormal if it measures 25% or more in anteroposterior diameter as compared to the diameter of the canal at the L1 level. If CT or conventional radiographs of the spine are available, immediately place them on the viewbox, because the diagnosis of spondylolysis can be made much more easily and confidently than with MRI.

Intraosseous Disk Herniations

Disk material not only projects into the spinal canal, but may directly herniate into the adjacent

vertebral bodies through the endplates, in which case it is known as a Schmorl's or cartilaginous node. These may occur because bone is weakened by osteoporosis, tumor, metabolic diseases, or congenital weak points in the endplates. Although usually asymptomatic, Schmorl's nodes may occur from trauma with axial loading forces and may be acutely painful in this latter situation. Multiple thoracic Schmorl's nodes can occur in very active teens from axial stresses and result in irregularity of several endplates, loss of disk height, as well as narrowing of the height of the affected anterior vertebral bodies from fractures, with a resultant kyphosis (Scheuermann's disease) (Fig. 13–47).

An inflammatory, foreign body-type response to intraosseous disk herniation may occur, with vascularization around the disk material and surrounding marrow edema, which may cause severe pain (Fig. 13–48).[40] Vascularized Schmorl's nodes on MRI tend to have large, dome-shaped regions of marrow edema surrounding them; marrow edema is low signal on T1W and high signal on T2W and contrast-enhanced T1W images. A rim of contrast enhancement around the periphery of the Schmorl's node is seen in addition to the surrounding marrow edema. These can have an aggressive look, similar to a tumor, and careful evaluation is necessary to make the proper diagnosis.

Major Trauma (Box 13–13)

MRI for evaluation of traumatic changes in the spine usually is performed to look for soft tissue

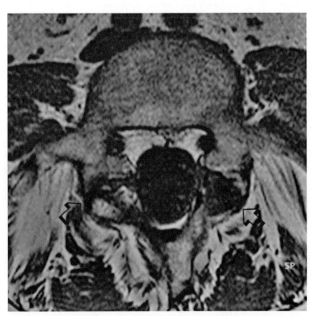

Figure 13–45. SPONDYLOLYSIS: Axial Plane.
T1 axial image, lumbar spine. Oblique, irregular defects *(open arrows)* are evident bilaterally in the posterior ring of L4 from spondylolysis. A cut through the mid-vertebral body at the inferior aspect of the pedicles should have a solid ring of bone, without any defects from facet joints, spondylolysis, or other entities. The anteroposterior diameter of the canal is elongated from displacement of bone as the result of the lysis.

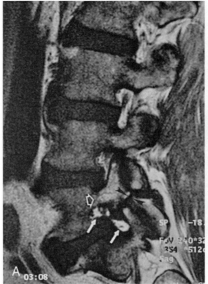
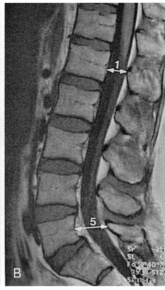

Figure 13–46. SPONDYLOLYSIS: Secondary Signs. *A,* T1 sagittal image, lumbar spine. A spondylolytic defect is seen between the *arrowheads* at L5. Secondary evidence includes the lobulated, oblique figure-of-eight L5-S1 neural foramen *(solid arrows)* and the high-signal fat from reactive type 2 marrow changes in the pedicle and superior articular process of L5 *(open arrow).* *B,* T1 sagittal image, lumbar spine. There is wedging of the posterior L5 vertebral body. The spinal canal at L5 *(arrows; 5)* is more than 25% wider compared to the anteroposterior diameter of the canal at L1 *(arrows; 1).*

injury; however, certain fractures in the spine are also well depicted with MRI. In general, ligament rupture, traumatic disk extrusions, cord injury, epidural hematomas, and paraspinous hematomas are shown better with MRI than other imaging techniques. There are some logistical difficulties in performing MRI examinations in critically injured spinal trauma patients, and these must be weighed against the potential benefits of the examination.

We use MRI (after conventional films and CT) in patients who have sustained major spine trauma for several different indications: radiographs suggesting ligamentous injury, some thoracolumbar burst fractures to look for intact ligaments, cervical facet dislocations to look for a disk extrusion or epidural hematoma prior to performing a closed reduction, incomplete neurologic deficits to assess the cord and ligaments in order to help determine what type of surgery will be done and the patient's prognosis, neurologic deficits in the face of no radiographic traumatic abnormalities (eg, central cord syndrome), if the neurologic deficit does not match with the level of a radiographic traumatic abnormality, and in obtunded trauma patients with no radiographic abnormalities in order to determine the need to keep them in a cervical collar. In general, there is no purpose in doing MRI in patients with a complete neurologic deficit, because the treatment and outcome are unlikely to be affected.[41]

Osseous. Osseous spinal injuries are well identified by radiographs and CT. Any fracture through cortical bone will be difficult to identify on MRI compared to CT; thus, many posterior element fractures definitely will be missed on MRI, and MRI should not be done as a replacement examination for detecting spinal fractures. Fractures of the vertebral bodies may be evident on MRI, however, when they are not identifiable on CT or radiographs, because of the marrow edema and hemorrhage in the trabecular bone, for which MRI is very sensitive (Fig. 13–49). Vertebral body fractures appear as amorphous regions of high signal intensity on T2W images and may be intermediate signal intensity on T1W images, if evident at all on this sequence; linear fracture lines are usually not evident.

Ligaments. The anterior and posterior longitudinal ligaments of the spine, the ligamentum flavum, the interspinous ligaments, and the supraspinous

Figure 13–47. SCHEUERMANN'S DISEASE. T1 sagittal image, lumbar spine. The endplates are irregular at multiple levels in the lower thoracic and throughout the lumbar spine from intraosseous disk herniations. There is also loss of the normal lumbar lordosis and loss of disk and vertebral body height.

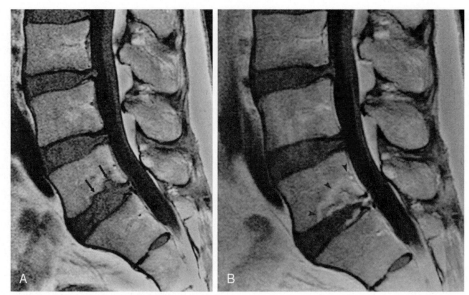

Figure 13–48. VASCULARIZED (PAINFUL) SCHMORL'S NODES.
A, T1 sagittal image, lumbar spine. The inferior endplate of L5 is irregular from intraosseous disk herniations *(arrows).* *B,* T1 contrast-enhanced sagittal image, lumbar spine. An enhancing rim is present in the marrow surrounding the Schmorl's node, and there is peripheral enhancement around the herniated intraosseous disk itself. This patient had disk surgery in the remote past, which accounts for the enhancing posterior periphery of the L5–S1 disk.

and nuchal ligaments must be carefully evaluated in trauma patients. These supporting ligaments of the spine are made of collagen and, therefore, appear (in general) as taut, low signal intensity bands on all pulse sequences on MRI (Fig. 13–50).[42] An exception to this MRI appearance involves the normal interspinous ligaments, which run vertically between adjacent spinous processes and may have a striated or patchy appearance with areas of intermediate signal intensity interspersed with large areas of high signal intensity fat on T1W images. An-

other exception involves the supraspinous and nuchal ligaments, which are not always taut and normally have areas that are wavy and may have high signal intensity within them from the magic angle phenomenon on short TE pulse sequences.

Ligaments may be partially or completely torn. Some type of T2W sequence, especially with fat suppression (such as STIR), is necessary for demonstrating high signal intensity edema and hemorrhage in and around an injured ligament (Fig. 13–51). Discontinuity of the ligament indicates a complete

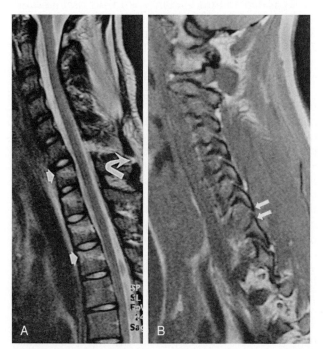

Figure 13–49. MAJOR TRAUMA: Osseous.
A, Fast T2 sagittal image, cervical spine. There is marrow edema from fractures of C7 through T3 (between *solid white arrows*); radiographs and CT were normal. The supraspinous ligament is discontinuous from a tear *(curved arrow)* at C6–7. *B,* T1 sagittal image, cervical spine (different patient than in *A*). Perched facets *(arrows)* are easy to see in the lower cervical spine because of the tomographic nature of MRI.

Osseous
- Posterior element (cortical) fractures, easily missed on MRI
- Vertebral body (marrow) fractures, easily detected

Ligaments
- ↑ Signal on T2 from hemorrhage/edema directs attention to sites of acute ligament injury
- Ligament partial tears: thickening and intrasubstance ↑ signal
- Complete tears: discontinuity of ligament

Disks
- Traumatic extrusions

Epidural Fluid
- Hematoma
- Pseudomeningocele

Vascular
- Vertebral artery occlusion

Cord
- Early
  —Transection
  —Hemorrhage
  —Hemorrhage surrounded by edema
  —Edema (contusion)
- Delayed
  —Myelomalacia
  —Intramedullary cysts
  —Syrinx
  —Infarction

Nerves
- Avulsion, contusion

Paraspinous Soft Tissues
- Hematoma, muscle strains

rupture, but partial tears with ligamentous thickening and intrasubstance high signal intensity also can be seen. Obliteration of the fat between spinous processes on T1W images, with high signal intensity on T2W images, indicates interspinous ligament sprain. The high signal intensity areas of edema and hemorrhage are extremely useful for directing one's attention to the sites of ligamentous injury, which otherwise may be subtle on MRI. It is for this reason that MRI should be performed as soon as possible after the trauma, before the edema resolves (preferably within 3 days).

Traumatic Disks. Acute traumatic disk extrusions are important in specific situations. An 11% incidence of increased neurologic compromise as a result of unrecognized disk extrusions was reported in patients who had reduction of cervical facet dislocations under anesthesia.[43] If a traumatic disk extrusion is demonstrated by MRI, careful consideration should be given to open reduction of the dislocated facets, or at least in not performing the reduction under general anesthesia, in order to pre-vent progressive neurologic deficits. Acute disk herniations also may be associated with traumatic cord abnormalities prior to reducing or manipulating the spine (Fig. 13–52).

T2W images of traumatic disk extrusions may show them as either low or high signal intensity, depending on whether or not there is hemorrhage involving the disk. Disks at the injured level have signal intensity identical to adjacent intact disks on T2W images if there is no hemorrhage; there is higher signal intensity than the normal disk in the presence of hemorrhage, and the disk height often is decreased.

Epidural Fluid Collections. Trauma may result in an epidural hematoma (Fig. 13–53) or a pseudomeningocele. Pseudomeningoceles occur from a rent in the dura (as from avulsion of a nerve root) with leakage of cerebrospinal fluid into the epidural space and beyond.

Vascular Abnormalities. The vertebral arteries of patients with cervical trauma have been reported as abnormal from occlusion in 24% of patients.[44] MRI shows vertebral artery asymmetry, with lack of the normal, low signal intensity from flow void in the vertebral artery on the abnormal side (Fig. 13–54). Asymmetry of signal intensity also may occur in

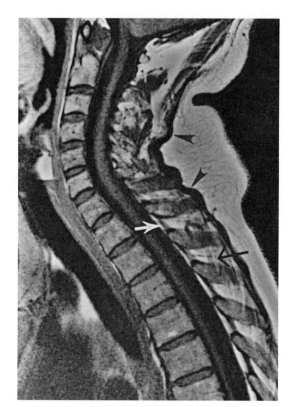

Figure 13–50. SPINOUS LIGAMENTS: Normal.
T1 sagittal image, cervical spine. The supraspinous ligament is shown *(arrowheads)*. The ligamentum flavum is a vertical, low-signal structure anterior to the spinous processes *(white arrow)*. The interspinous ligaments are difficult to see and the presence of fat between spinous processes is the best indication of normal *(black arrow)*. The normal anterior and posterior longitudinal ligaments are not seen on this sequence because they blend with adjacent cortical bone and other low-signal structures.

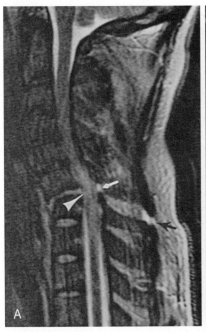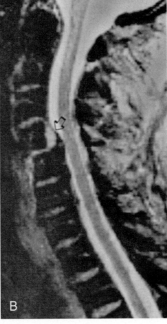

Figure 13–51. MAJOR TRAUMA: Ligaments.
A, STIR sagittal image, cervical spine. The supraspinous ligament is torn *(black arrow)*, as is the ligamentum flavum *(white arrow)* and posterior longitudinal ligament at the C6–7 level *(arrowhead).* There is high signal in the cord from contusion at the same level. *B,* T2* sagittal image, cervical spine (different patient than in *A*). There is subluxation of C4 on C5. The linear, low-signal posterior longitudinal ligament *(open arrow)* is displaced from the adjacent vertebral body by blood or disk material but remains intact, which significantly impacts on management.

asymptomatic, nontraumatized patients because of asymmetry in size and of flow in the arteries. This may be evaluated best on the axial images, but also on sagittal cervical spine MRI.

Treatment for this entity is controversial for patients with a concomitant spinal cord injury, because it is undesirable to give anticoagulants to these patients and because the frequency of vertebrobasilar ischemia in trauma patients is low.

Cord Injuries. Three abnormal patterns may occur in the cord from trauma: (1) contusion (edema), (2) hemorrhage, or (3) a combination of central hemorrhage with peripheral, surrounding edema (Fig. 13–55).[45] Cord transection may occur with hemorrhage in the gap between the segments. The cord may be either enlarged or normal in size.

The appearance of hemorrhage in the cord is a function of the chronicity of the lesion.[46] The signal characteristics listed in Box 13–14 are based on conventional spin echo techniques, but recall that gradient echo sequences also may be valuable in demonstrating blood because it shows blooming. The mnemonic we use to help remember the progression of MRI changes from hemorrhage is dis-

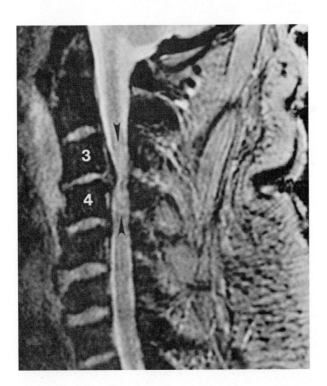

Figure 13–52. MAJOR TRAUMA: Disks.
T2* sagittal image, cervical spine. There is a traumatic disk herniation at C3–4. The posterior longitudinal ligament remains intact, draped over the displaced disk material. There is abnormal signal in the cord *(arrowheads),* centered at the level of the abnormal disk from hemorrhage/edema.

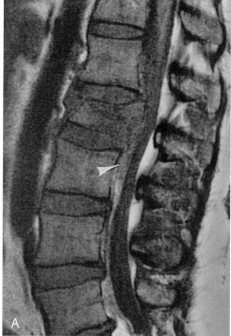
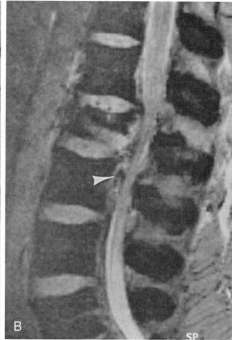

Figure 13–53. MAJOR TRAUMA: Epidural Hematoma.
A, T1 sagittal image, lumbar spine. A burst fracture of L2 protrudes into the spinal canal. Intermediate signal in the anterior epidural space *(arrowhead)* is from blood. *B,* T2* sagittal image, lumbar spine. There is very low signal and blooming in the epidural hematoma *(arrowhead)* from blood. The canal is narrowed secondary to the retropulsed fracture and the epidural hematoma.

cussed in detail in the chapter on Tendons and Muscles ("It Be IdDy BidDy BaBy Doo Doo" mnemonic—see Box 13–14).

Cord edema without hemorrhage or fractures is a common manifestation of the central cord syndrome, which occurs with a hyperextension injury, usually in older people with degenerative changes in the cervical spine that cause spinal stenosis. The osteophytes and bulging disks impinge against the cord during the injury, resulting in central cord edema. Patients have symptoms of weakness or paralysis of the upper limbs and sparing of the lower extremities. Edema is manifest on MRI as being isointense to the cord on T1W images and high signal intensity on T2W images (Fig. 13–56).[43]

There is a better prognosis with contusion of the cord than with hemorrhage; recuperation of neurologic function is unlikely with cord hemorrhage. Other possible sequelae of trauma to the cord include myelomalacia, intramedullary cysts, syrinx, or infarction.

Other Soft Tissues. Muscles, nerves, and prevertebral and other paraspinous soft tissues may show evidence of injury on MRI after trauma. The paraspinous muscles may be strained and demonstrate high signal intensity on T2W images from edema, or hemorrhage into muscle may have variable signal depending on the age of the injury (Fig. 13–57). Nerves may be injured, either avulsed or contused, and leakage of cerebrospinal fluid may be seen with

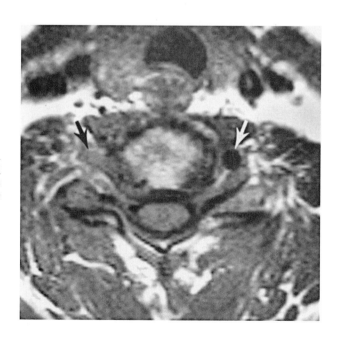

Figure 13–54. MAJOR TRAUMA: Vascular.
T1 axial image, cervical spine. There is asymmetry in the appearance of the vertebral arteries bilaterally. The left side is normal *(white arrow)* with low signal from flow void. The right side has abnormal increased signal in the vertebral artery *(black arrow)* due to decreased flow from occlusion.

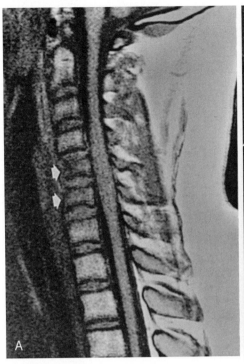
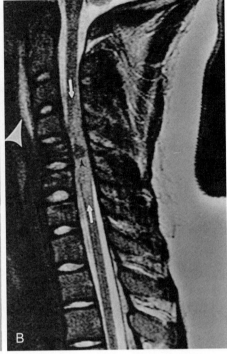

Figure 13–55. MAJOR TRAUMA: Cord Injury.
A, T1 sagittal image, cervical spine. Vague decreased signal in the C5 and C6 vertebral bodies *(arrows)* is from fractures (not evident on radiography or CT). The cord has normal signal, but is increased in caliber posterior to the abnormal vertebral bodies. The patient had a significant neurologic deficit. *B,* Fast T2 sagittal image, cervical spine. There is a focal area of low signal *(black arrowhead)* in the cord from hemorrhage. There is diffuse increased signal from edema *(arrows)* surrounding the hemorrhage. There is a small, high-signal prevertebral hematoma *(white arrowhead).*

nerve avulsions (Fig. 13–58). A contused nerve demonstrates high signal intensity, usually with enlargement, on T2W images in the injured segment.

Osseous Spine Tumors (Box 13–15)

Benign Bone Tumors

The most common benign osseous tumors of the spine are hemangiomas, osteoid osteoma, osteoblastoma, giant cell tumor, osteochondroma, and an-

eurysmal bone cyst. Prior to the age of 30 years, tumors of the spine are fairly uncommon and generally benign.

Hemangiomas in the vertebral bodies are so common, that they are discussed separately. Otherwise, suffice it to say that a few simple rules, such as the location of spine lesions, help to narrow the differential diagnosis on MRI. Osteoid osteomas, osteoblastomas, and aneurysmal bone cysts are most likely to occur in the posterior spinal elements. In addition, aneurysmal bone cysts are expansile and

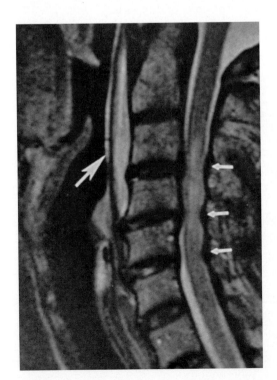

Figure 13–56. MAJOR TRAUMA: Central Cord Syndrome.
Fast T2 sagittal image, cervical spine. The central spinal canal is stenotic from bulging disks and ligamentum flavum *(small arrows)* at several levels. There is increased signal in the cord at the level of the stenosis from contusion. There are no fractures or traumatic disk herniations. There is also prevertebral soft tissue hemorrhage/edema *(large arrow).*

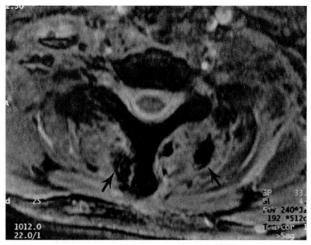

Figure 13–57. MAJOR TRAUMA: Muscle Strain.
T2* axial image, cervical spine. This patient had severe neck pain, but negative radiographs and CT. MR shows muscle strains in the paraspinous muscles with areas of high signal and focal areas of low signal with blooming *(arrows)* from hemorrhage in torn muscle.

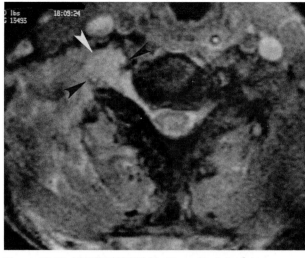

Figure 13–58. MAJOR TRAUMA: Nerve Root Avulsion.
T2* axial image, cervical spine. The right neural foramen is high signal and appears empty compared to the normal left side. There is a bulbous collection *(arrowheads)* of high signal just outside of the neural foramen, compatible with a pseudomeningocele associated with nerve root avulsion and leak of spinal fluid.

usually have fluid–fluid levels within them, whereas osteoid osteomas are small and usually have a target appearance because of the calcified central nidus, as well as large surrounding areas of edema in the marrow and soft tissue structures adjacent to the lesion (Fig. 13–59). Giant cell tumors of the spine are rare and nonspecific in appearance, but when they occur in the spine, they most frequently involve the sacrum.

Intraosseous Hemangiomas. Spinal hemangiomas are common and frequently multiple. The vertebral bodies are more commonly affected than the posterior elements.

Most garden-variety hemangiomas have a classic appearance and are asymptomatic (Fig. 13–60). On T1W images, they are round lesions of high signal intensity, caused by the large fat component of typical hemangiomas; on T2W images, they are also high signal intensity (higher than fat) because of the slow-flowing blood in the lesions. Thick, low signal intensity, vertical trabecular struts may be seen within the lesions. The high signal intensity of hemangiomas on T2W sequences distinguishes them from focal areas of marrow conversion, which consist almost entirely of fat and have a lower signal intensity than hemangiomas on T2W images. Fast T2W sequences without fat saturation show fat as high signal intensity, which may make it difficult to distinguish hemangiomas from focal areas of marrow fat conversion.

A small percentage of hemangiomas have a completely different appearance than the fatty lesions described above; these are referred to as aggressive or atypical hemangiomas.[47] These have diffuse low signal intensity on T1W images, enhance with contrast, and are high signal on T2W images. Aggressive

	BOX 13–14: CORD HEMORRHAGE*			
AGE	**Blood Products**	**T1 Signal**	**T2 Signal**	**Mnemonic**
Hyperacute (0–1 day)	Oxyhemoglobin/ Serum	Isointense to cord	Bright	It Be **(IB)**
Acute (1–3 days)	Deoxyhemoglobin	Isointense to cord	Dark	IdDy **(ID)**
Early subacute (4–7 days)	Intracellular Methemoglobin	Bright	Dark	BiDdy **(BD)**
Late subacute (>7 days)	Extracellular Methemoglobin	Bright	Bright	BaBy **(BB)**
Chronic (>2 weeks)	Hemosiderin	Dark	Dark	Doo Doo **(DD)**

*Hemorrhage into soft tissues other than the cord and brain goes through the same sequence of changes, but often slower and in a less predictable fashion, because of the lower oxygen tension.

BOX 13–15: OSSEOUS SPINE TUMORS:
Decreasing Order of Frequency

Benign
- Hemangiomas (↑ signal T1 and T2)
- Osteoid osteoma (posterior elements)
- Osteoblastoma (posterior elements)
- Giant cell tumor (sacrum)
- Osteochondroma (protrude from bone)
- Aneurysmal bone cyst (posterior elements)

Malignant
- Metastases (multiple)
- Myeloma (multiple)
- Lymphoma (multiple)
- Chordoma (sacrum)
- Sarcomas
  —Ewing's, osteosarcoma, chondrosarcoma

Most tumors discovered before the age of 30 years are benign.

Most tumors discovered after the age of 30 years are malignant.

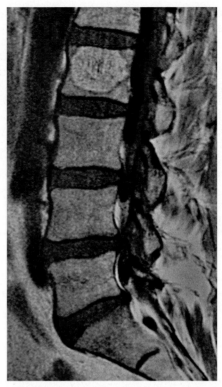

Figure 13–60. BENIGN BONE TUMORS: Hemangioma.
T1 sagittal image, lumbar spine. There is a large, round, high-signal fat lesion in the L2 vertebral body with thick, low-signal vertical struts in its center, typical of a hemangioma.

hemangiomas are composed predominantly of vessels, rather than fat. These lesions tend to be symptomatic because of fracture and collapse of the vertebral body, or extension of the hemangioma into the epidural space, with mass effect that may result in neurologic symptoms as well as pain. These have an appearance like that of metastatic disease or other aggressive lesions of bone.

Malignant Bone Tumors

The most common malignant osseous lesions to affect the spine usually occur after the age of 30 years and include metastases, multiple myeloma, lymphoma, chordoma, and sarcomas (Ewing's, osteosarcoma, and chondrosarcoma, in decreasing order of frequency). Ewing's sarcoma and osteosarcoma occur at a younger age than any of the other malignant lesions, usually during the second decade.

Metastases and Multiple Myeloma. These lesions are common and are covered in detail in Chapter 2. The spine is the site of most bone metastases and myeloma because of its high red marrow content; the thoracolumbar spine in particular is affected. In the spine, MRI is extremely useful not only to demonstrate the presence and location of lesions, but also to depict any epidural spread and its effect on the cord or nerves. Gadolinium frequently is used to better demonstrate epidural extension of tumor arising from bone.

Metastases are usually focal and multiple, but may cause diffuse homogeneous marrow disease, or occasionally be a solitary focal lesion. Lytic metastases are generally low signal intensity on T1W im-

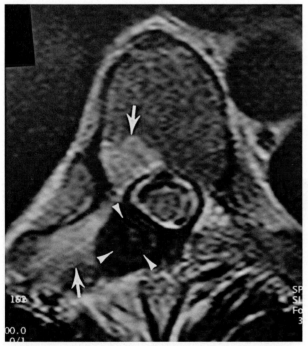

Figure 13–59. BENIGN BONE TUMORS: Osteoid Osteoma.
Fast T2 axial image, T10. A target lesion (*small arrowheads* indicate the inner circle of the lesion) in the right lamina represents the osteoid osteoma, which is surrounded by high-signal edema in the posterior vertebral body, pedicle, transverse process, and soft tissues (*arrows*). There is mild central canal narrowing from the lesion. The low signal in the cerebrospinal fluid that surrounds the cord is simply flow artifact from the normal motion of the fluid.

ages and become bright on T2W images, especially if untreated. Most sclerotic metastases have low signal on both T1W and T2W sequences. Myeloma has the following patterns on MRI with increasing severity of disease: normal marrow appearance, focal lesions (the "mini brain" appearance is characteristic if present, but otherwise they look like metastases), variegated pattern, diffuse pattern.

There is a pitfall to be aware of in the thoracic spine that may mimic a metastasis or myeloma. Sagittal T1W images through the costovertebral joint may give the appearance of a focal low signal lesion in the posterosuperior vertebral body, extending into the pedical (Fig. 13–61). The location on the lateral margin of the vertebral body, and in its posterosuperior aspect, makes the true nature of this finding obvious. This may be seen at multiple levels, mimicking multiple lesions.

Acute osteoporotic compression fractures in the spine may have features similar to metastatic disease, and it is a common problem to try to differentiate the two on spine MRI examinations of elderly individuals. This is discussed in Chapter 2, but also is briefly reviewed here. A fractured vertebral body is statistically more likely to be from metastatic disease than from an acute osteoporotic fracture with surrounding hemorrhage and edema if: (1) the pedicles and posterior elements have abnormal signal intensity; (2) there is an associated soft tissue mass; (3) there are multiple lesions in other bones, especially round, focal lesions; (4) the entire vertebral body has abnormal signal intensity, without any areas of fatty marrow; (5) the posterior vertebral body wall has a convex rather than an angled appearance; and (6) no linear fracture line is present. Follow-up MRI (in 6 to 8 weeks) or biopsy is generally necessary to make a definitive distinction between acute osteoporotic fractures and pathologic fractures from metastases.

Chordomas. This and the other primary bone tumors that may arise in the spine are exceedingly uncommon. Chordomas arise from notochordal remnants, and most spinal chordomas are located in the sacrum or coccyx (the differential diagnosis includes metastases, plasmacytoma, or giant cell tumor). Rarely, chordomas are present in vertebral bodies elsewhere in the spine. It is not uncommon for more than one adjacent vertebral segment to be involved by this tumor. The MRI appearance is nonspecific, showing a mass that is heterogeneous, low signal intensity on T1W images, hyperintense on T2W images, and which may involve more than one adjacent level (Fig. 13–62).

Primary Bone Tumors. Bone sarcomas that arise in the spine have features identical to their appearance in any other bone.

Spinal Canal Contents

The vast majority of abnormalities affecting the spine were described in earlier sections. The osseous structures and joints are the sites of origin for the bulk of spine abnormalities; indeed, many abnormalities of the structures within the spinal canal are secondary to abnormalities of the adjacent bones and joints of the spine.

As musculoskeletal radiologists, our goals in evaluating the spinal canal contents are (1) not to miss anything of importance, and (2) to be able to make the diagnosis or to have a reasonable list of differential diagnostic possibilities for the abnormal findings, without crowding too much of our brain with erudite details of spinal canal pathology. Abnormalities involving the contents of the canal are covered accordingly in this chapter, and additional information can be obtained from other texts devoted to these topics.

The classic division of spinal structures into intramedullary, intradural extramedullary, and extradural is not used here. These terms are ingrained in the literature from work initially done with myelography, but we find it easier with MRI to discuss the precise location of a lesion, because that is virtually

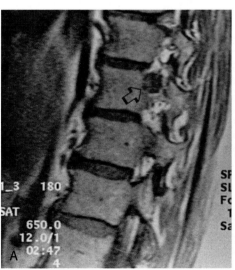 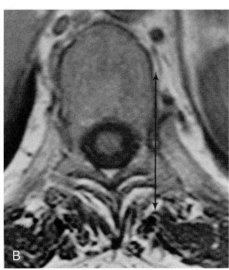

Figure 13–61. MALIGNANT BONE TUMORS: A Pitfall.
A, T1 sagittal image, thoracic spine. A focal, low-signal round lesion in the posterosuperior vertebral body and pedicle *(open arrow)* resembles a metastatic lesion. *B*, T1 axial image, thoracic spine. A sagittal slice obtained through the costovertebral joint *(double-headed arrow)* shows the focal "lesion" in the sagittal plane, but it is simply due to volume averaging.

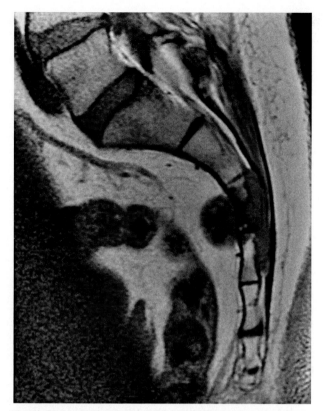

Figure 13–62. MALIGNANT BONE TUMORS: Chordoma.
T1 sagittal image, sacrum. There is destruction of the S3 and S4 vertebral bodies with extension of tumor into the spinal canal and presacral space. The sacral location and involvement of adjacent segments is typical of a chordoma.

always possible to ascertain with MRI. For instance, why use the vague term "extradural," which includes everything from the dural sac to the Atlantic ocean? We do not refer to an osteoid osteoma in the shaft of a femur as being an intracortical, extramedullary, subperiosteal lesion; it is simply a cortical lesion, a medullary lesion, or a subperiosteal lesion. The same simplicity should apply to the spine; therefore, we use the terms cord, intradural space, and epidural space to define the location of lesions within the spinal canal.

Epidural Space (Box 13–16)

The epidural space extends from the foramen magnum to the sacral hiatus in the craniocaudal direction; it lies external to the thecal sac and deep to the osseous structures and ligaments of the spine within the spinal canal. It is composed mainly of fat and blood vessels. MRI shows the normal epidural space with signal characteristics that follow fat on all pulse sequences.

Lesions that occur in the epidural space include epidural lipomatosis, epidural hematoma, epidural abscess, and certain kinds of cysts. Many lesions from the adjacent bones, disks, and ligaments may secondarily encroach upon the epidural space.[48] Masses within the epidural space often are sur-

rounded by a rim of epidural fat, which helps to place the lesions within this anatomic compartment.

Epidural Abscess. This was discussed under the infection section earlier. It is a localized fluid collection with rim enhancement that usually is associated with adjacent spondylodiskitis (Fig. 13–37 and 13–38).

Epidural Hematoma. Focal collections of blood in the epidural space occur from acute trauma (Fig. 13–53), as a complication of surgery (Fig. 13–35), from anticoagulaton, or spontaneously (Fig. 13–13). The appearance of a hematoma on MRI depends on its age; this was described in the trauma section earlier.

Spontaneous epidural hematomas are believed to occur from tearing of fragile epidural veins at the time of an acute disk disruption. Annular tears or focal disk herniations usually are present at the level of a spontaneous epidural hematoma; symptoms are those of an acute disk herniation, but resolve more rapidly. Spontaneous epidural hematomas are largest in the anteroposterior diameter at the mid-vertebral body level (adjacent to the basivertebral venous plexus) and taper as they extend to the adjacent disk level. Spontaneous epidural hematomas are often quite small and may be difficult to distinguish from a sequestered disk or extrusion, depending on their signal intensity at the time of imaging.

Epidural Lipomatosis. Deposition of excessive quantities of fat in the epidural space usually affects patients who are taking steroids or who have endogenous hypercorticalism, but also may occur in obese individuals or for no apparent reason. This entity is often an incidental finding on MRI and causes no symptoms. Only the thoracic or lumbar spine, or both, are involved (Fig. 13–63). Symptoms of spinal stenosis may exist. MRI shows large amounts of epidural fat that follow the signal intensity of fat on all pulse sequences, and a decreased thecal sac size caused by compression by the fat.

Epidural Cysts. Several different cystic structures may be found in the epidural space. *Synovial cysts* that arise from degenerative facet joint disease may impinge upon the epidural space (Fig. 13–20). They may be located deep to the ligamentum flavum, or break through the ligament so that they are directly within the epidural space and may compress nerves. The MRI appearance was discussed in the section on degenerative changes earlier.

Arachnoid cysts occur when the arachnoid protrudes into the epidural space through a congenital or traumatic defect in the dura and is filled with cerebrospinal fluid. The mass effect may cause neurologic symptoms by compressing adjacent soft tissue structures in the canal (cord and nerves). There may be pressure erosions of adjacent osseous structures (posterior vertebral bodies or inner aspects of pedicles). MRI shows an epidural mass that is low signal intensity on T1W and high signal intensity on T2W images (Fig. 13–64).

Sacral meningoceles are arachnoid cysts that oc-

BOX 13–16: EPIDURAL ABNORMALITIES

Abscess
• Usually associated with spondylodiskitis
Hematoma
• Trauma, surgery, anticoagulation, or spontaneous
—Spontaneous, probably secondary to disk disruption
Lipomatosis
• ↑ Fat in thoracic/lumbar spine may cause stenosis symptoms
Cysts
• Synovial cysts
—Facet joint degeneration
• Arachnoid cysts (includes sacral meningoceles)
—Defect in dura allows arachnoid and CSF herniation
—May compress nerves or displace cord
—May erode bone
—Often have static flow, therefore ↑ signal on T2 relative to CSF
• Arachnoid diverticulae
—Dilatation of nerve root sleeves
—Common, multiple, may erode bone
—Occur above sacral level
—Asymptomatic or mimic disk extrusion
—Signal follows CSF; no enhancement differentiates from nerve sheath tumors
• Perineural (Tarlov cysts)
—Dorsal nerve root fibers involved with cyst
—Affect sacral nerve roots usually
—Asymptomatic, or may cause nerve compression symptoms
—May erode bone. Cysts present in central canal and/or neural foramina
—Signal follows CSF, or higher than CSF on T2 (static flow)
• Pseudomeningoceles
—Traumatic, nerve root avulsion often associated
—Rent in dura and arachnoid with CSF collection in epidural space and beyond
• Lateral thoracic meningoceles
—Associated with neurofibromatosis; other manifestations usually present (dural ectasia)
Miscellaneous
• Any bone or disk abnormality extending into epidural space
• Ossification, posterior longitudinal ligament

CSF, cerebrospinal fluid.

cur in a specific location. They protrude through a developmental dural defect and may erode the sacrum (intraosseous or intrasacral meningoceles); these may or may not be symptomatic. Cyst size does not seem to relate to the presence of symptoms, but cysts that communicate with the subarachnoid space are usually asymptomatic, whereas those that do not communicate are symptomatic. Compression of nerves by the cystic mass may cause symptoms. These cysts are similar in signal intensity to cerebrospinal fluid, but often have slightly higher signal intensity on T2W images, caused by static flow (Fig. 13–65).

Arachnoid diverticulae are very common cysts, formed by dilatation of nerve root sleeves (Fig. 13–66). These are commonly multiple, bulbous dilatations of the dura and arachnoid that are filled with cerebrospinal fluid and can clinically mimic disk extrusions or compression by other masses. These diverticulae may erode bone. Arachnoid diverticulae typically affect nerve root sleeves above the sacral level. There is no contrast enhancement, which differentiates them from tumor, and the signal intensity follows that of the fluid in the subarachnoid space on all pulse sequences, allowing differentiation from most disk herniations.

Perineural cysts, or Tarlov cysts, occur in the sacral region and have nerve fibers within the wall of the cyst or coursing through the cyst (Fig. 13–67). They may cause nerve compression or bone erosion, but usually are asymptomatic. They have no direct connection to the thecal sac, but are continuous with the dura and arachnoid of the posterior nerve roots in the sacral region. The signal intensity follows that of cerebrospinal fluid or, because of an increased protein content or absence of flow, they often have higher signal intensity on T2W images than cerebrospinal fluid.

Other cystic lesions that may occur in the epidural space are *lateral thoracic meningoceles*

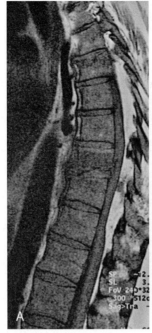

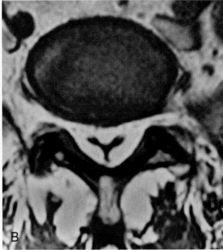

Figure 13–63. EPIDURAL SPACE: Epidural Lipomatosis.
A, T1 sagittal image, thoracic spine. There is a large amount of high-signal fat in the posterior epidural space of the thoracic spine. It causes compression of the dural sac anteriorly. The sac widens distally, where the fat becomes thinner. *B,* T1 axial image, lumbar spine (different patient than in *A*). High-signal fat is filling the central canal, and the dural sac is compressed into a small triangular structure.

(which typically occur in neurofibromatosis, but other spinal abnormalities such as dural ectasia will be present to help make the diagnosis), and *traumatic pseudomeningoceles* (which tend to extend out of the epidural space through neural foramina and are large).

Scalloping of posterior vertebral bodies may occur from the different epidural cysts described above, as well as from dural ectasia seen in neurofibromatosis, Marfan syndrome, and Ehlers-Danlos syndrome and, of course, from erosion by any soft tissue tumor mass and in patients with acromegaly and achondroplasia.

Miscellaneous. Many different abnormalities can secondarily affect the epidural space from the adjacent ligaments, bones, and joints. Most of these entities have been discussed elsewhere (disk herniations, osteophytes, bone tumors, etc). These lesions are directly visible on MRI, so that it is clear from where they arose.

Ossification of the posterior longitudinal ligament of the spine (OPLL) usually affects the cervical spine, resulting in thickening of the posterior longitudinal ligament, which impinges on the epidural space and may cause symptoms relating to spinal stenosis. This entity is very common in patients with diffuse idiopathic skeletal hyperostosis (DISH) and should be looked for closely in this disorder.

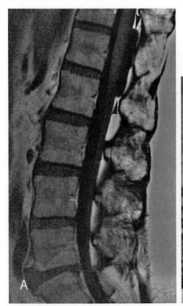

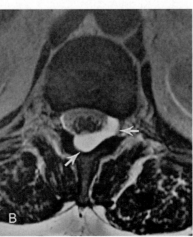

Figure 13–64. EPIDURAL SPACE: Arachnoid Cyst.
A, T1 sagittal image, lumbar spine. A low-signal mass *(arrowheads)* replaces the posterior epidural fat posterior to L1. *B,* Spin echo-T2 axial image, L1. The high-signal cystic mass in the posterior epidural space *(arrows)* compresses the dural sac.

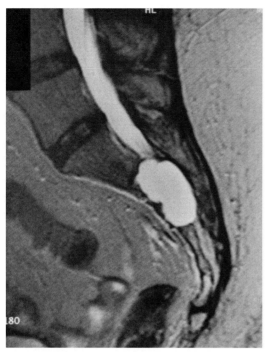

Figure 13–65. EPIDURAL SPACE: Sacral Meningocele.
Fast T2 sagittal image, lumbar spine. There is a large, high-signal, cystic mass in the sacral canal that is eroding the bone of the sacrum from pressure. This is a sacral meningocele that has higher signal than the cerebrospinal fluid because of the relatively slower flow within it.

Intradural Space (Box 13–17)

This is the cerebrospinal fluid-filled subarachnoid space between the dura and the spinal cord; nerve roots are included in this space.

Benign intradural lesions include nerve sheath tumors, meningiomas, paragangliomas, and assorted cysts. Nerve sheath tumors and spinal meningiomas make up about 90% of all intradural tumors, both benign and malignant. The most common malignant abnormality to affect this space is metastases. A common artifact in the intradural space on MRI occurs from turbulent flow of the cerebrospinal fluid, which must not be mistaken for a true mass in this region. It appears as elongated, oblong regions of low signal within the spinal fluid on all pulse sequences, best seen on the T2W images (Fig. 13–68).

Nerve Sheath Tumors. Pathologic and MRI features of these tumors were discussed in detail in Chapter 4 and are not repeated here. Nerve sheath tumors consist of neurofibromas and Schwannomas (neurilemomas). Most nerve sheath tumors (75%) arise within the dura, but a few are located both intradurally and in the epidural space ("dumbbell" lesions), whereas a few more are located completely outside the dura (either epidural or paraspinous) (Fig. 13–69). They may be solitary or multiple.

Meningioma. Most spinal meningiomas are benign, occur in the thoracic spine or, less commonly, the cervical spine, usually in women. They have a broad attachment to the dura, and on MRI studies show signal intensity similar to the cord on all pulse sequences and diffuse homogenous enhancement with contrast (Fig. 13–70). Some meningiomas may show areas of dense calcification, which have low signal intensity on all pulse sequences.

Other Tumors. *Paragangliomas* are rare lesions that may occur in several locations in the body. Pheochromocytomas of the adrenal glands are the most common paraganglioma. In the spine, paragangliomas occur in the filum terminale and the cauda equina. MRI shows a mass that is isointense to cord on T1W images and becomes slightly hyperintense to cord on T2W images (Fig. 13–71). Paragangliomas

Figure 13–66. EPIDURAL SPACE: Arachnoid Diverticulum.
A, T1 sagittal image, thoracolumbar spine. There is a rounded, low-signal mass in the right neural foramen at T8–9 *(arrow).* Smaller, but similar-appearing low-signal masses are evident in several neural foramina below T9. There are hemangiomas in T10 and L3 (focal fat within the vertebral bodies). *B,* Fast T2 axial image through T8–9 neural foramen. The high-signal arachnoid diverticulum is evident in the right foramen *(arrow),* separate from the dural sac. There is pressure erosion of the anterior aspect of the transverse process and the posterior vertebral body.

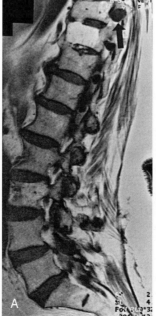

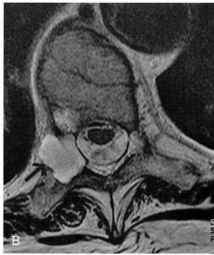

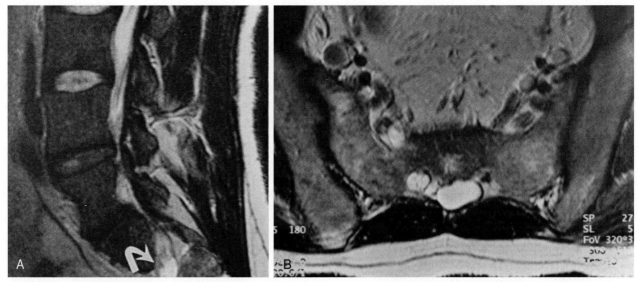

Figure 13–67. EPIDURAL SPACE: Perineural (Tarlov Cyst).
A, Fast T2 sagittal image, lumbar spine. There is a high-signal cyst surrounding the right S2 nerve in the neural foramen *(curved arrow). B,* Fast T2 axial image, S2. The perineural cyst is evident in the right sacral foramen as well as in the central canal as high-signal intensity.

are vascular and show marked contrast enhancement; they may have a heterogeneous appearance from hemorrhage. *Ependymomas* often arise from the filum terminale or conus medullaris and should be considered along with paragangliomas and the much more common nerve sheath tumors or metastases in the differential diagnosis for masses in this anatomic region.

Lipomas. Fatty masses that have signal characteristics typical of fat on all pulse sequences occur in

several locations and forms in the spine, including an intradural location (Fig. 13–72). Intradural lipomas most commonly are found on the dorsal surface of the cord. This is a congenital abnormality associated with occult spinal dysraphism. Much more common than the intradural lipoma are lipomas associated with myelomeningoceles (lipomyelomeningoceles) and tethered cords. Another lipomatous lesion is the filum terminale fibrolipoma, or "fatty filum." The fatty filum is a common MRI finding of

---

BOX 13–17: INTRADURAL ABNORMALITIES

Nerve sheath tumors
• Neurofibroma or schwannoma
• Most are intradural; dumbbell lesions are intra- and extradural
Meningiomas
• Usually women
• Thoracic > cervical
⎱ 90% of intradural lesions

Ependymomas ⎱ Conus/filum terminale/cauda equina region
Paragangliomas ⎰ (include nerve sheath tumor and metastasis in differential for this area)

Cysts
• Epidermoid (lumbar usually)
• Dermoid (lumbar usually, signal resembles fat)
• Arachnoid (posterior thoracic, usually)
Metastases
• Multiple nodules or sheet-like pattern involving leptomeninges in
   conus/cauda equina region
• Contrast enhancement essential to make diagnosis
Lipomas

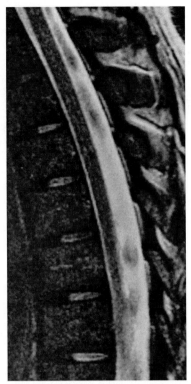

Figure 13–68. INTRADURAL SPACE: Pitfall.
Fast T2 sagittal image, thoracic spine. There are multiple low-signal, oblong regions in the cerebrospinal fluid (CSF) posterior to the thoracic cord secondary to turbulent CSF flow. These are not true masses, and they would remain low signal on T1 sequences also.

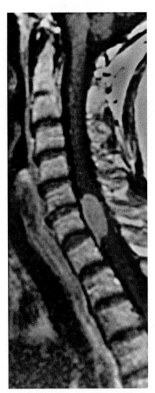

Figure 13–70. INTRADURAL SPACE: Meningioma.
T1 contrast-enhanced sagittal image, cervical spine. There is an enhancing mass in the anterior intradural space with a broad-based attachment to the anterior dura. This is a typical appearance for a meningioma.

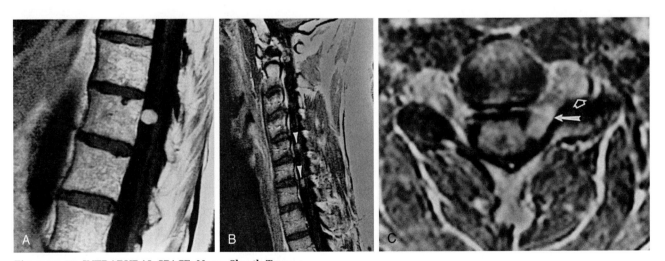

Figure 13–69. INTRADURAL SPACE: Nerve Sheath Tumors.
A, T1 contrast-enhanced sagittal image, lumbar spine. There is a round, enhancing mass posterior to an upper lumbar vertebral body within the dural sac. This was a schwannoma at surgery. *B,* T1 contrast-enhanced sagittal image, cervical spine (different patient than in *A*). Two enhancing lesions are present in the anterior dural sac *(arrowheads),* surrounded by cerebrospinal fluid. These were neurofibromas. *C,* T1 contrast-enhanced axial image, cervical spine (same patient as in *B*). A neurofibroma is present in the intradural space *(solid arrow)* and extends into the epidural space in the neural foramen *(open arrow).* This is a dumbbell neurofibroma that is both intra- and extradural.

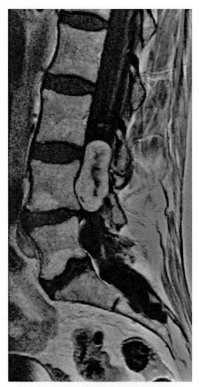

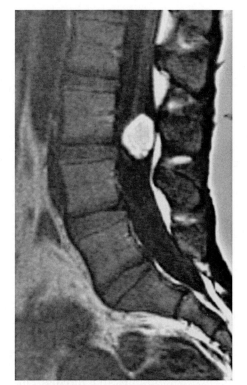

Figure 13–71. INTRADURAL SPACE: Paraganglioma.
T1 contrast-enhanced sagittal image, lumbar spine. There is a large mass involving the cauda equina that fills the dural sac and erodes the posterior L4 vertebral body, indicating it is a long-standing lesion. The center of the mass is low signal from necrosis or hemorrhage. This was a paraganglioma at surgery; the differential diagnosis should include ependymoma, metastasis, and nerve sheath tumor.

Figure 13–72. INTRADURAL SPACE: Lipoma.
T1 sagittal image, lumbar spine. There is a high-signal mass in the dural sac from an intradural lipoma. The patient presented with atrophy in one of the lower extremities from nerve compression.

no clinical significance. It consists of a filum that has a normal size and shape, but is infiltrated with fat and follows the signal of fat on all pulse sequences (Fig. 13–73).

Intradural Cystic Lesions. These include epidermoid, dermoid, and arachnoid cysts.

Epidermoid cysts are either congenital, in which case they occur in the cauda equina or conus, or acquired from lumbar punctures and occur in the lower lumbar region. MRI features are variable and nonspecific, but generally show a mass of low signal intensity on T1W and high signal intensity on T2W images (higher than spinal fluid).

Dermoid cysts are congenital tumors that arise from epithelial inclusions in the neural groove during development. They may either be located intradurally or within the cord in equal numbers. They usually are found in the lumbar spine, and signal characteristics on MRI are similar to fat.

Arachnoid cysts are rare lesions that usually arise in the posterior aspect of the thoracic spine. Their cause is uncertain. Adhesions in the subarachnoid space from previous trauma and bleeding may be a cause of these cysts. They communicate with the subarachnoid space and have the signal characteristics of cerebrospinal fluid on MRI examinations, so that they may be difficult or impossible to see except

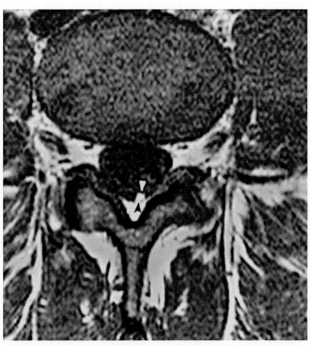

Figure 13–73. INTRADURAL SPACE: Fatty Filum Terminale.
T1 axial image, lumbar spine. When fat infiltrates a normal-sized filum terminale, it is of no consequence and is known as a lipoma of the filum, or simply as a fatty filum *(arrowheads)*.

for the mass effect they have on the cord by displacing it.

Metastases. Metastases to the subarachnoid space usually involve the lumbosacral spine. They are multiple and are deposited in the arachnoid and pia mater. The conus and cauda equina may be diffusely involved, with a sheet-like infiltrative pattern or with multiple nodules. The leptomeninges (the arachnoid that lines the dural sac and the pia that covers the cord and nerve roots) may be involved by metastases from primary tumors arising in the central nervous system or from any other primary carcinoma, lymphoma, or leukemia. MRI may not show these lesions unless intravenous contrast is used. There may be thickened nerve roots or multiple small intradural nodules that are high signal intensity from contrast enhancement on T1W images. Contrast enhancement of the leptomeninges also can be seen in inflammatory causes of meningitis.

Spinal Cord Lesions
(Boxes 13–18 and 13–19)

Lesions arising within the cord are varied and numerous, but their MRI appearance is as limited as abnormalities of tendons. In a nutshell, just about all that can happen with abnormalities in the cord is that there is signal intensity different from the normal cord (usually, high signal intensity on T2W or contrast-enhanced T1W images) and the caliber of the cord may increase, decrease, or remain normal.

Lesions most commonly found in the spinal cord generally are caused by **D**emyelinating diseases, **C**ysts, **I**nfarction, or **T**umor; thus, our mnemonic **DCIT: D**amn **C**ord **I**s **T**rouble. This obviously is not an exhaustive list of all abnormalities that can affect the cord, but it covers the vast majority and the most common entities.

Demyelination Abnormalities. Myelomalacia, multiple sclerosis, transverse myelitis (usually from infection or postvaccination), compressive myelopathy (as from a disk extrusion or spinal stenosis), and radiation myelopathy fall into this category. These lesions usually are difficult to identify on T1 unenhanced images, have high signal intensity on T2W images, and may have diffuse or patchy increased signal or no enhancement on T1W enhanced images. The margins of these lesions may not be as distinct as compared with a syrinx. The cord caliber is usually normal, but may be enlarged or atrophic. Plaques from multiple sclerosis usually are located in the posterior and lateral regions of the cord, and posttraumatic myelomalacia occurs at the site of previous spinal trauma; other demyelinating lesions have no predilection for a specific site. Myelomalacia is discussed further in the section on cysts of the cord (below), because posttraumatic myelomalacia may lead to cyst or syrinx formation, and it may be difficult or impossible to differentiate among these entities by MRI.

Cysts. Hematomyelia and hydrosyringomyelia

BOX 13–18: SPINAL CORD:
Abnormalities within the Cord

Mnemonic: **D**amn **C**ord **I**s **T**rouble
Demyelination
- Myelomalacia
- Multiple sclerosis
- Transverse myelitis
- Compressive myelopathy (disks, osteophytes)
- Radiation myelopathy

Cysts
- Hematomyelia
  —Signal varies with age of lesion
- Intramedullary cysts in area of posttraumatic myelomalacia
  —Round, may progress to typical syrinx
- Syrinx
  —Trauma and congenital lesions (Chiari malformation) associated
  —Elongated with ↓ signal on T1 and proton density; ↑ signal on T2

Infarction
- Causes
  —Arteriosclerotic disease
  —Arteriovenous malformations
  —Aortic dissection

Tumors
- Ependymoma
  —Conus or filum, most common
- Astrocytoma
  —Cysts often associated
- Hemangioblastoma
- Metastases

---

cause cysts in the cord that are unrelated to underlying neoplasm. Hematomyelia was described earlier in the trauma section, and the appearance of blood varies with its age. After trauma, myelomalacia may develop at the site of trauma. Eventually, small cysts may form in the area of myelomalacia and coalesce into an apparent rounded, posttraumatic intramedullary cyst, which is known as progressive posttraumatic myelomalacic myelopathy (Fig. 13–74). The cavities that form in the areas of myelomalacia may then progress to a typical elongated syrinx.

A syrinx may be the sequela of trauma, occurring several months to many years after the traumatic event, and it occurs at the site of the trauma. Posttraumatic syringomyelia probably occurs from bleeding, which leads to arachnoid adhesions, tethering of the cord to the dura (usually dorsally, where blood pools with the patient supine), and consequent turbulent flow of cerebrospinal fluid, which initiates cord cavitation. Syringomyelia also occurs in association with several congenital abnormalities, in particular the Chiari malformation.

A syrinx has sharply demarcated margins from the cord and usually has signal intensity that is

BOX 13–19: SPINAL CORD LESIONS: MRI Features

	Cord Contour	T2 Signal	Contrast-enhanced T1 Signal
Demyelination	↑, normal, ↓	↑ (or sometimes normal with cord atrophy)	↑ (diffuse or patchy), or none
Cysts	↑ usually	↑	None
Infarction	↑, normal, ↓	↑ H pattern in gray matter	↑ (patchy or diffuse), or none
Tumors	↑ usually	↑	↑ (patchy or diffuse), or none

isointense to cerebrospinal fluid on all pulse sequences (Fig. 13–75). The cystic lesions do not demonstrate contrast enhancement. The cord caliber often appears increased, but actually is reduced from atrophy, and the intramedullary cyst or syrinx causes focal expansion of the cord contour. Myelomalacia and a posttraumatic cyst or syrinx can look very similar on MRI (Fig. 13–76). Proton density images may be useful in the differentiation, because myelomalacia has intermediate to high signal intensity on this sequence, whereas a syrinx has low signal intensity. In general, however, a syrinx follows the signal intensity of cerebrospinal fluid, whereas myelomalacia is slightly different in appearance even on standard T1W and T2W images. Differentiating between myelomalacia and syringomyelia on standard spine MR examinations is usually impossible. Cord atrophy without signal abnormalities is another manifestation of myelomalacia that will clearly not be confused with a syrinx.

Infarction. Arteriosclerotic disease, arteriovenous malformations, aortic dissection, and disk extrusions or other masses all may cause cord infarction. The MRI appearance is high signal intensity on T2W

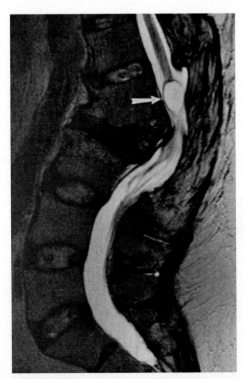

Figure 13–74. CORD: Progressive Posttraumatic Myelomalacic Myelopathy.
Fast T2 sagittal image, thoracolumbar spine. There is an old healed fracture in the upper lumbar spine with a secondary acute angle kyphosis. A rounded, high-signal, cystic cord lesion *(arrow)* is present posterior to the fracture site. This is compatible with an area of previous myelomalacia in the cord that developed cysts, which coalesced into a rounded cyst, known as progressive posttraumatic myelomalacic myelopathy. This will probably progress proximally into a typical elongated syrinx.

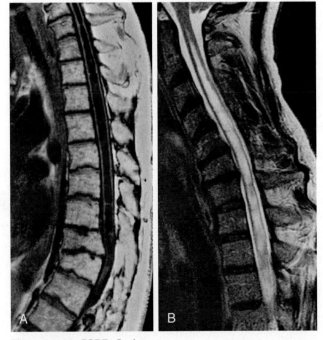

Figure 13–75. CORD: Syrinx.
A, T1 sagittal image, thoracic spine. Old fracture of the lower thoracic spine is evident with retropulsion into the spinal canal. There is very low signal throughout the thoracic cord proximal to the site of previous injury, compatible with a syrinx. *B,* Fast T2 sagittal, cervicothoracic spine (same patient as in *A*). The abnormality within the cord follows the signal of cerebrospinal fluid, is elongated, and progresses proximally from the site of trauma, typical of a syrinx. The cord is markedly atrophic, but the overall contour of the cord is increased in size because of the syrinx.

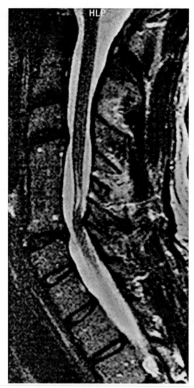

Figure 13–76. CORD: Myelomalacia.
Fast T2 sagittal image, cervical spine. There was previous trauma to the spine with fusion of the mid-cervical vertebral bodies. The cord posterior to the site of the trauma and fusion is atrophied and has linear high signal within it. The atrophy allows the diagnosis of myelomalacia to be made, but the high signal within the cord could otherwise be from a syrinx, as well as from malacia.

images, and shows contrast enhancement as either diffuse or patchy or not at all. The high signal may occur in an H pattern in the central cord because the gray matter is affected preferentially as a result

of the blood supply to the cord (Fig. 13–77). The cord is enlarged initially, but later may be atrophic. Arteriovenous malformations may be seen on MRI as punctate or serpentine areas of low signal intensity from flow void in vessels in or on the surface of the cord. This appearance should not be confused with the much more commonly encountered areas of signal intensity loss in the cerebrospinal fluid from turbulent flow artifact.

Tumors. Ependymomas and astrocytomas comprise about 95% of all cord gliomas. Hemangioblastomas and metastases (especially from lung or breast primaries) are other tumors occurring in the cord. Ependymomas are more common than astrocytomas and usually affect the conus or filum. Ependymomas often become necrotic or hemorrhagic. Astrocytomas often have associated cysts and are long lesions. However, cysts also may be seen with ependymomas (Fig. 13–78) and are frequent with hemangioblastomas. Metastases often have edema surrounding them that is out of proportion to the size of the lesion. Neoplasms usually cause enlargement of the caliber of the cord. Lesions are low signal intensity on T1W images and diffuse or patchy high signal intensity on T2W and T1W enhanced images, with heterogeneous areas present if there has been hemorrhage.

Tethered Cord (Box 13–20)

There are many congenital abnormalities affecting the spine, but only a few are discussed in this chapter. Many of the osseous abnormalities are evaluated best using CT or conventional radiography. Lesions that are manifest at birth or shortly thereafter are not diagnostic dilemmas for us, because they have been thoroughly worked up by the time we see them in our practice, which consists mainly of adults. Thus, congenital lesions such as myeloceles, menin-

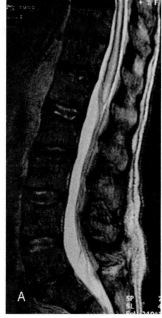
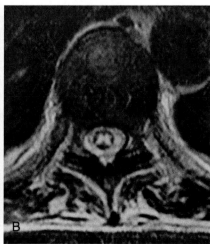

Figure 13–77. CORD: Infarction.
A, Fast T2 sagittal image, lumbar spine. There is increased signal throughout the distal cord in this diabetic patient with severe atherosclerotic disease. *B,* Fast T2 axial image, thoracic spine (same patient as in *A*). The high signal in the center of the cord has an H shape, which is typical of a cord infarction.

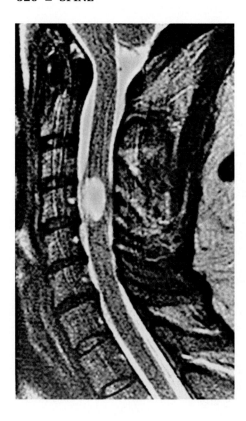

Figure 13–78. CORD: Ependymoma.
Fast T2 sagittal image, cervical spine. There is a cystic mass in the cervical cord with focal increase in caliber of the cord. The findings are good for a glioma, but nonspecific as to which type. This happened to be an ependymoma, although these are typically more common in the conus and without a cystic component.

goceles, myelomeningoceles, and lipomyelomeningoceles (among other congenital lesions) are not described here. One category of congenital spinal abnormalities that may not become manifest until adulthood is that of the tethered cord.

The conus of the spinal cord ends normally at or above the L1–2 disk level; if it exists below this level, it is considered an abnormal *tethered cord*.

An abnormally low (tethered) cord is a common feature of many congenital spinal malformations, and a thickened filum terminale usually is associated with it. Symptoms may become manifest in childhood or adulthood and consist of pain, dysesthesias, spasticity, or loss of bowel and bladder control.

Abnormalities that are associated with a tethered

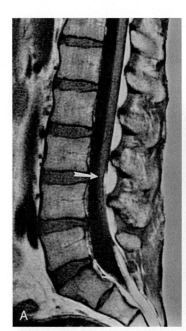
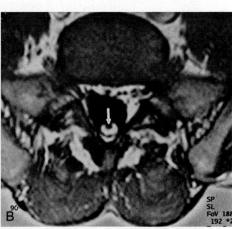

Figure 13–79. TETHERED CORD: Associated Dorsal Lipoma.
A, T1 sagittal image, lumbar spine. The cord is abnormally low, extending at least as far as the L4 vertebra *(arrow). B,* T1 axial image, L5 (same patient as in *A*). There is a high-signal intradural lipoma in the dorsal aspect of the lower lumbar spine, which is surrounding a thickened filum terminale *(arrow).*

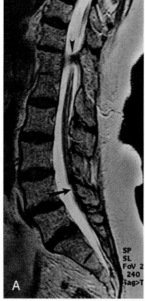
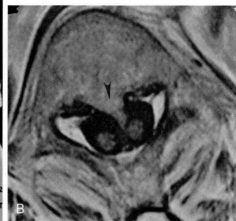

Figure 13–80. TETHERED CORD: Associated Diastematomyelia.
A, Fast T2 sagittal image, lumbar spine. The cord terminates at approximately the L4 level *(arrow).* There is congenital fusion of the T12–L1 vertebrae, with a spike of bone running through the spinal canal at that level *(arrowhead).* *B,* T1 axial image, T12. The bone spike *(arrowhead)* separates the spinal canal and cord into two halves.

cord include, in descending order of frequency, lipoma (a tethered cord often terminates in a dorsally located lipoma) (Fig. 13–79), tight filum terminale, diastematomyelia (Fig. 13–80), and myelomeningocele.[48]

MRI of a tethered cord shows the conus located caudal to the L1–2 level and lack of a sharp transition between the conus and filum (the conus appears elongated). It is essential to evaluate the axial images when a tethered cord is suspected, because the nerve roots of the cauda equina that layer posteriorly in the thecal sac may mimic a low-lying conus on sagittal MR images. There may be associated findings of scoliosis, spinal dysraphism, lipoma, diastematomyelia, or myelomeningocele also present on the imaging study.

References

1. Boden S, Davis D, Dina T, et al. Abnormal magnetic resonance scans of the lumber spine in asymptomatic subjects: a prospective investigation. *J Bone Joint Surg [Am]* 1990; 72:403–408.
2. Yu S, Haughton V, Sether LA. Anulus fibrosus in bulging intervertebral disks. *Radiology* 1988; 169:761–763.
3. Yu S, Haughton VM, Sether LA, et al. Criteria for classifying normal and degenerated intervertebral disks. *Radiology* 1989; 170:523–526.
4. McCarron R, Wimpee M, Hudkins P, et al. The inflammatory effect of nucleus pulposus: a possible element in the pathogenesis of low back pain. *Spine* 1987; 12:760–764.
5. Schellhas KP, Pollei SR, Gundry CR, Heithoff KB. Lumbar disc high-intensity zone: correlation of magnetic resonance imaging and discography. *Spine* 1996; 21:79–86.
6. Jensen M, Brant-Zawadzki M, Obuchowski N, et al. Magnetic resonance imaging of the lumbar spine in people without back pain. *N Engl J Med* 1995; 331:69–73.
7. Saal JA, Saal JS. The non-operative treatment of herniated nucleus pulposus with radiculopathy: an outcome study. *Spine* 1989; 14:431–437.
8. Bozzao A, Gallucci M, Masciocchi C. Lumbar disk herniation: MR imaging assessment of natural history in patients treated without surgery. *Radiology* 1992; 185:135–141.
9. Guinto FC, Hashim H, Stuner M. CT demonstration of disc regression after conservative therapy. *AJNR* 1984; 5:632–657.
10. Pardatscher K, Fiore D, Barbiero A. The natural history of lumbar disc herniations assessed by a CT follow-up study. *Neuroradiology* 1991; 33:84.
11. Saal JA, Saal JS, Herzog RJ. The natural history of lumbar intervertebral disc extrusions treated non-operatively. *Spine* 1990; 15:683–687.
12. Teplick J, Haskin M. Spontaneous regression of herniated nucleus pulposus. *AJNR* 1985; 6:331–335.
13. Modic M. Degenerative disorders of the spine. In Modic M, Masaryk T, Ross J (eds). *Magnetic Resonance Imaging of the Spine.* Chicago: Year Book; 1989.
14. Modic M, Masaryk T, Boymphrey F. Lumbar herniated disc

BOX 13–20: TETHERED CORD

Clinical
• Presents in children or adults
• Pain, dysesthesias, spasticity, loss of bowel and bladder control

Possible Associations
• Scoliosis
• Dysraphic spine
• Thickened filum terminale
• Lipoma
• Diastematomyelia
• Myelomeningocele

MRI Findings
• Conus distal to L1–2 disk
• No sharp transition between conus and filum (conus appears elongated)
• Pitfall: Layering of cauda equina may mimic low-lying cord; must depend on axial images for diagnosis.
• May see associated findings listed above (eg, lipoma)

disease and canal stenosis: prospective evaluation by surface coil MR, CT, and myelography. *AJNR* 1986; 7:709–717.

15. Brown B, Schwartz R, Frank E, et al. Preoperative evaluation of cervical radiculopathy and myelopathy by surface coil MR imaging. *AJR* 1988; 151:1205–1212.

16. Modic M, Masaryk T, Mulopulos G, et al. Cervical radiculopathy: prospective evaluation with surface coil MR imaging, CT with metrizamide, and metrizamide myelography. *Radiology* 1986; 161:753–759.

17. Vanharanta H, Scahs B, Ohnnmeiss D, et al. Pain provocation and disc deterioration by age: a CT/discography study in a low back pain population. *Spine* 1989; 14:420–423.

18. Franson R, Saal JA, Saal JS. Human disc phospholipase A2 is inflammatory. *Spine* 1992; 17:129–132.

19. Olmarker K, Rydenik B, Nordborg C. Autologous nucleus pulposus induces neurophysiologic and histologic changes in procine cauda equina nerve roots. *Spine* 1993; 18:1425–1432.

20. Takahashi M, Jameshita Y, Sakamoto Y, Kojima R. Chronic cervical cord compression: clinical significance of increased signal intensity on MR images. *Radiology* 1989; 173:219–224.

21. Helms CA, Dorwart RH, Gray M. The CT appearance of conjoined nerve roots and differentiation from a herniated nucleus pulposus. *Radiology* 1982; 144:803–807.

22. Schweitzer ME, El-Noueam KI. Vacuum disc: frequency of high signal intensity on T2-weighted MR images. *Skeletal Radiol* 1998; 27:83–86.

23. Malghem J, Maldague B, Labaisse M-A, et al. Intravertebral vacuum cleft: changes in content after supine positioning. *Radiology* 1993; 187:483–487.

24. Dupuy DE, Palmer WE, Rosenthal DI. Vertebral fluid collection associated with vertebral collapse. *AJR* 1996; 167:1535–1538.

25. Lafforgue P, Chagnaud C, Daumen-Legré V, et al. The intravertebral vacuum phenomenon ("vertebral osteonecrosis"): migration of intradiscal gas in a fractured vertebral body? *Spine* 1997; 22:1885–1891.

26. Major NM, Helms CA, Genant HK. Calcification demonstrated as high signal intensity on T1-weighted MR images of the disks of the lumbar spine. *Radiology* 1993; 189:494–496.

27. Modic MT, Steinberg PM, Ross JS, et al. Degenerative disk disease: assessment of changes in vertebral body marrow with MR imaging. *Radiology* 1988; 166:193–199.

28. Dussault RG, Kaplan PA. Facet joint injection: diagnosis and therapy. *Appl Radiol* 1994; 23:35–39.

29. Dussault RG, Kaplan PA, Anderson MW, Whitehill R. Interventional musculoskeletal radiology of the spine. In Taveras JM, Ferrucci JT (eds): *Radiology: Diagnosis–Imaging–Intervention.* Philadelphia: Lippincott-Raven; 1998.

30. Sartoris DJ, Resnick D, Tyson R, Haghighi P. Age-related alterations in the vertebral spinous processes and intervening soft tissues: radiologic-pathologic correlation. *AJR* 1985; 145:1025–1030.

31. Boden S, Davis D, Dina T. Contrast enhanced MR imaging performed after successful lumbar disc surgery: prospective study. *Radiology* 1992; 182:59–64.

32. Ross J, Masaryk T, Modic M. Lumbar spine: postoperative assessment with surface coil MR imaging. *Radiology* 1987; 164:851–860.

33. Deutsch A, Howard M, Dawson E, et al. Lumbar spine following successful surgical discectomy: magnetic resonance imaging features and implications. *Spine* 1993; 18:1054–1060.

34. Ross TS, Masaryk TJ, Schrader M, et al. MR imaging of the postoperative lumbar spine: assessment with gadopentetate dimeglumine. *AJR* 1990; 155:867–872.

35. Dagirmanjian A, Schils J, McHenry M, Modic MT. MR imaging of vertebral osteomyelitis revisited. *AJR* 1996; 167:1539–1543.

36. Roos AE, Meerten EL, Bloem JL, Bluemm RG. MRI of tuberculous spondylitis. *AJR* 1986; 147:79–82.

37. Numaguchi Y, Rigamonti D, Rothman MI, et al. Spinal epidural abscess: evaluation with gadolinium-enhanced MR imaging. *Radiographics* 1993; 13:545–559.

38. Johnson CE, Sze G. Benign lumbar arachnoiditis: MR imaging with gadopentetate dimeglumine. *AJR* 1990; 155:873–880.

39. Ulmer JL, Mathews VP, Elster AD, et al. MR imaging of lumbar spondylolysis: the importance of ancillary observations. *AJR* 1997; 169:233–239.

40. Stäbler A, Bellan M, Weiss M, et al. MR imaging of enhancing intraosseous disk herniation (Schmorl's nodes). *AJR* 1997; 168:933–938.

41. Slucky AV, Potter HG. Use of magnetic resonance imaging in spinal trauma: indications, techniques, and utility. *JAAOS* 1998; 6:134–145.

42. Grenier N, Greselle J-F, Vital J-M, et al. Normal and disrupted lumbar longitudinal ligaments: correlative MR and anatomic study. *Radiology* 1989; 171:197–205.

43. El-Khoury GY, Kathol MH, Daniel WW. Imaging of acute injuries of the cervical spine: value of plain radiography, CT, and MR imaging. *AJR* 1995; 164:43–50.

44. Millar W. Vertebral artery injury after acute cervical spine trauma: rate of occurrence as detected by MR angiography and assessment of clinical consequences. *AJR* 1995; 164:443–447.

45. Kulkarni MV, McArdle CB, Kopanicky D, et al. Acute spinal cord injury: MR imaging at 1.5 T. *Radiology* 1987; 164:837–843.

46. Bradley WG Jr. MR appearance of hemorrhage in the brain. *Radiology* 1993; 189:15–26.

47. Friedman DP. Symptomatic vertebral hemangiomas: MR findings. *AJR* 1996; 167:359–364.

48. Raghavan N, Barkovich AJ, Edwards M, Norman D. MR imaging in the tethered spinal cord syndrome. *AJR* 1989; 152:843–852.

49. Munday TL, Johnson MH, Hayes CT, et al. Musculoskeletal causes of spinal axis compromise: beyond the usual suspects. *Radiographics* 1994; 14:1225–1245.

SPINE PROTOCOLS

This is one set of suggested protocols; there are many variations that would work equally well.

Sequence #	1	2	3	4	5	6
			CERVICAL SPINE: DEGENERATIVE			
Sequence Type	T1	Fast T2	T1	T2*		
Orientation	Sagittal	Sagittal	Axial	Axial		
Field of View (cm)	14	14	11	11		
Slice Thickness (mm)	4	4	4	2		
Contrast	No	No	No	No		
			Stacked	Angle through disks		

THORACIC SPINE: DEGENERATIVE						
Sequence #	1	2	3	4	5	6
Sequence Type	T1	Fast T2	T1	T2*		
Orientation	Sagittal	Sagittal	Axial	Axial		
Field of View (cm)	16	16	12	12		
Slice Thickness (mm)	3	3	9	4		
Contrast	No	No	No	No		
			Stacked	Angle through disks		

LUMBAR SPINE: DEGENERATIVE						
Sequence #	1	2	3	4	5	6
Sequence Type	T1	Fast T2	T1	Fast T2		
Orientation	Sagittal	Sagittal	Axial	Axial		
Field of View (cm)	16	16	14	14		
Slice Thickness (mm)	4	4	4	4		
Contrast	No	No	No	No		
			Angle through disks	Stacked mid L3 to mid S1		

SPINE: POSTOPERATIVE						
Sequence #	1	2	3	4	5	6
Sequence Type	T1	Fast T2	T1	T1	T1	
Orientation	Sagittal	Axial	Axial	Axial	Sagittal	
Field of View (cm)	Depends on site (same as for degenerative protocols)					
Slice Thickness (mm)						
Contrast	No	No	No	Yes	Yes	
		Stacked	Stacked	Stacked		

May also routinely do a fast T2 sagittal sequence if you have time to spare on the scanner.

SPINE: TRAUMA						
Sequence #	1	2	3	4	5	6
Sequence Type	T1	Fast T2*	T2*	T2*	T1	Fast STIR
Orientation	Sagittal	Sagittal	Sagittal	Axial	Axial	Sagittal
Field of View (cm)	Depends on site (same as for degenerative spine protocols)					
Slice Thickness (mm)	4	4	4	4	4	4
Contrast	No	No	No	No	No	No
				Stacked	Stacked	

OSSEOUS SPINE METASTASES/CORD COMPRESSION					
Sequence #	1	2	3	4	5	6
Sequence Type	T1	STIR	T1	Fast T2	***	
Orientation	Sagittal	Sagittal	Axial	Axial		
Field of View (cm)	Depends on site covered (same as for degenerative spine protocols)					
Slice Thickness (mm)	4	4	8	8		
Contrast	No	No	No	No		
			Stacked	Stacked		

***If mass is seen in epidural space or cord, give intravenous contrast and repeat sagittal and axial T1 sequences through abnormal region(s).

SPINE: INFECTION/INTRADURAL LESIONS					
Sequence #	1	2	3	4	5	6
Sequence Type	T1	Fast T2	T1	Fast T2	T1	T1
Orientation	Sagittal	Sagittal	Axial	Axial	Sagittal	Axial
Field of View (cm)	Depends on site covered (same as for degenerative spine protocols)					
Slice Thickness (mm)	4	4	4	4	4	4
Contrast	No	No	No	No	Yes	Yes
			Stacked	Stacked		Stacked

Scout

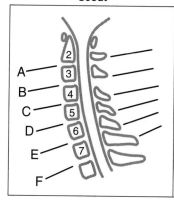

A
B
C
D
E
F

2
3
4
5
6
7

- Sagittal scout

- Obtain images angled through disks from C2-3 through C7-T1 (lines A-F)

- 2-3 slices at each disk, depending on disk height

Final Image

Axials angled through disks

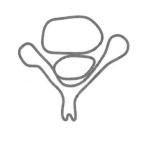

Scout

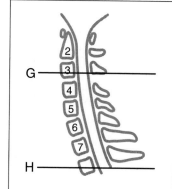

G

H

2
3
4
5
6
7

- Sagittal scout

- Obtain axials in a block with no angulation from line G to line H

- Final image should fill frame, and not include entire neck

Final Image

Stacked axials (no angulation)

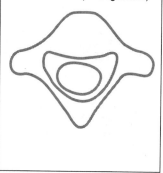

Scout

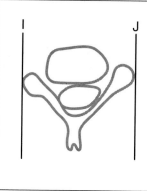

I   J

- Axial or coronal scout

- Obtain sagittal images from line I to line J

- Cover entire osseous spine from skull base through at least T1

Final Image

Sagittals

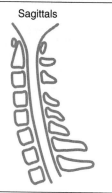

Scout		Final Image
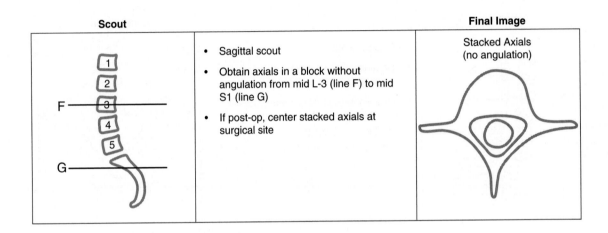	• Sagittal scout • Obtain images angled with disks from L1-2 through L5-S1 (lines A-E) • 2-4 slices at each level, depending on disk height	Axials angled through disks

Scout		Final Image
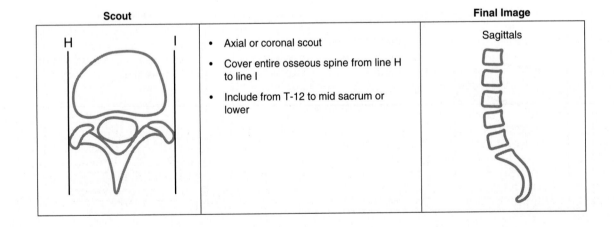	• Sagittal scout • Obtain axials in a block without angulation from mid L-3 (line F) to mid S1 (line G) • If post-op, center stacked axials at surgical site	Stacked Axials (no angulation)

Scout		Final Image
	• Axial or coronal scout • Cover entire osseous spine from line H to line I • Include from T-12 to mid sacrum or lower	Sagittals

14 HIPS AND PELVIS

HOW TO IMAGE THE HIPS AND
PELVIS
NORMAL AND ABNORMAL
Osseous Structures
Normal Osseous Structures
Vascular Abnormalities of Bone
Osteonecrosis (avascular necrosis)
Idiopathic transient osteoporosis
of the hip
Fractures
Fatigue fractures
Insufficiency fractures
Salter fractures
Herniation Pits
Osseous Tumors
Benign osseous lesions
Malignant osseous lesions

Soft Tissues
Muscle/Tendon Abnormalities
Normal capsule/ligaments
Normal muscles
Muscle strains
Gluteus medius tendon tears
Other muscles and tendons
Piriformis syndrome
Nerves
Normal nerves
Abnormal sciatic nerve
Bursae
Iliopsoas bursa
Greater trochanteric bursitis
Soft Tissue Tumors
Benign soft tissue tumors
Malignant soft tissue tumors

Joints
Normal Ligamentum Teres
Labrum
Labral tears
Normal Articular Cartilage
Inflammatory Arthritides
Degenerative Joint Disease
Developmental Dysplasia
Intraarticular Tumors
Pigmented villonodular synovitis
Primary synovial
osteochondromatosis
Amyloid arthropathy
HIP AND PELVIS PROTOCOLS

HOW TO IMAGE THE HIPS AND PELVIS

See the hip and pelvis protocols at the end of the chapter.

Coils/Patient Position. Generally, when evaluating the hips for such entities as avascular necrosis (AVN) or fractures it is possible in many patients to use a torso phased array coil. For larger patients, the body coil is necessary. Both hips and the entire pelvis are imaged simultaneously for most clinical indications. The patient is placed supine in the magnet. For evaluation of smaller structures in the hip joint, such as the labrum or cartilage, a surface coil such as a flexible wrap coil is recommended, and then only the symptomatic hip is evaluated.

Image Orientation (Box 14–1). The most useful information for evaluating hip pathology can be obtained in the axial and coronal planes. Sagittal images sometimes can be difficult to interpret because the fovea centralis may mimic pathology and these images generally give no additional information.

Pulse Sequences/Regions of Interest. A large field of view (24 to 30 cm) is necessary when evaluating both hips and the pelvis simultaneously, as is done for AVN or trauma. Especially in the setting of trauma, the entire osseous pelvis should be evaluated. We routinely scan from the iliac crest to the lesser trochanter. In order to scan the pelvis in a timely fashion, a slice thickness of 6 or 7 mm with an interslice gap of about 3 mm is reasonable. How-ever, when assessing joint pathology such as labral detail, a smaller field of view is recommended (14 to 24 cm), with a smaller slice thickness. We have found that 4 mm slice thickness with a 10% interslice gap (0.4 mm for those who do not wish to do the math) is satisfactory. The coverage for a dedicated hip MR examination should include the supraacetabular location through the bottom of the lesser trochanter.

A T1W sequence is necessary for demonstrating anatomic detail. Some type of T2W image in the same planes also is recommended. The T2W images show edema or fluid that is not necessarily appreciated on the T1W images. Keep in mind that fast spin echo T2W images and (fast) STIR images show fluid and edema with increased conspicuity as compared to other types of T2 sequences. Additionally, (fast) STIR and fast spin echo T2 with fat suppression are marrow-sensitive sequences and are superb for assessing bone marrow edema.

Contrast. Intravenous contrast is generally not necessary, except to differentiate a cystic from solid mass. However, intraarticular contrast is of great benefit when assessing labral pathology. The dilution technique is the same as for the shoulder or any other joint. A 1/200 dilution of gadolinium in normal saline is injected into the joint after confirmation with a small amount of radioopaque contrast material. The high signal contrast (gadolinium) compared with the low signal labrum makes identification of tears easier. Additionally, we recommend fat

---

BOX 14–1: STRUCTURES TO EVALUATE IN DIFFERENT PLANES

Coronal
  Osseous Structures
  • Acetabulum
  • Femoral head, neck
  • Greater, lesser trochanter
  • Sacrum
  • Ilium
  • Sacroiliac joints
  Muscles
  • Gluteal muscles
  • Adductors
  • Abductors
  • Hamstrings
  • Quadriceps
  Labrum
  Pulvinar
Axial
  Osseous Structures
  • Acetabulum
  • Femoral head, neck
  • Greater, lesser trochanter
  • Sacrum
  • Ilium
  • Sacroiliac joints
  Muscles
  • Gluteus maximus, medius, and minimus
  • Sartorius, rectus femoris
  • Gracilis, pectineus, adductor longus, brevis, and magnus
  • Tensor fascia lata
  • Piriformis
  • Obturator internus, externus
  • Gemelli superior and inferior
  • Quadratus femoris
  Labrum
  Pulvinar
Sagittal—Not standard or necessary to perform

---

suppression with T1 and T2W images after intraarticular contrast injection to make the gadolinium more conspicuous.

NORMAL AND ABNORMAL

Osseous Structures

Normal Osseous Structures

The hip is a ball-and-socket joint, allowing for considerable motion with flexion, extension, internal and external rotation, as well as abduction and adduction.

The acetabulum covers 40% of the femoral head and is formed from ilium, ischium, and pubic bones. At birth, these three bones are separated by the triradiate cartilage, a Y-shaped physeal plate. The acetabulum is tilted anteriorly, which explains the greater potential for flexion as compared with extension. Because of the concave shape of the acetabulum, the hip is inherently stable. The depth of the acetabulum is increased by the dense fibrocartilagenous labrum that surrounds it. The combination of the labrum and transverse acetabular ligament makes a complete ring around the acetabulum.

The femur is the longest and strongest bone in the body. The proximal femur is comprised of a head, neck, and greater and lesser trochanters. The femoral head is spherical in shape, but is slightly flattened both anteriorly and posteriorly. With the exception of the fovea, it is covered by articular cartilage that ends approximately at the level of the epiphyseal plate at the femoral head–neck junction. The fovea is seen as an indentation in the normal round contour of the femoral head on its medial aspect, and is the site of attachment of the ligamentum teres.

The trochanters are apophyses, which add to the width of bone and not its length. The greater trochanter serves as the insertion site for the tendons of the gluteus medius and minimus, the obturator internus and externus, and the piriformis muscles. The lesser trochanter receives the iliopsoas tendon (Fig. 14–1).

The bone marrow of the pelvis and hips is generally diffuse or patchy intermediate signal (but higher signal than muscle on T1W images) because of the large amount of red marrow that persists in this region throughout life. The epiphyses and apophyses should have high signal fatty marrow on T1W images. Occasionally, a small rim of red marrow may parallel the subchondral bone of the femoral epiphysis; this is considered normal. Thick stress trabeculae in the femoral neck can be seen as low signal lines on MRI, as can linear physeal scars at the femoral head–neck junction.

Vascular Abnormalities of Bone

Osteonecrosis (Avascular Necrosis) (Box 14–2). One of the major indications for MRI of the hip is for detection of osteonecrosis of the femoral head. The presumed mechanism of mechanical failure of the femoral head is accumulated stress fractures of necrotic trabeculae that are not repaired. MRI is capable of detecting the early stages of ischemic necrosis, which is important clinically so that therapy can be instituted before the onset of femoral head collapse, fragmentation, degenerative change, and hip replacement. Early diagnosis can lead to joint-sparing techniques such as core decompression, rotational osteotomy, or free vascularized fibular graft.

Numerous causes of AVN have been proposed, including trauma, steroids, hemoglobinopathies, al-

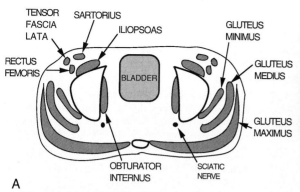

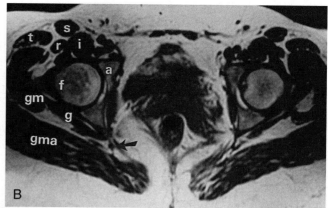

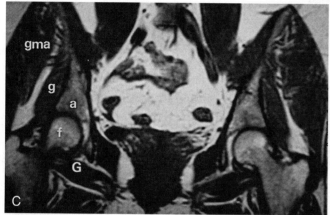

Figure 14–1. NORMAL ANATOMY OF THE PELVIS.
A, Sketch showing normal anatomy. *B,* Axial and *C,* coronal T1W images through a normal pelvis. a—acetabulum; f—femoral head; g—gluteus minimus; gm—gluteus medius; gma—gluteus maximus; r—rectus femoris; t—tensor fascia lata; s—sartorius; I—iliopsoas; G—gemella. *Arrow* points to the sciatic nerve.

coholism, pancreatitis, Gaucher's disease, radiation, and idiopathic when no cause can be identified. Keep in mind that both anabolic and catabolic steroid use can result in AVN.

AVN is bilateral in 40% of hips, so both hips should be imaged simultaneously for this indication. The classification scheme for AVN observed on radiographs cannot be used for MRI. MR proves most useful when plain films are negative.[1] It is also more sensitive than computed tomography (CT) or radionuclide bone scintigraphy.[2] Additionally, MR can provide information regarding articular cartilage, marrow conversion, joint fluid, and associated insufficiency fractures, which are also common in patients taking steroids.

The appearance of AVN on MRI includes a diffuse pattern of bone marrow edema early (identical in appearance to transient bone marrow edema), subsequently becoming more focal in the femoral head; a serpiginous line of low signal intensity surrounding an area of fatty marrow in the femoral head between the 10 o'clock and 2 o'clock positions on coronal images (usually anterior in the femoral head) is characteristic for AVN (Figs. 14–2 and 14–3). This is the typical geographic pattern of AVN that is seen most often. Collapse of bone and sclerosis may result in a focal area of low signal on T1W images that is variable signal on T2W images (Fig. 14–4)—in other words, not a fatty center. This latter appearance is not common and is less specific than the geographic pattern. On spin echo T2W images, the double-line sign has been described as an appearance typical of ischemic necrosis. The double line is a line of low signal that surrounds an inner line of high signal on T2W images. The double-line sign is not present in many cases of AVN. MR signal abnormalities such as the double-line sign initially were thought to be helpful in staging osteonecrosis because they corresponded to histologic findings;[3]

BOX 14–2: AVASCULAR NECROSIS

Cause
Trauma, steroids, hemoglobinopathies, alcoholism, pancreatitis, Gaucher's disease, radiation therapy, idiopathic
MRI
• Diffuse edema (low T1, ↑ T2) early
• Focal serpiginous low signal line with fatty center (most common appearance)
• Double-line sign
• Focal subchondral low signal lesion on T1 with variable signal on T2
Location
• 10 o'clock to 2 o'clock position on coronal images
• Anterior femoral head affected first

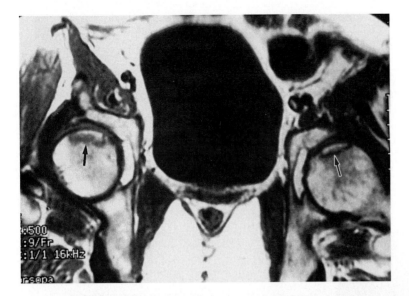

Figure 14–2. AVASCULAR NECROSIS.
Coronal T1W image in 51-year-old man with left hip pain and normal bone scintigraphy. Serpiginous low-signal area in the subchondral location is noted in both femoral heads *(arrows)* with fat in center. A small amount of edema is noted in the left hip, as demonstrated by surrounding low signal.

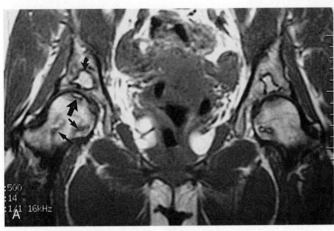
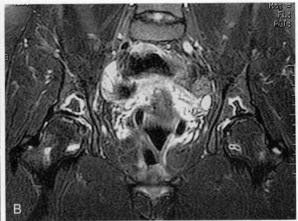

Figure 14–3. AVASCULAR NECROSIS (AVN).
A, Coronal T1W image demonstrating serpiginous, low-signal areas in the proximal femur *(small arrows)* and acetabulae *(curved arrow)*. Note the curvilinear low signal in the subchondral location of the femora *(large arrow)* compatible with AVN. *B,* Fast spin echo, fat suppressed T2W image shows serpiginous high signal with fat in the center in the areas of infarcts and AVN.

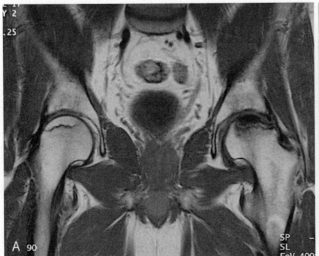
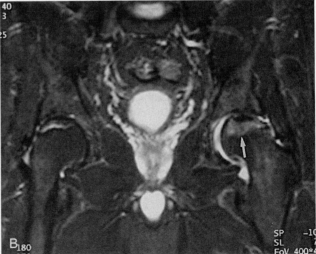

Figure 14–4. AVASCULAR NECROSIS (AVN).
A, Coronal T1W image shows curvilinear, serpiginous low-signal intensity in the femoral heads bilaterally. The articular surface of the left femoral head is slightly collapsed and irregular; the lesion is diffusely low signal. *B,* Coronal fast T2 image with fat suppression shows the changes of AVN with surrounding edema in the left femoral head *(arrow)*, and the double-line sign on the right side.

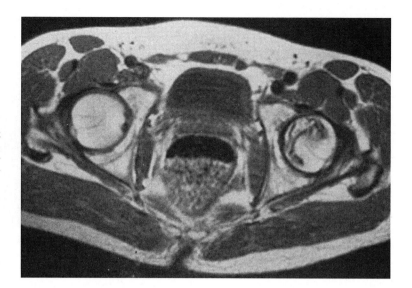

Figure 14–5. AVASCULAR NECROSIS (AVN).
Axial T1W image in a 35-year-old man with left hip pain and no risk factors for AVN. Low-signal, serpiginous areas in subchondral location characteristic for AVN are well demonstrated. Note the typical anterior involvement of the femoral head.

however, because the prognostic significance is not clear, staging based on signal characteristics generally is not recommended.

Important additional findings necessary to report to the clinician include the volume of the head that is involved with AVN. This is best determined with axial imaging (Fig. 14–5). Additionally, findings of degenerative disease such as joint space narrowing and osteophytes are important to report, because this helps with staging of the disease. Similarly, it is important to report collapse of the femoral head (Fig. 14–4). The presence and amount of a joint effusion often correspond to the severity of clinical pain symptoms.

Misinterpretation of osteonecrosis may occur if one is not familiar with a few potential pitfalls (Box 14–3). Occasionally, normal hematopoietic marrow can be identified in the femoral head. A synovial herniation pit, which represents a tiny defect in the bone that allows joint fluid to fill this space (analogous to a subchondral cyst, but removed from the articular surface), can erroneously be interpreted as an area of AVN (Fig. 14–6).[4] The fovea centralis, a normal anatomic finding, inadvertently may be diagnosed as a site of AVN with subchondral collapse (Fig. 14–7). Subchondral cysts from degenerative joint disease of the hip may appear similar to AVN, but the low signal margins of the cyst are smooth and regular, rather than serpiginous as with AVN. Also, abnormalities on both sides of the joint usually are present, with evidence of degenerative cysts and degenerative cartilage loss and osteophytes. Metastases occasionally may have an appearance similar to AVN that is diffusely low signal on the T1W images.

Legg-Calvé-Perthes disease is an idiopathic avascular necrosis of the growing femoral epiphysis that results in a progressive deformity and outward displacement of the femoral head; it occurs in children 4 to 10 years of age (Box 14–4). MRI has been reported to be useful for assessing Legg-Calvé-Perthes. Diffuse low signal in the femoral head on the T1 and T2W images is the most common finding. Collapse of the femoral epiphysis also can occur.[5, 6] Jaramillo and associates showed that physeal bridging and deformity of the femoral head with abnormal low signal in the head on MRI were statistically significant predictors of growth arrest.[6, 7] Abnormalities of the epiphysis did not relate to growth arrest. Depiction of physeal bridging at MRI was the best predictor of growth arrest in their study. MRI allows earlier diagnosis and diagnosis of coexistent contralateral disease, as well as monitoring of therapy (Figs. 14–8 and 14–9).

Idiopathic Transient Osteoporosis of the Hip (ITOH) (Box 14–5). Transient osteoporosis of the hip also has been referred to as transient painful bone marrow edema. The first well-documented description was reported in three women during the last trimester of pregnancy.[8] It is an uncommon and

---

BOX 14–3: AVASCULAR NECROSIS

Pitfalls for focal avascular necrosis
• Hematopoietic marrow
• Synovial herniation pit
• Fovea centralis

BOX 14–4: LEGG-CALVÉ-PERTHES DISEASE

• Idiopathic avascular necrosis of femoral head
• 4 to 10 years of age
• May lead to growth arrest
• MR findings: diffuse low signal on T1 and T2W images ± collapse of femoral head
• MR predictors of growth arrest:
  Physeal bridging
  Signal change in physis/metaphysis

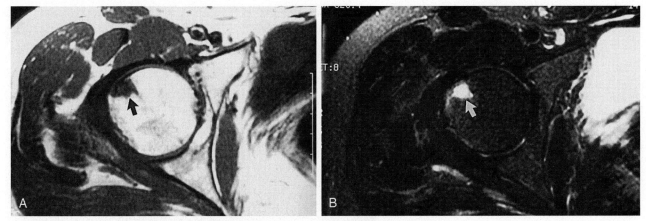

Figure 14–6. AVASCULAR NECROSIS (AVN) PITFALLS: Synovial Herniation Pit.
A, Axial T1W image shows a wedge-shaped area of low signal at the 10 o'clock position *(arrow).* *B,* Axial fast spin echo with fat suppression shows high signal *(arrow)* (similar to that of fluid in the bladder). This is a characteristic location for a synovial herniation pit.

usually self-limited clinical entity of unknown cause that primarily affects middle-aged men (40 to 55 years of age). Although the underlying cause is uncertain, a vascular basis almost certainly exists. When women are affected, it is usually during the third trimester of pregnancy. There are anecdotal reports of ITOH occurring in early pregnancy with resolving hip pain after spontaneous or therapeutic abortions. The male to female ratio is 3:1. This condition is rare in children,[9] and there are no known predisposing factors except pregnancy.[10–12] Generally, only one hip is affected at a time. Recurrence in the same hip can occur.[12] Regional migratory osteoporosis is the name given to this entity when joints other than the hip are subsequently affected.[12]

Clinically, patients present with disabling pain without a history of trauma. The conventional radiograph demonstrates osteopenia isolated to the affected hip. It is important to make the proper diagnosis so correct treatment can be instituted. ITOH generally resolves spontaneously in 6 to 8 months after protected weight-bearing and symptomatic support. Fractures of the hip may occur without protected weight-bearing because of the severity of the localized osteoporosis. Because early AVN can have a similar appearance on imaging and the treatments are different, it becomes important to try and differentiate ITOH from AVN. In fact, there is some controversy as to whether ITOH represents a very early, reversible stage of AVN.[10–12] VandeBerg and colleagues developed criteria to increase sensitivity and specificity of irreversible changes of ITOH that would lead to a diagnosis of AVN.[13] They suggested that the absence of a subchondral low signal intensity on T2W images or postcontrast T1W images suggests a favorable outcome (reversible disease). The presence of a low signal subchondral area measuring more than 4 mm in thickness and greater than 12.5 mm in length on T2W images or postcontrast T1W images suggests an irreversible lesion (AVN). MRI in ITOH shows decreased signal on T1W images and increased signal on the T2W im-

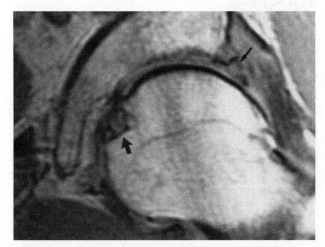

Figure 14–7. AVASCULAR NECROSIS (AVN) PITFALLS: Fovea Centralis.
Coronal T1W image shows a low-signal area medial in location *(arrow).* This represents a prominent fovea centralis (a normal structure). Incidentally, a superior labral tear also is noted *(small arrow).*

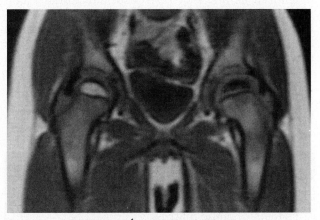

Figure 14–8. LEGG-CALVÉ-PERTHES DISEASE.
Coronal T1W image of a 4-year-old girl. Left hip shows low signal involving the femoral head. The right hip is normal.

BOX 14–5: IDIOPATHIC TRANSIENT OSTEOPOROSIS OF THE HIP (ITOH)

Middle-aged men
Pregnant women
Male:female ratio, 3:1
No history of trauma
Spontaneous resolution (6 to 8 mo)
MR: low signal T1; ↑ T2 signal femoral head
   to intertrochanteric region
Differential: septic hip, avascular necrosis
   (early), osteoid osteoma (younger age group)

BOX 14–6: FRACTURES

Stress fractures—abnormal stress across
   normal bone
Insufficiency fractures—normal stress across
   abnormal bone
   • Femoral neck
   • Sacrum
   • Supraacetabular
   • Pubic bones, superior and inferior pubic
     rami
MR appearance:
   Linear low signal T1 with low-signal edema
   Increased signal (edema) T2 with linear low
     signal (fracture line)
Salter fracture, hip—medial, inferior, posterior
   slip of femoral head
   • Widened physis with edema

ages extending from the femoral head to the intertrochanteric region (Fig. 14–10). These findings have been attributed to bone marrow edema. Joint effusions can be large (Fig. 14–11). Importantly, the signal intensity in the acetabulum is normal. These characteristics have been reported within 48 hours after the onset of symptoms of ITOH.[10] An intraarticular osteoid osteoma of the hip can cause marrow edema in a similar distribution as ITOH, and a cortically based, small, round lesion should be carefully searched for in order to exclude this; however, different age groups generally are affected by these two disease processes. Infection of the proximal femur with a septic joint also should be considered in the differential diagnosis on MRI.

Fractures (Box 14–6)

Fatigue Fractures. Stress fractures occur commonly about the hips and in the pelvis. Stress fractures are divided into fatigue fractures and insufficiency fractures. Fatigue fractures result from increased or abnormal stress applied to normal bone. MRI is superb for evaluating this abnormality and may be positive when the conventional radiograph is negative.[14] Bone scintigraphy is sensitive but not specific for stress fractures or stress reactions. MRI is both sensitive and specific because it can show the linear fracture or marrow edema from a stress reaction (Figs. 14–12 through 14–14). Because of the exquisite contrast and intrinsic spatial resolution of MRI, this abnormality can be diagnosed early, leading to early and appropriate treatment.

Stress reactions occur typically in the femoral neck along the medial aspect (compressive surface) or the superior surface (tensile surface). Additional locations of stress fractures in the pelvis include the pubic rami (superior and inferior) and sacrum. Stress fractures image as linear low signal surrounded by bone marrow edema.

Insufficiency Fractures. Insufficiency fractures may occur in the osteoporotic population. These are fractures that occur from physiologic stresses on bone weakened by osteoporosis. In the clinical setting of a painful hip in an osteoporotic patient (even with no significant history of trauma, and despite the fact that the patient may be able to bear weight),

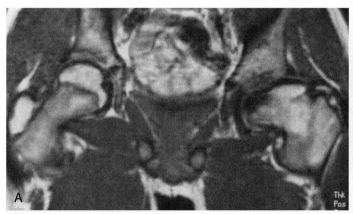
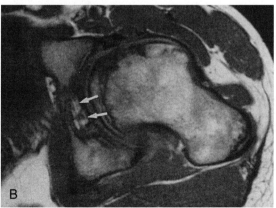

Figure 14–9. LEGG-CALVÉ-PERTHES DISEASE.
A, Coronal T1W image shows irregularity of left femoral head with widening of the femoral neck. *B,* Axial T1W image in the same patient shows the amount of femoral head involved with irregular surface. Note normal pulvinar *(small arrows).*

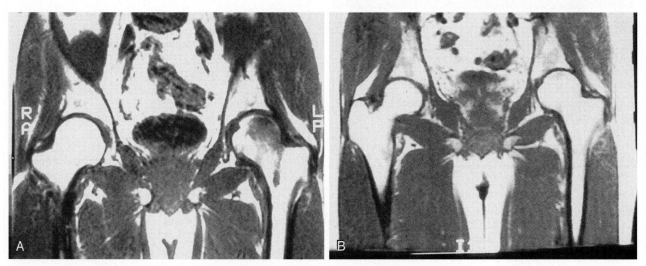

Figure 14–10. IDIOPATHIC TRANSIENT OSTEOPOROSIS OF THE HIP.
A, Coronal T1W image of a 54-year-old man with left hip pain shows low signal involving the left femoral head and neck. *B,* Coronal T1W image 6 months later shows normal hips bilaterally.

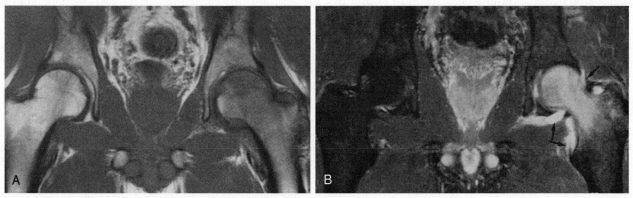

Figure 14–11. IDIOPATHIC TRANSIENT OSTEOPOROSIS OF THE HIP.
A, Coronal T1W image shows low signal involving the left femoral head and neck to the intertrochanteric line. *B,* Coronal fat-suppressed T2W image shows high signal in the femoral head and neck, representing bone marrow edema from hyperemia. Note the large joint effusion *(arrows).*

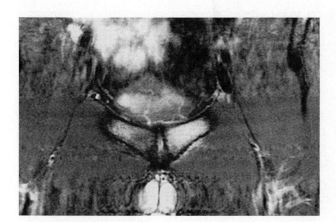

Figure 14–12. STRESS REACTION: Pubic Symphysis.
Coronal fat-suppressed T2W image shows high signal in the pubic bones bilaterally, compatible with stress reaction.

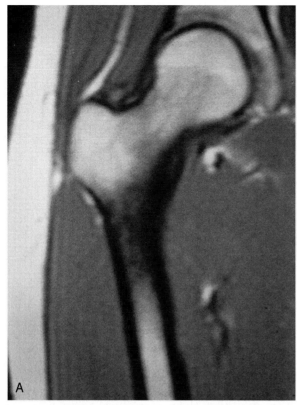

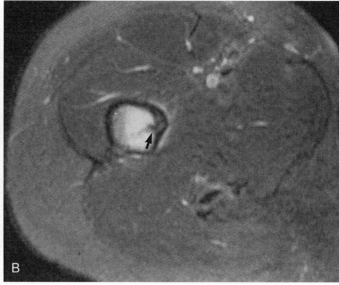

Figure 14–13. STRESS (FATIGUE) FRACTURE.
A, Coronal T1W image in a 33-year-old woman with groin pain while training for a marathon. Low signal extends along medial aspect of femoral neck. Periosteal thickening is evident. *B,* Axial fast spin echo image with fat suppression shows linear, low-signal fracture line *(arrow)* with surrounding edema and edema adjacent to periosteum.

a radiographically occult fracture may exist.[15] MRI is the fastest, most cost effective, and most sensitive and specific method for making the diagnosis in this setting. A limited MR examination consisting of coronal and axial images of the entire pelvis using T1 and fat-suppressed T2W sequences can be done to evaluate for this entity. Any marrow sequence will do. MR demonstrates linear low signal with surrounding bone marrow edema on T1W images. The fracture remains low in signal on T2W images, but surrounding bone marrow edema is high in signal intensity (Fig. 14–15). The reason we recommend including the entire pelvis in the field of view is that pain in the hip may be referred from abnormalities outside of the hip, such as sacral insufficiency fractures. Multiple fractures often coex-

Figure 14–14. FEMORAL NECK (FATIGUE) FRACTURE.
A, Coronal T1W image shows low signal in femoral neck with focal linear low signal (fracture). *B,* Coronal STIR image shows marrow edema with low-signal fracture line.

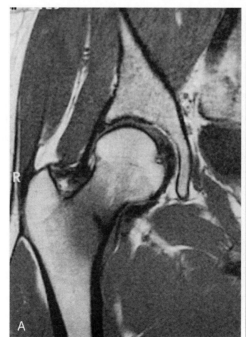

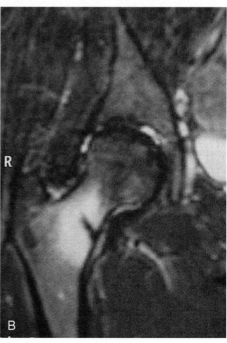

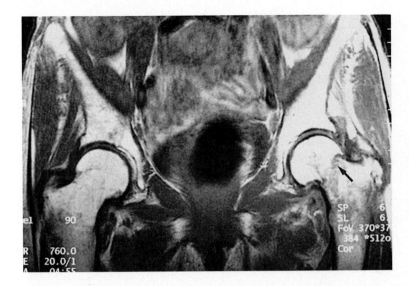

Figure 14–15. INSUFFICIENCY FRACTURE, FEMORAL NECK.
Elderly female with left hip pain and normal plain films. Coronal T1W image shows linear low signal in the femoral neck *(arrow).*

ist. The most common locations for insufficiency fractures of the hips and pelvis are subcapital, intertrochanteric, sacral, supraacetabular, pubic bones, and superior or inferior pubic rami.

A *sacral insufficiency fracture* has a pathognomonic appearance on MR. The T1W images show linear low signal (representing the fracture), usually paralleling the sacroiliac joint with surrounding bone marrow edema (low signal on T1W images and high signal on T2W images). Generally, the bone marrow edema is confined to the sacral ala with the fracture and does not extend across the midline unless the fracture is bilateral (Figs. 14–16 and 14–17). If the linear component of the fracture is not evident, the abnormality of the sacral marrow may mimic metastatic disease.

Supraacetabular insufficiency fractures are reliably diagnosed with MRI by noting a curvilinear (eyebrow-shaped) low signal fracture line that parallels the roof of the acetabulum, accompanied by surrounding bone marrow edema (low in signal on the T1W images that becomes high in signal on the T2W images) (Fig. 14–18).[16] These fractures are seen in the same patient population that suffers from sacral insufficiency fractures; ie, patients with osteoporosis and especially patients who had previous pelvic radiation, which very significantly weakens the bone. The characteristic curvilinear low signal fracture line should be identified, along with the geographic appearance of the bone marrow edema, so that insufficiency fractures are not confused with metastatic disease, which generally has diffuse edema and perhaps an associated soft tissue mass with destruction of the acetabulum.

Both insufficiency and fatigue fractures have a predilection for the femoral neck and pubic bones (although they have been reported in the sacrum), whereas supraacetabular and sacral fractures are almost exclusively of the insufficiency type in osteoporotic individuals.

Salter Fractures (Box 14–7). Traumatic epiphyseal slip can occur in skeletally immature individu-

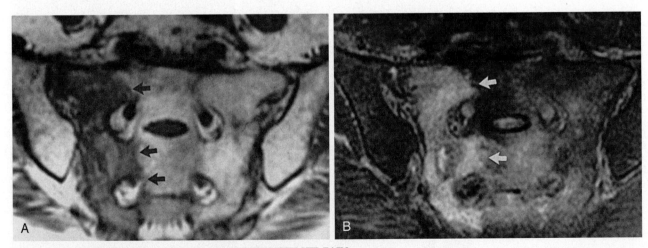

Figure 14–16. SACRAL INSUFFICIENCY FRACTURE WITH HIP PAIN.
A, Axial T1W image in a 57-year-old woman with a history of breast cancer and right hip pain. Low signal is identified in a linear orientation through the right sacral ala *(arrows). B,* Axial fast spin echo image with fat suppression shows high signal from a sacral insufficiency fracture in the same area *(arrows).*

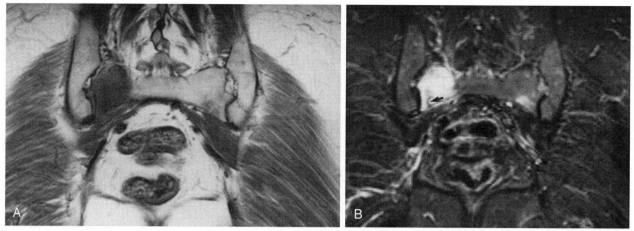

Figure 14–17. SACRAL INSUFFICIENCY FRACTURE.
A, Coronal T1W image shows linear low signal in the right sacral ala with surrounding poorly defined, low-signal edema that does not cross the midline. A small left sacral insufficiency fracture is beginning. *B,* Coronal STIR image shows bone marrow edema (high signal) bilaterally with linear low signal, representing the fracture line on the right side *(arrow).*

als in the setting of infant abuse and even as a result of birth trauma. If the femoral head ossification center is not mineralized, conventional radiography may suggest developmental dysplasia of the hip (due to lateral displacement of the femoral shaft). A T2W sequence, particularly fast spin echo with fat suppression or (fast) STIR imaging, shows edema and hemorrhage through the physis, and is diagnostic of a shear injury.

Slipped capital femoral epiphysis is predominantly an adolescent occurrence, typically observed between 10 to 17 years of age in boys and 8 to 15 years of age in girls. Boys generally are more frequently affected than girls, and this entity is more common in blacks than whites. The incidence is especially high in overweight children. Proposed causes include adolescent growth spurt, hormonal influences, increased weight and activity that result in repetitive stresses, and a Salter 1 fracture of the proximal femoral growthplate.

If conventional radiography is equivocal, MRI can be used to assess the relationship of the femoral head and neck. MR shows a widened growthplate with abnormal high signal on the T2W image through the growthplate, with medial and posteriorly located femoral epiphysis with respect to the metaphysis. On the coronal T1W image, the growthplate appears wider than normal, as evidenced by increased width of the low signal physis (Fig. 14–19). These findings can aid the surgeon with operative planning. An additional important advantage of MRI is its ability to identify early osteonecrosis, which can be seen in up to 15% of children afflicted with this entity.

Herniation Pits

A commonly encountered aperture in the femoral neck cortex is termed a herniation pit. It is seen on the anterior surface of the femoral neck. Ingrowth

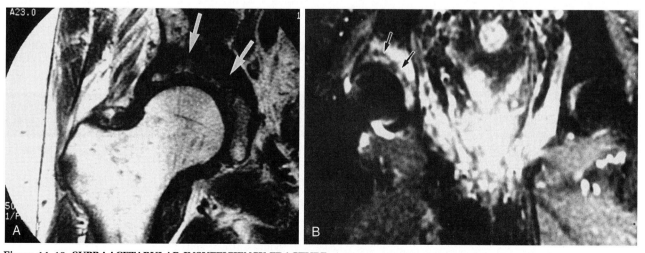

Figure 14–18. SUPRAACETABULAR INSUFFICIENCY FRACTURE.
A, Coronal T1W image in an 80-year-old man with prostate carcinoma and right hip pain. Curvilinear low signal is identified paralleling the roof of the acetabulum *(arrows).* Surrounding edema also is present. *B,* Coronal (fast) STIR image shows edema pattern and curvilinear signal diagnostic of supraacetabular insufficiency fracture *(arrows).*

BOX 14–7: SLIPPED CAPITAL FEMORAL EPIPHYSIS (SCFE)

- 10 to 17 yr (males), 8 to 15 yr (females)
- Male > female
- ↑ Incidence in overweight children
- MR: widened growth plate with ↑ T2 signal
  Epiphyseal slip

of fibrous and cartilaginous elements occurs through a perforation in the cortex, resulting in unilateral or bilateral, small, rounded radiolucent areas in the anterolateral aspect of the femoral neck (in the upper outer quadrant of the femoral neck in the coronal plane). Generally, these lesions are unchanging and asymptomatic, although they may enlarge in individuals of all ages, perhaps related to changing mechanics such as the pressure and abrasive effect of the overlying hip capsule and anterior muscles. MRI generally shows a focus of low signal intensity on T1W images and high signal intensity of T2W images consistent with that of fluid (Fig. 14–20) in the typical location, as described earlier.

Osseous Tumors

Benign Osseous Lesions (Box 14–8). The hip is not a site unique to any particular bone tumor. A benign lesion that can be found incidentally is an enchondroma. As in other long bones, it is well defined, lobular in contour, and low in signal intensity on T1W images and high in signal intensity on T2W images. The stippled calcification seen on conventional radiography is low signal on all imaging sequences (Fig. 14–21).

Another lesion that can be seen in the epiphysis, trochanters (apophysis), or flat bones of the pelvis is

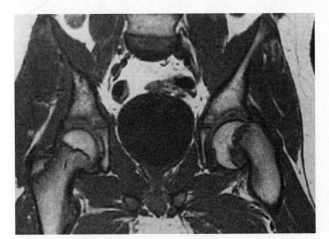

Figure 14–19. SLIPPED CAPITAL FEMORAL EPIPHYSIS. Coronal T1W image shows marked inferior slip of femoral head from the growthplate in the left hip. Note normal relationship of right femoral head and neck.

a giant cell tumor. The appearance on conventional radiographs is usually characteristic. MRI is helpful if the conventional imaging is not diagnostic. Giant cell tumor is low in signal on T1W images and is intermediate on T2W images. This tumor usually does not get very bright on the T2W images. MR can show areas of cortical destruction and the extent of the soft tissue component.

In children and young adults, a chondroblastoma occasionally is encountered around the hip. As with giant cell tumor, chondroblastoma also has a predilection for the epiphysis or apophysis. MR demonstrates a rounded lesion with low signal on the T1W image; the T2W image also shows low to intermediate signal intensity, generally with a large area of surrounding marrow edema (low signal on T1 and high signal on T2W images). Calcified chondroid matrix may be identified as punctate areas of low signal within the lesion, but is better appreciated on computed tomography (CT) than with MR. Periosteal elevation also can be seen occasionally with this lesion. It is not unusual to have a small soft tissue component with this benign lesion (Fig. 14–22).

Occasionally, a subchondral cyst in the femoral head or acetabulum can get very large, mimicking an aggressive lesion, AVN, or something more sinister than what it is. It is not unusual to see subchondral cysts enlarge over time. A search for associated abnormalities, such as joint space narrowing, osteophyte formation (osteoarthritis), or pannus formation (rheumatoid arthritis), can help make the diagnosis of a subchondral cyst. Subchondral cysts image as low signal intensity on T1W images that becomes high in signal (fluid-like) on T2W images.

Malignant Osseous Lesions. There is no primary malignant tumor of bone that is site-specific for the hip or pelvis. Chondrosarcoma does occur in this location more than other malignant tumors of bone. As mentioned in Chapters 7 and 10, it can sometimes be difficult to differentiate an enchondroma from a chondrosarcoma. A soft tissue mass, bone marrow edema, and significant endosteal scalloping are helpful signs that indicate the more aggressive chondrosarcoma. Metastatic lesions and myeloma (plasmacytoma) are the most common malignant

BOX 14–8: COMMON OSSEOUS TUMORS OF THE HIP AND PELVIS

Benign
  Enchondroma
  Chondroblastoma
  Giant cell tumor
  Geode
Malignant
  Metastatic disease
  Myeloma (plasmacytoma)
  Chondrosarcoma

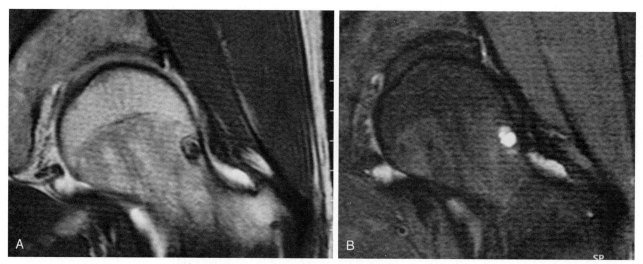

Figure 14–20. SYNOVIAL HERNIATION PIT.
A, Coronal T1W image shows well-defined round area of low signal along the cortical surface in the femoral neck. *B,* Coronal fast T2 image with fat suppression shows high signal in the lesion characteristic of synovial herniation pit.

processes that affect the hip and pelvis and are discussed in detail in Chapter 2.

Soft Tissues

Muscle/Tendon Abnormalities

Normal Capsule/Ligaments. The capsule of the joint attaches to the margin of the acetabular rim and extends distally to cover the femoral neck, inserting anteriorly along the intertrochanteric line and posteriorly halfway down the femoral neck. The greater and lesser trochanters are, therefore, extra-capsular structures. The capsule is lined by synovium, which is not evident on MR when it is normal. The capsule is reinforced externally by three ligaments: the iliofemoral (the strongest), pubofemoral, and ischiofemoral. The iliofemoral ligament inserts on the intertrochanteric line and explains why almost the entire femoral neck is intracapsular. In approximately 15% of individuals, there is a hiatus between the iliofemoral and pubofemoral ligaments; this hiatus allows connection between the hip joint and the adjacent iliopsoas bursa. The capsule is more easily identified when the joint is distended (either with joint fluid or intraarticular contrast), and images as a thin, low-signal structure. Occasion-

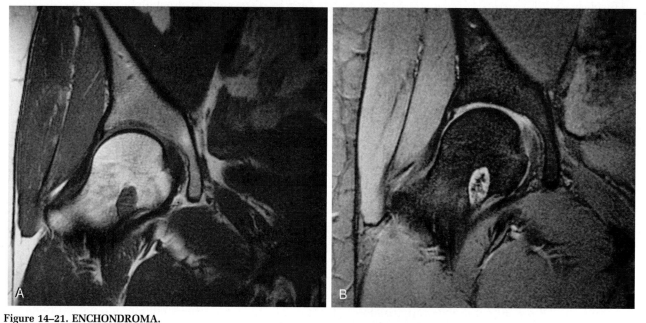

Figure 14–21. ENCHONDROMA.
A, Coronal T1W image shows lobular contour of low signal in the femoral neck. *B,* Coronal T2 image shows high signal chondroid with some areas of punctate low signal consistent with calcification seen on the conventional radiograph.

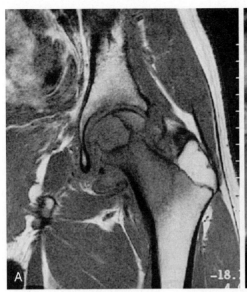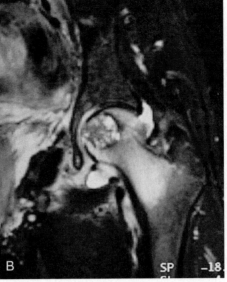

Figure 14–22. CHONDROBLAS-TOMA.
A, Coronal T1W image shows round, low-signal abnormality in the epiphysis of this child, with surrounding bone marrow edema. *B,* Coronal STIR image shows the lesion in the femoral epiphysis with some low-signal areas. This appearance is typical for chondroid matrix; without the low signal foci on T2, this could just as easily be osteomyelitis with a septic joint. Bone marrow edema is noted as high signal in the femoral neck and surrounding the lesion.

ally, capsular thickening can occur in the setting of recurrent joint effusions, which can lead to adhesions and fibrotic thickening of the capsule.

Normal Muscles (Box 14–9). Four muscle groups that affect hip motion can be identified. The anterior femoral muscles—including the sartorius and the rectus femoris—flex, abduct, and externally rotate the thigh. The medial group, including the gracilis, pectineus, adductor longus, adductor brevis, and adductor magnus, act as adductors but also internally rotate and flex the hip. The lateral muscles— the tensor fascia lata and the gluteus maximus, medius, and minimus—extend and abduct the hip; the piriformis, the obturator internus and externus, the gemelli superior and inferior, and the quadratus femoris produce external rotation. The posterior femoral muscles (the hamstring muscles) include the biceps femoris, semimembranosus, and semitendinosus, which integrate hip extension and knee flexion. The iliopsoas (comprised of the iliacus and the psoas major and minor) flexes the hip and externally rotates the thigh.

Muscle Strains (Box 14–10). Injuries to the thigh muscles and their pelvic attachments are common in trained and untrained athletes.[17] The injury pattern is discussed in great detail in Chapter 3. Patients may have an MRI for evaluation of pain after a fall when conventional radiography is normal (shows no fracture). Muscle abnormalities may account for the symptoms, but MRI is also very valuable in assessing the underlying bone for an occult fracture. The hamstring muscles are injured most

---

BOX 14–9: NORMAL SOFT TISSUE STRUCTURES OF THE HIP AND PELVIS

Muscles
  Anterior (flex and abduct)
    Sartorius
    Rectus femoris
  Medial (adduct, internally rotate, flex)
    Gracilis
    Pectineus
    Adductor longus, brevis, magnus
  Lateral (extend, abduct)
    Tensor fascia lata
    Gluteus maximus, medius, minimus
  External rotators
    Piriformis
    Obturator internus, externus
    Gemelli superior, inferior
    Quadratus femoris
  Posterior—hip extension, knee flexion (hamstrings)
    Biceps femoris
    Semimembranosus
    Semitendinosus
  Iliopsoas—flexes hip and externally rotates thigh

BOX 14–10: MUSCLE ABNORMALITIES

Muscle strains
  Hamstring strain, avulsion
  Gluteus medius tendon tears (greater trochanter pain syndrome)
MR findings: isointense to muscle T1W image
    ↑ signal T2W image in the tendon
    disruption of tendon fibers (may have edema in adjacent bone and muscle)

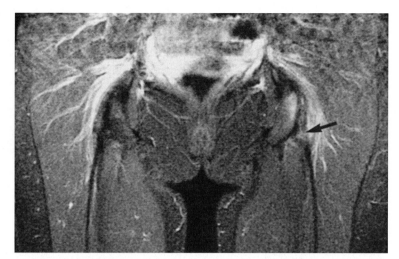

Figure 14–23. PARTIAL TEAR, HAMSTRING.
Coronal fast T2W, fat-suppressed image shows abnormal high signal in the origin of the left hamstring *(arrow),* with high signal in the adjacent ischial tuberosity. The findings are consistent with a partial tear of the hamstring. Note the low-signal, triangular-shaped hamstring tendon on the right side for comparison.

frequently, but tears in quadriceps and adductor muscles also occur (Figs. 14–23 and 14–24).

Gluteus Medius Tendon Tears. This entity also has been referred to as greater trochanter pain syndrome. Patients complain of chronic pain around the hip or groin region. The symptoms often mimic intraarticular hip pathology. It is associated with tendinopathy or tears of the gluteus medius or minimus tendons and associated muscle. This entity more commonly affects middle-aged to elderly women (Fig. 14–25).[18, 19] MR examinations show abnormal high signal in the gluteus medius or minimus muscles on the T2W images; discontinuity of the tendons may be evident, without their normal attachment to the greater trochanter. The signal intensity on the T1W images is isointense to musculature; therefore, it is not appreciated as abnormal. T2W images must be performed to make this diagnosis. The coronal images are by far the most valuable for making this diagnosis.

Other Muscles and Tendons. Injuries also can oc-

cur to the other muscle groups around the hip. The findings on MRI are the same for injured tendons located anywhere. Fat-suppressed T2W or STIR images show the abnormal fluid/edema with increased conspicuity and are recommended for evaluation of these structures. Tendons may be thinned or thickened, have abnormal high signal within them on any pulse sequence, or be discontinuous or avulsed from their osseous attachments. In the setting of hip pain and evaluation for an occult fracture, muscle strain or hematoma may account for pain when no fracture is identified. One study showed a 27% incidence of occult pelvic fractures and a 50% incidence of soft tissue injury demonstrated on MRI as a cause of pain (Fig. 14–26).[15] Appropriate therapy then can be instituted to address the source of pain.

Piriformis Syndrome. The sciatic nerve exits the pelvis at the greater sciatic notch and is intimately associated with the piriformis muscle. The nerve usually is located immediately anterior to the piriformis muscle. There can be variations in the rela-

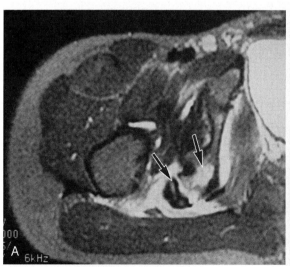
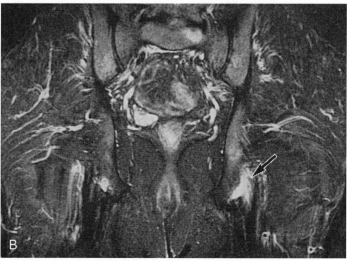

Figure 14–24. HAMSTRING AVULSION.
A, Axial fast T2W image with fat suppression shows abnormal signal in the hamstring tendon origin, as well as in the bone *(arrows).*
B, Coronal image shows abnormal high signal at the origin of the hamstring tendon *(arrow).*

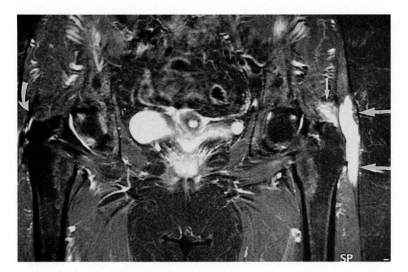

Figure 14–25. TORN GLUTEUS MEDIUS TENDON AND TROCHANTERIC BURSITIS.
Coronal STIR image shows abnormal high signal in the location of gluteus medius muscle and tendon *(short arrow)*. *Curved arrow* points to normal gluteal insertion on the right. Note also the high-signal fluid collection adjacent to the greater trochanter, representing greater trochanteric bursitis *(large arrows)*.

tionship between these structures: the sciatic nerve can split through the piriformis muscle, the nerve itself can split and a portion of the split nerve can go through the piriformis muscle, or the nerve can be split and a portion of the nerve can be superficial to the piriformis muscle. Because of this variation in location of the sciatic nerve, compression, hypertrophy, or injury to the piriformis muscle can cause irritation to the sciatic nerve, mimicking radicular symptoms from disc disease.

MRI may show asymmetry in the size of one piriformis muscle compared to the contralateral side. There usually is no abnormal signal or size of the piriformis muscle in those with the piriformis syndrome, unless there has been direct trauma. In the case of trauma to the piriformis muscle, high signal may be identified on the T2W images, caused by edema and hematoma.

Nerves

Normal Nerves. The largest nerve adjacent to the hip joint is the sciatic nerve. It is located immediately posterior to the posterior column of the acetabulum and lateral to the ischial tuberosity. It generally arises from the ventral L4–S3 nerve roots, exits the infrapiriform portion of the greater sciatic foramen, and courses between the ischial tuberosity and the greater trochanter. It is surrounded by fat and located between the quadratus femoris muscle anteriorly and the gluteus maximus muscle posteriorly. On MRI, the sciatic nerve is easiest to identify as an intermediate signal intensity stippled structure surrounded by fat just lateral to the hamstring origin (ischial tuberosity) on axial images (see Fig. 14–1).

Abnormal Sciatic Nerve. The sciatic nerve can be compressed by a nearby mass or can be traumatized

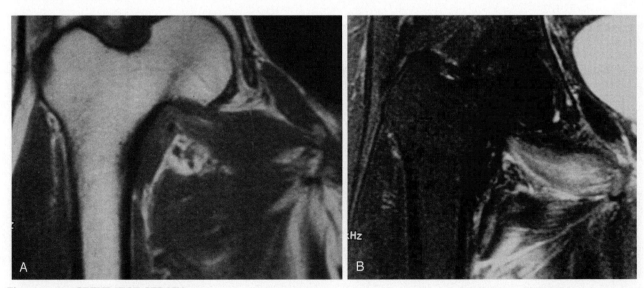

Figure 14–26. OBTURATOR STRAIN.
A, Coronal T1W image in a 71-year-old man with right hip pain after a fall. No fracture is identified. *B,* Coronal fast spin echo-T2 image with fat suppression reveals abnormal high signal throughout the obturator externus and adductors, consistent with a strain.

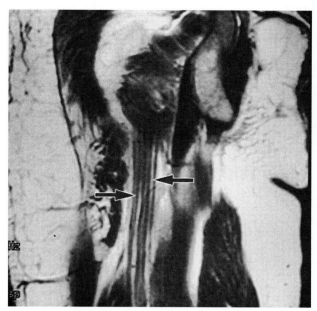

Figure 14–27. FIBROLIPOMATOUS HAMARTOMA OF SCI-ATIC NERVE.
Coronal T1W image shows multiple fascicles of sciatic nerve surrounded by fat *(arrows)* in this patient with sciatic nerve symptoms.

from a direct blow; this may result in swelling of the nerve. The location of the nerve around the hip joint makes it susceptible to traumatic injury. The appearance of the nerve is not unlike any other nerve injury, where the nerve may be enlarged focally or diffusely and has increased signal on the T2W images. For a more comprehensive discussion, refer to Chapter 4. Another entity that can affect the sciatic nerve is fibrolipomatous hamartoma (Fig. 14–27).

Bursae (Box 14–11)

Iliopsoas Bursa. The iliopsoas bursa is the largest bursa of the hip (and of the entire body). The ilio-

BOX 14–11: BURSAE

Iliopsoas
• Largest bursa in body
• 15% communicate with hip joint
• Distended in inflammatory/infection/ degenerative disease
• May have groin pain, palpable mass
• Anterior to hip joint
Greater trochanteric bursitis
• Repetitive hip flexion
• Lateral hip pain
• Lateral to greater trochanter
MR findings
• T1 isointense to muscle
• ↑ T2 isointense to joint fluid

psoas bursa can be distended and cause groin pain. It communicates with the joint in up to 15% of the population and can become distended when the joint is distended, when there is no significant joint effusion, or even when it does not communicate with the hip joint. It usually becomes distended in patients with rheumatoid or osteoarthritis (Fig. 14–28).[20] Distention of this bursa can help explain the patient's pain.

The ilipsoas bursa is located immediately anterior to the hip joint and adjacent to the femoral vessels, femoral nerve, and the iliopsoas muscle. It is not seen unless distended with fluid, which is isointense to joint fluid (Fig. 14–28); that is, it is low in signal on T1W images and high in signal intensity on T2W images. After the administration of intravenous contrast, the bursa is more readily diagnosed because the fluid does not enhance, but the lining of the bursa does. This helps to distinguish a potentially confusing anterior groin mass from the fluid-filled bursa (Fig. 14–29). These bursae can be treated short term with direct intrabursal steroid injections, but if they are inflamed because they are in communication with an abnormal hip joint, they cannot be treated permanently without addressing the joint problem.

Greater Trochanteric Bursitis. Trochanteric bursitis is another cause of hip pain. Patients usually localize the pain to the lateral aspect of the hip. Often this entity results from repetitive hip flexion. It can be impossible to distinguish it on clinical grounds from a torn gluteus medius or minimus tendon/muscle, which occurs in a similar middle-aged and elderly population. Patients generally are treated with anti-inflammatory medications. If pain is refractory to anti-inflammatory medications, a steroid injection into the bursa can be beneficial.

The findings on MR for trochanteric bursitis consist of no perceptible abnormality on the T1W image because the fluid is isointense to surrounding musculature. However, the T2W images show increased signal intensity paralleling the greater trochanter. This does not have to be a well-defined fluid collection, but rather a focus of high signal interdigitating around the tendons of the greater trochanter (Fig. 14–30).

Soft Tissue Tumors (Box 14–12)

Benign Soft Tissue Tumors. There are no soft tissue tumors that are particularly unique to the hip region. A lesion that occurs with some frequency is a lipoma, which can occur in the subcutaneous tissues or can be intramuscular. Lipoma is easily identified on MRI because the signal intensity of the lesion follows that of fat on all imaging sequences; it is high in signal intensity on the T1W images and suppresses on the fat-suppressed images. Another soft tissue mass that can occur around the pelvis is a desmoid, which is benign fibrous tumor that is locally aggressive. In general, the imaging features of desmoids are like most soft tissue tumors, low in

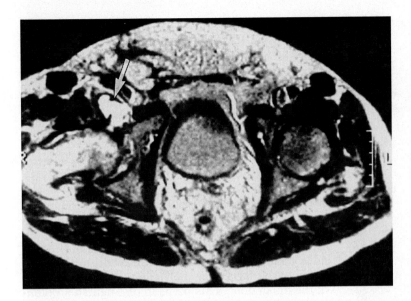

Figure 14–28. ILIOPSOAS BURSITIS.
Axial T2W image in a 67-year-old woman with rheumatoid arthritis and right hip pain. High-signal mass is noted adjacent to the iliopsoas muscle *(arrow)*, consistent with an iliopsoas bursitis.

signal intensity on a T1W image and increased signal intensity on a T2W image. However, because of the predominant fibrous component in this tumor, it can remain low in signal on the T2W images. This is a useful sign, when present.

Malignant Soft Tissue Tumors (Box 14–12). The most common malignant soft tissue tumor is malignant fibrohistiocytoma. This is a tumor that is not unique to the hip and pelvis area, but should be considered in the differential diagnosis for a mass that occurs in the soft tissues that is low in signal on T1W images. T2W images may show some high signal intensity, but because of the fibrous component may have some intermediate- to low-signal elements on T2W images.

Other soft tissue sarcomas such as liposarcoma and synovial cell sarcoma also can occur and are fairly nonspecific in their imaging characteristics (low in signal on T1W images and high in signal on T2W images). Occasionally, synovial cell sarcoma resembles fluid-like signal on the T2W image—that is, very intense signal. Gadolinium is helpful in differentiating a cystic collection from a solid mass. Liposarcomas have a variable fat content and, therefore, may not be high in signal on the T1W images, as would be expected for a lipoma.

Joints

Normal Ligamentum Teres

The ligamentum teres and the pulvinar (extrasynovial fibrofatty tissue) are contained within the acetabular fossa—the nonarticular medial wall of the acetabulum. The ligamentum teres runs from the acetabular fossa to the fovea centralis of the femoral head. Although the ligamentum teres does not normally contribute to hip joint stability, it does carry the artery of the ligamentum teres that supplies blood to the femoral head in children. In

adults, the blood supply associated with the ligamentum teres tends to involute.

Labrum (Box 14–13)

The acetabular labrum is a rim of fibrocartilaginous tissue around the margin of the acetabulum that deepens the acetabular fossa and provides additional coverage for the femoral head. The labrum is innervated by nerves that play a role in proprioception and pain production. The normal labrum is a triangular structure on axial and coronal imaging that is attached to the rim of the acetabulum.[21, 22] The normal labrum is low in signal on all imaging sequences (Fig. 14–31). Using surface coils, the labrum can be imaged in exquisite detail. If a labral abnormality is the clinical question, we always do a MR arthrogram with a dedicated hip MR rather than imaging the entire pelvis and hips at once.

Labral Tears. Symptoms of labral tears include persistent pain, clicking, or decreased range of motion.[21] Those affected by labral tears have sustained a single traumatic event that led to a subluxation of the femoral head (usually a motor vehicle accident), chronic stress as from athletic events such as cheerleading and running, or have developmental dysplasia of the hip.

The MR appearance of an abnormal labrum is that of linear or diffuse high signal in the labrum, a deformity in the contour of the labrum (loss of the normal triangular-shaped structure) (Fig. 14–32), or the labrum can be detached from the acetabulum (Figs. 14–33 and 14–34). Amorphous, round high signal within the substance of the labrum is a result of degeneration of the labrum, which is not thought to be clinically significant.[22] As in the shoulder, a small paraarticular cyst can form as a result of a labral tear (Fig. 14–35). The presence of a paraarticular cyst is a strong indicator of an associated labral tear.

One pitfall in imaging is the extension of the

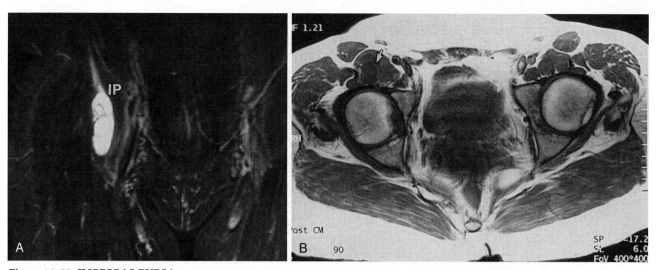

Figure 14–29. ILIOPSOAS BURSA.
A, Coronal STIR image shows a high-signal mass adjacent to iliopsoas muscle (IP). *B,* Axial T1W image after contrast shows peripheral enhancement of the mass *(arrow),* confirming the fluid nature of this mass.

Figure 14–30. GREATER TROCHANTERIC BURSITIS AND TORN GLUTEUS MEDIUS TENDON.
A, Coronal STIR image shows focal high signal around the greater trochanter (gt; *arrow*). The torn and retracted gluteus medius tendon also is seen *(small arrow).* *B,* Axial image shows the well-defined fluid collection, compatible with greater trochanteric bursitis. The gluteus medius tendon is torn *(arrows).* Greater trochanteric bursitis often is seen in association with gluteus medius tendon tears.

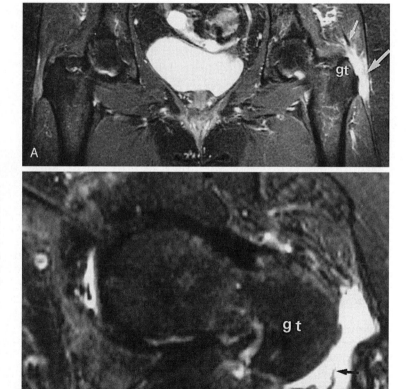

BOX 14–12: SOFT TISSUE TUMORS OF THE HIP AND PELVIS

Benign—Lipoma (follows fat signal on MR imaging)
  Desmoid
      Locally aggressive (low signal on T1W, usually low signal T2W)
    No tumors unique to hip/pelvis
Malignant
  Malignant fibrous histiocytoma (MFH)
  MR features: Low signal T1W
                Low to intermediate signal T2W
  Liposarcoma may have fat
  MR features: May have some high signal on T1W (fat)
                Otherwise: low signal T1W; ↑ T2W
  Synovial cell sarcoma
  MR features: Occasionally can be very intense on T2W (mimics fluid)
                Otherwise; low signal T1W; ↑ T2W

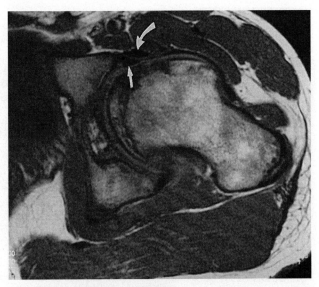

Figure 14–31. NORMAL LABRUM.
Axial T1W image shows a triangular, low-signal structure, representing normal appearance of the labrum *(small arrow)*. The low-signal structure adjacent to the labrum is the iliopsoas tendon *(curved arrow)*. The normal relationship between the labrum and iliopsoas tendon should be understood so that a tear in the labrum is not erroneously diagnosed. The abnormal contour of femoral head is due to Legg-Calvé-Perthes disease.

acetabular cartilage along the medial aspect of the labrum, which should not be confused with a labral tear or detachment. The iliopsoas tendon crosses anterior to the labrum. It is important to understand this relationship, because the high signal between these two low signal structures could mimic a tear of the labrum (Fig. 14–31). As opposed to the labrum of the shoulder with its many normal variations, the acetabular labrum is relatively straightforward to evaluate, with no other pitfalls yet described. In the United States, most labral tears generally are anterior and superior in location, whereas in Asian countries the defect is more commonly found posteriorly. A possible explanation for this disparity is the squatting position many Asians

assume for relaxation. Surgery generally is indicated to repair labral defects.

Normal Articular Cartilage

The acetabulum is not entirely covered by articular cartilage. Surrounding the nonarticular medial aspect of the acetabulum (acetabular fossa) is the

BOX 14–13: LABRUM

Normal
• Best imaged with surface coil and intraarticular contrast
• Triangular, low signal on all sequences
Abnormal
  Patients complain of clicking, pain, ± decreased range of motion
MR Appearance
• High signal in or through labrum (diffuse or linear high signal)
• Deformed contour
• Detached from acetabulum

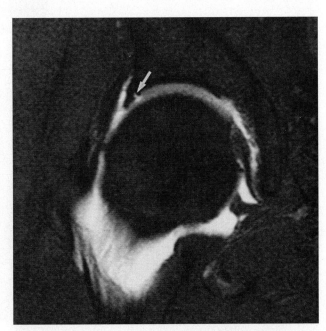

Figure 14–32. LINEAR DEGENERATIVE LABRAL TEAR.
Coronal T1W image with fat suppression and intraarticular contrast. Linear high signal is identified through the undersurface of the labrum *(arrow)*.

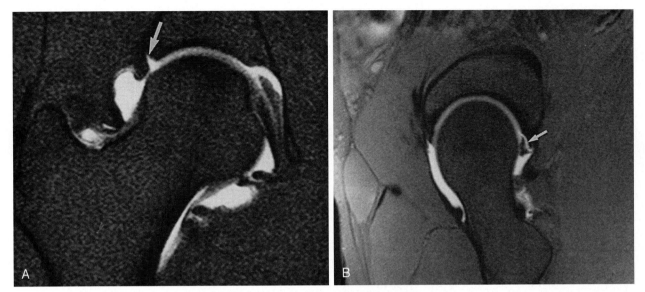

Figure 14–33. AVULSION (DETACHED) POSTERIOR SUPERIOR LABRUM.
A, Coronal T1W image with fat suppression and intraarticular saline shows triangular labrum avulsed from acetabular attachment *(arrow)*. Fluid is identified around labral detachment. *B,* Sagittal image showing labrum avulsed from attachment *(arrow)* (anterior is to the left).

articulating portion of the acetabulum, which is covered by articular cartilage. The cartilage is relatively thin, measuring no more than 3 mm.

The sacroiliac joints are composed of two parts, the true joint and a strong ligamentous attachment between the two bones (Fig. 14–36). The true joint, a synovial joint, comprises the anteroinferior half to two thirds of the joint. The articular surfaces are covered with cartilage and separated by a joint space. Hyaline cartilage exclusively lines the sacral surface, whereas a thinner mixture of hyaline and fibrocartilage lines the iliac surface. This discrepancy likely accounts for why disease processes be-

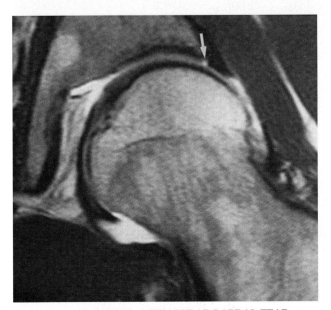

Figure 14–34. SUPERIOR ACETABULAR LABRAL TEAR.
Coronal T1W image shows partial detachment of superior labrum *(arrow)*.

gin along the iliac margin first. Many joint abnormalities may affect the articular cartilage, as described below.

Inflammatory Arthritides

Arthritis affecting the hip joint can be from a variety of causes. Rheumatoid arthritis can affect the hip, most often symmetrically bilaterally with axial joint space narrowing. Differentiating an inflammatory arthritis from a septic joint generally is not possible when only a single joint is known to be involved. Subchondral cyst formation, pannus, and joint effusion are common findings.

Sacroilitis is a nonspecific term suggesting an inflammatory process involving the sacroiliac joints. A variety of disease processes can affect the sacroiliac joint. These include the human leukocyte antigen (HLA) B-27 spondyloarthropathies, such as ankylosing spondylitis, inflammatory bowel disease, psoriasis, and Reiter's syndrome. Other common entities that affect these joints include osteoarthritis, gout, rheumatoid arthritis, and infection. The appearance on MRI is similar for each of these entities. The joint space may show erosions that image as foci of high signal along the joint space on the T2W images. Bone marrow edema may be seen immediately adjacent to the joint within the iliac bone and sacral ala. Erosions can be seen with any of the aforementioned abnormalities. The symmetry of the appearance may help with the differential diagnosis, because ankylosing spondylitis and inflammatory bowel disease are nearly always bilateral and symmetric. Psoriasis and Reiter's syndrome are bilateral and symmetric about 40% of the time.

Infection of the sacroiliac joint may show fluid that appears high in signal on the T2W image within

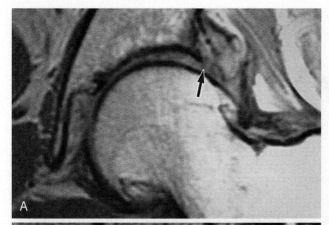

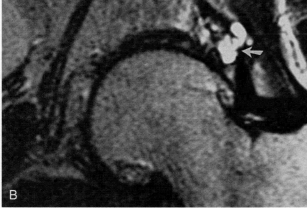

Figure 14–35. LABRAL TEAR WITH PARALABRAL CYST.
A, Coronal T1W image shows abnormal-appearing superior labrum *(arrow)* with no low-signal triangular structure seen. Large osteophytes from degenerative joint disease are seen. *B,* Coronal fast spin echo-T2 image with fat suppression shows a fluid collection adjacent to the labrum, compatible with a paralabral cyst *(arrow).*

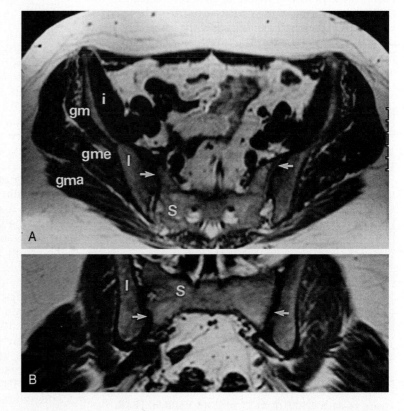

Figure 14–36. NORMAL SACROILIAC JOINTS.
A, Axial and *B,* coronal T1W images of the sacroiliac joints. True synovial portion *(arrows).* I—ilium; S—sacrum; i—iliacus; gm—gluteus minimus; gme—gluteus medius; gma—gluteus maximus.

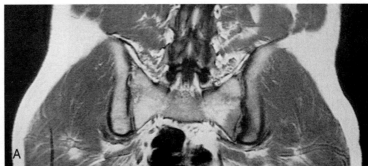

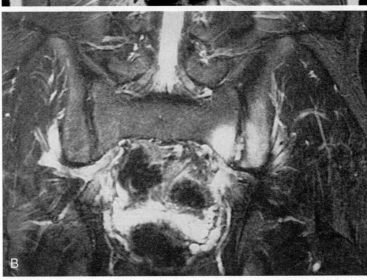

Figure 14–37. SACROILIITIS FROM INFECTION.
A, Coronal T1W image demonstrates low signal in the left sacral and iliac bones with low signal in a slightly widened irregular joint space. **B,** Fast T2W fat-suppressed image shows abnormal signal in the bones, as well as fluid in the joint space. The findings are consistent with sacroiliitis.

the joint space, but which does not enhance after the administration of contrast. The inflammatory reaction (phlegmon) may enhance, but the abscess collection or associated joint fluid does not enhance (Fig. 14–37). The appearance of a septic joint may be impossible to differentiate by MRI from an uninfected inflammatory arthritis (seronegative spondyloarthropathy or rheumatoid arthritis). Obviously, if the process is bilateral, it is highly unlikely to be from infection.

Degenerative Joint Disease

Osteoarthritis also affects the hip and is much more common than rheumatoid arthritis. The find-

ings of joint space narrowing (superolateral and anteriorly), osteophyte formation, and subchondral cysts can easily be noted on MRI. Often, the only finding initially is a nonspecific joint effusion or marrow edema in the subchondral bone (Fig. 14–38). It can be useful to have conventional radiographs of the hip available when evaluating the MR for suspected arthritis, because they can be complementary studies.[23]

Developmental Dysplasia
(Box 14–14)

Developmental dysplasia of the hip (DDH), formerly called congenital dislocation of the hip

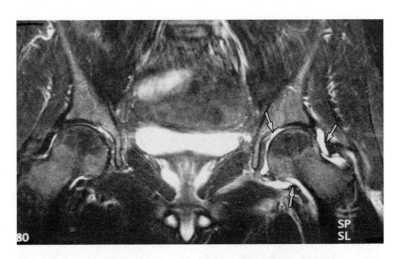

Figure 14–38. HIP JOINT EFFUSION.
Coronal fast T2W image with fat suppression shows a distended joint as demonstrated by high signal surrounded by joint capsule *(arrows).*

BOX 14–14: DEVELOPMENTAL DYSPLASIA OF THE HIP (DDH)

- 1% newborns
- Females slightly more affected than males
- Left hip more often affected than right
- Up to 95% normal development after intervention
- If undetected, early hip degeneration ensues (in patient's 30s)

MR useful in cases refractory to reduction attempts

- Possible causes: redundant labrum, excess pulvinar, transverse acetabular ligament, capsular hypertrophy, constriction of iliopsoas tendon, deformities of acetabulum or femoral head
- Femoral head located superior to acetabulum, upturned lateral aspect of acetabular roof, shallow/steep acetabulum

Common associated findings in adults

- Labral tears
- Degenerative joint disease

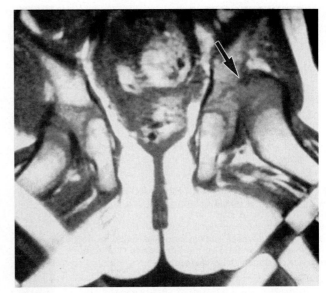

Figure 14–39. DEVELOPMENTAL DYSPLASIA OF THE HIP. Coronal T1W image demonstrating superior, posterior location of the left femoral head *(arrow)*.

(CDH), occurs in 1% of newborns. The disorder is more common in newborn girls, as well as newborns with a positive family history. The left hip is more commonly affected.[24] Early intervention can lead to normal hip development in up to 95% of patients with DDH. DDH has been classified according to the configuration of the acetabulum and labrum.[25] Type 1 is characterized by positional instability; type 2 as subluxation of femoral head and eversion of the labrum; type 3 by frank dislocation of the femoral head posterosuperiorly.

DDH ideally is diagnosed at birth by physical examination; however, the diagnosis can be missed and therapy delayed. These infants present for evaluation and treatment at several months to years of age. Ultrasound still should be regarded as the principal means of investigation in the newborn.[26] However, MRI should be considered for DDH when

reduction has been attempted but is not successful. Because of MRI's ability to resolve tissue types, structures that may prevent reduction of the femoral head can be identified. These include an abnormal labrum, pulvinar, transverse acetabular ligament (connects anterior with posterior labrum), capsular hypertrophy, constriction of iliopsoas tendon, and deformities of the acetabulum or femoral head.[25] The fact that the child can be imaged in cast material is another advantage of MRI. Sedation is necessary to perform the MRI on most younger patients.

Young adults, usually in their 30s, may develop severe hip pain from DDH that was never diagnosed as a child. The DDH leads to early degenerative joint disease and labral tears, both of which are a source of pain. Degenerative joint disease in the hip, whether or not it is caused by DDH, usually begins in the far anterior aspect of the hip joint. MRI shows edema in the subchondral bone of the acetabular region or femoral head early in the process; this progresses to subchondral cysts in the same loca-

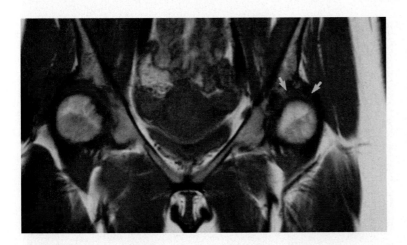

Figure 14–40. BILATERAL DEVELOPMENTAL DYSPLASIA OF THE HIPS. Coronal T1W image shows bilateral irregular articular surface, likely representing early degenerative disease, and shallow acetabulae *(arrows)*. Also note the femoral heads are slightly laterally located with respect to the acetabulae.

tions. A careful search for the typical abnormal configuration of the osseous structures of the hip can be made on both MRI and radiographs when degenerative changes are seen at a young age; the degenerative changes generally are easier to identify than the DDH on MR images. On MR examination, the abnormal hip is located superiorly to the acetabulum (Fig. 14–39). Irregular shape and shallow acetabulum also can be identified (Fig. 14–40). Instead of the lateral aspect of the roof of the acetabulum turning downward, as normal, it is directed superiorly (like a raised eyebrow). Careful inspection of the joint space should be performed to identify if the pulvinar (fat; high signal on T1W images) is trapped in the joint space, preventing reduction. A redundant labrum also can prevent reduction. This structure images as low signal on all sequences and also should be evaluated as a cause of nonreducible hip.

Intraarticular Tumors (Box 14–15)

Pigmented Villonodular Synovitis (PVNS). This is an uncommon disorder characterized by synovial proliferation with hemosiderin deposition in the involved synovial tissue. Pressure erosions of bone by the synovial masses may occur. PVNS occurs most commonly in the second through fifth decades and is usually monoarticular. The hip is among the joints most commonly affected by this disease process. Synovial involvement may be localized, although a diffuse form of synovial involvement is evident in up to 75% of cases. Because incomplete excision of PVNS guarantees recurrence, the entire joint must be carefully evaluated on MRI. A complete synovectomy is necessary for successful treatment.

Both T1 and T2W images are necessary to evaluate hemosiderin deposition, which is demonstrated as large, globular areas of low signal intensity on all imaging sequences. Gradient echo imaging demonstrates blooming of the hemosiderin elements, making them more prominent.[27] The presence of hemosiderin makes the diagnosis of PVNS on MRI virtually pathognomonic.

Primary Synovial Osteochondromatosis. This is the result of metaplastic proliferation of the synovium, resulting in multiple cartilagenous or osseous loose bodies (Fig. 14–41). Secondary osteochondromatosis also is referred to as degenerative due to loose body formation as a result of cartilage fragments being knocked off in the joint from degenerative disease. Primary synovial chondromatosis is not associated with degenerative changes until very late in the disease process. It is not possible to distinguish PVNS from synovial chondromatosis (nonos-

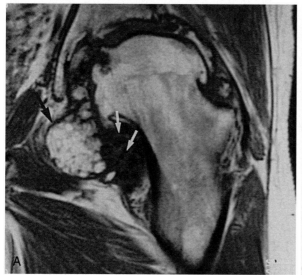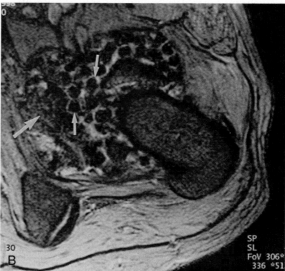

Figure 14–41. SYNOVIAL OSTEOCHONDROMATOSIS.
A, Coronal T1W image shows multiple intraarticular loose bodies of similar size *(arrows)* around the hip joint. *B,* Axial T2* image conspicuously demonstrates low signal (sclerotic) loose bodies. T2* has magnetic susceptibility properties, causing a blooming effect of the sclerotic loose bodies. A large, marrow-filled loose body also is identified *(large arrow)*. This patient has secondary degenerative joint disease.

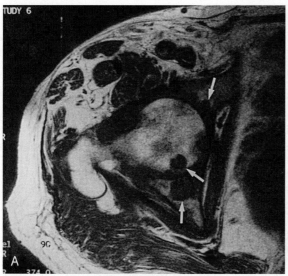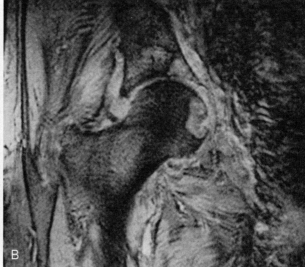

Figure 14–42. AMYLOID ARTHROPATHY.
A, Axial T1W image shows multiple low-signal erosions in the femoral head and acetabulum *(arrows).* *B,* Coronal T2* image shows that the erosions do not become significantly increased in signal. This finding is compatible with amyloid arthropathy.

sified) with conventional radiography. MRI makes the differentiation between these two processes possible. As stated earlier, the hemosiderin deposits characteristic of PVNS are low in signal on all imaging sequences. Synovial chondromatosis, however, follows the signal characteristics of cartilage. Cartilagenous loose bodies are low in signal on T1 and higher in signal on T2W images, following the signal of the articular cartilage.[28] Ossified loose bodies allow the diagnosis of synovial osteochondromatosis to be made on conventional radiography. On MRI, the ossified bodies may have low-signal cortical margins with a fatty (chewy nougat) center that follows the appearance of fat on all pulse sequences. Some ossified bodies are diffusely dense and sclerotic (low signal on all pulse sequences) throughout. Often, a mix of cartilagenous and ossified bodies is present.

Amyloid Arthropathy. This is a rare entity in terms of the hip. Typically, patients have renal failure and present with hip pain clinically similar to that of rheumatoid arthritis. Conventional radiography may show erosions within the acetabulum and femoral head or neck. MRI shows the erosions to be low in signal on T1W images that become low to intermediate signal on T2W images. This arthropathy often presents as mass lesions within the joint space. The radiographic features of this entity can be confused with PVNS on both conventional radiography and MRI. History and a careful search for hemosiderin (PVNS) should allow the two diagnoses to be distinguished (Fig. 14–42).

References

1. Coleman B, Kressel H, Dalinka M, et al. Radiographically negative avascular necrosis: detection with MR imaging. *Radiology* 1988; 168:525–528.

2. Beltran J, Herman L, Burk J. Femoral head avascular necrosis: MR imaging with clinical-pathological and radionuclide correlations. *Radiology* 1988; 166:215–220.
3. Mitchell D, Rao V, Dalinka M. Femoral head avascular necrosis: correlation of MR imaging, radiographic staging, radionuclide imaging, and clinical findings. *Radiology* 1987; 162:709–715.
4. Nokes SR, Vogler JB, Spritzer CE, et al. Herniation pits of the femoral neck: appearance at MR imaging. *Radiology* 1989; 172:231–234.
5. Rush B, Bramson R, Ogden J. Legg-Calvé-Perthes disease: detection of cartilaginous and synovial changes with MR imaging. *Radiology* 1988; 167:473–476.
6. Bluemm R, Falke T, des Plantes B, Steiner R. Early Legg-Perthes disease (ischemic necrosis of the femoral head) demonstrated by magnetic resonance imaging. *Skeletal Radiol* 1985; 14:95–98.
7. Jaramillo D, Galen TA, Winalski CS, et al. Legg-Calvé-Perthes disease: MR imaging evaluation during manual positioning of the hip—comparison with conventional arthrography. *Radiology* 1999; 212:519–525.
8. Curtiss P, Kincaid W. Transitory demineralization of the hip in pregnancy: a report of three cases. *J Bone Joint Surg [Am]* 1959; 41:1327–1333.
9. Nishiyama K, Sakamaki T. Transient osteopenia of the hip joint in children. *Clin Orthop* 1992; 275:199–203.
10. Guerra J, Steinberg M. Distinguishing transient osteoporosis from avascular necrosis of the hip. *J Bone Joint Surg [Am]* 1995; 77:616–624.
11. Yamamoto T, Kubo T, Hirasawa Y. A clinicopathologic study of transient osteoporosis of the hip. *Skeletal Radiol* 1999; 28:621–627.
12. Major NM, Helms CA. Idiopathic transient osteoporosis of the hip. *Arthritis Rheum* 1997; 40:1178–1179.
13. VandeBerg BC, Malghem JJ, Lecourt FE, et al. Idiopathic bone marrow edema lesions of the femoral head: predictive value of MR imaging findings. *Radiology* 1999; 212:527–535.
14. Stafford S, Rosenthal D, Gebhardt M, et al. MRI in stress fracture. *AJR* 1986; 147:553–556.
15. Bogost GA, Lizerbram EK, Crues JR. MR imaging in evaluation of suspected hip fracture: frequency of unsuspected bone and soft-tissue injury. *Radiology* 1995; 197:263–267.
16. Otte MT, Helms CA, Fritz RC. MR imaging of supra-acetabular insufficiency fractures. *Skeletal Radiol* 1997; 26:279–283.
17. Ishikawa K, Kai K, Mizuta H. Avulsion of the hamstring muscles from the ischial tuberosity: a report of two cases. *Clin Orthop* 1988; 232:153–155.

18. Chung CB, Robertson JE, Cho G, et al. Gluteus medius tendon tears and avulsive injuries in elderly women: imaging findings in six patients. *AJR* 1999; 173:351–353.
19. Kingzett-Taylor A, Tirman PFJ, Feller J, et al. Tendinosis and tears of gluteus medium and minimus muscles as a cause of hip pain: MR imaging findings. *AJR* 1999; 173:1123–1126.
20. Pritchard R, Shah H, Nelson C, FitzRandolph R. MR and CT appearance of iliopsoas bursal distention secondary to diseased hips. *J Comput Assist Tomogr* 1990; 14:797–800.
21. Fitzgerald R. Acetabular labrum tears: diagnosis and treatment. *Clin Orthop* 1995; 311:60–68.
22. Czerny C, Hoffman S, Urban M, et al. MR arthrography of the adult acetabular capsular-labral complex: correlation with surgery and anatomy. *AJR* 1999; 173:345–349.
23. Sanchez R, Quinn S. MRI of inflammatory synovial processes. *Magn Reson Imaging* 1989; 7:529–540.
24. Johnson N, Wood B, Jackman K. Complex infantile and congenital hip dislocation: assessment with MR imaging. *Radiology* 1988; 168:151–156.
25. Guidera K, Einbecker M, Berman C, et al. Magnetic resonance imaging evaluation of congenital dislocation of the hips. *Clin Orthop* 1990; 261:96–101.
26. Terjesen T, Runden T, Johnsen H. Ultrasound in the diagnosis of dislocation of the hip joints in children older than two years. *Clin Orthop* 1991; 262:159–169.
27. Flandry F, Hughston J, McCann S, Kurtz D. Diagnostic features of diffuse pigmented villonodular synovitis of the knee. *Clin Orthop* 1994; 298:212–220.
28. Hermann G, Abdelwahab IF, Klein M, et al. Synovial chondromatosis. *Skeletal Radiol* 1995; 24:298–300.

HIP AND PELVIS PROTOCOLS
This is one set of suggested protocols; there are many variations that would work equally well.

	DEDICATED HIP MRI (NOT ARTHROGRAM)			
Sequence #	**1**	**2**	**3**	**4**
Sequence Type	T1	Fast spin echo with fat saturation	T1	Fast spin echo with fat saturation
Orientation	Axial	Axial	Coronal	Coronal
Field of View (cm)	14	14	14	14
Slice Thickness (mm)	4	4	4	4
Contrast	No	No	No	No

	DEDICATED HIP MRI (ARTHROGRAM)			
Sequence #	**1**	**2**	**3**	**4**
Sequence Type	T1 with fat saturation	Fast spin echo T2 with fat saturation	T1 with fat saturation	Fast spin echo T2 with fat saturation
Orientation	Coronal	Coronal	Axial	Axial
Field of View (cm)	14	14	14	14
Slice Thickness (mm)	4	4	4	4
Contrast	(Intraarticular done in fluoro)*			

*Same solution as used for shoulders (see Chapter 10). Inject about 12 to 15 mL.

	PELVIS MRI (FRACTURES/AVASCULAR NECROSIS)			
Sequence #	**1**	**2**	**3**	**4**
Sequence Type	T1	Fast spin echo with fat saturation	T1	Fast spin echo with fat saturation
Orientation	Coronal	Coronal	Axial	Axial
Field of View (cm)	32	32	32	32
Slice Thickness (mm)	7	7	7	7
Contrast	No	No	No	No

Scout

Final Image

- Axial scout
- Obtain coronal images from line A to line B to cover joint

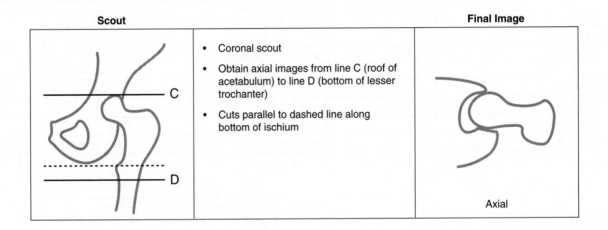

Coronal

Scout

Final Image

- Coronal scout
- Obtain axial images from line C (roof of acetabulum) to line D (bottom of lesser trochanter)
- Cuts parallel to dashed line along bottom of ischium

Axial

Scout

Final Image

- Coronal scout
- Obtain sagittal images perpendicular to dashed line along bottom of ischium
- Cover from line E (medial to hip joint) to line F (lateral to greater trochanter).

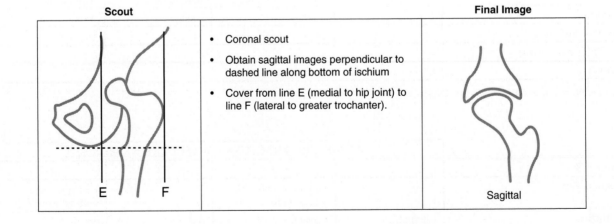

Sagittal

Scout		Final Image
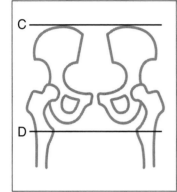	• Axial scout • Obtain coronal images • Cover from line A (pubic symphysis) to line B (posterior sacrum)	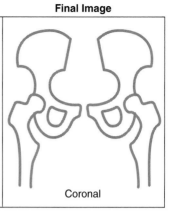 Coronal

Scout		Final Image
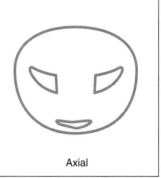	• Coronal scout • Obtain axial images parallel to line C, which connects iliac wings • Cover from line C (iliac crests) to line D (lesser trochanters)	Axial

HOW TO IMAGE THE KNEE
NORMAL AND ABNORMAL
Menisci
  Tears
    Oblique or horizontal tears
    Bucket-handle tears
    Radial or free-edge tears
    Medial flipped meniscus
  Cysts
  Discoid Meniscus
  Pitfalls
    Transverse ligament
    Speckled anterior horn lateral
      meniscus

  Meniscofemoral ligament
    insertion
  Pulsation from popliteal artery
  Magic-angle phenomenon
  Popliteus tendon pseudotear
Ligaments
  Anterior Cruciate Ligament
  Posterior Cruciate Ligament
  Medial Collateral Ligament
  Lateral Collateral Ligament
Patella
Synovial Plicae
Patellar Tendon

Bursae
  Popliteal (Baker's Cyst)
  Prepatellar Bursa
  Pes Anserinus Bursa
  Semimembranosus Tibial Collateral
    Ligament Bursa
  Tibial Collateral Ligament Bursa
Bones
Soft Tissues
KNEE PROTOCOLS

HOW TO IMAGE THE KNEE

See the protocols for knee MRI at the end of this chapter.

MRI of the knee is the most frequently requested MR joint study in musculoskeletal radiology. The reasons for this are quite simple: it works, and orthopedic surgeons therefore request it. MRI gives a comprehensive examination of the knee, providing surgeons with information they cannot obtain clinically or noninvasively. It also provides a road map for the surgeon who takes the patient to arthroscopic or open surgery. It has proven to be very accurate, with sensitivity/specificity in the 90% to 95% range for the menisci and close to 100% for the cruciate ligaments. This chapter shows how that kind of accuracy can be obtained.

Coils/Patient Position/Pulse Sequences. There are many ways to adequately image the knee, with different centers having differing imaging protocols based solely on personal preferences. We give not only what recipes work but, more importantly, try to stress what should not be used.

As with all joint imaging, a dedicated surface coil must be used. Most centers have a knee coil of some sort, and one seems to work as well as another (at a cost of $10,000 to $20,000 each, they should!). A small field of view should be used to maximize resolution. We usually use 14 to 16 cm, depending on the size of the patient. Slice thickness can be anywhere from 3 to 5 mm, with 4 mm being the standard in most centers. A small interslice gap (0.4 mm) is used to reduce crosstalk, unless volume imaging is employed. Having slice thickness thinner than 4 mm does not seem to increase accuracy and

leads to more images to interpret, or information overload. A matrix of 256 x 192 or 256 x 256 is fairly standard, with neither being necessarily better than the other. We try to have the knee in about 5 degrees of external rotation so that the anterior cruciate ligament (ACL) is orthogonal to the sagittal plane of imaging. This is typically the position of the knee in the relaxed state, and no effort at externally rotating the knee needs to be made in the majority of patients.

The menisci are best evaluated using sagittal images. It is necessary to have a short TE to effectively see meniscal tears. This can be in the form of conventional spin echo T1W images, proton density, or gradient echo sequences. It has been shown conclusively that fast spin echo (FSE) proton density (PD) images are unacceptable. Although there seems to be conflicting data on this subject, with several articles touting FSE-PD[1, 2] and others condemning it,[3, 4] we strongly believe that many meniscal tears are missed using FSE-PD sequences. We compared conventional PD sequences and FSE-PD sequences in 216 consecutive knees and found that the FSE-PD examination missed 42 tears that were seen on the conventional PD sequences (Fig. 15–1). Our overall sensitivity for interpreting the menisci using conventional PD sequences is 90% to 95%; using FSE-PD, our sensitivity was 80%. Why would we dream of using FSE-PD when our sensitivity would be so low? We wouldn't! Why is there such a difference in our results and in those of other investigators? In fact, there is not much difference. If one calculates the sensitivity for meniscal tears in the papers published on this subject, one would find that every paper has a sensitivity of around 80%. It seems all

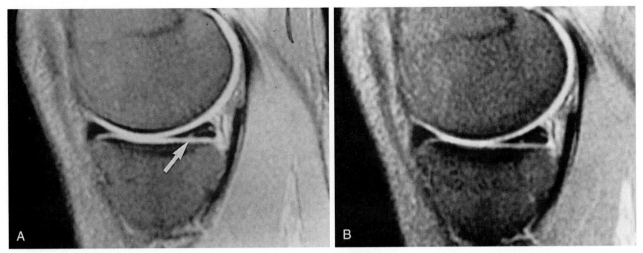

Figure 15–1. MENISCUS TEAR NOT SEEN WITH FAST SPIN ECHO SEQUENCE.
A, A sagittal conventional spin echo-proton density (TR/TE 2000/20) image with fat suppression shows an oblique tear of the posterior horn of the medial meniscus *(arrow)*. **B,** A sagittal fast spin echo-proton density (TR/TE 3000/16; ETL 4) image with fat suppression prospectively was called normal.

of the papers have the same results; however, the conclusions differ. It makes no sense to us to sacrifice accuracy in finding meniscus tears for the small decrease in imaging time that FSE sequences give. The savings in time do not allow enough of a savings to increase patient throughput, and even if it did, it would not justify missing about 10% of the meniscal tears, which is exactly what happens with FSE-PD sequences.

For evaluating the menisci we use a 4-mm-thick sagittal spin echo proton density sequence that has fat suppression. Fat suppression makes a more aesthetic-looking image when looking at the menisci (Fig. 15–2). It increases the range of signal in the menisci and makes tears more conspicuous than without fat suppression. It has not been shown that it increases accuracy (in fact, in side-to-side comparison of hundreds of cases with and without fat sup-

pression, we have found no examples of tears seen on one sequence and not on the other). Nevertheless, it gives the reader more confidence and makes for a pretty image, which is not all bad.

We also use a 4-mm-thick sagittal fast spin echo T2W image with fat suppression which is excellent for examining the cruciate ligaments, cartilage, and bones. A sagittal conventional spin echo T2W image would suffice similarly, but does not have the same high signal-to-noise ratio or resolution as fast spin echo and takes more time. A STIR image also would suffice. A gradient echo sagittal (volume or single slice) also would do nicely for the cartilage and cruciates, but is not acceptable for examining the bones. Some centers use sagittal gradient echo to replace both the T1W and the T2W image in the sagittal plane. This is a considerable time-saving technique. The marrow signal is then examined

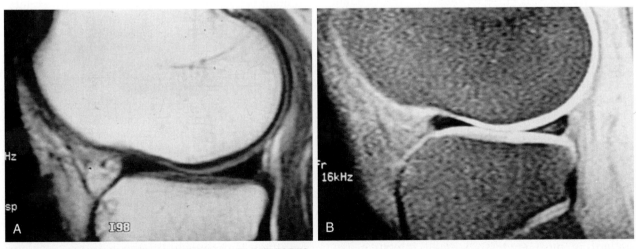

Figure 15–2. USE OF FAT SUPPRESSION FOR THE MENISCUS.
A, A sagittal conventional spin echo-T1W image of the lateral meniscus without fat suppression shows most of the signal emanating from the marrow in the femur and tibia. **B,** The same sequence with fat suppression shows the meniscus to better advantage due to the suppression of signal from the marrow.

with a marrow-sensitive sequence in the coronal or axial planes.

The coronal plane is used to examine the collateral ligaments and serves as another plane to examine the cruciate ligaments if doubt exists on the sagittal plane. The coronal plane also is used to inspect the cartilage. It has not been shown to be a useful plane for the menisci. It is rare to see a meniscus tear on the coronal plane that is not seen on the sagittal images. We compiled the results of over 200 consecutive knees in which we repeated our meniscus-sensitive sagittal sequence in the coronal plane and interpreted the coronal images separately from the sagittal images. In over 400 menisci (two menisci/knee, over 200 knees) we had only two menisci in which we saw tears that were not seen on the sagittal images. One of those had arthroscopy and no tear was found. Therefore, we believe that a meniscus-sensitive sequence is not necessary in the coronal plane.

The coronal plane should have some sort of T2W image. If fast spin echo sequences are employed, then fat suppression is recommended. It can be difficult to differentiate fat from fluid on high field-strength magnets with fast spin echo. It is important to determine if fluid lies between the medial meniscus and the medial collateral ligament to diagnose a meniscocapsular separation. A small fat pad often separates those structures and can be mistaken for fluid unless fat suppression is used.

For many years, the coronal plane images were solely T1W. It took us years to realize that little, if any, information was gained using this sequence, but gradually we all moved to coronal T2W images. Only in hindsight do we see how foolish we were not to question why we were using T1W images in the coronal plane when we never saw any abnormalities. Most of us used T1W images in the coronal plane because everyone else did. Talk about the emperor's new clothes!

The axial plane also should be imaged with some sort of T2 sequence. As in the coronal plane, nothing is gained using a T1W image, and much can be overlooked. This is the best plane to examine the patellar cartilage. The trochlear cartilage also is well seen on this sequence. Medial patellar plica are best seen in this plane. A second (or third) look at the cruciate ligaments can be made on the axial images and, similarly, the collateral ligaments can be re-inspected.

A knee protocol that works well consists of three planes of fast spin echo T2W images with fat suppression and a sagittal sequence that is conventional proton density with fat suppression. That's right, fat suppression on all four sequences, leaving us open to missing the dreaded lipoma of the knee. In 3 years of monitoring our accuracy using our MR interpretations against the arthroscopy reports, we are satisfied that this is a solid imaging protocol that allows us a high accuracy for menisci, cruciate ligaments, collateral ligaments, and cartilage.

Contrast. There is no place for gadolinium in routine imaging of the knee. MR arthrography has been advocated as useful in the postoperative knee to help differentiate between a repaired meniscus and a torn meniscus, but we have little experience with this.

NORMAL AND ABNORMAL

Menisci

Normal

The menisci in the knee are C-shaped, fibrocartilagenous structures that are thick peripherally and thin centrally. A sagittal slice through the body segment should show the meniscus as an elongated rectangle or a bowtie, depending on how peripheral the sagittal slice is (Fig. 15–3). Both the medial and lateral menisci should have two contiguous images of the body of the meniscus if 4- or 5-mm-thick slices are obtained. Three or four sagittal images should be seen through the anterior and posterior horns of the menisci (Fig. 15–4), with the posterior horn of the medial meniscus usually larger than the anterior horn. The anterior and posterior horns of the lateral meniscus are equal in size. The posterior horn of either meniscus should never be smaller than the anterior horn if it is normal.

The normal meniscus is devoid of signal on all imaging sequences, with the exception of children and young adults, who typically have some intermediate to high signal in the posterior horns near the meniscal attachment to the capsule. This signal represents normal vascularity and should not be misinterpreted as meniscus degeneration. The vascularity of the meniscus is greatest near the periphery and is almost nonexistent near the free edge. Therefore, peripheral tears can be repaired, whereas more central tears cannot.

Abnormal

Several grading schemes for abnormal meniscus signal have been developed. They are not generally in widespread use because the only abnormal signal that has any real significance is that which disrupts the articular surface of a meniscus, representing a tear. Any signal that does not disrupt an articular surface, with one exception, which will be covered in detail, is intrasubstance or myxoid degeneration (Fig. 15–5). Presumably, myxoid degeneration is a result of aging or wear and tear, but its cause remains unknown. It is not a source of symptoms, does not necessarily lead to meniscus tears, and is not treated clinically or surgically. Therefore, why mention it? If myxoid degeneration is prominent, it can be mentioned so that anyone else looking at the study will know we saw it but judged the signal not to be a tear, rather than thinking it was simply overlooked. Also, if it is especially prominent, there is a possibility that it might represent a meniscal cyst. More about meniscal cysts later.

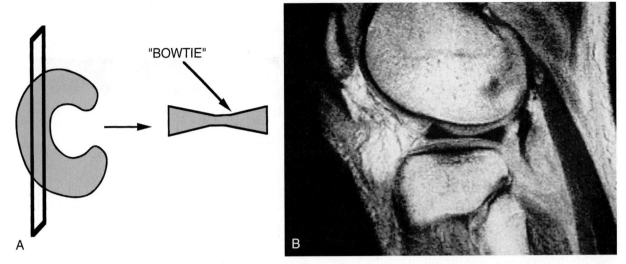

Figure 15–3. NORMAL BODY SEGMENT OF MENISCUS.
A, This schematic shows how a sagittal slice through the body of the meniscus gives an image of the meniscus that resembles a bowtie. *B,* A sagittal T1W image through the body of the lateral meniscus shows the normal bowtie appearance.

Tears

If high signal clearly disrupts an articular surface of the meniscus, it is an easy call: it is a torn meniscus. If high signal comes close to the articular surface but does not quite reach the articular surface, it is an easy call: it is not a tear, it is intrasubstance degeneration. Unfortunately, it is not always that clear cut. In many cases, it is too close to call. What should one do in these situations? Do the same thing radiologists do all the time—hedge. We are not being facetious. If you tell your orthopedic surgeons that when you call a tear or when you call no tear they can count on a correct diagnosis in more than 90% of the cases, they will find MR examinations and your readings to be very helpful. You will be able to give a definitive diagnosis in about 90% of cases. You should explain that about 10% of the time you will be unable to definitely discern if the meniscus is torn or not. In those cases, the clinical examination is paramount. If the patient gets better with conservative care, it was probably not a torn meniscus. If the patient does not improve, the surgeon may decide to perform an arthroscopic procedure, in which case you will have told him or her where to look for a possible meniscus tear. It seems that 10% is the hedge rate for the menisci.[5, 6]

It has been shown that sensitivity for meniscal tears decreases considerably if there is an associated ACL tear.[7] There are several reasons for this. First, the meniscal tears that seem to occur when the ACL is torn are located in two places: the posterior horn of the lateral meniscus and in the periphery of the menisci (both medial and lateral menisci). These are not the usual locations for meniscus tears and consequently often are overlooked. Also, several pit-

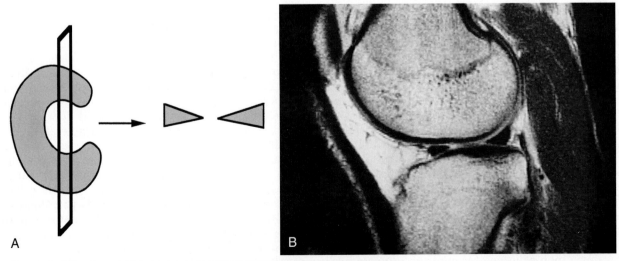

Figure 15–4. NORMAL ANTERIOR AND POSTERIOR HORNS OF THE MENISCUS.
A, This schematic shows the appearance of a sagittal slice through the anterior and posterior horns of the meniscus. *B,* A sagittal T1W image through the anterior and posterior horns of the lateral meniscus.

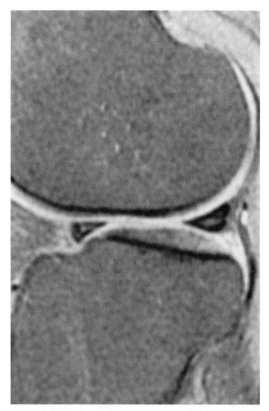

Figure 15–5. MYXOID OR INTRASUBSTANCE DEGENERATION. A sagittal proton density image with fat suppression through the lateral meniscus shows some high signal in both the anterior and posterior horns that does not disrupt an articular margin of the meniscus. This is myxoid degeneration.

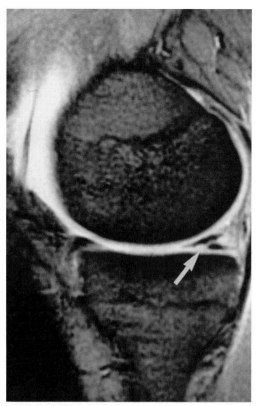

Figure 15–6. MENISCUS TEAR. A sagittal image through the medial meniscus reveals an oblique tear of the posterior horn *(arrow)*.

falls occur in the posterior horn of the lateral meniscus that can be confused with meniscal tears, all of which are mentioned later in this chapter. Suffice it to say that when the ACL is torn, close inspection should be made for a peripheral tear or for a tear in the posterior horn of the lateral meniscus.

Oblique or Horizontal Tears. There are many types of meniscal tears (Box 15–1). The most common is an oblique or horizontal tear (these are synonymous terms; some surgeons prefer one term over the other, and others use them interchangeably) that affects the undersurface of the posterior horn of the medial meniscus (Fig. 15–6). These commonly are

---

BOX 15–1: TYPES OF MENISCAL TEARS

    Oblique or horizontal
    Vertical
        Flap
        Bucket handle
    Peripheral
    Medially flipped flap tear
    Radial (parrot beak tear)
    Meniscocapsular separation

---

degenerative in nature, rather than as a result of trauma.

Bucket-Handle Tears. Vertical longitudinal tears (Fig. 15–7) make up the common bucket-handle tear that occurs in about 10% of meniscal tears. The normal meniscus has a body width of about 9 mm, which is seen on two consecutive sagittal images as a single slab of meniscal tissue that has a shape similar to a bowtie. When the inner edge of the meniscus displaces, a bucket-handle tear is easily diagnosed by noting only one instead of the normal two body segments present on the outermost sagittal images through the meniscus (Fig. 15–8). This is called the "absent bowtie sign," because the body segments have a bowtie appearance on the sagittal images.[8] Often, this is the only indication of a bucket-handle tear. A displaced meniscal fragment usually, but not always, can be found, especially in the intercondylar notch (Fig. 15–9), and a careful inspection for a fragment should be made when only one body segment is seen on the sagittal images. The displaced meniscal fragment can lie in front of the posterior cruciate ligament (PCL), which is called a double PCL sign (Fig. 15–10). The displaced fragment also may flip over the anterior horn of the affected meniscus, which is called an anterior flipped meniscus sign (Fig. 15–11). In any case, the absent bowtie sign is a very sensitive sign for a bucket-handle tear.

Radial or Free-Edge Tears. The absent bowtie sign

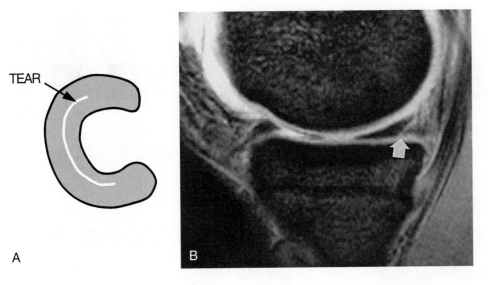

Figure 15–7. VERTICAL LONGI-TUDINAL MENISCUS TEAR.
A, This schematic shows a meniscus with a vertical longitudinal tear. If the inner edge displaces, it would be called a bucket-handle tear. **B,** A sagittal image through a meniscus with a vertical tear *(arrow).*

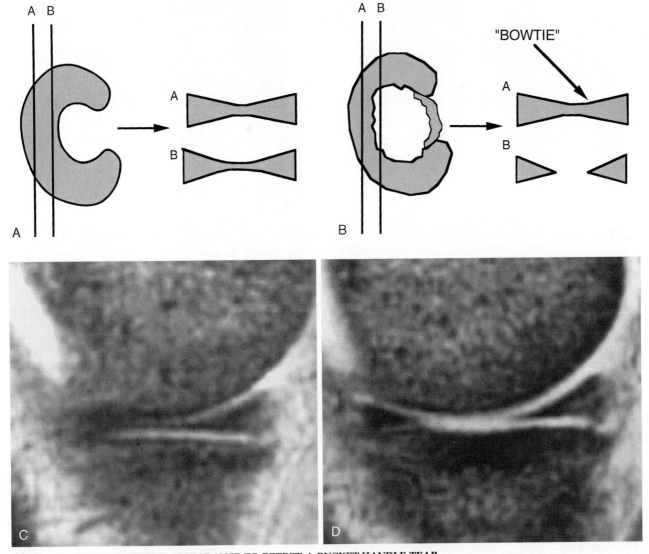

Figure 15–8. USE OF "BOWTIE" APPEARANCE TO DETECT A BUCKET-HANDLE TEAR.
A, This schematic shows how two sagittal images through the body normally produce two images of the meniscus that have a bowtie appearance. **B,** This schematic shows how, in a bucket-handle tear with the free edge of the meniscus displaced, only one sagittal image has a bowtie appearance. **C,** The first sagittal image through the medial meniscus in a patient with a bucket-handle tear shows the normal bowtie appearance. **D,** The next sagittal image in the same patient shows anterior and posterior horns, rather than another bowtie. This appearance is characteristic of a bucket-handle tear of the meniscus.

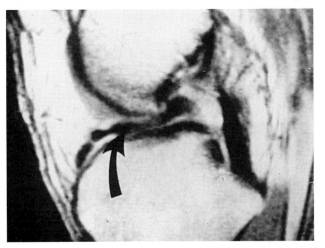

Figure 15–9. DISPLACED FRAGMENT IN A BUCKET-HANDLE TEAR.
A sagittal image through the intercondylar notch in a patient with a bucket-handle tear shows the displaced fragment *(arrow)*.

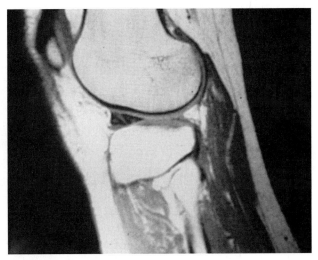

Figure 15–11. ANTERIOR FLIPPED MENISCUS.
A sagittal image of the lateral meniscus in a patient with a bucket-handle tear shows the displaced fragment flipped onto the anterior horn—the anterior flipped meniscus sign.

is also positive in free-edge tears (also called radial tears or parrot beak tears). Free-edge tears are quite common and are an unusual source of symptoms unless they are large. Again, the absent bowtie sign is useful in recognizing these tears. They are easily differentiated from bucket-handle tears because the second body segment, or bowtie, has only a small gap, rather than the large gap as seen in bucket-handle tears (Fig. 15–12). A recent investigation of around 200 knees that underwent arthroscopy by a single surgeon showed a 15% incidence of radial tears. At surgery, the free edge of a meniscus with a radial tear is treated with debridement and smoothing.

Medial Flipped Meniscus. A recently described meniscus tear that can be seen with MRI and can be overlooked at arthroscopy is a flap tear of the medial meniscus with the flap of meniscus flipped into the medial gutter underneath the meniscus.[9] It can be missed at surgery if the surgeon fails to probe the medial gutter and deliver the flipped fragment. These are not uncommon tears and should be considered when the body segments look somewhat thinner than normal or have a piece of meniscus missing from the undersurface (Fig. 15–13). The medial flipped fragment can be seen on the coronal images lying just below and medial to the medial meniscus.

Cysts

Meniscal cysts occasionally are seen that involve a meniscus without the meniscus having a tear that extends to the articular surface. With weight-bearing, the fluid in the cyst can be expressed into the adjacent soft tissues, where it is called a parameniscal cyst (Fig. 15–14). It is important to advise the surgeon of the presence of such a cyst, because without a meniscal tear the cyst can be missed at arthroscopy. Also, many surgeons decompress a meniscal cyst that does not have a meniscal tear by an extraarticular approach rather than via arthroscopy.[10] Most meniscal cysts do not exhibit marked high signal with T2W images, yet the parameniscal component usually is very high in signal. When the cyst is confined to the meniscus, the signal resembles intrasubstance degeneration, only it is much more pronounced (Fig. 15–15). If a mass effect makes the meniscus appear swollen, it is an easy diagnosis; otherwise, it is a difficult call. These cases are handled by suggesting a meniscal cyst versus severe intrasubstance degeneration—at least the surgeon is aware of the possibility of a meniscal cyst. A meniscal cyst often is first noticed by seeing on the most medial or lateral sagittal images through

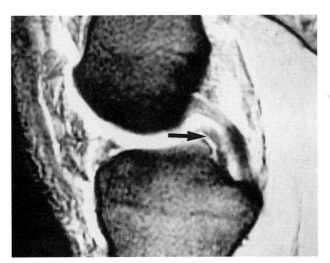

Figure 15–10. DOUBLE POSTERIOR CRUCIATE LIGAMENT (PCL) SIGN.
A sagittal image through the intercondylar notch in a patient with a bucket-handle tear shows the displaced fragment anterior to the PCL *(arrow)*—the double PCL sign.

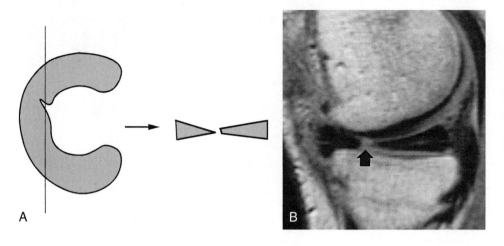

Figure 15–12. RADIAL TEAR.
A, This schematic of a free edge or radial tear shows how the sagittal image has a small gap in the expected bowtie appearance. **B,** The sagittal image in a meniscus with a free edge or radial tear shows a small gap in the bowtie *(arrow)*.

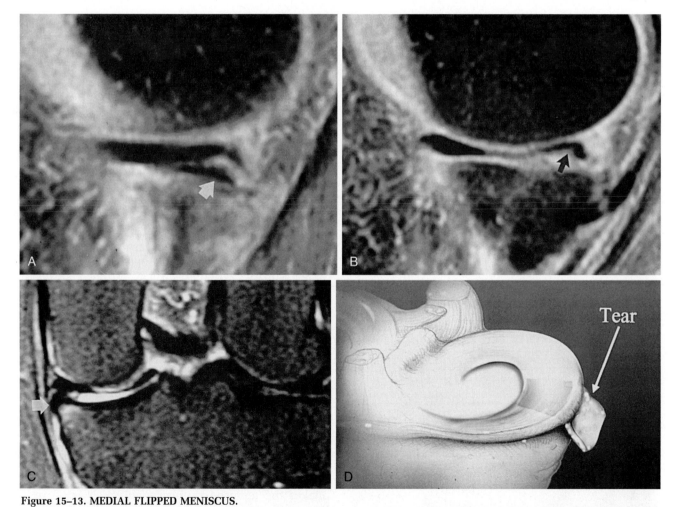

Figure 15–13. MEDIAL FLIPPED MENISCUS.
A, The first sagittal image through the body of the medial meniscus in a patient with a medially displaced flap tear shows a small fragment of meniscus inferiorly displaced *(arrow)*. **B,** The next adjacent sagittal image reveals a defect in the undersurface of the posterior portion of the body of the meniscus *(arrow)*. This defect is the donor site for the displaced flap of meniscus seen in A. **C,** A coronal image shows the medially displaced flap of meniscus inferior to the body of the meniscus *(arrow)*. **D,** An artist's depiction of a medially displaced flap tear.

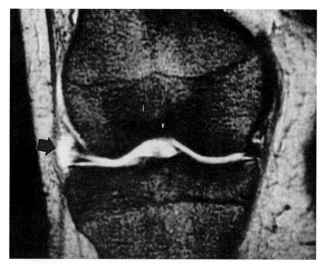

Figure 15–14. MENISCAL CYST.
A coronal gradient echo image in a patient with a meniscal cyst of the lateral meniscus. A small parameniscal cyst *(arrow)* has resulted from the fluid in the meniscus being expressed into the adjacent soft tissues.

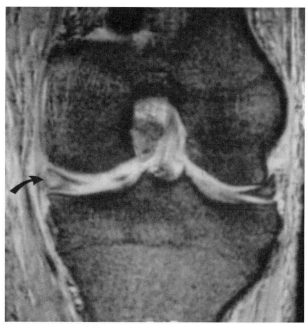

Figure 15–15. MENISCAL CYST.
A medial meniscal cyst is noted *(arrow)*, which gives a slightly swollen appearance to the meniscus. The lateral meniscus has marked intrasubstance degeneration, which should not be mistaken for a meniscal cyst.

the body of the meniscus that the normal bowtie appearance has a horizontal stripe, which represents the collapsed meniscal cyst (Fig. 15–16). This often is called a horizontal cleavage tear, but that term is not appropriate, because a true meniscal tear is not always present.

Discoid Meniscus

If more than two body segments are present on the sagittal images, a discoid meniscus should be considered (Fig. 15–17). A discoid meniscus is most likely a congenital (although some insist it is acquired) malformation of the meniscus in which the meniscus, in the most extreme form, is disc shaped rather than C shaped. In fact, most discoid menisci are not completely disc shaped, but have a wider

than normal body of the meniscus. The lateral meniscus is most commonly affected, with an incidence reported of around 3%, whereas the medial meniscus is uncommonly affected. Often a discoid meniscus is enlarged and affects the anterior or posterior horns of the meniscus asymmetrically. In such a case, the anterior or posterior horn is much larger than its counterpart. Although often encountered incidentally, discoid menisci are more prone to undergo cystic degeneration with subsequent tears than a normal meniscus. Even without cystic changes or a tear, a discoid meniscus can cause symptoms and require surgery.[11]

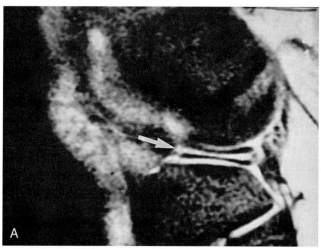
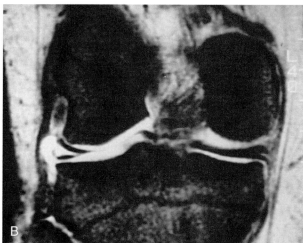

Figure 15–16. MENISCAL CYST.
A, A sagittal gradient echo image through the body of the lateral meniscus shows a high-signal stripe bisecting the meniscus *(arrow).*
B, A coronal image reveals a meniscal cyst with a small parameniscal cyst attached.

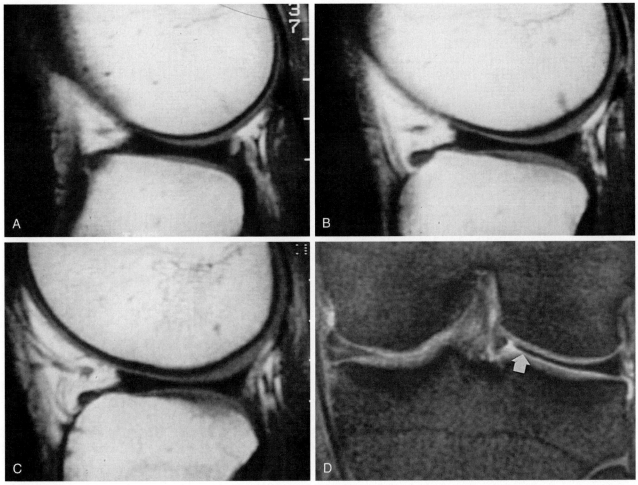

Figure 15–17. DISCOID LATERAL MENISCUS.
A through *C,* Successive sagittal images through the lateral meniscus show a bowtie appearance, indicating the body segment is present on more than two images. This should suggest a discoid meniscus. *D,* A coronal image reveals that the meniscus extends almost into the intercondylar notch *(arrow),* indicative of a discoid lateral meniscus.

It is extremely valuable to recognize the normal bowtie appearance of the body segments in both the medial and lateral menisci as seen on sagittal images on every examination. Many of the aforementioned abnormalities can be recognized easily by noting the absence of the normal two body segments. This includes the bucket-handle tear, radial tear, medially flipped flap tear, and the meniscal cyst (Box 15–2). A discoid meniscus exhibits more than two body segments. Our routine search pattern on the sagittal images includes a close inspection of the body segments to be certain there are two, and only two, bowties that are not deformed in any way.

Exceptions to this would include a large patient (Shaquille O'Neal would undoubtedly have three or four bowties), or very thin slices (the two bowtie rule applies only to slice thicknesses of 4 or 5 mm) and, as mentioned previously, a discoid meniscus.

Exceptions to the two bowtie rule that can mimic a bucket-handle tear (Box 15–3) can be seen in children or small adults in whom the menisci are small—only one bowtie is seen, but this is followed by only two or three images showing the anterior and posterior horns, rather than the usual three or four images; also, it occurs in both menisci. Simultaneous medial and lateral bucket-handle tears are

BOX 15–2: ABNORMALITIES WITH ABSENT BOWTIE SIGN
Bucket-handle tear Radial tear Medially flipped flap tear Meniscal cyst

BOX 15–3: PITFALLS IN ABSENT BOWTIE SIGN
Children or small adults Postoperative Severe osteoarthritis Older patients (over the age of 65 years)

rare. Another exception is in the postoperative knee where the free edge of the meniscus has been debrided. To recognize this, we have every patient fill out a form prior to the MR examination that asks about prior surgery. The two bowtie rule can be broken if severe osteoarthritis is present or in older patients (over the age of 65 years). These patients can wear down the free edge of the meniscus, leaving a very thin body segment that can be confused with a bucket-handle tear.

Pitfalls

A few pitfalls involving the menisci deserve mention.

Transverse Ligament. An easy pitfall to recognize is the insertion of the transverse ligament on the anterior horns of the menisci. The transverse ligament runs across the anterior aspect of the knee in Hoffa's fat pad from the anterior horn of the medial meniscus to the anterior horn of the lateral meniscus. Its function is unknown, and it is not present in every knee. At its insertion on the anterior horn of the lateral meniscus, it often has the appearance of a meniscus tear (Fig. 15–18). It can reliably be differentiated from a tear by following it across the knee in Hoffa's fat pad on sequential sagittal images. It only uncommonly causes a similar pseudotear appearance on the medial meniscus.

Speckled Anterior Horn Lateral Meniscus. The anterior horn of the lateral meniscus occasionally has a speckled appearance, which can resemble a macerated or torn anterior horn (Fig. 15–19). This is caused by fibers of the anterior cruciate ligament inserting into the meniscus. It is reported to be seen in up to 60% of normal patients.[12]

Meniscofemoral Ligament Insertion. The posterior horn of the lateral meniscus has several pitfalls that mimic tears. Insertion of the meniscofemoral

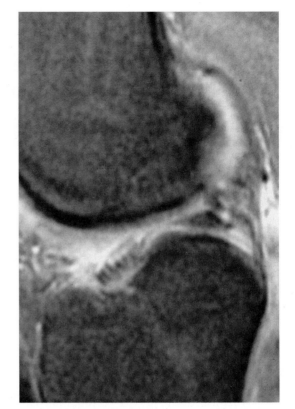

Figure 15–19. SPECKLED ANTERIOR HORN LATERAL MENISCUS.
A sagittal image through the lateral meniscus shows the anterior horn with a speckled appearance. This is a normal variant created by fibers of the anterior cruciate ligament inserting into the meniscus.

ligament of Humphry or Wrisberg can give the appearance of a meniscal tear (Fig. 15–20). A meniscofemoral ligament is present in about 75% of knees. It originates on the medial femoral condyle and runs obliquely across the knee in the intercondylar notch

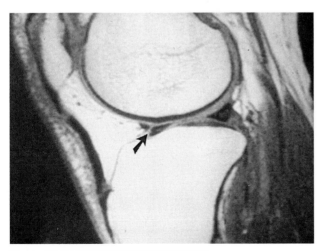

Figure 15–18. TRANSVERSE LIGAMENT.
A sagittal image through the lateral meniscus shows a transverse ligament inserting onto the anterior horn *(arrow),* creating a pseudotear.

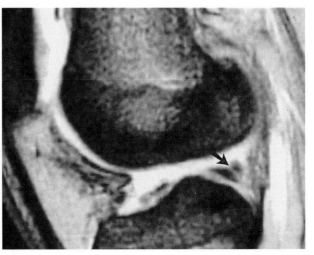

Figure 15–20. PSEUDOTEAR FROM MENISCOFEMORAL LIGAMENT.
A sagittal image through the lateral meniscus shows the posterior horn with a pseudotear *(arrow)* caused by the insertion of one of the meniscofemoral ligaments.

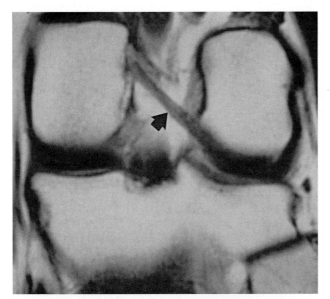

Figure 15–21. MENISCOFEMORAL LIGAMENT.
A coronal image shows a meniscofemoral ligament *(arrow)* extending obliquely across the intercondylar notch.

(Fig. 15–21), anterior (ligament of Humphry) or posterior (ligament of Wrisberg) to the posterior cruciate ligament (Fig. 15–22), and inserts into the posterior horn of the lateral meniscus. When considering a pseudotear from the insertion of one of the meniscofemoral ligaments, be sure to follow the ligament through the intercondylar notch to the PCL on sequential sagittal images. In 2% to 3% of knees both ligaments (Humphry and Wrisberg) are present. The function of the meniscofemoral ligament has not been clearly established, and no injury to it has been described.

Pulsation from Popliteal Artery. The popliteal artery is just posterior to the posterior horn of the lateral meniscus, and pulsation artifact can extend through the meniscus, making it difficult to examine or, in some instances, giving the appearance of a torn meniscus (Fig. 15–23). This is easily rectified by swapping the phase and frequency direction prior to scanning, so that the vessel pulsation extends superior to inferior rather than anterior to posterior.

Magic-Angle Phenomenon. On occasion, the posterior horn of the lateral meniscus has an ill-defined, hazy appearance with diffuse intermediate signal seen on proton density or T1W images (Fig. 15–24 *A* & *B*). This is due to the magic-angle phenomenon.[13] The posterior horn of the lateral meniscus slopes upward at around 55 degrees, which is the angle at which high signal begins to be seen in certain collagen-containing structures if the TE is short.[14] It will disappear on the T2W sequences or if the 55-degree angle is changed (Fig. 15–24 *C* & *D*). This has not proved to be a big problem in hiding meniscus tears, so imaging with the knee abducted has not been recommended.

Popliteus Tendon Pseudotear. The popliteus ten-

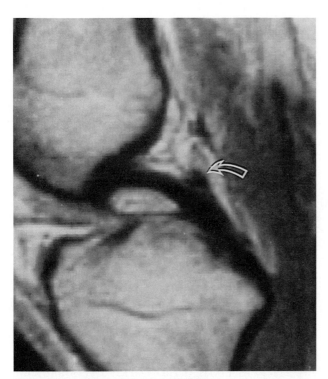

Figure 15–22. LIGAMENT OF WRISBERG.
A sagittal image through the intercondylar notch shows a ligament of Wrisberg *(arrow)* just posterior to the posterior cruciate ligament.

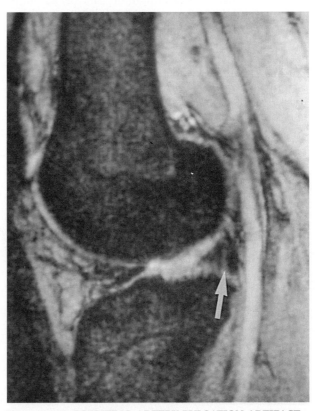

Figure 15–23. POPLITEAL ARTERY PULSATION ARTIFACT.
This sagittal gradient echo image through the lateral meniscus has a pulsation artifact from the popliteal artery that mimics a tear of the posterior horn *(arrow)*.

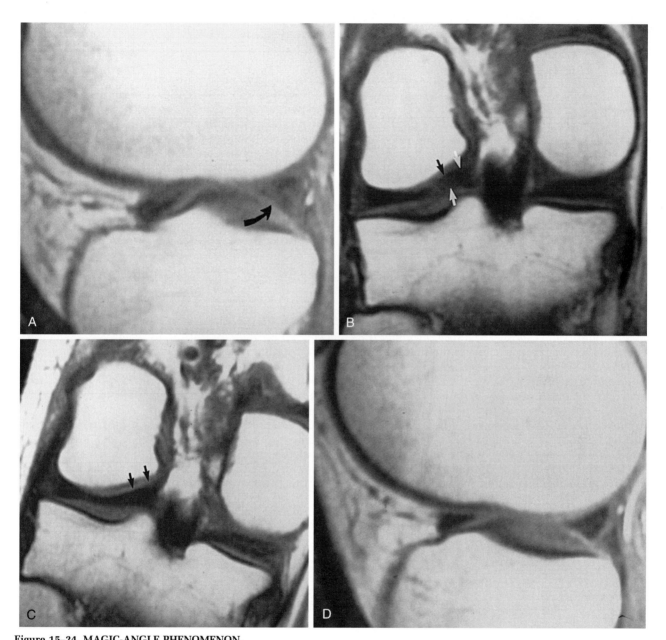

Figure 15–24. MAGIC-ANGLE PHENOMENON.
A, This sagittal T1W image shows the posterior horn of the lateral meniscus *(arrow)* as ill defined and intermediate in signal. *B,* A coronal T1W image in the same knee again shows the posterior horn to be ill-defined and intermediate in signal *(arrows).* Note that the posterior horn slopes upward at an angle of about 55 degrees. *C,* The same knee with a coronal T1W image taken with the knee abducted to flatten out the angle of the posterior horn now shows the meniscus sharply and without signal *(arrows).* *D,* A sagittal T1W image through the abducted lateral meniscus shows the posterior horn sharply and without intermediate signal. The signal and hazy appearance in *A* and *B* are from the magic-angle effect.

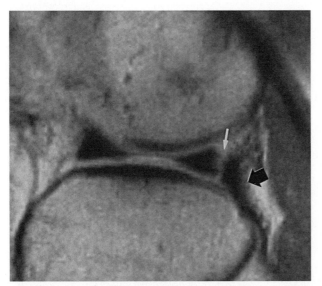

Figure 15–25. POPLITEUS TENDON PSEUDOTEAR.
This sagittal image through the lateral meniscus shows the popliteus tendon *(black arrow)* passing close to the posterior horn of the meniscus, creating a pseudotear *(white arrow)* appearance.

don originates on the lateral femoral condyle and extends inferiorly between the posterior horn of the lateral meniscus and the joint capsule. It runs obliquely and extends posteriorly to join its muscle belly, which lies just posterior to the proximal tibia. Where the tendon passes between the meniscus and the capsule, it can give the appearance of a meniscus tear (Fig. 15–25). This should be recognized as a normal structure and not confused with a tear. Further, a vertical tear of the posterior horn of the lateral meniscus should not be confused with the popliteus tendon (Fig. 15–26). This type of tear often occurs when there is an ACL tear, and care should be taken to account for the normal popliteus tendon so that a meniscus tear is not overlooked.

> **BOX 15–4: PITFALLS INVOLVING THE POSTERIOR HORN OF THE LATERAL MENISCUS**
>
> Meniscofemoral ligament insertion
> Pulsation artifact from popliteal artery
> Magic-angle phenomenon
> Popliteus tendon

Because the sensitivity for meniscal tears is known to decrease when the ACL is torn and many of the missed tears occur in the posterior horn of the lateral meniscus, close attention should be paid to this area when an ACL tear is present. Knowing the pitfalls that involve the posterior horn of the lateral meniscus is therefore imperative to a high accuracy rate (Box 15–4).

Ligaments

Anterior Cruciate Ligament

The normal ACL has straight, taut fibers that run parallel to the roof of the intercondylar notch (Fig. 15–27). It typically has a striated appearance with some high signal within it, especially at its insertion on the tibia. T2W sagittal images are recommended for evaluating the ACL. If the ACL is not clearly seen as normal or as torn on sagittal images, axial and coronal images should be used to further examine the ACL, but this is not necessary except in rare instances. Accuracy of MRI for the ACL is extremely high, approaching 95% to 100% in almost all reported series.[15–17]

A torn ACL usually is obvious by the fact that no normal-appearing fibers of the ACL can be identified

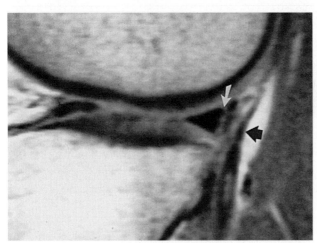

Figure 15–26. POPLITEUS TENDON PSEUDOTEAR.
This sagittal image through the lateral meniscus shows a peripheral vertical tear of the posterior horn *(arrow)*, which erroneously was thought to be the popliteus tendon. The popliteus tendon can be seen just posterior to the meniscus *(large arrow)*.

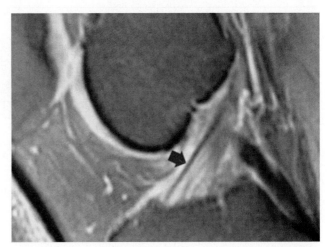

Figure 15–27. NORMAL ANTERIOR CRUCIATE LIGAMENT (ACL).
A sagittal fast spin echo-T2W image through the intercondylar notch shows a normal ACL *(arrow)*, with the anterior band parallel to the roof of the notch.

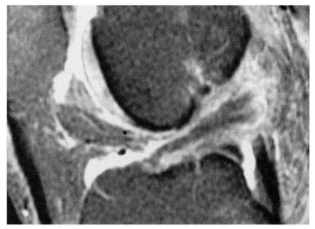

Figure 15–29. TORN ANTERIOR CRUCIATE LIGAMENT (ACL). This sagittal image through the intercondylar notch shows the ACL to be flatter than the roof of the notch. Also, its origin off the femur could not be identified. This is a torn ACL.

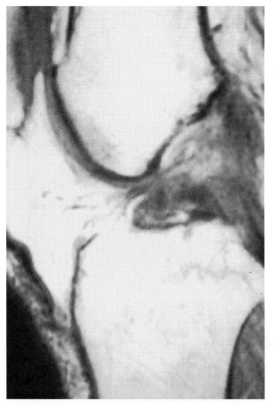

Figure 15–28. TORN ANTERIOR CRUCIATE LIGAMENT (ACL). This sagittal image through the intercondylar notch shows the ACL to be disrupted, with no normal fibers identified.

(Fig. 15–28). When it tears, it literally explodes, leaving nothing with which the surgeon can do a primary repair. A tendon graft (usually from the patella) is used to reconstruct the ACL when necessary. Occasionally, an ACL tear is seen in which the fibers of the torn ACL are seemingly intact but the angle is flatter than normal (Fig. 15–29). As mentioned, the fibers should be parallel to the roof of the intercondylar notch.

A partial tear of the ACL is treated nonoperatively, and the imaging literature has very little concerning our accuracy in diagnosing partial tears of the ACL.

A sprain or partial tear of the ACL can be mentioned when focal or diffuse high signal or laxity of the ACL is present. Unfortunately, there is no way of determining the validity of these findings, because surgeons are equally unable to confidently diagnose partial tears. Partial tears are not treated, so it is not worth getting bothered with this diagnosis.

A pitfall that can lead the unwary to call an ACL tear when it is, in fact, essentially normal is an ACL cyst. An ACL cyst is an entity of unknown cause in which the ACL is distended with mucinous fluid (Fig. 15–30). The normal ACL fibers are not clearly identified and appear to be disrupted; however, these patients have no instability and usually are asymptomatic. At most, they have a feeling of swelling or fullness in the knee and are unable to fully flex the knee because of the mass effect. The ACL has a drumstick appearance on sagittal images and appears cystic on coronal or axial images. We have seen this in about 1% of all our knee MR examinations. One report in the surgery literature tells of mistaking an ACL cyst for a tumor, with subsequent resection of the normal ACL.[18]

Figure 15–30. ANTERIOR CRUCIATE LIGAMENT (ACL) CYST. *A,* This sagittal proton density image through the intercondylar notch shows the ACL as a cystic, drumstick-shaped structure without clearly identifiable fibers. *B,* A coronal fast spin echo-T2W image shows the ACL to have a cystic appearance *(arrows).* This is characteristic of an ACL cyst.

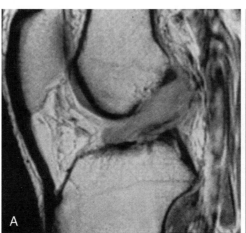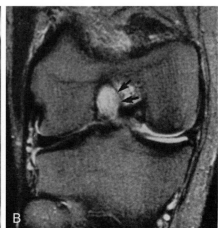

After surgery to reconstruct the ACL, we occasionally are asked to re-image a patient because of pain or instability. The ACL graft should be present as a taut structure, usually with some increased signal on T2W sagittal images (Fig. 15–31). If the graft is disrupted or absent, it has obviously failed. The tibial tunnel should be parallel to the roof of the femoral intercondylar notch. If it is too steep, the graft will be impinged by the femur on extension of the knee (Fig. 15–32). If it is too flat, it may be too lax and not give the needed stability.

One of the most common reasons for pain after knee arthroscopy is the presence of arthrofibrosis (scar) in Hoffa's fat pad. This can have several appearances and may require reoperation. A round mass of scar in Hoffa's fat pad, called a cyclops lesion, can interfere with knee extension and often needs to be resected (Fig. 15–33). A linear scar that extends to the inferior pole of the patella can restrict patellar motion and cause pain (Fig. 15–34).[19]

Posterior Cruciate Ligament

The PCL normally is seen as a low signal structure in the intercondylar notch, gently curving between the posterior tibia and the femur (Fig. 15–35). It is infrequently torn and even less frequently surgically repaired. When it tears, it typically does not have an actual disruption of the fibers, as is seen with other ligaments, but rather it stretches and is not structurally competent, more like overstretching the elastic in one's socks. On MRI it most commonly has a fat, gray appearance on proton density or T1W images (Fig. 15–36) and does not get high in signal on T2W images (Fig. 15–37) (although PCL tears have been reported to be high in signal on STIR

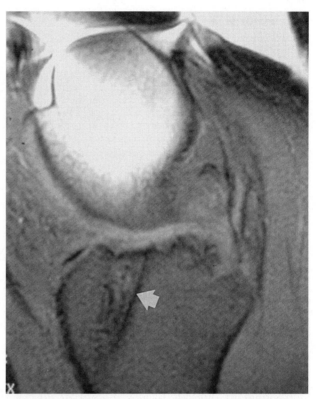

Figure 15–32. TORN ANTERIOR CRUCIATE LIGAMENT (ACL) GRAFT.
This sagittal fast spin echo-T2W image in a patient with a prior ACL reconstruction fails to show the ACL graft because it is disrupted. Note that the tibial tunnel *(arrow)* is steeper than the roof of the intercondylar notch, allowing the femur to impinge on the graft when the knee is in extension.

sequences). Because this is contrary to most injured structures, it has been our experience that tears of the PCL frequently are missed. If the PCL avulses from its tibial attachment it is easily diagnosed, but this is not a common presentation. Orthopedic surgeons are repairing the PCL more frequently than in the past, but in most cases a torn PCL is not repaired. Hence, for most cases it does not matter what you say about the PCL—the surgeon will not even inspect it at arthroscopy. However, we should be able to tell the surgeon with a high degree of accuracy if the PCL is torn or not.

Medial Collateral Ligament

The medial collateral ligament (MCL) originates on the medial aspect of the distal femur and inserts on the medial aspect of the proximal tibia. Its fibers are intimately interlaced with the joint capsule at the level of the joint, and the medial meniscus is attached directly to it. It is not an intrasynovial structure; therefore, it is not seen or repaired arthroscopically. Accuracy of MRI has therefore not been established, but it is generally agreed that MRI is highly accurate in depicting the MCL.

The three grades of injury described clinically correspond to three appearances of the MCL seen

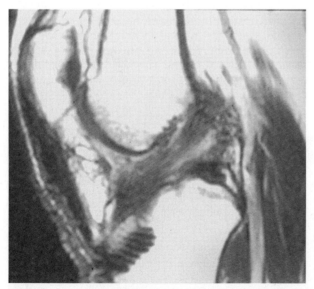

Figure 15–31. ANTERIOR CRUCIATE LIGAMENT (ACL) GRAFT INTACT.
A sagittal T1W image through the intercondylar notch in a patient with a prior ACL reconstruction shows the ACL graft to be intact. It has some increased signal, which is normal in reconstructions.

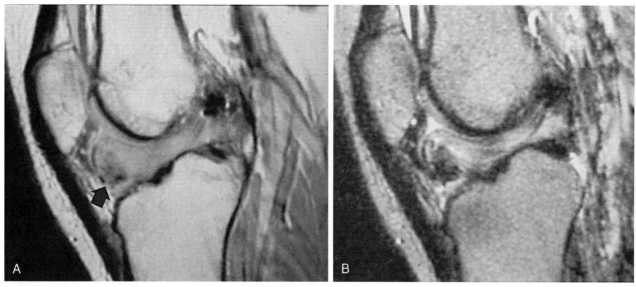

Figure 15–33. CYCLOPS LESION.
A, This sagittal proton density image in a patient with a prior anterior cruciate ligament (ACL) reconstruction shows scar tissue in Hoffa's fat pad *(arrow).* *B,* On a sagittal T2W image, the scar stays low in signal. It has a rounded configuration, which has been termed a cyclops lesion. This is arthrofibrosis secondary to the surgery.

with T2W coronal images. Grade 1, a sprain, shows high signal in the soft tissues medial to the MCL (Fig. 15–38). Grade 2, a severe sprain or partial tear, shows high signal in the soft tissues medial to the MCL, but also has high signal or partial disruption of the MCL itself (Fig. 15–39). A grade 3, or complete tear, shows disruption of the MCL (Fig. 15–40). The MCL is seldom repaired even if it is completely disrupted, unless multiple other ligaments are torn. Grade 1 and 2 sprains usually are treated conservatively with bracing and continuance of athletic ac-

tivities as pain allows. High signal medial to the MCL may occur from causes unrelated to an MCL sprain, such as subcutaneous edema.

A meniscocapsular separation is easily diagnosed on T2W coronal images by noting fluid between the MCL and the medial meniscus. This can be overlooked on T1W coronal images (Fig. 15–41). Because these patients present clinically in an identical manner to a patient with a sprained MCL, they often are allowed to continue their activities with a brace. This is not acceptable treatment for a menis-

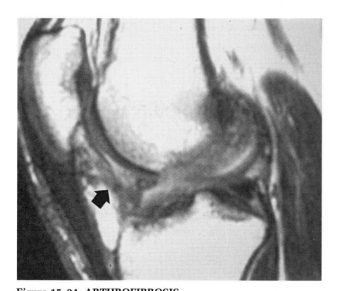

Figure 15–34. ARTHROFIBROSIS.
This sagittal proton density image in a patient with a prior anterior cruciate ligament (ACL) reconstruction shows scar tissue in Hoffa's fat pad *(arrow),* which is linear in configuration and extends to the inferior pole of the patella. This form of arthrofibrosis can cause patellar pain and patellar tracking abnormalities.

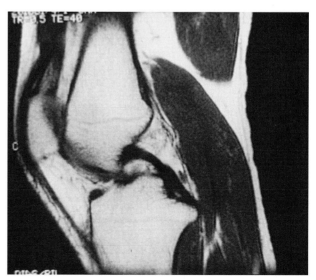

Figure 15–35. NORMAL POSTERIOR CRUCIATE LIGAMENT (PCL).
This sagittal T1W image through the intercondylar notch shows a normal PCL with uniform low signal.

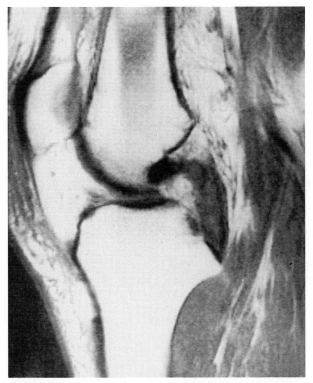

Figure 15–36. TORN POSTERIOR CRUCIATE LIGAMENT (PCL).
This sagittal proton density image through the intercondylar notch shows a torn PCL that is thicker than normal and has uniform intermediate signal, rather than low signal.

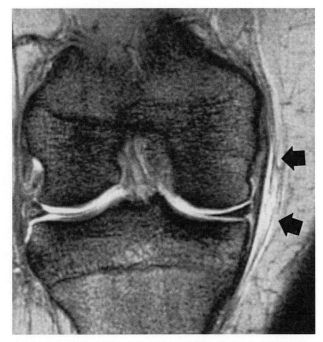

Figure 15–38. GRADE 1 MEDIAL COLLATERAL LIGAMENT (MCL) SPRAIN.
A coronal gradient echo image in a patient with an injury to the MCL shows increased signal in the soft tissues medial to the MCL *(arrows)* with a normal-appearing MCL. This is a grade 1 MCL sprain.

cocapsular separation. The vascular interface between the MCL and the meniscus can become avascular with continued activity, resulting in a meniscus that does not heal to the capsule. These patients need either immobilization or surgical repair. If the meniscocapsular separation is isolated solely to the area of the MCL, it can be considered a partial tear of the deep fibers of the MCL. If the separation is only over a short portion of the meniscal attachment, it is unlikely to be significant. A meniscocapsular separation that extends posteriorly, involving the posterior oblique ligament (a thickening of the capsule at the joint line posterior to the MCL), seems to be more significant in terms of stability than one that is solely medial or anterior (Fig. 15–42).

Lateral Collateral Ligament

The lateral collateral ligament (LCL) complex is composed of many structures, but only three that

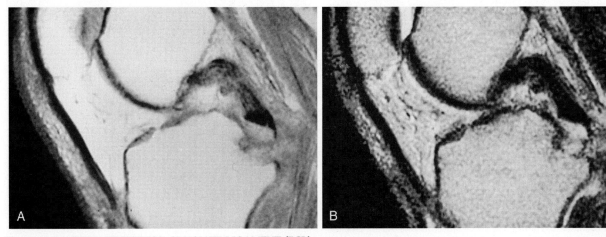

Figure 15–37. TORN POSTERIOR CRUCIATE LIGAMENT (PCL).
A, This sagittal proton density image through the intercondylar notch shows a PCL that has torn off its insertion on the posterior tibia. Note that the body of the PCL is thicker than normal and has intermediate signal throughout. *B,* A fast spin echo-T2W image in the same knee demonstrates how the PCL does not have increased signal even though it is torn.

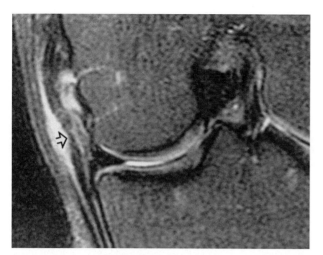

Figure 15–39. GRADE 2 MEDIAL COLLATERAL LIGAMENT (MCL) SPRAIN.
This coronal fast spin echo-T2W image shows increased signal in a thinned but otherwise intact MCL *(arrow)*—a grade 2 sprain.

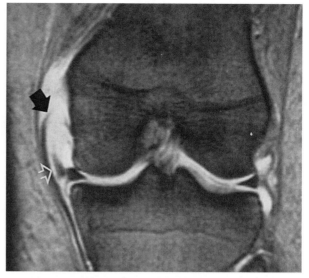

Figure 15–40. TORN MEDIAL COLLATERAL LIGAMENT (MCL) AND MENISCOCAPSULAR SEPARATION.
This coronal gradient echo image reveals a complete tear of the MCL *(arrow)*. Note also the fluid tracking between the MCL and the meniscus *(open arrow)*. This indicates a meniscocapsular separation, because it could be seen on multiple adjacent images.

are easily evaluated with MRI: posterior to anterior, they are the biceps femoris tendon, the fibulocollateral ligament (the true lateral collateral ligament) (Fig. 15–43*A*), and the iliotibial band. The biceps and the fibulocollateral ligament insert onto the proximal fibula, whereas the iliotibial band inserts onto Gerdy's tubercle on the anterior tibia. Tears of the lateral ligament (Fig. 15–43*B*) are not nearly as common as those of the MCL. LCL tears often are associated with injury to other structures in the posterolateral corner of the knee, as this area is called. Injury to a component of the LCL in association with tears of the popliteus tendon, arcuate ligament (a thickening of the capsule at the joint line posterolaterally), and either the ACL or the PCL are termed posterolateral corner injury. Such injury results in pain and instability with knee hyperextension if not surgically corrected. It is one of the few

knee injuries that is considered a near emergency. Failure to surgically treat a posterolateral corner injury in 3 to 4 days is said to have a high incidence of a poor result.[20] These are therefore operated on almost immediately.

The popliteus tendon can tear as an isolated injury, but usually tears in conjunction with other structures, as in posterolateral corner injuries or complete knee dislocations. A popliteus tear usually occurs at the musculotendinous junction and results in a large amount of fluid in the popliteus tendon sheath, a lax popliteus tendon, and high signal in or around the popliteus muscle (Fig. 15–44).[21]

Pain in the anterolateral knee often is found in

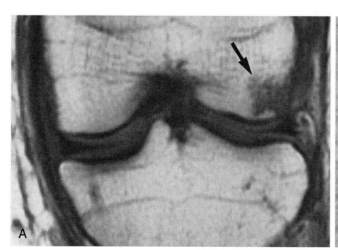

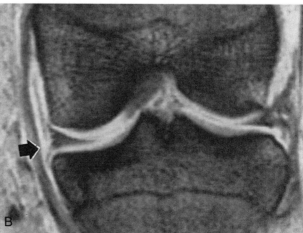

Figure 15–41. MENISCOCAPSULAR SEPARATION.
A, A coronal T1W image in a patient with a blow to the lateral side of the knee shows a contusion on the lateral femoral condyle *(arrow).* *B,* A coronal gradient echo image in the same knee shows fluid tracking between the medial meniscus and the medial collateral ligament (MCL; *arrow*), which indicates a meniscocapsular separation. Note that in *A,* a meniscocapsular separation cannot be diagnosed.

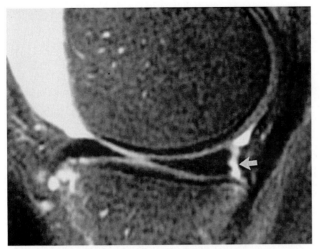

Figure 15–42. MENISCOCAPSULAR SEPARATION.
A sagittal fast spin echo-T2W image through the medial meniscus shows fluid between the posterior horn attachment and the capsule *(arrow)*. This indicates a meniscocapsular separation.

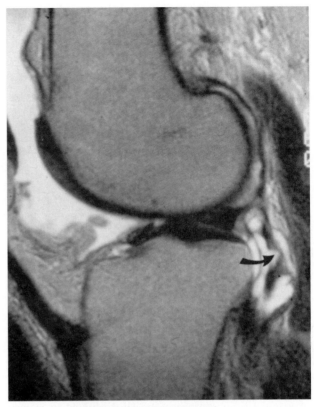

Figure 15–44. TORN POPLITEUS TENDON.
This sagittal fast spin echo-T2W image shows a marked amount of fluid around the popliteus tendon. The tendon is wavy and lax, rather than taut *(arrow)*. These findings are typical for a torn popliteus tendon.

runners because of the iliotibial (IT) band rubbing on the lateral femoral condyle. This is called IT band friction syndrome or IT band syndrome.[22] It is easily diagnosed on MRI by noting fluid on both sides of the IT band (Fig. 15–45). It is seen most easily on the axial images. The IT band may have thickening or high signal within its fibers, but in our experience it usually has high signal around it.

Patella

Dislocation of the patella frequently is diagnosed with MRI, to the surprise of the referring physician. Because the dislocated patella often rapidly reduces on its own, only about half of the patients with patella dislocations are aware of what really occurred. They get referred for imaging with the nebulous "rule out internal derangement" history. The MR examination usually is easily interpreted as a patella dislocation.[23] A contusion characteristically occurs on the anterior lateral femoral condyle (Fig. 15–46A). The contusion is from the impaction of the patella as it either dislocates or as it reduces. There may or may not be a kissing contusion on the medial side of the patella. The medial retinaculum is always injured, although a frank tear can be difficult to appreciate. The key finding is the patellar cartilage. If a piece of cartilage is missing, it usually means an arthroscopic procedure is necessary (Fig.

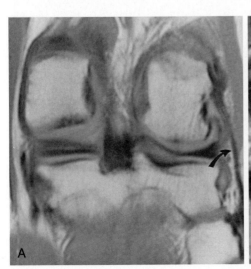

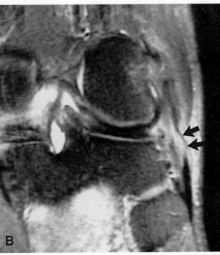

Figure 15–43. NORMAL AND TORN FIBULOCOLLATERAL LIGAMENT.
A, A coronal T1W image shows a normal fibulocollateral ligament *(arrow)*. *B,* This coronal fast spin echo-T2W image shows a torn fibulocollateral ligament *(arrows)*.

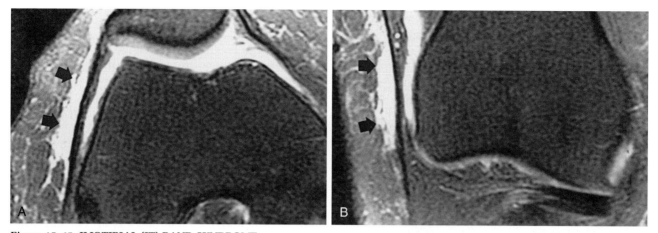

Figure 15–45. ILIOTIBIAL (IT) BAND SYNDROME.
A, This axial fast spin echo-T2W image in a patient with lateral knee pain shows fluid around the IT band *(arrows),* indicative of IT band syndrome. *B,* A coronal fast spin echo-T2W image again shows fluid around the IT band *(arrows).*

15–46*B*), whereas if the cartilage is normal, the patient usually is treated conservatively. Therefore, the main role of the radiologist is to carefully examine the patellar cartilage. One should also evaluate the depth of the trochlear notch, which often is hypoplastic in those with dislocating patellae and is a predisposing factor to subsequent dislocations.

Synovial Plicae

A thin, fibrous band frequently is seen on the axial images that extends from the medial joint capsule toward the medial facet of the patella (Fig. 15–47). This is a normal structure, the medial patella plica, which is a remnant of the embryologic development of the knee.[24] Embryologically, the knee is divided into compartments by a superior, inferior, and medial patella plica. About half of all normal knees demonstrate one or more of the plicae on MRI. The medial patella plica can get thickened, stiff, and trapped between the patella and the femur, causing pain, clicking, and locking, similar to a torn meniscus. There are no measurements used to diagnose a thickened medial patellar plica. With experience, it becomes obvious when the plica appears to be too thick (Fig. 15–48). An axial T2W image and joint fluid are both required to visualize the medial plica. An inflamed plica is easily removed at arthroscopy, but plica syndrome is an uncommon diagnosis.

The other plicae found in the knee are the suprapatellar plica and the infrapatellar plica. They commonly are seen on MR images but do not cause plica

Figure 15–46. PATELLAR DISLOCATION.
A, A coronal fast spin echo-T2W image shows a large contusion on the anterior lateral femoral condyle. *B,* An axial fast spin echo-T2W image through the patella shows a large defect in the patellar cartilage *(arrow).* Whereas the contusion pattern seen in *A* is virtually diagnostic of a patellar dislocation, the cartilage defect usually means this is a surgical case.

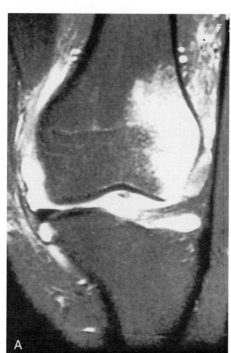

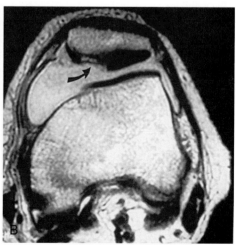

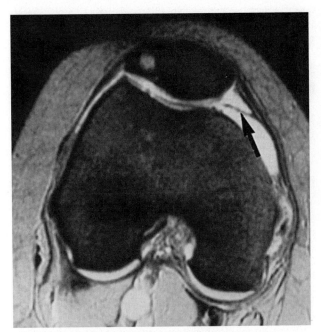

Figure 15–47. MEDIAL PATELLAR PLICA.
An axial gradient echo image through the patella shows a thin fibrous band extending off the medial capsule *(arrow)*, which is a normal medial patellar plica.

syndrome, as does the medial patellar plica; hence, they will not be discussed further.

Patellar Tendon

Pain in the inferior patella region in athletes, so-called jumper's knee, is often seen on MRI as thickening of the proximal patellar tendon with high signal in and around it on T2W images[25] (Fig. 15–49). Jumper's knee can be a debilitating entity for athletes and can require surgery to remove the focus of myxoid degeneration in the tendon.

Bursae

Several bursae are present around the knee that can become inflamed and cause symptoms which, in some cases, can mimic intraarticular pathology and result in inappropriate therapy, including surgery. It is important to recognize these and correctly report their occurrence so that the orthopaedic surgeon can institute the appropriate treatment.

Popliteal (Baker's Cyst)

The most common knee bursa is a popliteal bursa or Baker's cyst, which extends from the knee joint posteriorly between the tendons of the medial head of the gastrocnemius and the semimembranosus. It can contain a small amount of fluid in normal individuals, but any more than 5 to 10 mL of fluid should be mentioned, because it could be a source

of symptoms. These bursae can get quite large and cause a compartment syndrome. They can extend far down the leg in some patients. They can rupture and cause inflammation to the surrounding musculature, which can be very symptomatic. They often mimic deep vein thrombosis clinically.

Prepatellar Bursa

Prepatellar bursitis is a common cause of anterior knee pain. It is caused from repetitive trauma from kneeling; hence, it has been termed housemaid's knee in the older, less politically correct literature. Because it is an easy clinical diagnosis, we do not usually see prepatellar bursitis as an isolated finding, but often we see it in addition to other abnormalities. On MRI it is seen as a fluid collection superficial to the patella (Fig. 15–50).

Pes Anserinus Bursa

A bursa that occurs on the anteromedial tibia, just below the joint line, is the pes anserinus bursa. *Pes anserinus* means "goose's foot" in Latin and refers to the configuration of the insertion of the pes tendons onto the tibia—it has a webbed foot appearance (it takes a little imagination). The pes tendons are the gracilis, sartorius, and the semitendinosus. The pes bursa lies beneath the tendons and, when inflamed, extends proximally toward the joint (Fig. 15–51).[26] We have seen several patients who had arthroscopy for a clicking, popping, painful knee that was thought to be a meniscus tear but was simply a pes anserinus bursitis. Bursae about the knee are not seen at arthroscopy; therefore, it is

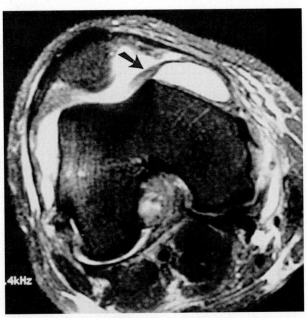

Figure 15–48. THICKENED MEDIAL PATELLAR PLICA.
This axial fast spin echo-T2W image through the patella shows an enlarged, thickened medial patellar plica *(arrow)* trapped between the patella and femur that extends well posterior to the patella.

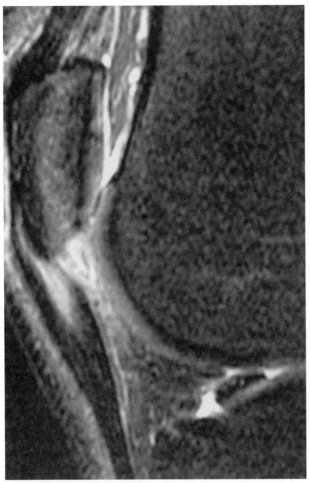

Figure 15–49. JUMPER'S KNEE.
A sagittal fast spin echo-T2W image through the patellar tendon demonstrates a thickened proximal portion of the tendon with high signal. This is diagnostic of jumper's knee.

imperative that MRI or physical diagnosis pick them up.

Semimembranosus Tibial Collateral Ligament Bursa

Another bursa about the knee that can mimic an internal derangement is the semimembranosus tibial collateral ligament bursa.[27] This commonly inflamed bursa has a characteristic appearance that makes it easily recognized with MRI. It occurs right on the joint line and drapes over the semimembranosus tendon like a horseshoe (Fig. 15–52). On both coronal and sagittal images (Fig. 15–53) it appears to arise at the meniscus and extend inferiorly, making the diagnosis of a meniscal cyst attractive. However, no connection to a meniscal tear is found.

Tibial Collateral Ligament Bursa

An uncommonly seen bursa is the tibial collateral ligament bursa. It lies just deep to the medial collateral ligament and extends vertically above and be-

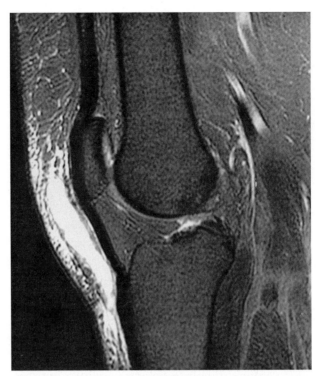

Figure 15–50. PREPATELLAR BURSITIS.
This sagittal fast spin echo-T2W image through the knee shows a well-contained fluid collection anterior to the patella. This is prepatellar bursitis.

low the joint line (Fig. 15–54). It can be confused for a meniscocapsular separation but, unlike a traumatic separation, the fluid is well contained and cyst-like, rather than diffusely distributed.

The four bursae described here all occur medially and are located in distinctly different locations (Fig. 15–55). On occasion, a bursa is so distended that it

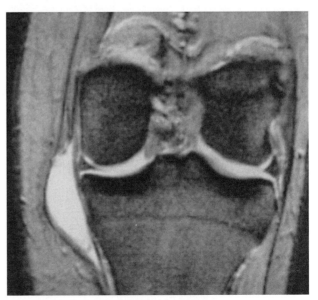

Figure 15–51. PES ANSERINUS BURSITIS.
This coronal gradient echo image shows a fluid collection medially, just inferior to the joint line. This is pes anserinus bursitis.

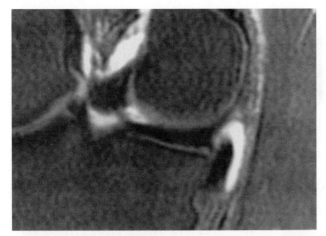

Figure 15–52. SEMIMEMBRANOSUS–TIBIAL COLLATERAL LIGAMENT BURSITIS.
A coronal fast spin echo-T2W image shows a fluid collection at the medial joint line that is adjacent to the medial meniscus and is draped over the semimembranosus tendon. This is the appearance of a semimembranosus–tibial collateral ligament bursa.

overlaps an area usually reserved for another bursa and it can be difficult to determine which bursa is present. The actual name of the bursa is not nearly as important as recognizing that there is a bursa and letting the surgeon know about it.

Bones

Bone contusions, seen as amorphous, subarticular high signal on T2W images, are commonly encountered on knee MR examination. They have significance in that they can be the sole source of pain, they can precede a focal area of bone necrosis (osteochondritis dissecans), and they can indicate ad-

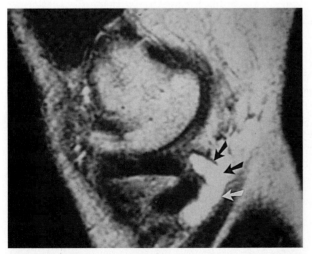

Figure 15–53. SEMIMEMBRANOSUS–TIBIAL COLLATERAL LIGAMENT BURSITIS.
This sagittal fast spin echo-T2W image shows the semimembranosus–tibial collateral ligament bursa *(arrows)* at the level of the medial meniscus and draping over the semimembranosus tendon.

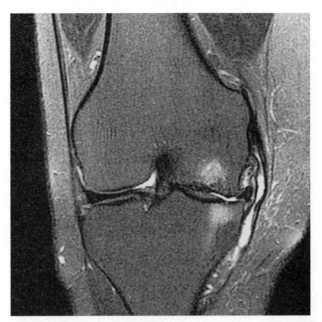

Figure 15–54. MEDIAL COLLATERAL LIGAMENT (MCL) BURSITIS.
This fast spin echo-T2W image shows a fluid collection just deep to the MCL, which is an MCL bursitis.

ditional internal derangements when they have a specific pattern. Bone contusions are basically microfractures. They invariably heal with rest, as would any fracture. However, if they are not protected, there is at least the potential that they can progress to osteochondritis dissecans. This is thought to be more frequently seen with the contusions that are more geographic in appearance (Fig. 15–56), as opposed to the reticular appearance of most contusions.[28]

A contusion pattern that is fairly specific for an ACL tear is one that involves the posterolateral aspect of the tibial plateau (Fig. 15–57). When the ACL tears, the tibia internally rotates on the femur, allowing the lateral femoral condyle to impact on the posterolateral tibial plateau. This has been termed the pivot-shift phenomenon. There is often a kissing contusion on the central to anterior lateral femoral condyle above the anterior horn of the lat-

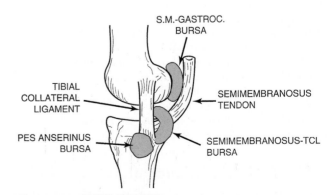

Figure 15–55. KNEE BURSAE.
This schematic shows the location of the common bursae on the medial side of the knee. S.M.-gastroc. bursa—Baker's cyst.

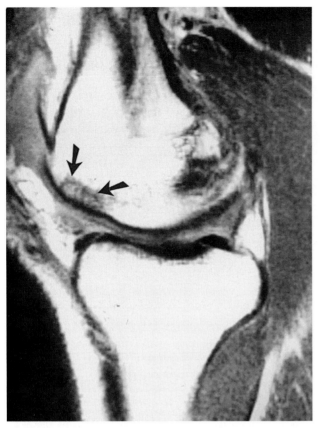

Figure 15–56. BONE CONTUSION.
This sagittal T1W image shows a well-defined, geographic contusion on the femoral condyle *(arrows)*. This type of contusion is thought to more likely develop into osteochondritis dissecans, as compared to an ill-defined, reticular contusion.

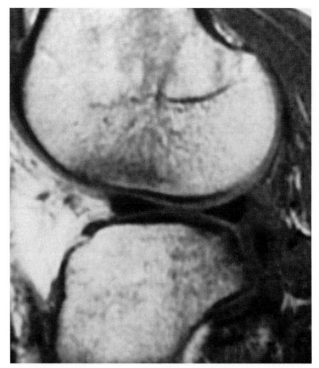

Figure 15–57. BONE CONTUSION.
This sagittal T1W image through the lateral side of the knee in a patient with a torn anterior cruciate ligament (ACL) shows reticular contusions in the posterior tibial plateau and centrally in the femoral condyle. This pattern typically is seen with an ACL tear.

eral meniscus. This contusion pattern occasionally is found in the absence of an ACL tear in children who have stretched the ACL, but their increased flexibility protects it from tearing.

Another contusion that frequently is seen with an ACL tear is found on the posteromedial tibial plateau and sometimes the medial femoral condyle just posterior to the MCL as well. Kaplan et al.[29] found this contusion in 25 of 215 knees (12%). All had an ACL tear, and 24 of 25 had meniscocapsular injuries, which they termed contrecoup injuries.

Soft Tissues

Tears of the plantaris tendon have been termed tennis leg because of its frequent association with that activity. The patient presents with acute calf pain and occasionally displays swelling with purplish skin discoloration caused by the hemorrhage. It can clinically resemble a torn medial head of the gastrocnemius (which requires different treatment than a torn plantaris tendon) or deep venous thrombosis. The plantaris muscle arises on the lateral femoral condyle and runs distally just deep to the lateral head of the gastrocnemius and superficial to the soleus muscle. Its tendon begins in the upper

part of the lower leg and courses medially deep to the medial head of the gastrocnemius and continues adjacent to the medial aspect of the achilles tendon to the calcaneus (Fig. 15–58). MRI through the calf shows a focal fluid collection between the soleus and the medial head of the gastrocnemius (Fig. 15–59). A torn, retracted tendon sometimes may be visualized. The fluid collection is often very tubular

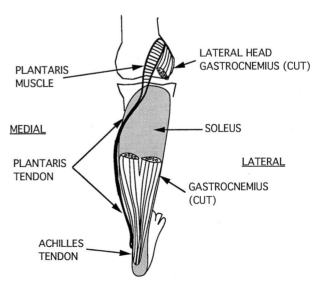

Figure 15–58. PLANTARIS MUSCLE AND TENDON.
This schematic shows the plantaris muscle and tendon from a posterior view.

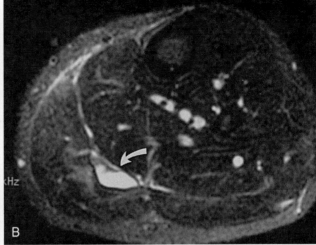

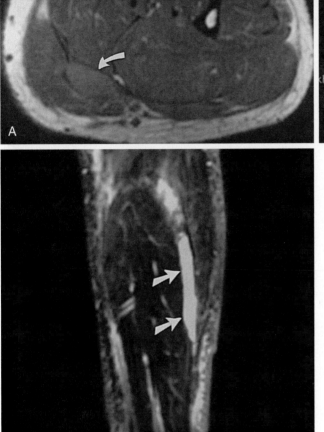

Figure 15–59. PLANTARIS TENDON TEAR.
A, An axial proton density and *B,* T2W image through the calf in a patient with sudden calf pain during tennis shows a fluid collection *(arrow)* between the soleus and the medial head of the gastrocnemius muscle. *C,* A sagittal T2W image shows a tubular fluid collection *(arrows)* just deep to the medial head of the gastrocnemius. This is characteristic of a torn plantaris tendon.

in configuration. An association between an injured plantaris muscle and a torn anterior cruciate ligament has been noted.[30]

References

1. Escobedo EM, Hunter JC, Zinkbrody GC, et al. Usefulness of turbo spin-echo MR imaging in the evaluation of meniscal tears — comparison with a conventional spin-echo sequence. *AJR* 1996; 167:1223–1227.
2. Cheung L, Li K, Hollett M, et al. Meniscal tears of the knee: accuracy of detection with fast spin-echo MR imaging and arthroscopic correlation in 293 patients. *Radiology* 1997; 203:508–512.
3. Rubin D, Kneeland J, Listerud J, et al. MR diagnosis of meniscal tears of the knee: value of fast spin-echo vs conventional spin-echo pulse sequences. *AJR* 1994; 162:1131–1136.
4. Anderson M, Raghavan N, Seidenwurm D, et al. Evaluation of meniscal tears: fast spin-echo versus conventional spin-echo MR imaging. *Acad Radiol* 1995; 2:209–214.
5. De Smet A, Norris M, Yandow D, et al. MR diagnosis of meniscal tears of the knee: importance of high signal in the meniscus that extends to the surface. *AJR* 1993; 161:101–107.
6. Kaplan PA, Nelson NL, Garvin KL, Brown DE. MR of the knee: the significance of high signal in the meniscus that does not clearly extend to the surface. *AJR* 1991; 156:333–336.
7. De Smet A, Graf B. Meniscal tears missed on MR imaging: relationship to meniscal tear patterns and anterior cruciate ligament tears. *AJR* 1994; 162:905–911.
8. Helms CA, Laorr A, Cannon WD. The absent bow tie sign in bucket-handle tears of the menisci in the knee. *AJR* 1998; 170:57–61.
9. Lecas L, Helms C, Kosarek F, Garrett W. Inferiorly displaced flap tears of the medial meniscus: MR appearance and clinical significance. *AJR* 2000; 174:161–164.
10. Pedowitz R, Feagin J, Rajagopalan S. A surgical algorithm for treatment of cystic degeneration of the meniscus. *Arthroscopy* 1996; 12:209–216.
11. Silverman J, Mink J, Deutsch A. Discoid menisci of the knee: MR imaging appearance. *Radiology* 1989; 173:351–354.
12. Shankman S, Beltran J, Melamed E, Rosenberg ZS. Anterior horn of the lateral meniscus — another potential pitfall in MR imaging of the knee. *Radiology* 1997; 204:181–184.
13. Peterfy C, Janzen D, Tirman P, et al. "Magic-angle" phenomenon: a cause of increased signal in the normal lateral meniscus on short-TE MR images of the knee. *Radiology* 1994; 163:149–154.
14. Erickson S, Cox I, Hyde J, et al. Effect of tendon orientation

on MR imaging signal intensity: a manifestation of the "magic angle" phenomenon. *Radiology* 1991; 181:389–392.

15. Ha T, Li K, Beaulieu CF, et al. Anterior cruciate ligament injury — fast spin-echo MR imaging with arthroscopic correlation in 217 examinations. *AJR* 1998; 170:1215–1219.

16. Mink J, Levy T, Crues JI. Tears of the anterior cruciate ligament and menisci of the knee: MR imaging evaluation. *Radiology* 1988; 167:769–774.

17. Lee J, Yao L, Phelps C, et al. Anterior cruciate ligament tears: MR imaging compared with arthroscopy and clinical tests. *Radiology* 1988; 166:861–864.

18. Kumar A, Bickerstaff DR, Grimwood JS, Suvarna SK. Mucoid cystic degeneration of the cruciate ligament. *J Bone Joint Surg [Br]* 1999; 1999:304–305.

19. Recht MP, Piraino DW, Cohen MA, et al. Localized anterior arthrofibrosis (cyclops lesion) after reconstruction of the anterior cruciate ligament: MR imaging findings. *AJR* 1995; 165:383–385.

20. Veltri D, Warren R. Posterolateral instability of the knee. *J Bone Joint Surg [Am]* 1994; 76:460–472.

21. Brown T, Quinn S, Wensel J, et al. Diagnosis of popliteus injuries with MR imaging. *Skeletal Radiol* 1995; 24:511–514.

22. Murphy B, Hechtman K, Uribe J, et al. Iliotibial band friction syndrome: MR imaging findings. *Radiology* 1992; 185:569–571.

23. Virolainen H, Visuri T, Kuusela T. Acute dislocation of the patella: MR findings. *Radiology* 1993; 189:243–246.

24. Deutsch AL, Resnick D, Dalinka MK, et al. Synovial plicae of the knee. *Radiology* 1981; 141:627–634.

25. Yu JS, Popp JE, Kaeding CC, Lucas J. Correlation of MR imaging and pathologic findings in athletes undergoing surgery for chronic patellar tendinitis. *AJR* 1995; 165:115–118.

26. Forbes JR, Helms CA, Janzen DL. Acute pes anserine bursitis: MR imaging. *Radiology* 1995; 194:525–527.

27. Rothstein CP, Laorr A, Helms CA, Tirman P. Semimembranosus-tibal collateral ligament bursitis — MR imaging findings. *AJR* 1996; 166:875–877.

28. Vellet A, Marks P, Fowler P, Munro T. Occult posttraumatic osteochondral lesions of the knee: prevalence, classification, and short-term sequelae evaluated with MR imaging. *Radiology* 1991; 178:271–276.

29. Kaplan PA, Gehl RH, Dussault RG, et al. Bone contusions of the posterior lip of the medial tibial plateau (contrecoup injury) and associated internal derangements of the knee at MR imaging. *Radiology* 1999; 211:747–753.

30. Helms CA, Fritz RC, Garvin GJ. Plantaris muscle injury: evaluation with MR imaging. *Radiology* 1995; 195:201–203.

DEDICATED KNEE MRI
This is one set of suggested protocols; there are many variations that would work equally well.

Sequence #	1	2	3	4
Sequence Type	Proton density with fat saturation	Fast spin echo with fat saturation	Fast spin echo with fat saturation	Fast spin echo with fat saturation
Orientation	Sagittal	Sagittal	Coronal	Axial
Field of View (cm)	14–16	14–16	14–16	14–16
Slice Thickness (mm)	4	4	4	4
Contrast	No	No	No	No

Scout

Final Image

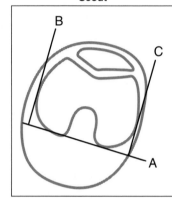

- Axial scout
- Obtain sagittal images perpendicular to line A, which is tangent to posterior aspect of femoral condyles
- Cover from line B to C through bones only

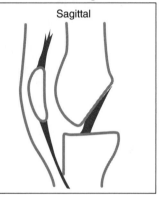
Sagittal

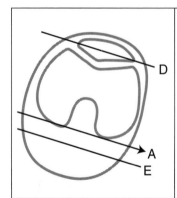

- Axial scout
- Obtain coronal images parallel to line A, which is tangent to posterior aspect of femoral condyles
- Cover from line D to E to include bones

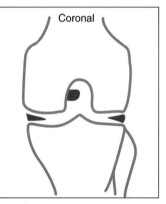
Coronal

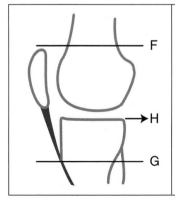

- Sagittal scout
- Obtain axial images parallel to tibial plateau (line H)
- Cover from just above patella (line F) to tibial attachment of patellar tendon (line G)

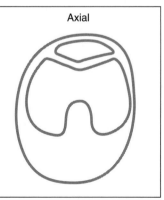
Axial

Coronal images (A-B)

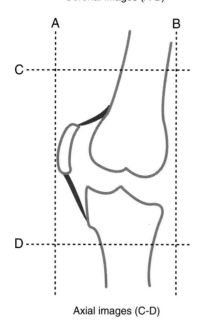

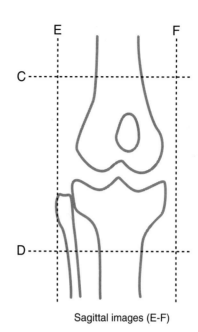

Axial images (C-D)

Sagittal images (E-F)

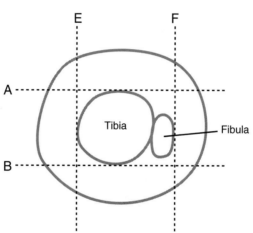

Tibia

Fibula

16 FOOT AND ANKLE

HOW TO IMAGE THE FOOT AND ANKLE
NORMAL AND ABNORMAL
Tendons
Posterior Ankle Tendons
  Achilles and Plantaris
Medial Ankle Tendons
  Posterior Tibial Tendon
  Flexor Digitorum Longus
  Flexor Hallucis Longus
Lateral Ankle Tendons
  Peroneal Tendons
Anterior Ankle Tendons
  Anterior Tibial Tendon
Ankle Ligaments

Medial Ankle Ligaments
Lateral Ankle Ligaments
Miscellaneous Inflammatory Conditions
  Anterolateral Impingement Syndrome in the Ankle
  Sinus Tarsi Syndrome
  Plantar Fasciitis
Nerve Abnormalities
  Tarsal Tunnel Syndrome
  Morton's Neuroma
Bone Abnormalities
  Tarsal Coalition
  Accessory Bones and Sesamoids
  Os Trigonum Syndrome

Accessory Navicular
Hallux Sesamoids
Fractures
  Osteonecrosis of the Foot and Ankle
  Osseous Tumors
Soft Tissue Tumors
  Benign
  Malignant
  Soft Tissue Tumor Mimickers
The Diabetic Foot
Foreign Bodies
FOOT AND ANKLE PROTOCOLS

HOW TO IMAGE THE FOOT AND ANKLE

See the protocols for foot and ankle MRI at the end of this chapter.

The foot and ankle are among the most difficult anatomic sites to image, simply because of the angle formed between the foot and ankle. Even the terminology for plane orientation in the foot and ankle is confusing and certainly not universal.

Coils and Patient Position. Ideally, imaging of the ankle and foot should be done with the foot at right angles to the lower leg with the patient in a supine position. This may require a support on the sole of the foot to maintain the alignment (special surface coils are now being made to accomplish this). A standard extremity coil generally is employed for the foot and ankle (the same one used for knee MRI), and such a precise position for the foot is not always possible to obtain or maintain. More importantly, the patient should be immobilized with padding and made comfortable so as not to move and degrade the images with motion, and the radiologist should know the anatomy well enough so that it is easily interpretable, regardless of slight variations in the angle of the foot with the ankle.

How to angle MR images properly with the anatomic planes of the foot and ankle in order to obtain images that are reproducible and most easily understood are shown in the protocols of how to image the foot and ankle. The lower extremity externally rotates when a patient is in a relaxed supine position, and the planes of imaging must be oriented to the anatomy of the foot, rather than to the magnet.

For example, true sagittal images of the foot and ankle are mandatory to show the Achilles tendon accurately. If a slice cuts through the tendon obliquely, it gives the false impression of abnormal thickening of the tendon.

Imaging the forefoot or toes often is done with the patient prone to allow the toes to be in a neutral position, more easily immobilized, and better centered in the coil.

Only the extremity suspected of being abnormal is imaged; the opposite normal side is never done simultaneously for comparison, because it is unnecessary and decreases the detail and resolution of the images owing to the larger field of view required.

Image Orientation (Box 16–1). Planes of imaging in the ankle are standard and identical to elsewhere in the body. The foot is more complicated. For purposes of this chapter, we will consider the images that run parallel with the long axis of the foot, and appear similar to an anteroposterior (AP) foot radiograph, as either *long axis axial* or *long axis coronal* images. Images obtained perpendicular to the long axis of the foot so that the metatarsals are seen as five circles of bone cut transversely are referred to as *short axis axials*. Sagittal images are self-explanatory and standard.

Pulse Sequences/Regions of Interest. Different pulse sequences are used, based on the clinical indications. Generally, we do a combination of T1W and some type of T2W sequences in all three orthogonal planes in order to demonstrate the different anatomic structures and pathologic entities well. The pulse sequences are chosen by selecting one of the following clinical categories: (1) "routine" (pain,

BOX 16–1: FOOT AND ANKLE STRUCTURES TO EVALUATE IN DIFFERENT PLANES

Sagittal
  Achilles tendon
  Sinus tarsi
  Plantar fascia
  Osseous structures (length of metatarsals)
  Ankle joint
Axials of Ankle and Long Axis Axials (Coronal) of Foot
  Ankle tendons
  Sinus tarsi
  Tibiofibular ligaments
  Anterior, posterior talofibular ligaments
  Osseous structures (length of metatarsals)
Coronal Ankle and Short Axis Axials of Foot
  Deltoid ligaments, deep and superficial
  Calcaneofibular ligament
  Tarsal tunnel
  Sinus tarsi
  Ankle joint
  Osseous structures (metatarsals in cross section)
  Plantar fascia in cross section

trauma), (2) infection/mass, and (3) Morton's neuroma. We select from four anatomic regions for imaging: (1) ankle/hindfoot/midfoot, (2) forefoot/toes, (3) entire foot, and (4) Achilles tendon (screening examination).

Contrast. Gadolinium is used only in cases of suspected infection, Morton's neuroma, or for differentiating a solid from a cystic mass.

NORMAL AND ABNORMAL

Tendons

Tendon abnormalities are among the most common abnormalities affecting the foot and, particularly, the ankle. This is because of the many tendons that are present, as well as their close relationship to adjacent osseous structures that may cause irritation, and the frequent stresses and trauma affecting this anatomic location.

Tendons generally are best evaluated on the short axis axial images of the foot, or axial images of the ankle where the tendons are depicted in cross section. Other imaging planes may help to substantiate findings in tendons, but do not demonstrate the tendons to greatest advantage, because the tendons, with the exception of the Achilles, run obliquely to these planes.

The general principles regarding the MRI appearance of normal and abnormal tendons can be found in Chapter 3. However, as a brief review, remember that the abnormalities that may affect tendons are tenosynovitis, tendon degeneration, partial or complete tendon tears, subluxation or dislocation of certain tendons from their normal locations, xanthomas from hyperlipidemia, calcific tendinitis, uric acid tophi from gout and, rarely, tumors. Tendons may tear as the result of chronic repetitive microtrauma; acute major trauma; and from weakening as the result of myxoid degeneration, rheumatoid arthritis, chronic renal failure, diabetes, gout, steroids, and other medications. Abnormalities on MRI consist of fluid completely surrounding a tendon (tenosynovitis), abnormal tendon size, intratendinous high signal intensity (from partial tears), abnormal position (from dislocation), or complete absence of a segment of tendon (complete tear).

Tendons of the ankle are conveniently divided

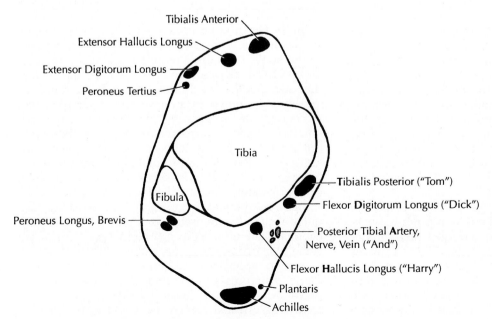

Figure 16–1. NORMAL ANKLE TENDONS.
Diagram of tendons about the ankle, which are divided into the anterior extensors, the medial flexors, the posterior Achilles and plantaris, and the lateral peroneals.

BOX 16–2: ACHILLES TENDON

- No sheath, but a posterior paratenon
- Xanthomas
- Tears at midpoint, and proximal or distal extremes
- Plantaris medially may simulate tear
- "Pump bumps" or Haglund's deformity
  —Retrocalcaneal bursitis
  —Tendo-Achilles bursitis
  —Thickened distal Achilles

into four groups, based on their location in the ankle: anterior, posterior, medial, and lateral (Fig. 16–1).

Posterior Ankle Tendons

Achilles and Plantaris (Box 16–2)

The Achilles tendon is located in the midline of the posterior ankle and is the largest tendon in the body, formed by the confluence of tendons from the gastrocnemius and the soleus muscles (Fig. 16–2). The Achilles tendon is normally low signal intensity diffusely; however, there is a vertically oriented line of high signal intensity in many Achilles tendons that probably represents a normal interface between the two components of the tendon (gastrocnemius and soleus) or else small vessels within the tendon. The Achilles does not have a tendon sheath because it does not come into close contact with other structures along its length; therefore, it cannot

have changes of tenosynovitis, but only of paratendinitis. There is a paratenon present on the dorsal, medial, and lateral aspects of the Achilles tendon that allows smooth gliding of the tendon in lieu of a tendon sheath. This may be seen on axial images as a thin line of intermediate signal intensity paralleling the posterior tendon. Anterior to the Achilles tendon is a triangular fat pad called Kager's triangle.

The Achilles tendon usually has a flat or concave anterior margin on axial images (Fig. 16–2); if it becomes diffusely convex, an abnormally thickened tendon exists.[1, 2] The anterior margin of the Achilles tendon normally may have a focal convexity that starts on the lateral side of the proximal tendon and shifts to the medial aspect of the distal tendon. This focal anterior contour convexity is caused by the fibers of the soleus merging with those of the gastrocnemius in a spiral configuration as they extend to insert on the calcaneus. The posterior margin of the Achilles has a convex contour. The normal tendon measures about 7 mm in the anteroposterior dimension, and the anterior and posterior margins are parallel on true sagittal images through the tendon.

Ninety percent of individuals have a small plantaris tendon lying anteromedial to the Achilles tendon, which inserts onto the Achilles tendon, or to the posterior calcaneus, or else to the flexor retinaculum (Fig. 16–3). The high signal intensity plane between the plantaris and the Achilles tendons can be mistaken for a partially torn Achilles when none exists, or else a completely torn Achilles may mistakenly be considered to have some remaining intact medial fibers, which are merely the fibers of the intact plantaris tendon. Evaluation of adjacent axial images distinguishes between a normal plantaris tendon and an abnormal Achilles tendon.

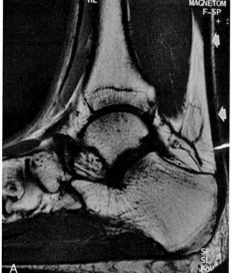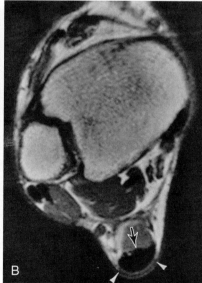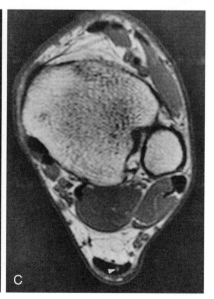

Figure 16–2. ACHILLES TENDON: Normal.
A, T1 sagittal image, ankle. The Achilles tendon *(arrows)* is low signal, taut, and with parallel straight anterior and posterior margins. *B,* T1 axial image, ankle. The Achilles tendon has a flat or concave anterior margin, but a focal convexity *(arrow)* is a normal finding in many people. The paratenon is demonstrated posterior to the tendon *(arrowheads)* as intermediate signal. *C,* T1 axial image, ankle. The Achilles tendon is thin, has a concave anterior margin, and has a focus of high signal *(arrowhead)* in the substance.

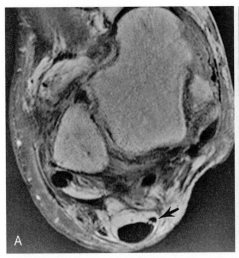

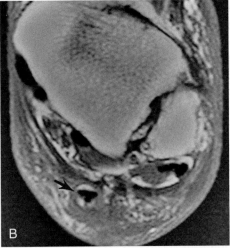

Figure 16–3. PLANTARIS TENDON.
A, T1 axial image, ankle. The small plantaris tendon *(arrow)* is located medial to the Achilles tendon and may mimic a partial tear of the Achilles tendon. **B,** T1 axial image, ankle (different patient than in *A*). The Achilles tendon is completely ruptured and no fibers are evident on this cut. The plantaris tendon *(arrow)* should not be mistaken for a partially intact Achilles tendon.

Degeneration and partial or complete tears of the Achilles tendon usually occur about 4 cm above its calcaneal insertion (Fig. 16–4), but may exist anywhere along the length of the tendon. Tears also may occur at the musculotendinous junction (Fig. 16–5), and the field of view must be large enough to include this region on sagittal images to look for hemorrhage and edema in the acute state, or muscle atrophy in the chronic setting.

Unconditioned, middle-aged athletes (weekend athletes) are most commonly affected with Achilles tendon abnormalities. Complete tears are usually easy to diagnose clinically, but some people believe that there is still a valuable role for imaging in these patients, in order to evaluate how close the tendon fragments are to one another and the condition of the tendon. This may be done with a cast in place, which serves to hold the ankle in plantar flexion

and cause increased apposition of tendon fragments. If there is a large gap between fragments, many orthopedists will perform surgery to repair the tendon, whereas close apposition of tendon fragments can be treated with casting only. As with all things orthopedic, there is debate regarding the ideal method of treating these injuries.

Xanthomas occur from familial hyperlipidemia types II and III (hypercholesterolemia and hypertriglyceridemia) and have a predilection for the Achilles tendon (as well as the extensor tendons of the hands). Infiltration between the low signal intensity tendon fibers by intermediate signal intensity lipid-laden foamy histiocytes causes a stippled pattern and either focal or diffuse enlargement of the tendon (Fig. 16–6). The findings often are bilateral and cannot be distinguished from partial tendon tears on MRI.[3] This must be remembered among the differen-

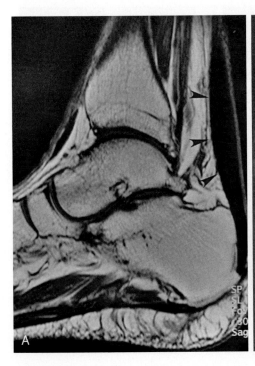

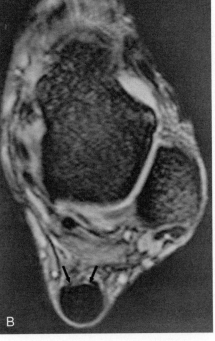

Figure 16–4. ACHILLES TENDON: Partial tears.
A, T1 sagittal image, ankle. The tendon has a fusiform thickening *(arrowheads)* with a convex anterior margin in its midsubstance, approximately 4 cm above the calcaneal insertion, from partial tears. **B,** T2* axial image, ankle. The tendon is thickened in the anteroposterior direction and has a diffusely convex anterior margin from the tears.

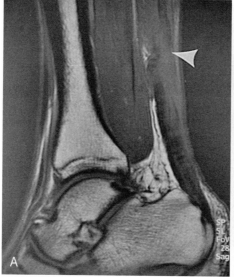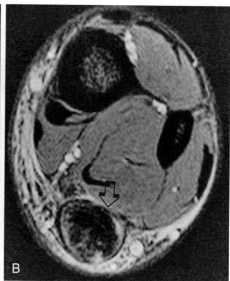

Figure 16–5. ACHILLES TEN-DON: Full-thickness tear.
A, T1 sagittal image, ankle. There is a complete-thickness tear of the Achilles tendon at the myotendinous junction *(arrowhead)*. The entire tendon is thickened and has abnormal high signal within it from partial tears as well. *B,* T2* axial image, ankle. A cut through the torn tendon *(open arrow)* shows the tendon to be markedly thick, with a diffusely convex anterior margin. There is a stippled appearance as the result of hemorrhage and edema separating the low-signal collagen fibers in the tendon.

tial diagnostic possibilities for the abnormal Achilles tendon, because the first manifestation of this deadly disease may be that of an Achilles xanthoma. The diagnosis may be proved with laboratory work-up.

There are two bursae that relate to the distal attachment of the Achilles tendon, the retrocalcaneal and tendo-Achilles bursae. The retrocalcaneal bursa is a teardrop-shaped structure that is normally located between the tendon and the posterior aspect of the upper calcaneus; it has little or no fluid within it when not inflamed. The tendo-Achilles (retro-Achilles) bursa is an acquired or adventitious bursa, located just posterior to the distal Achilles tendon in the subcutaneous fat. Distention of these bursae with fluid or inflammatory thickening of the

synovial linings indicates bursitis. If these bursae become inflamed, they may be a source of heel pain. Inflammation occurs with chronic overuse, especially from ill-fitting footwear, and from inflammatory arthropathies. The triad of retro-Achilles bursitis, retrocalcaneal bursitis, and thickening of the distal Achilles tendon is known as Haglund's deformity or as "pump bumps," because wearing high-heeled or ill-fitting shoes is considered a predisposing factor (Fig. 16–7).[4]

Medial Ankle Tendons

The flexor tendons are located on the medial side of the ankle (see Fig. 16–1). The position and names

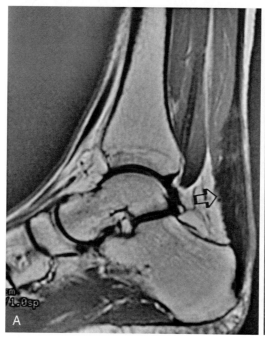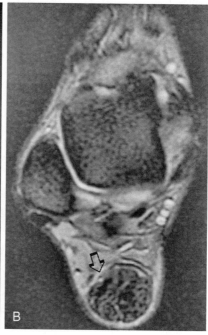

Figure 16–6. ACHILLES TEN-DON: Xanthoma.
A, T1 sagittal image, ankle. The Achilles tendon *(open arrow)* is diffusely thickened, with linear areas of high signal in the substance. *B,* T2* axial image, ankle. The Achilles *(open arrow)* has a stippled appearance, with the focal low-signal regions representing collagen fibers and the higher signal being the xanthoma from hyperlipidemia. The appearance on MR is indistinguishable from the much more common tendon tear.

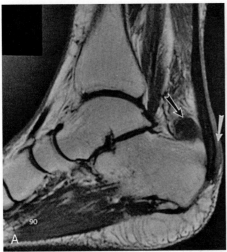

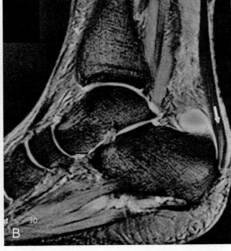

Figure 16–7. HAGLUND'S DE-FORMITY.
A, T1 sagittal image, ankle. The Achilles tendon is mildly thickened and has high signal in it from partial tears. Anterior to the tendon is a rounded mass *(black arrow),* representing the enlarged and inflamed retrocalcaneal bursa. Posterior to the tendon is an inflamed tendo-Achilles bursa *(white arrow).* *B,* T2* sagittal image, ankle. The triad of Haglund's deformity is evident as high signal in the retrocalcaneal and tendo-Achilles bursae, and in the partially torn Achilles tendon *(arrow).*

of these tendons can be easily remembered by using the mnemonic "Tom, Dick, And Harry" to represent the structures running from medial to lateral. "Tom" represents the posterior **T**ibial tendon; "Dick" is the flexor **D**igitorum longus tendon; "And" is the posterior tibial **A**rtery, nerve, and vein; and "Harry" depicts the flexor **H**allucis longus tendon. The tendons are surrounded by separate tendon sheaths, and they pass through the tarsal tunnel, discussed subsequently.

Posterior Tibial Tendon ("Tom")

(Box 16–3)

The posterior tibial tendon is the largest of the three medial flexor tendons. It has an oval shape and is approximately twice as large as the adjacent round flexor digitorum and flexor hallucis longus tendons. The posterior tibial tendon passes beneath the medial malleolus, which it uses as a pulley, and attaches to the medial navicular bone, the three cuneiforms, and the bases of the first to fourth metatarsals. The attachment to the navicular bone is generally the only portion of the attachment identified by MRI. Because of the orientation of the tendinous attachment and the multiple tendon slips that attach to the bone, the attachment often has the appearance of a thickened tendon with high signal intensity within it; this normal appearance must not be confused with a partial tendon tear. Most posterior tibial tendon tears occur at the level of the medial malleolus rather than more distally. In general, we

---

BOX 16–3: POSTERIOR TIBIAL TENDON

- Most commonly abnormal medial tendon
- May tear or dislocate
- Tears lead to flat foot
- Tears associated with sinus tarsi syndrome
- Tears more common with accessory navicular

---

disregard high signal in this tendon at its attachment site to the navicular, because it typically is seen as a normal variant. High signal intensity or tendon thickening elsewhere in the length of the tendon is considered pathologic. It is not uncommon to see a longitudinal split tear of this tendon, in which case the axial images appear to show two posterior tibial tendons.

The posterior tibial tendon is the most common abnormal tendon on the medial side of the ankle (Fig. 16–8). This tendon provides a significant amount of support to the arch of the foot, and tears of the tendon can cause loss of the longitudinal arch, resulting in a flat foot deformity. Middle-aged or older women and rheumatoid arthritis patients often suffer from this abnormality. There is a much higher incidence of posterior tibial tendon tears in people with accessory navicular bones or those with large medial tubercles of the navicular bone (the cornuate process), which result in altered stresses and premature tendon degeneration.[5]

Secondary signs of a posterior tibial tendon tear have been reported and include loss of the longitudinal arch of the foot and a small spur or periosteal reaction along the posterior aspect of the medial malleolus (Figs. 16–8 and 16–9).[6] Tears of this tendon also are associated with the sinus tarsi syndrome and degenerative joint disease of the posterior subtalar joint, which may serve as sources of pain.

The posterior tibial tendon rarely can sublux or dislocate in a medial and anterior direction relative to the medial malleolus (Fig. 16–9).

Flexor Digitorum Longus ("Dick")

The flexor digitorum longus tendon is rarely involved with abnormalities. It passes just lateral to the posterior tibial tendon and divides to send insertions to the plantar aspects of the distal phalanges of the second through fifth toes.

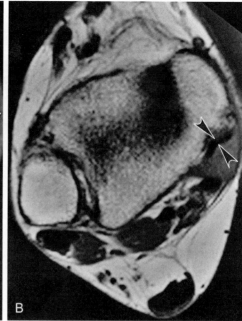

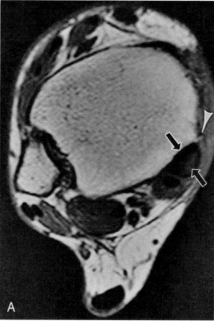

Figure 16–8. POSTERIOR TIBIAL TENDON: Partial tears.
A, T1 axial image, ankle. The posterior tibial tendon is markedly enlarged (between *arrows*) and has abnormal high signal within it. It is more than twice the size of the adjacent flexor digitorum and flexor hallucis tendons. There is a small bone spur *(arrowhead)*, which is a sign of a chronic tendon abnormality. **B,** T1 axial image, ankle (different patient than in *A*). The posterior tibial tendon in this patient is very attenuated (between *arrowheads*) with surrounding fluid from tenosynovitis. A thin tendon is closer to a complete tear than is a thick tendon.

Flexor Hallucis Longus ("Harry")

(Box 16–4)

The flexor hallucis longus tendon is the most lateral of the three medial flexor tendons (see Fig. 16–1). It passes in a groove on the medial side of the posterior process of the talus, and then beneath the sustentaculum tali, which it uses as a pulley. It passes along the plantar aspect of the foot, between the hallux sesamoids at the head of the first metatarsal, to attach to the base of the distal phalanx of the great toe.[7] The flexor hallucis longus synovial tendon sheath is in communication with the ankle joint in 20% of people; fluid surrounding the tendon is common and may have no significance if an ankle joint effusion also is present (Fig. 16–10). This tendon tends to normally have more fluid in its sheath than do the adjacent two tendons.

Focal, asymmetric pooling of fluid within the tendon sheath is indicative of stenosing tenosynovitis, which occurs as the result of focal areas of synovitis or fibrosis within the tendon sheath, interrupting normal synovial fluid flow (Fig. 16–11). Stenosing tenosynovitis of the flexor hallucis longus often is associated with the os trigonum syndrome, which occurs with extreme plantar flexion and causes the os trigonum as well as the flexor hallucis longus tendon to be trapped between the posterior malleolus of the tibia and the calcaneus.[8] Tears of the flexor hallucis longus tendon at the level of the ankle are rare, and tenosynovitis is far more common. Repeated plantar flexion of the ankle and foot, as occurs in ballet dancers and basketball players, results in inflammatory changes to the sheath of this tendon.

The distal end of the flexor hallucis longus tendon

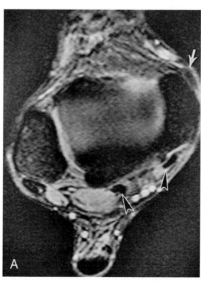

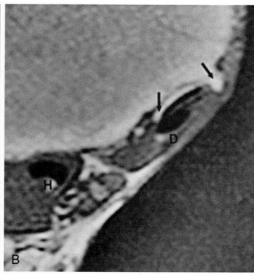

Figure 16–9. POSTERIOR TIBIAL TENDON: Dislocation.
A, T2* axial image, ankle. Only two flexor tendons *(arrowheads)* are present medial to the ankle. The posterior tibial tendon is dislocated anterior to the medial malleolus *(white arrow)* and is thinned from partial tears. **B,** T1 axial image, ankle. A close-up of the posterior aspect of the medial malleolus shows only the flexor digitorum (D) and flexor hallucis (H) tendons; the posterior tibial tendon is absent. There are large spurs on the malleolus *(arrows)* from chronic tendinopathy.

BOX 16–4: FLEXOR HALLUCIS LONGUS TENDON

- Rarely tears
- Sheath communicates with ankle (20%)
  —Asymptomatic tendon sheath fluid common
- Proximal tenosynovitis
  —Repeated plantar flexion (ballet, basketball)
  —Os trigonum syndrome
- Distal tenosynovitis/partial tears
  —Running, ballet

---

may be partially torn or may develop tenosynovitis where it passes through the confined space between the hallux sesamoid bones (Fig. 16–12). These distal tendon injuries are common in runners and in ballet dancers who dance en pointe.

Lateral Ankle Tendons

Peroneal Tendons (Boxes 16–5 and 16–6)

The peroneus brevis and longus tendons are located on the posterolateral aspect of the ankle and serve as the major everters of the foot (see Fig. 16–1). These tendons pass posterior and inferior to the lateral malleolus, which they use as a pulley. The

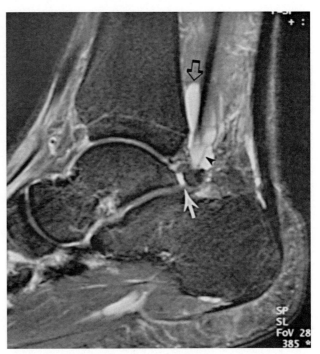

Figure 16–11. FLEXOR HALLUCIS LONGUS TENDON: Stenosing tenosynovitis and os trigonum syndrome.
STIR sagittal image, ankle. The tendon sheath of the flexor hallucis is distended with fluid proximally *(open arrow)*. There is a septation in the fluid *(arrowhead)*, indicating this is a stenosing tenosynovitis. There also is very high signal between the os trigonum and the talus *(white arrow)* because of disruption of the normal synchondrosis between the two structures (posterior impingement) syndrome, which often is associated with stenosing tenosynovitis of the flexor hallucis.

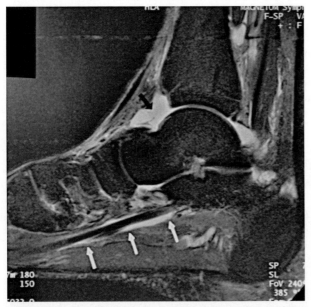

Figure 16–10. FLEXOR HALLUCIS LONGUS TENDON: Communication between ankle and tendon sheath.
STIR sagittal image, ankle. There is a large ankle joint effusion *(black arrow)*. There also is fluid surrounding the flexor hallucis longus tendon *(white arrows)*, which runs beneath the sustentaculum tali. Fluid in this tendon sheath has no significance and cannot be called tenosynovitis when an ankle joint effusion is present, because the two structures communicate in about 20% of people.

tendons share a common tendon sheath proximally, but have separate sheaths distally. The brevis usually is located anterior to the longus (although the brevis may sometimes lie medial to the longus) and runs in a shallow retromalleolar groove on the back of the lateral malleolus (Fig. 16–13). The peroneal tendons are held in place relative to the lateral malleolus by the superior peroneal retinaculum. The tendons often are separated by the small peroneal tubercle on the lateral aspect of the calcaneus, with the brevis passing anterior to the tubercle (Fig. 16–13), or both tendons may pass anterior to the peroneal tubercle. The brevis eventually attaches to the base of the fifth metatarsal. The longus has a broad-based insertion on the plantar surface of the base of the first metatarsal and medial cuneiform, after traversing the plantar aspect of the foot.

The peroneus brevis and longus tendons may be difficult to distinguish as separate structures at the level of the lateral malleolus on MRI. The brevis generally is much flatter and broader than the longus, which has a more rounded appearance (Fig. 16–13). Flat is acceptable (for many things), but if the brevis becomes C-shaped, it is considered abnormal.

Calcaneal fractures can be associated with peroneal tendon abnormalities, including entrapment of

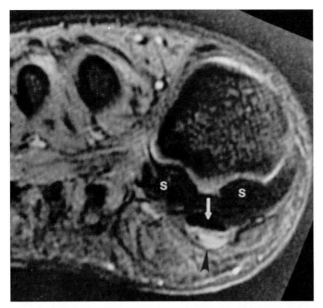

Figure 16–12. FLEXOR HALLUCIS LONGUS TENDON: Distal tenosynovitis.
T2* axial image, forefoot. The distal flexor hallucis longus tendon *(arrow)* is positioned between the hallux sesamoids (S) beneath the first metatarsal head. There is high-signal fluid *(arrowhead)* from tenosynovitis in this long-distance runner with pain.

BOX 16–6: PERONEUS BREVIS SPLITS

- Vertical tendon tear at level of tip of lateral malleolus
    Elderly: often asymptomatic
    Young: lateral pain, swelling
- Caused by increased wear and tear of tendon
  —Entrapment between peroneus longus and fibula in dorsiflexion
  —Chronic tendon subluxation from torn retinaculum
  —Flat or convex posterior aspect of lateral malleolus (predisposes to subluxation)
  —Low-lying brevis muscle belly or peroneus quartus accessory muscle (cause compression of brevis)
- Pitfalls
  —Bifurcate brevis tendon or peroneus quartus may simulate
  —Distinguish by: split tendon has one muscle belly with two tendons coming from it

---

the peroneal tendons between bone fragments, tendon tears, tendon displacement, or impingement on tendons by fracture fragments.[9] Complete and partial tears also occur in the absence of calcaneal fractures (Fig. 16–14).[10, 11]

Peroneus brevis splits is a term used for longitudinal or vertical tears of the peroneus brevis tendon that can occur in all ages and in athletes (Fig. 16–15). Those occurring in the elderly may be asymptomatic, whereas younger patients usually have pain and swelling along the lateral malleolus and the course of the peroneal tendons. A history of recurrent inversion injuries and ankle sprains is common. The diagnosis is difficult or impossible clinically, and overlaps with chronic ankle instability symptoms. Those who do not respond to conservative management may benefit from surgery with anastomosis of fragments or tenodesis to the peroneus longus tendon.

Peroneus brevis longitudinal tears occur during dorsiflexion, when the brevis tendon is wedged between the lateral malleolus and the peroneus longus tendon. The tear originates at the distal tip of the lateral malleolus, but may propagate variable distances proximally and distally. The peroneus longus tendon also is partially torn in about 30% of those individuals with a brevis tear, because it becomes directly exposed to the lateral malleolus and subjected to abnormal stresses. A sharp posterolateral fibular spur may be seen with the peroneus brevis splits, representing a reactive periostitis.[12, 13]

Certain conditions are associated with peroneus brevis longitudinal tears. Anything that causes compression or subluxation of the peroneal tendons may predispose to this abnormality by causing increased wear and tear on the tendons. Such conditions include a torn or lax superior peroneal retinaculum, a flat or convex (rather than normal concave) posterior aspect of the lateral malleolus, low-lying peroneus brevis muscle belly (extending to the tip of the lateral malleolus), and the presence of an accessory muscle called the peroneus quartus.

The diagnosis of a longitudinal split of the peroneus brevis tendon may be simulated by the presence of a bifurcated distal peroneus brevis tendon or by the peroneus quartus accessory muscle and tendon (Fig. 16–16). A brevis tendon tear can be distinguished from these two muscle variants, owing to the fact that separate muscle bellies surround each of the tendon slips in the case of a bifurcate brevis tendon, and a muscle belly separate from the peroneus brevis muscle is seen when a peroneus quartus is present. With a peroneus brevis split, there is one muscle belly and two tendons coming from it.[13]

The peroneal tendons are among the few tendons that can sublux or dislocate. This usually occurs when the superior retinaculum has been disrupted.

BOX 16–5: PERONEUS TENDONS

- Brevis anterior or medial to longus
- Brevis: flat or oval is normal; curved (boomerang-shape) is abnormal
- Tear or dislocate laterally
- Calcaneal fractures cause
  —Entrapment, displacement, tenosynovitis

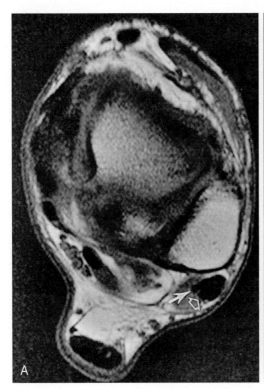
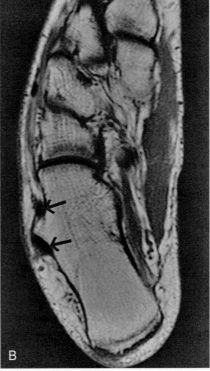

Figure 16–13. PERONEAL TENDONS: Normal.
A, T1 axial image, ankle. The peroneus brevis tendon *(solid arrow)* is flat and sandwiched between the posterior aspect of the lateral malleolus and the peroneus longus tendon *(open arrow).* The longus is more round than the brevis and located posteriorly. The intermediate-signal muscle adjacent to the tendons is the peroneal muscle. *B,* T1 long-axis coronal image, foot. The peroneus brevis and longus tendons *(arrows)* are located anterior and posterior, respectively, to the peroneal tubercle of the calcaneus.

Figure 16–14. PERONEAL TENDONS: Partial tears.
T1 axial image, ankle. The peroneal tendons are held in place by the peroneal retinaculum *(arrowheads).* The longus *(white arrow)* is lateral to the brevis *(black arrow).* Both tendons are enlarged and have high signal within them from partial tears.

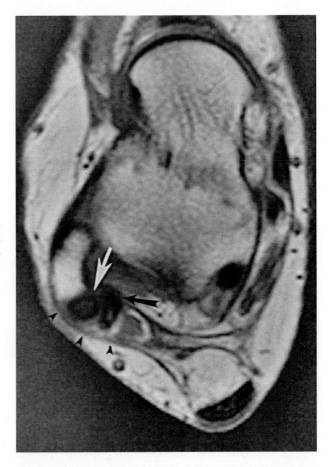

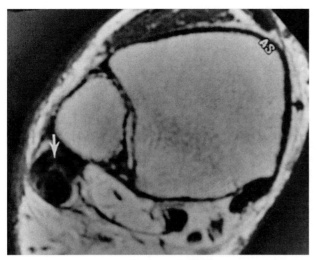

Figure 16–15. PERONEUS BREVIS SPLITS.
T1 axial image, ankle. There is a longitudinal tear or split of the **C**-shaped peroneus brevis *(arrow)*. The peroneus longus is thickened.

The retinaculum becomes disrupted from a forced inversion injury with plantar flexion, typically occurring in skiing, basketball, or soccer injuries. The diagnosis is made on MRI if the tendons are located lateral to the distal fibula, instead of posterior to it, or if the torn retinaculum is identified (Fig. 16–17). A shallow or hypoplastic retromalleolar groove of the fibula may predispose to subluxation of the peroneal tendons.

Anterior Ankle Tendons

There are four tendons that can be found anterior to the ankle (see Fig. 16–1). From medial to lateral these are the anterior tibial, extensor hallucis longus, extensor digitorum longus, and peroneus tertius tendons. These tendons serve to dorsiflex the ankle and foot. These tendons seldom are affected with pathology in comparison to the flexor tendons; therefore, little attention is paid to those structures.

Anterior Tibial Tendon (Box 16–7)

The anterior tibial tendon is the most likely of all of the anterior tendons to be abnormal. This tendon is the most medial and the largest of the anterior tendons. Tears are uncommon, but may be seen with increasing age and in people who run on hills. Many patients with a partial or complete tear of this tendon present with a mass suspected of being a tumor, rather than with symptoms of a tendon abnormality (Fig. 16–18).[14, 15]

Ankle Ligaments

MRI is not routinely used to diagnose ligamentous injuries, because they usually can be easily and less

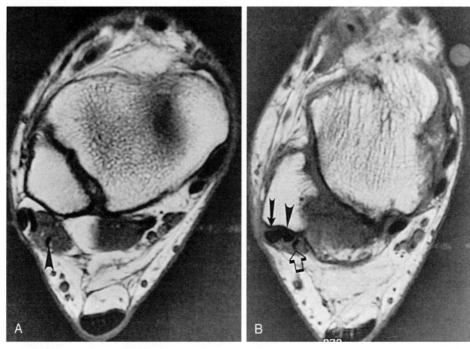

Figure 16–16. ACCESSORY PERONEUS QUARTUS.
A, T1 axial image, ankle. There are three tendons posterior to the lateral malleolus. The peroneus longus and brevis are the two most lateral tendons. The most posteromedial tendon *(arrowhead)* is surrounded by muscle, and this is the peroneus quartus accessory muscle and tendon. The peroneal retinaculum is stretched because of the increased volume in the confined space, and this may predispose to peroneus brevis splits. *B,* T1 axial image, ankle (different patient than in *A*). There are three tendons posterior to the lateral malleolus: the peroneus longus *(solid arrow)*, the peroneus brevis *(arrowhead)*, and the most medial tendon is the peroneus quartus *(open arrow)*. The peroneus quartus simulates the appearance of a split peroneus brevis tendon. Each tendon has its own muscle belly on more proximal cuts, allowing differentiation.

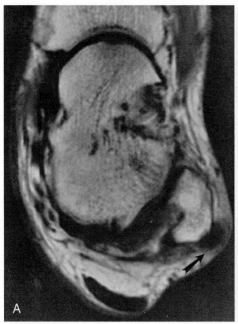

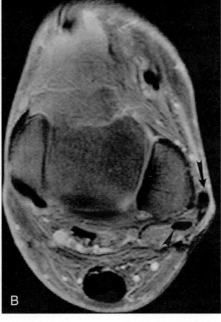

Figure 16–17. PERONEAL TENDONS: Dislocation.
A, T1 axial image, ankle. Both peroneal tendons are dislocated laterally *(arrow)*. The flexor retinaculum is not evident. ***B,*** T1 contrast-enhanced with fat suppression axial image, ankle. One of the peroneal tendons is dislocated laterally *(arrow)*, whereas the other remains in normal position posterior to the lateral malleoleus *(arrowhead)*. The Achilles tendon is thickened and convex anteriorly from partial tears.

expensively determined by clinical examination. However, in patients who have persistent pain or who may be imaged for seemingly unrelated reasons, the ligaments need to be evaluated and well understood, because abnormalities can be identified and may have clinical significance.[16–19] Also, it is becoming apparent that many ligament abnormalities are associated with other causes of chronic ankle pain (eg, sinus tarsi syndrome). Therefore, one must be able to identify ligament pathology on MRI. In general, the ligaments are thin, taut, low signal intensity structures; however, the thick bands of collagen may predictably create a striated appearance in certain ligaments: the anterior tibiofibular, the posterior talofibular, and the deep (tibiotalar) and superficial (tibiocalcaneal) layers of the deltoid. The striated appearance in these ligaments must not be confused with partial tears.

Medial Ankle Ligaments

The medial collateral ligamentous complex (deltoid ligament) lies deep to the medial flexor tendons. It has several components: tibiotalar, tibiocalcaneal, talonavicular, and the spring ligament (between the sustentaculum of the calcaneus and navicular bone); it is the first two of these components that routinely are seen well on coronal MR

images (Fig. 16–19). The deep tibiotalar portion of the deltoid ligament is seen as a striated structure coursing obliquely between the medial malleolus and the talus on both coronal and axial images, usually best on the coronal images. The tibiocalcaneal component of the deltoid runs vertically, just deep to the flexor retinaculum and superficial to the tibiotalar component of the ligament.[19] The deltoid

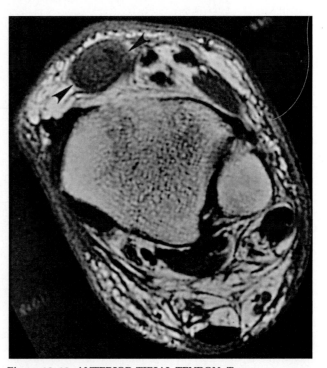

Figure 16–18. ANTERIOR TIBIAL TENDON: Tear.
T1 axial image, ankle. There is a large, round intermediate-signal structure *(arrowheads)* anterior to the ankle from a complete tear of the tibialis anterior tendon.

BOX 16–7: ANTERIOR TIBIAL TENDON

—Most commonly abnormal anterior tendon
—Tears occur from age or running hills
—Tears often present as a mass

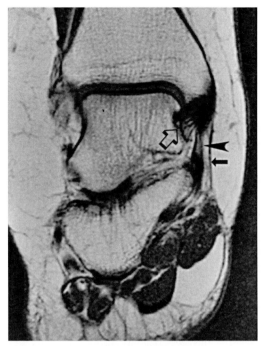

Figure 16–19. MEDIAL ANKLE LIGAMENTS: Normal.
T1 coronal image, ankle. Two layers of the deltoid (medial) ligament are seen on routine MRI. The deep tibiotalar ligament is striated *(open arrow)*. The more superficial tibiocalcaneal ligament *(arrowhead)* may have vertical striations also. The thin, vertical, low-signal structure superficial to the tibiocalcaneal ligament is the flexor retinaculum *(solid arrow)*.

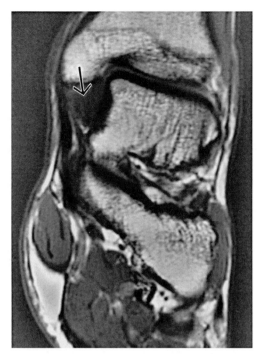

Figure 16–20. MEDIAL ANKLE LIGAMENTS: Tears.
T1 coronal image, ankle. The deep tibiotalar ligament *(arrow)* has lost its striated appearance secondary to tears/contusion.

ligament is only infrequently injured as compared to the lateral ankle ligaments.

The MRI appearance of a deltoid ligament injury depends on which components were injured and to what extent (Fig. 16–20). The tibiotalar component often loses its striated appearance and shows high signal intensity on both T1W and T2W images. This may indicate either a contusion or tear of the ligament. The tibiocalcaneal portion may be discontinuous and have high signal intensity hemorrhage and edema acutely; a chronic tear may appear as a thickened or discontinuous ligament.

Lateral Ankle Ligaments (Box 16–8)

The lateral collateral ligamentous complex is affected in 80% to 90% of all ankle ligament injuries. In general, these ligaments are best evaluated on axial images. The superiorly located lateral ligaments include the *anterior and posterior tibiofibular ligaments*, which are located just above the tibiotalar joint (Fig. 16–21). These ligaments course superiorly from the fibula to the tibia (or inferiorly from the tibia to the fibula). The anterior and posterior tibiofibular ligaments, along with the interosseous membrane between the tibia and fibula, make up the syndesmosis. These ligaments are seen well on axial images and often are seen on coronal images also (Fig. 16–21). These ligaments often are best identified on an axial cut that passes through the dome of the talus. This should not cause confusion

in thinking that the cut is too distal to be the tibiofibular ligaments. On sagittal images through the ankle, the posterior tibiofibular ligament cut in cross section may resemble an intraarticular loose body in the ankle, because it is surrounded by ankle joint fluid (Fig. 16–21). Following the structure on adja-

---

BOX 16–8: LATERAL ANKLE LIGAMENTS

Superior group
- Anterior and posterior tibiofibular ligaments
  —Seen at top of ankle joint on axial images
  —Posterior tibiofibular ligament mimics ankle loose body on sagittal images

Inferior group
- Anterior to posterior: anterior talofibular, calcaneofibular, posterior talofibular
  —Calcaneofibular: best seen on coronal images, but seen inconsistently
  —Anterior and posterior talofibular: seen on axial images at level of malleolar fossa of fibula
  —Usually tear in sequence from anterior to posterior
  —Tears associated with
    Osteochondral fractures
    Long-term instability
    Sinus tarsi syndrome

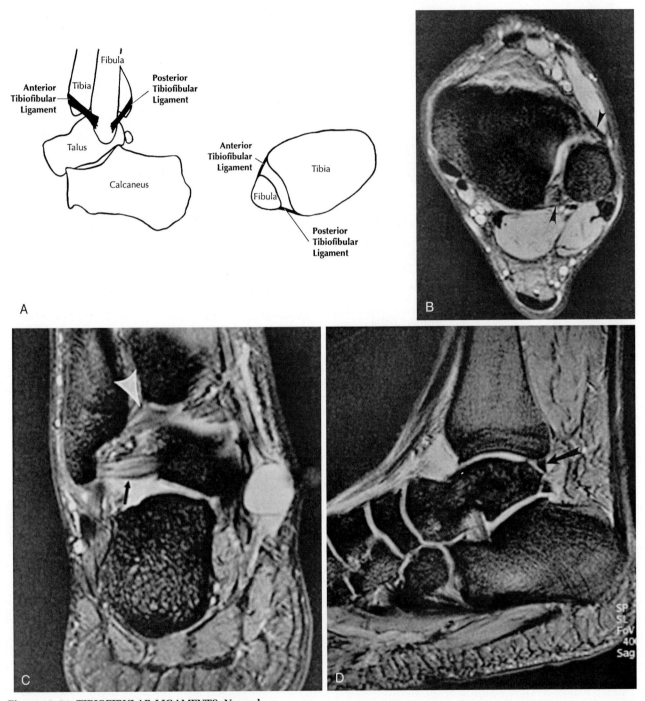

Figure 16–21. TIBIOFIBULAR LIGAMENTS: Normal.
A, Diagram of the anterior and posterior tibiofibular ligaments from sagittal and axial perspectives. These ligaments run inferiorly from the tibia to the fibula. *B,* T2* axial image, ankle. Intact anterior and posterior tibiofibular ligaments *(arrowheads).* *C,* T2* coronal image, ankle. The posterior tibiofibular ligament *(white arrowhead)* and the posterior talofibular ligament *(arrow)* both are seen as striated structures on this image. There is a ganglion cyst medially. *D,* T2* sagittal image, ankle. The posterior tibiofibular ligament is seen in cross section *(arrow)* at the ankle joint line. This must not be confused with an intraarticular loose body. There is an os trigonum below the ligament with a very similar size and appearance.

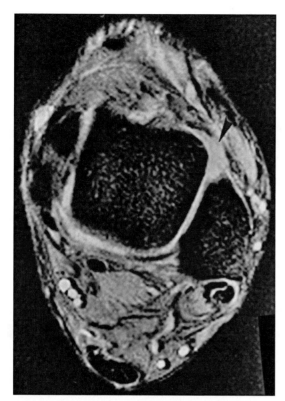

Figure 16–22. TIBIOFIBULAR LIGAMENT: Tear.
T2* axial image, ankle. The anterior tibiofibular ligament is absent *(arrowhead)* and there is high-signal edema in the region.

the concavity in the medial aspect of the lateral malleolus, called the malleolar fossa (Fig. 16–24). The calcaneofibular ligament is the most difficult ligament to identify routinely and may be best seen on coronal images (Fig. 16–24).[16]

The anterior talofibular ligament is the most commonly torn of the ankle ligaments. It usually is an isolated tear, but if the traumatic forces are great enough, the other ligaments may tear in a sequential fashion. That is, after the anterior talofibular ligament tears, the calcaneofibular ligament tears, followed, only rarely, by the posterior talofibular ligament. The anterior talofibular ligament is a thickening of the ankle joint capsule. Thus, an acute ligament tear results in a capsular tear with leakage of fluid into the soft tissues around the ligament (Fig. 16–25). An acute tear is seen as a discontinuous ligament with surrounding edema/hemorrhage. A chronic tear may show discontinuity of the ligament, but often scarring forms so that the ligament appears intact but irregular, with thickening, thinning, or detachment from the associated osseous structures (Fig. 16–25).[17, 18]

Approximately 15% of ankle sprains result in instability, either mechanical (objective instability on physical examination) or functional (subjective feeling that the ankle is giving way). Several entities have an association with lateral ankle ligament tears, including sinus tarsi syndrome, anterolateral impingement syndrome, and longitudinal split tears of the peroneus brevis tendon. Finally, bone contusions and osteochondral fractures of the talar dome are common complicating features, often impossible to identify by conventional radiography, but easily identified on MRI.

cent cuts and its predictable location at the level of the tibiotalar joint make the differentiation between pathology and normal anatomy possible.[16] The tibiofibular ligaments can be torn, and this is recognized by discontinuity of the low signal structures on axial MR images (Fig. 16–22).

The second set of lateral ligaments is located just distal to the tibiotalar joint. This inferior set of ligaments is made of the *anterior talofibular, calcaneofibular, and the posterior talofibular ligaments*, from anterior to posterior (Fig. 16–23). The anterior and posterior talofibular ligaments are seen best on axial images just below the tibiotalar joint at the level of

Miscellaneous Inflammatory Conditions

Anterolateral Impingement Syndrome in the Ankle (Box 16–9)

Anterolateral impingement syndrome in the ankle is produced by entrapment of abnormal soft tissue

Figure 16–23. INFERIOR SET OF LATERAL ANKLE LIGAMENTS.
Diagram of anterior talofibular, calcaneofibular, and posterior talofibular ligaments from sagittal and axial perspectives.

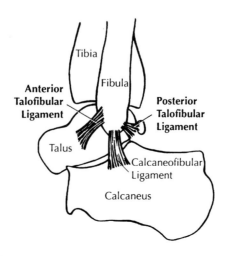

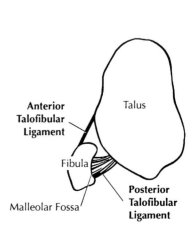

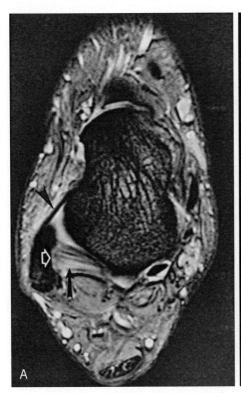
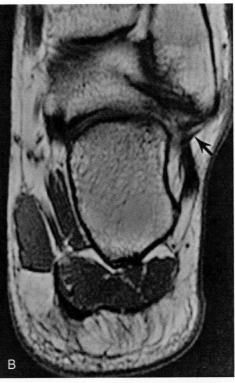

Figure 16–24. INFERIOR LATERAL ANKLE LIGAMENTS: Normal.
A, T2* axial image, ankle. The anterior talofibular ligament *(arrowhead)* and striated posterior talofibular ligament *(arrow)* are well seen at the level of the malleolar fossa *(open arrow)*. *B,* T1 coronal image, ankle. The calcaneofibular ligament *(arrow)* is best seen on this view. The posterior talofibular ligament is seen above.

in the anterolateral gutter of the ankle. The gutter is the space bounded by the anterior tibiofibular and anterior talofibular ligaments anteriorly, by the talus medially, and by the fibula laterally. The space extends superiorly to the tibial plafond and tibiofibular syndesmosis, and distally to the calcaneofibular ligament (Fig. 16–26).[20] This is also a common location for intraarticular loose bodies to lodge.

Patients with the impingement syndrome have anterolateral ankle pain, swelling, and limited dorsiflexion that is clinically indistinguishable from symptoms caused by several other abnormalities. The soft tissue lesions that may cause the problems are hypertrophic synovium, fibrotic scar, or an accessory fascicle of the anterior tibiofibular ligament. Most cases result from trauma or surgery, and the lesion can be removed arthroscopically. Patients often give a history of an inversion injury, and there

is probably an injury to the anterior tibiofibular and talofibular ligaments at the time of the injury that leads to synovitis and scarring with resultant anterolateral joint line tenderness and the sensation of the ankle giving way.

The diagnosis is made on MRI by identifying soft tissue deep to the anterior tibiofibular or anterior talofibular ligament where normally none is present (Fig. 16–27). A joint effusion can aid in the recognition of the soft tissue mass in this region. Instability related to a disrupted ligament can cause clinical features identical to that of the anterior impingement syndrome.[20]

Sinus Tarsi Syndrome (Box 16–10)

The sinus tarsi, or tarsal sinus, is a cone-shaped space formed between the calcaneus and talus (Figs. 16–28 and 16–29). The narrow end of the cone is located medially, whereas the large end is located laterally, beneath the lateral malleolus. The sinus tarsi contains fat, several ligaments, neurovascular structures, and portions of the joint capsule of the posterior subtalar joint. Nerve endings in the sinus tarsi are important for proprioception of the hindfoot. Hindfoot stability is partially maintained by the talocalcaneal ligaments located within the sinus tarsi. The most lateral of the ligaments are slips from the lateral extensor retinaculum; medial to these slips are the cervical ligament, and most medial is the interosseous ligament.[21, 22]

The sinus tarsi syndrome is a pain syndrome characterized by lateral foot pain and the subjective feeling of hindfoot instability. There may be tenderness over the area on physical examination. Pathologi-

---

BOX 16–9: ANTEROLATERAL IMPINGEMENT SYNDROME

Clinical
Anterolateral pain, swelling, limited dorsiflexion
Etiology
Posttraumatic (inversion)
Pathology
Synovitis, fibrosis in anterolateral gutter
MRI
Low-signal soft tissue mass deep to anterior tibiofibular and talofibular ligaments

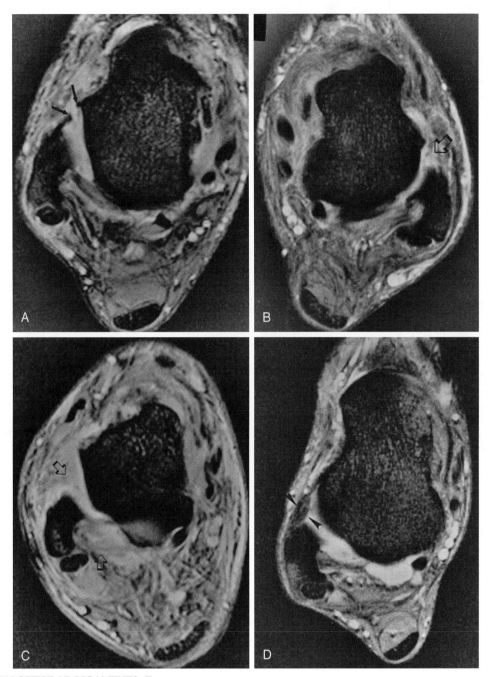

Figure 16–25. TALOFIBULAR LIGAMENTS: Tears.
A, T2* axial image, ankle. Torn fragments of the anterior talofibular ligament are seen *(arrows)*, with hemorrhage/edema leaking from the ankle joint into the soft tissues. The striated posterior talofibular ligament remains intact. **B,** T2* axial image, ankle (different patient than in *A*). The open arrow points to edema in the soft tissues, but no anterior talofibular ligament is evident because of a tear. The posterior ligament is not torn. **C,** T2* axial image, ankle (different patient than *A* or *B*). Both the anterior and posterior talofibular ligaments *(open arrows)* are not identified, indicating they are torn. By definition, the intervening calcaneofibular ligament also must be torn. The space between the talus and fibula is widened. **D,** T2* axial image, ankle (different patient than any of the above). The lateral aspect of the anterior talofibular ligament is markedly thickened *(arrowheads)* and low signal. This indicates a previous rupture with scarring and fibrosis that mimics an intact ligament.

cally, the sinus tarsi is found to contain inflammatory tissue or fibrosis, depending on the chronicity of the changes. Disruption of the interosseous and cervical ligaments also is often found. The major cause of this syndrome (up to 70%) is related to trauma, with lateral injuries and tears of the anterior talofibular and calcaneofibular ligaments usually present. The cervical and interosseous ligaments of the sinus tarsi are injured by an inversion injury, along with the lateral ankle ligaments. So up to 70% of patients with sinus tarsi syndrome may have a torn lateral ligament. Disruption of the ligaments in the sinus tarsi as well as injury to the proprioceptive nerve fibers are thought to account for the sensation of instability.

Other conditions are related to this syndrome besides ligamentous injury from trauma. Inflammatory arthropathies with extension of pannus from the subtalar joint and chronic posterior tibial tendon tears also are associated with the syndrome in about 30% of cases.

MRI often does not consistently show the ligaments of the sinus tarsi even when they are present and intact, so not identifying these ligaments has no significance. Abnormalities of the sinus tarsi on MRI include obliteration of the fat by low signal intensity material on T1W images and either high or low signal intensity (or a combination) on T2W images (Fig. 16–30). Acute abnormalities have inflammatory tissue that is high signal intensity on T2W images, whereas chronic lesions have fibrosis that is often low signal intensity on T2W images. People with symptoms of sinus tarsi syndrome usually have obliteration of all of the fat in the sinus tarsi. If only part of the fat has been replaced, it is unlikely to be associated with the sinus tarsi syndrome. Associated findings of lateral ligament tears, inflammatory arthritis, and posterior tibial tendon tears should be searched for.[23] One must not confuse a large joint effusion of the ankle or subtalar joint extending into the sinus tarsi as evidence of an abnormal sinus tarsi (Fig. 16–31). The fat in the sinus tarsi can be obscured by fluid or hemorrhage in acute ankle sprains; hence, a diagnosis of sinus tarsi syndrome should not be made in the setting of acute trauma (Fig. 16–31).

Abnormalities of the fat in the sinus tarsi on MRI

BOX 16–10: SINUS TARSI SYNDROME

Clinical
   Lateral foot pain, relieved by anesthetic injection
   Subjective hindfoot instability
Etiology
   Inflammatory arthritis (30%)
   Trauma from inversion (70%)
   • Torn lateral ankle and sinus tarsi ligaments
   • Disruption of proprioceptive nerves
Pathology
   Inflammatory tissue leads to fibrosis
   Disrupted ankle and sinus tarsi ligaments
   Posterior tibial tendon tears associated
MRI
   Obliteration of sinus tarsi fat
   • Low signal on T1
   • High or low signal on T2 (inflammatory versus fibrosis)
   Tears of calcaneofibular and anterior talofibular ligaments, and of posterior tibial tendon associated

---

do not always correlate with clinical features of the sinus tarsi syndrome. Thus, it is important to describe the abnormalities seen on MRI and state that this may indicate the patient has symptoms of the sinus tarsi syndrome, rather than making the dogmatic diagnosis of sinus tarsi syndrome based on the MRI features only. This syndrome can be treated by steroid injection, reconstruction of the ligaments of the sinus tarsi, surgical debridement and, rarely, triple arthrodesis.

Plantar Fasciitis (Box 16–11)

The plantar fascia or aponeurosis is a longitudinal fibrous condensation that originates from the plantar aspect of the calcaneal tuberosity. It is composed of a thick, cord-like central portion and thinner, membrane-like lateral and medial expansions. The central cord of the fascia arises from the medial

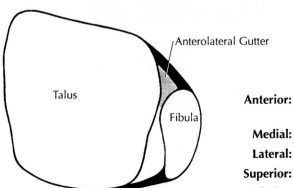

Anterolateral Gutter

Talus

Fibula

BOUNDARIES

Anterior:	Anterior Tibiofibular and Talofibular Ligaments
Medial:	Talus
Lateral:	Fibula
Superior:	Tibial Plafond, Syndesmosis
Inferior:	Calcaneofibular Ligament

Figure 16–26. ANTEROLATERAL IMPINGEMENT: Anatomy.
Diagram of the boundaries of the anterolateral gutter of the ankle. Soft tissue in the shaded area of the anterolateral gutter may be a source of pain.

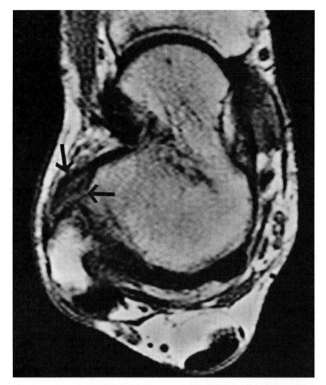

Figure 16–27. ANTEROLATERAL IMPINGEMENT SYNDROME. T1 axial image, ankle. There is abnormal heterogeneous soft tissue *(arrows)* deep to the anterior talofibular ligament in the anterolateral gutter, compatible with the anterolateral impingement syndrome. This area remained heterogeneously low signal on T2W images.

BOX 16–11: PLANTAR FASCIITIS/RUPTURE

Fasciitis
Clinical
- Obese women, runners, or seronegative arthritis with heel pain

Etiology
  Chronic, repetitive stresses or inflammation

Pathology
  Tears, myxoid degeneration, inflammation

MRI
- Thickened with high signal (T1, T2) at calcaneal attachment
- Perifasciitis (edema around thickened fascia)
- Marrow edema/erosions, plantar aspect of calcaneal tuberosity

Rupture
Clinical
- Forced dorsiflexion
- Thickened, disruption in mid-portion (distal to calcaneal attachment)

---

aspect of the calcaneus and attaches distally to the plantar surfaces of the phalanges and superficially into the skin. It is normally a low signal intensity structure on all pulse sequences that should not measure more than 4 mm in thickness at its thickest proximal attachment to the calcaneus (Fig. 16–32).

Plantar fasciitis is an inflammatory condition of the plantar fascia that causes pain and tenderness, usually near its attachment to the anteromedial calcaneal tuberosity. The two groups most commonly affected by this condition are running athletes and

obese, middle-aged women, because of chronic repetitive microtrauma and overuse. The seronegative spondyloarthropathies have a high incidence of plantar fasciitis as well, and it usually is bilateral in these patients. The clinical diagnosis of plantar fasciitis is often straightforward, without the necessity for performing MRI, but this is not always the case, especially if conservative management fails. Rarely, the plantar fascia can rupture completely, which is usually the result of forced dorsiflexion of the foot. This is clinically difficult to diagnose, but can be well seen on MRI.

MRI of plantar fasciitis shows thickening of the fascia, usually near the attachment to the calcaneus, with intermediate signal on T1 and high signal on T2W images. Edema often is seen surrounding the

Figure 16–28. SINUS TARSI: Anatomy.
Diagram of the sinus tarsi (tarsal sinus) between the talus and calcaneus from sagittal and axial perspectives. The different talocalcaneal ligaments are shown.

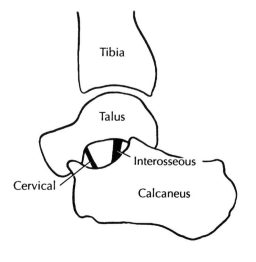

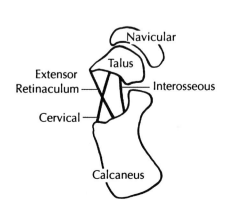

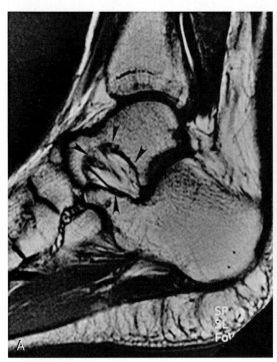

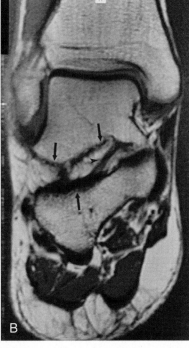

Figure 16–29. SINUS TARSI: Normal.
A, T1 sagittal image, ankle. The sinus tarsi *(arrowheads)* is filled with high-signal fat except for the linear, low-signal talocalcaneal ligaments coursing through it. *B,* T1 coronal image, ankle. Another perspective of the fat-filled space between the talus and calcaneus *(arrows)* with a talocalcaneal ligament *(arrowhead)* passing through it.

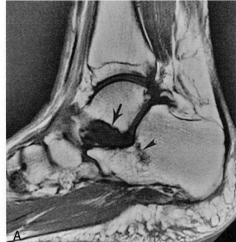

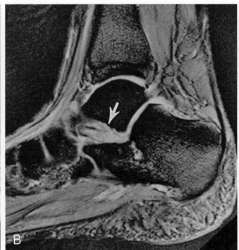

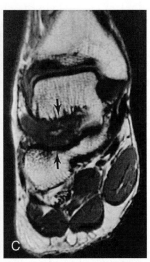

Figure 16–30. SINUS TARSI: Abnormal.
A, T1 sagittal image, ankle. The fat in the sinus tarsi is obliterated with intermediate-signal material *(arrow).* There is a cyst in the calcaneus *(arrowhead).* *B,* T2* sagittal image, ankle. The sinus tarsi is high signal, indicating inflammatory tissue that has not yet become fibrotic *(arrow).* *C,* T1 coronal image, ankle. Sinus tarsi fat obliteration *(arrows)* between the talus and calcaneus from another perspective.

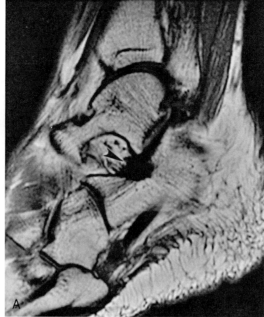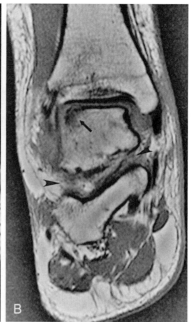

Figure 16–31. SINUS TARSI: Partial obliteration unrelated to sinus tarsi syndrome.
A, T1 sagittal image, ankle. There is a focus of low signal in the posterior sinus tarsi *(arrowhead).* This is an outpouching or recess of the posterior subtalar joint with fluid within it. *B,* T1 coronal image, ankle (different patient than in *A*). This was an acute ankle injury with fluid from hemorrhage/edema in the sinus tarsi, causing partial obliteration of the fat *(arrowheads).* There is an osteochondral injury in the lateral dome of the talus *(arrow).* Partial obliteration of the sinus tarsi is not associated with the sinus tarsi syndrome.

fascia, and adjacent bone marrow edema or erosions are common in the plantar aspect of the calcaneal tuberosity (Fig. 16–33). Plantar fascia rupture usually occurs in the midportion of the fascia, distal to the typical location of fasciitis at the calcaneal attachment (Fig. 16–34). A ruptured fascia appears as discontinuity of the fascia with surrounding high signal in the soft tissues on T2W images, secondary to the hemorrhage and edema.[23, 24]

Plantar fasciitis is treated conservatively with rest, modified footwear, nonsteroidal anti-inflammatory drugs (NSAIDs), and sometimes steroid injections. Surgery only rarely is performed for purposes of a fascial release or excision of damaged fascia.

Nerve Abnormalities

Tarsal Tunnel Syndrome (Boxes 16–12 and 16–13)

The tarsal tunnel is a fibro-osseous tunnel located on the medial side of the ankle and hindfoot, extending from the medial malleolus to the navicular bone. The talus and calcaneus, including the sustentaculum tali, form the lateral side of the tunnel, whereas the medial side is bordered by the flexor retinaculum and abductor hallucis muscle. Within the confines of these structures is the tunnel, which contains the posterior tibial nerve and its divisions,

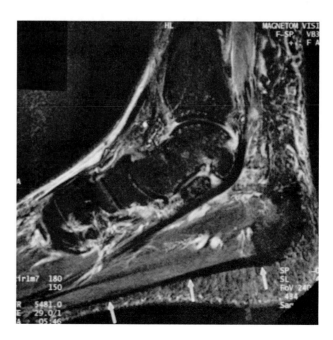

Figure 16–32. PLANTAR FASCIA: Normal.
STIR sagittal image, ankle. The low-signal plantar fascia *(arrows)* attaches to the calcaneal tuberosity proximally and gradually tapers as it extends distally. It originates medially (note the flexor hallucis longus tendon passing beneath the sustentaculum tali, indicating the medial side of the foot).

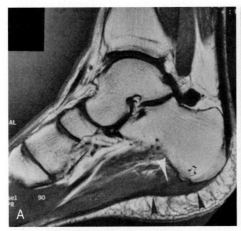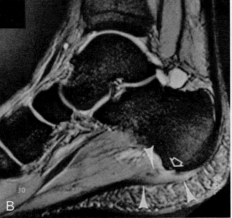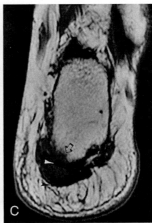

Figure 16–33. PLANTAR FASCIITIS.
A, T1 sagittal image, hindfoot. The proximal plantar fascia is thickened and high signal (between *arrowheads*). There is an erosion of the adjacent calcaneal tuberosity *(open arrow).* *B,* T2* sagittal image, hindfoot. The same findings are seen as in *A,* but the signal in the fascia is higher and the abnormality easier to identify. *C,* T1 coronal image, hindfoot. The calcaneal erosion and marrow edema are evident *(open arrow).* The plantar fascia on the medial side of the calcaneus is about four times its normal thickness (between *arrowheads*) and higher signal than normal.

the posterior tibial artery and vein, the posterior tibial tendon, flexor digitorum longus tendon, and the flexor hallucis longus tendon (Fig. 16–35).[25]

The tarsal tunnel syndrome consists of a constellation of symptoms that are secondary to compression of the posterior tibial nerve or its branches. The precise location of the compression determines exactly what the symptoms are, because different nerve branches will be affected. The symptoms consist of burning and paresthesias along the sole of the foot and to the toes, often worse with activity. Motor symptoms usually are absent until late.

Tarsal tunnel syndrome may arise from abnormalities intrinsic or extrinsic to the tunnel that cause compression of the nerves in the tunnel. Among the most common causes are ganglion cysts and nerve sheath tumors arising within the tunnel (Figs. 16–36 and 16–37). Other reported causes of the syndrome

are tenosynovitis of the flexor hallucis longus tendon, tarsal coalition with bone hypertrophy of the middle facet of the subtalar joint, anomalous muscles (either the accessory soleus or flexor digitorum longus), venous varices, pannus, hemangioma, and posttraumatic fibrosis, among others (Fig. 16–38).

MRI is valuable in showing the presence and precise location of the abnormality responsible for the compressive neuropathy. Ganglion cysts and nerve sheath tumors are the two most common causes of this syndrome seen on MRI, and it must be remembered that these masses can look identical with very homogenous low signal on T1W images and high signal intensity on T2W images. This is a good indication for giving contrast in order to differentiate between the two entities, because surgery for each is significantly different. Even if MRI shows no abnormality affecting the tarsal tunnel, it is valuable

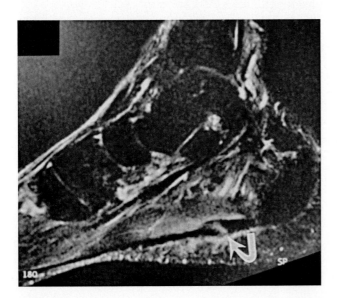

Figure 16–34. PLANTAR FASCIA: Rupture.
STIR sagittal image, hindfoot. There is disruption of the plantar fascia *(curved arrow)* about 2 cm from its origin on the calcaneus. There is surrounding high-signal edema/hemorrhage.

BOX 16–12: TARSAL TUNNEL ANATOMY

Confines
- Craniocaudal: medial malleolus to navicular
- Lateral: talus and calcaneus
- Medial: flexor retinaculum, abductor hallucis muscle

Contents
- Posterior tibial, flexor hallicus longus, flexor digitorum longus tendons
- Posterior tibial nerve, artery, and veins

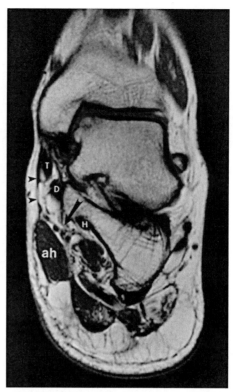

Figure 16–35. TARSAL TUNNEL: Normal.
T1 coronal image, hindfoot. The tarsal tunnel is located between the flexor retinaculum *(arrowheads)* and the abductor hallucis muscle (ah) medially, and the osseous structures laterally. The flexor tendons are located in this tunnel (T—tibialis posterior; D—flexor digitorum; H—flexor hallucis). The posterior tibial nerve, artery, and vein *(arrow)* pass through the tunnel.

because it means that surgery is not indicated and will not benefit the patient. In the latter situation, the nerve generally is affected by scarring and fibrosis, which MRI cannot detect.

Morton's Neuroma (Box 16–14)

Morton's neuroma, or interdigital neuroma, was once believed to represent a neoplastic process of the nerve, but now is thought to be secondary to chronic nerve entrapment with subsequent perineural fibrosis, neural degeneration, and often with adjacent intermetatarsal bursitis. The usual location is around the plantar digital nerve of the second or third intermetatarsal spaces (Fig. 16–39).

Symptoms are those of pain, often electrical in nature, and throbbing in the affected web space, radiating to the toes. Young and middle-aged women most commonly are afflicted; this may be due to chronic trauma to the nerve from wearing high-heeled shoes. Morton's neuromas and intermetatarsal bursitis may be present on MRI in patients who are asymptomatic.[26, 27]

Some people advocate performing only T1W short axis axial images through the metatarsal heads to screen for Morton's neuroma. This presumes that the diagnosis is clear cut clinically. That is not our experience, so we do a routine examination with all imaging planes, both T1W and T2W sequences, and give contrast. T1W images usually do not demonstrate Morton's neuromas with near the conspicuity as contrast-enhanced images.[28] Contrast enhancement can elucidate this entity very clearly with intense, diffuse uptake throughout the mass in most cases; however, it is our experience that not all Morton's neuromas demonstrate enhancement. The MRI appearance is of a teardrop-shaped soft tissue mass between the metatarsal heads that projects inferiorly into the plantar subcutaneous fat (Figs. 16–40 and 16–41). The signal intensity is intermediate on T1W and usually relatively low signal intensity on T2W images because of the abundant fibrosis present. Fluid in the adjacent intermetatarsal bursa secondary to inflammation often is present as well (Fig. 16–42). The intermetatarsal bursa runs in a vertical direction between (not beneath) metatarsal heads; bursitis shows low signal intensity on T1W images and high signal intensity on T2W images.

BOX 16–13: TARSAL TUNNEL SYNDROME

Clinical
    Burning, paresthesias in sole and into toes

Etiology/Pathology
    Compression of posterior tibial nerve or its branches from:
        Ganglion cyst
        Nerve sheath tumors
        Tenosynovitis
        Varices
        Pannus
        Hemangioma
        Tarsal coalition
        Fibrosis

MRI
    Shows presence of a mass (or not), which determines surgery (or not)
    MRI features dependent on underlying pathology

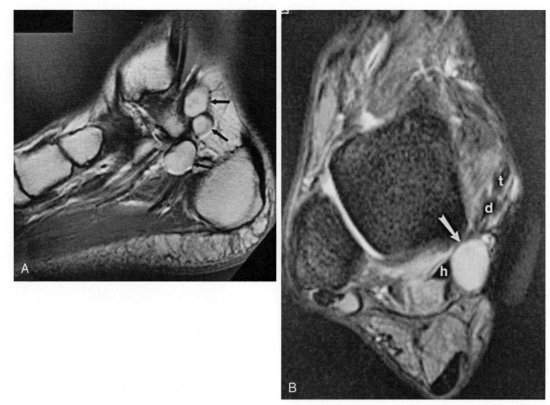

Figure 16–36. TARSAL TUNNEL SYNDROME: From schwannomas.
A, T1 contrast-enhanced sagittal image, hindfoot. Three round masses *(arrows)* that show enhancement are running through the tarsal tunnel. **B,** T2* axial image, hindfoot. One of the schwannomas is shown as a high-signal mass *(arrow)* in the space normally occupied by the posterior tibial nerve, artery, and vein. t—tibialis posterior tendon; d—flexor digitorum tendon; h—flexor hallucis tendon.

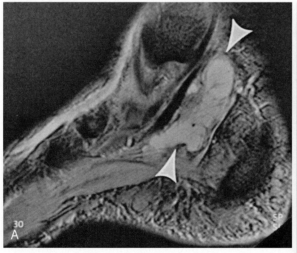

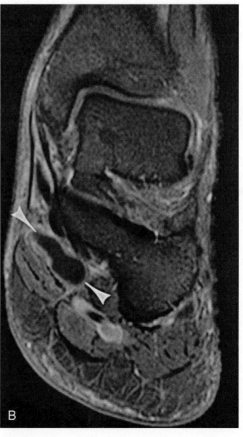

Figure 16–37. TARSAL TUNNEL SYNDROME: From ganglion cyst.
A, T2* sagittal image, hindfoot. There is a long, septated mass *(arrowheads)* posterior to the flexor digitorum tendon in the tarsal tunnel. **B,** T1 contrast-enhanced with fat suppression coronal image, hindfoot. The mass in the tarsal tunnel *(arrowheads)* shows enhancement only at its periphery, indicating this is a cystic lesion. The ganglion cyst lies adjacent to the posterior tibial nerve in the tunnel.

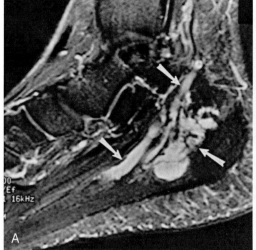
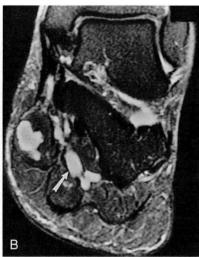

Figure 16–38. TARSAL TUNNEL SYNDROME: From hemangioma. *A,* Fast T2 with fat suppression sagittal image, hindfoot. High-signal linear structures *(arrows)* course through the tarsal tunnel. These are vessels from a hemangioma. *B,* Fast T2 with fat suppression coronal image, hindfoot. The tortuous vessels are evident in the tarsal tunnel *(arrow),* as well as within the abductor hallucis muscle.

Treatment may consist of modification of footwear, percutaneous neurolysis, surgical release by dividing the transverse metatarsal ligament, or excision.

Other entities that can occur in the intermatatarsal interspace include a true plantar nerve neuroma, synovial cysts, and intermetatarsal bursitis unrelated to Morton's neuroma. True neuromas are all high signal on T2W images and after the administration of gadolinium.

Bone Abnormalities

Tarsal Coalition

Tarsal coalition is a relatively common abnormality, occurring in about 6% of the population, and is thought to represent a failure of proper segmentation of the tarsal bones; it also can be acquired secondary to rheumatoid arthritis or trauma. Males are affected approximately four times more frequently than females, and it is bilateral in about 50% of individuals. The two most common types are calcaneonavicular (which often is asymptomatic and diagnosed on medial oblique foot films rather than MRI) and talocalcaneal, which usually occurs between the sustentaculum tali process of the calcaneus and the adjacent talus at the middle facet of the subtalar joint.

Symptoms generally occur because of limited motion in the subtalar joint, which places increased stresses elsewhere in the tarsus, leading to spasm of the peroneals and extensors, with an associated flat foot deformity. Coalitions may be osseous, fibrous, cartilaginous, or a combination.

MRI can be used to demonstrate the presence of the coalition, which type, and how extensive it is (Fig. 16–43 through 16–45). In addition, MRI can assess surrounding structures for impingement by the hypertrophic bony mass, such as displacement of the tibialis posterior and flexor hallucis longus tendons in the tarsal tunnel. Secondary degenerative joint disease in the posterior subtalar joint is common and can be documented with MRI. MRI shows narrowing and irregularity, or osseous fusion, of the middle facet of the subtalar joint. The angle of this joint is often abnormal, with a coalition being directed inferiorly.

Accessory Bones and Sesamoids
(Box 16–15)

Accessory ossicles may result in painful syndromes and associated soft tissue abnormalities. The most common syndromes in the foot are the os trigonum syndrome and abnormalities associated with an accessory navicular bone or the hallux sesamoids.

Os Trigonum Syndrome. The os trigonum syndrome (also known as the posterior ankle impinge-

---

BOX 16–14: MORTON'S NEUROMA

Clinical
- Pain in second or third web spaces, radiating to toes
- Women or others wearing high-heeled, poorly fitting shoes

Etiology/Pathology
- Chronic plantar digital nerve entrapment leading to perineural fibrosis, neural degeneration, adjacent intermetatarsal bursitis

MRI
- Teardrop-shaped soft tissue mass between and plantar to metatarsal heads
- T1: low signal
  T2: high or low signal, depending on quantity of fibrosis
  Gadolinium: usually enhances
- Fluid in the adjacent intermetatarsal bursa and surrounding soft tissue edema is common (low signal on T1; high signal on T2)

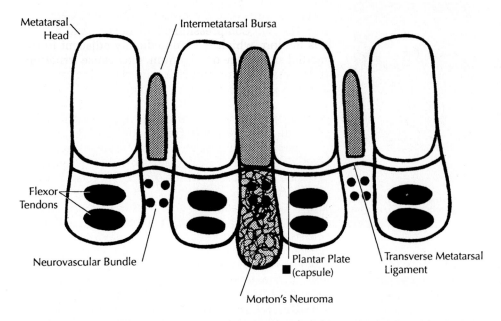

Figure 16–39. MORTON'S NEU-ROMA: Anatomy.
Diagram of the forefoot in cross section. The plantar digital nerves are located deep to the transverse metatarsal ligament between metatarsal heads. Above the nerves are the intermetatarsal bursae. Entrapment of the plantar digital nerve may lead to perineural fibrosis and neural degeneration (Morton's neuroma). Intermetatarsal bursitis is a common accompaniment.

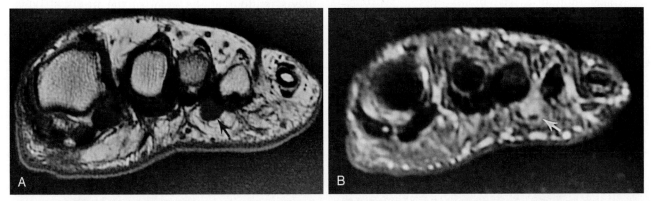

Figure 16–40. MORTON'S NEUROMA.
A, T1 short-axis axial image, forefoot. A low-signal, teardrop-shaped mass *(arrow)* from a Morton's neuroma is seen below the metatarsal heads in the third web space. *B*, STIR short-axis axial image, forefoot. The Morton's neuroma *(arrow)* becomes somewhat high signal, but is more difficult to see than on the T1 image.

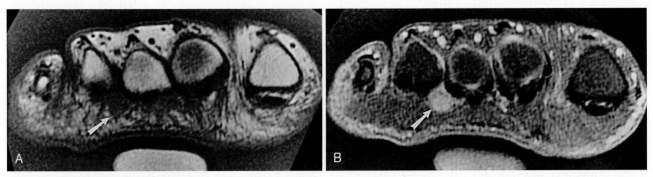

Figure 16–41. MORTON'S NEUROMA.
A, T1 short-axis axial image, forefoot. There is a mass *(arrow)* in the third web space beneath the metatarsal heads that is difficult to detect on this sequence. *B*, T1 contrast-enhanced with fat suppression short-axis axial image, forefoot. The mass enhances diffusely *(arrow)* and is an easy diagnosis on this image.

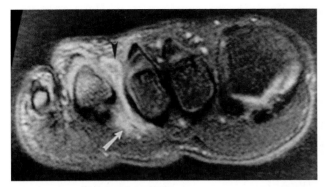

Figure 16–42. MORTON'S NEUROMA.
T1 contrast-enhanced with fat suppression short-axis axial image, forefoot. A teardrop-shaped mass *(arrow)* is diagnostic of a Morton's neuroma in the third web space. The lining of the inflamed intermetatarsal bursa also enhances *(arrowhead)* between the metatarsal heads.

chondrosis appears as high signal intensity fluid between the os trigonum and the rest of the talus on T2W images, where cartilage normally exists (see Fig. 16–11).[8] Compression of the flexor hallucis longus tendon, which lies immediately adjacent to the medial side of the os trigonum, may cause irritation, inflammation, tenosynovitis, and stenosing tenosynovitis with abnormal high signal intensity within the tendon or surrounding it (see Fig. 16–11). Loose bodies may be seen in the ankle joint secondary to the bone impaction and fragmentation.

Accessory Navicular. The accessory navicular bone or prominent medial tuberosity of the navicular bone can cause pain for several reasons. Painful degenerative changes between the accessory ossicle and the navicular can occur with marrow edema within the ossicle, a painful bursa can develop in the soft tissues superficial to the navicular prominence, and there is a much higher incidence of posterior tibial tendon tears in the presence of an accessory navicular bone, caused by altered stresses (Fig. 16–47).[29]

Hallux Sesamoids. The medial and lateral hallux sesamoids, which are located in the flexor hallucis brevis tendons at the level of the first metatarsal head, provide mechanical advantage during flexion of the great toe and serve to reduce friction. They may be abnormal for several reasons: acute fractures, stress fractures, osteonecrosis, infection, sesamoiditis, dislocation, and they participate in degenerative and inflammatory arthritides. In general, the medial sesamoid is more likely to be involved with

ment syndrome) occurs when the trigonal process of the talus or the os trigonum is compressed between the posterior tibia and the posterior calcaneus during forced plantar flexion, resulting in posterior ankle pain. Recurrent plantar flexion of the foot is required in ballet, running down hills, and kicking a football. Posterior talar compression can result in a stress reaction with marrow edema in the trigonal process or os trigonum (Fig. 16–46), an acute fracture or a chronic stress fracture of the trigonal process of the talus, or fracture through the synchondrosis that normally exists between the talus and the os trigonum. Disruption of the syn-

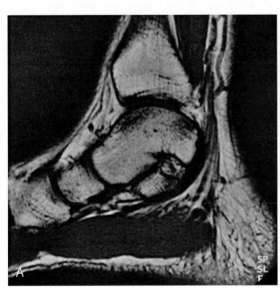
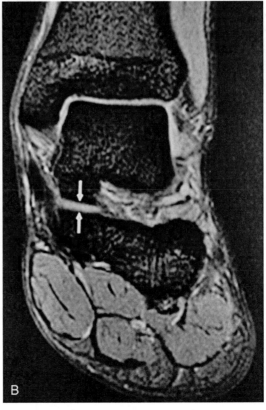

Figure 16–43. MIDDLE FACET OF THE SUBTALAR JOINT: Normal.
A, T1 sagittal image, hindfoot. The joint between the sustentaculum tali and talus is straight and uniform, without features of coalition. *B,* T2* coronal image, hindfoot. Uniform high-signal cartilage is present in the middle facet of the subtalar joint (between *arrows*).

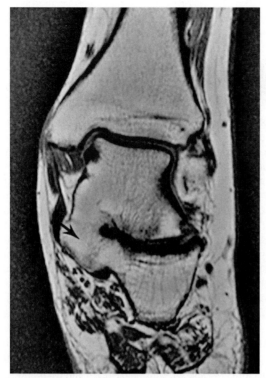

Figure 16–44. TARSAL COALITION: Osseous.
T1 coronal image, hindfoot. There is complete osseous ankylosis with no joint in the expected location *(arrow)* for the middle facet. This hypertrophic bone mass placed pressure on the adjacent posterior tibial nerve; the patient presented with tarsal tunnel syndrome.

traumatic abnormalities, whereas the lateral sesamoid more commonly is affected by ischemic changes with osteonecrosis (Fig. 16–48).

The MRI appearance of all of these varied abnormalities of the sesamoids is usually identical, regardless of the underlying pathology.[30] A differential diagnosis is necessary in most instances, because the findings are not specific. However, if a fracture line is evident, or if subchondral bone lesions are seen in both a sesamoid and the adjacent metatarsal head, a specific diagnosis of fracture or arthritis, respectively, can be made (Fig. 16–48).

The most common soft tissue abnormality to occur in the region of the hallux sesamoids is turf toe. Turf toe is the result of hyperdorsiflexion of the first metatarsophalangeal joint with disruption of the plantar capsular tissues. Sesamoid dislocation or subluxation may occur in conjunction with turf toe.

Fractures

MRI generally is only used to diagnose fractures when conventional radiographs are normal or inconclusive. The ability of MRI to demonstrate fractures is exquisite and is particularly useful for osteochondral fractures of the talar dome and stress and insufficiency fractures throughout the foot and ankle. At the same time, any soft tissue abnormalities are evident also.

BOX 16–15: ACCESSORY OSSICLES

Os Trigonum Syndrome (Posterior Impingement Syndrome)
Clinical:
Repetitive plantar flexion (ballet, basketball, kicking football, running on hills)
Etiology:
Os trigonum/trigonal process and flexor hallucis tendon trapped between calcaneus and tibia
Pathology:
Marrow edema/fracture of trigonal process or synchondrosis of os trigonum; flexor hallucis longus irritation (stenosing tenosynovitis)
MRI:
T1:—low signal in marrow of posterior talus
T2:—high signal marrow in talus
—high signal fracture of synchondrosis, os trigonum
—focal, loculated high signal fluid around flexor hallucis (stenosing tenosynovitis)
Navicular Bone
• Large cornuate process of navicular or accessory navicular bone
• Marrow edema, overlying bursitis, degenerative joint disease between accessory bone and navicular, associated posterior tibial tendon tears
• T2 MRI shows high signal of all abnormalities
Hallux Sesamoids
• Located in flexor hallucis brevis tendons at first metatarsal head
• Abnormalities: acute or stress fractures, osteonecrosis, infection, sesamoiditis (inflammation), dislocation, participate in inflammatory and degenerative joint disease
• MRI is sensitive, but nonspecific. Low signal on medial sesamoid more likely to be traumatic in origin; lateral sesamoid is more likely osteonecrosis

Bone contusions or osteochondral fractures usually are seen with inversion or eversion injuries of the ankle; associated ligamentous injury virtually is always present. The term osteochondritis dissecans has been used for this same entity, suggesting spontaneous osteonecrosis as the cause, but osteochondral fracture is probably the most accurate reflection of the pathology. The medial or lateral aspects of the dome of the talus are affected with equal frequency by these fractures. The fractures may be mere bone contusions or true linear fractures, either with or without overlying cartilaginous involvement. Sometimes a crack in the cartilage can lead to

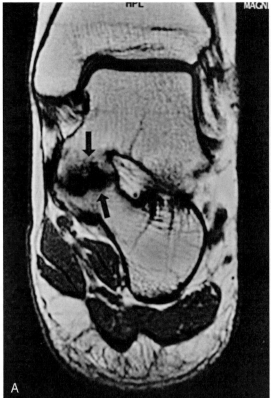

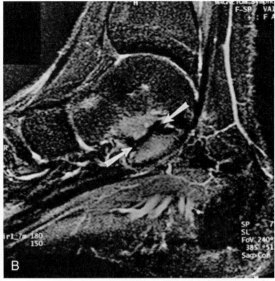

Figure 16–45. TARSAL COALITION: Fibrocartilaginous.
A, T1 coronal image, hindfoot. The joint between the sustentaculum tali and the talus is narrowed and irregular (between *arrows*). *B,* STIR sagittal image, hindfoot. The joint of the middle facet is again noted to be irregular and narrowed from fibrocartilaginous coalition *(arrows).* There is high-signal bone marrow edema on both sides of the abnormal joint.

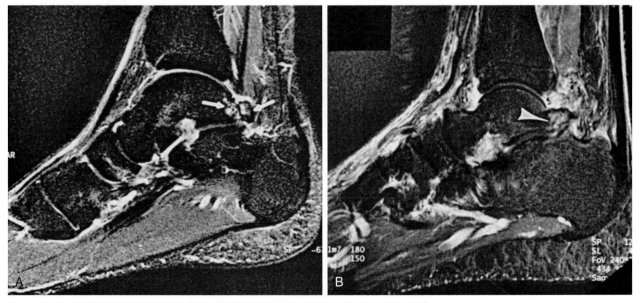

Figure 16–46. OS TRIGONUM SYNDROME (POSTERIOR IMPINGEMENT SYNDROME).
A, STIR sagittal image, hindfoot. There is high-signal marrow edema in the os trigonum as well as the adjacent posterior talus *(arrows).*
B, STIR sagittal image, hindfoot (different patient than in *A*). There is no os trigonum in this individual; instead, there is a trigonal process of the posterior talus that has abnormal high-signal marrow edema *(arrowhead)* from impingement during repeated plantar flexion.

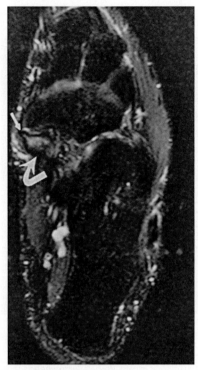

Figure 16–47. ACCESSORY NAVICULAR.
STIR long-axis coronal image, hindfoot. There is an accessory navicular bone *(curved arrow)* with degenerative changes between it and the navicular, as manifested by an osteophyte *(straight arrow)* at the joint line. The accessory navicular has diffuse high signal from marrow edema.

intrusion of joint fluid with development of large subchondral cysts in the talar dome that may resemble a bone tumor.

MRI of osteochondral fractures (Box 16–16) is useful to show their presence and to demonstrate if the fragment is loose (stable) or not. MRI features to indicate a loose osteochondral fragment are high signal surrounding the fragment on T2W images, large subchondral cysts deep to the fragment, cracks in the overlying cartilage, or absence of the fragment with or without an intraarticular loose body seen (Fig. 16–49). The commonly associated ligamentous injuries also can be identified.

BOX 16–16: OSTEOCHONDRAL FRACTURES (Osteochondritis Dissecans)

- Dome of talus affected from injury as talus impacts against tibia. Medial or lateral aspect of talar dome involved.
- Ligamentous injuries commonly are associated.
- MRI shows if fragment is unstable (loose):
  —High signal surrounding fragment on T2
  —Absent or displaced fragment
  —Crack in overlying cartilage
  —Large subchondral cysts deep to fragment

Stress fractures are seen on MRI as linear areas of low signal intensity on T1W images with high or low signal intensity on T2W images. The fractures generally run perpendicular to the long axis of the affected bone; however, stress fractures of the medial malleolus usually are vertically oriented (Fig. 16–50). The findings on MRI are specific, unlike bone scans done for the same indications. Just as anywhere else in the skeleton, traumatic fractures can be found in any of the bones of the foot and ankle with great sensitivity by MRI when conventional radiographs are negative and bone scans are negative or nonspecific.

Osteonecrosis of the Foot and Ankle
(Box 16–17)

Osteonecrosis may occur anywhere in the foot and ankle if the patient is taking steroids or has other predisposing systemic risk factors; however, the most common locations for osteonecrosis secondary to trauma include (1) the navicular bone, which may have an unrecognized fracture, causing the bone fragments to develop osteonecrosis; (2) the heads of the metatarsals, especially the second, in individuals who wear high-heeled shoes (Freiberg's infraction); (3) the lateral hallux sesamoid at the level of the head of the first metatarsal; and (4) osteonecrosis of the dome of the talus, a well-known sequela of a previous talar neck fracture with disruption of the blood supply to the proximal portion of the bone (Fig. 16–51).[23, 31]

The MRI appearance of osteonecrosis in the foot and ankle is identical to other bones in the skeleton: serpiginous low signal intensity lines creating a geographic pattern, or diffuse low signal on T1W images that may or may not become higher signal on T2W images. The differential diagnosis for the marrow changes in osteonecrosis, other than the pathognomonic serpiginous lines, include occult fractures, abnormal increased stresses, osteomyelitis, and regional migratory osteoporosis with bone marrow edema.

Osseous Tumors (Box 16–18)

A few tumors of bone have a predilection for the foot and ankle, but both malignant primary and metastatic lesions are rare in the foot and ankle.

BOX 16–17: OSTEONECROSIS IN THE FOOT

Navicular (unrecognized fracture)
Metatarsal heads, especially 2nd and 3rd (repetitive stresses, high-heeled shoes)
Talar dome (talar neck fracture)
Lateral hallux sesamoid
Anywhere else (steroids)

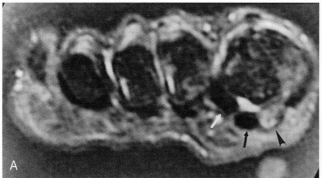

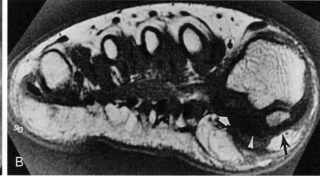

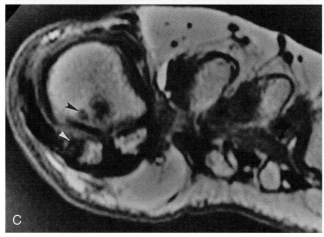

Figure 16–48. HALLUX SESAMOIDS.
A, STIR short-axis axial image, forefoot. There is abnormal high signal in the medial hallux sesamoid *(arrowhead).* This was a runner and is most likely a stress reaction. The normal lateral hallux sesamoid is shown with a *white arrow;* it is low signal because of fat suppression. The flexor hallucis longus tendon *(black arrow)* runs between the sesamoids. *B,* T1 short-axis axial image, forefoot (different patient than in *A*). There is low signal throughout the lateral sesamoid *(white arrow).* This contrasts to the high-signal fat in the normal medial sesamoid *(black arrow).* The flexor hallucis tendon is shown with an *arrowhead.* An abnormal lateral sesamoid is more likely to be the result of ischemia than other causes. *C,* T1 short-axis axial image, forefoot (different patient than in *A* and *B*). There is focal low signal in the medial hallux sesamoid *(white arrowhead).* Similar focal low-signal areas are seen in the adjacent first metatarsal head *(black arrowhead),* which makes the diagnosis of degenerative joint disease.

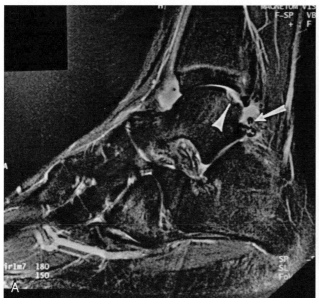

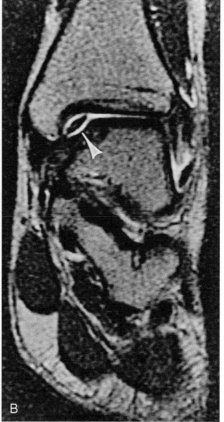

Figure 16–49. OSTEOCHONDRAL INJURIES OF THE TALUS.
A, STIR sagittal image, ankle. There is a focal osteochondral defect in the dome of the talus *(arrowhead),* with no fragment in the defect. The fragment has become loose and is an intraarticular loose body *(arrow)* in the posterior ankle. *B,* Spin echo-T2 coronal image, ankle (different patient than in *A*). There is an osteochondral fracture of the medial dome of the talus. The fragment remains in the bed of the defect. The high signal between the fragment and the talus *(arrowhead)* indicates that this is an unstable fragment.

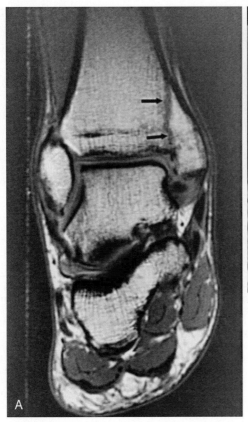

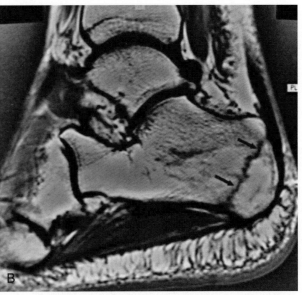

Figure 16–50. FRACTURES.
A, T1 coronal image, ankle. There is a vertical stress fracture *(arrows)* of the medial malleolus in a college basketball player with pain. Radiographs were normal. *B,* T1 sagittal image, hindfoot (different patient than in *A*). There is a low-signal linear stress fracture *(arrows)* in the posterior calcaneal tuberosity, running perpendicular to the long axis of the bone. This was not evident on radiographs.

MRI does not generally add to our ability to make the diagnosis, but is useful for demonstrating the extent of disease within the bone and for assessing for any soft tissue component.

The distal tibia and fibula most commonly may be affected by nonossifying fibromas, aneurysmal bone cysts, and giant cell tumors.

The calcaneus is a common site for intraosseous lipomas and simple bone cysts, both usually occurring in the mid-portion or neck of the calcaneus. This portion of the calcaneus has sparse trabeculae, caused by a paucity of stresses in this area, and normally often is filled with fat. An intraosseous lipoma can be distinguished from normal fat in the area of sparse trabeculae because in the lipoma, the fat is well circumscribed, whereas the pseudolesion is not circumscribed and blends with surrounding marrow fat (Fig. 16–52). Intraosseous lipomas often have an area of central fat necrosis that ossifies; this helps to make the diagnosis. Intraosseous lipomas may develop where simple bone cysts originally existed; fat fills in the cyst from the periphery toward its center. Other lesions that have a predilection for the calcaneus include chondroblastoma, an-

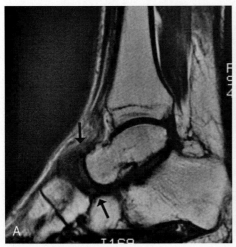

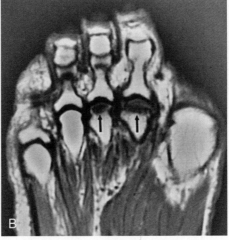

Figure 16–51. OSTEONECROSIS.
A, T1 sagittal image, hindfoot. There is diffuse low signal throughout the navicular bone *(arrows)* from osteonecrosis. This was a former basketball player with pain. *B,* T1 long-axis coronal image, forefoot. Focal areas of low signal *(arrows)* are evident in the second and third metatarsal heads from osteonecrosis (Freiberg's infraction).

BOX 16–18: COMMON BONE TUMORS, FOOT AND ANKLE

Distal Tibia and Fibula
Nonossifying fibroma, giant cell tumor, aneurysmal bone cyst
Calcaneus
Neck: simple bone cyst, lipoma
Tuberosity: aneurysmal bone cyst, chondroblastoma, giant cell tumor
Talus
Osteoid osteoma
Bone Tumor Mimickers
Medial malleolus: intraosseous ganglion cyst
Talar dome: posttraumatic large subchondral cyst

eurysmal bone cyst, and giant cell tumors, all of which usually are located posteriorly in the apophysis of the calcaneal tuberosity.

The talus is a site of predilection for osteoid osteomas, which classically occur in a subperiosteal location and involve the neck of the talus, where they produce periosteal reaction and may show extensive bone marrow edema of the talus, and edema in the surrounding soft tissues on MRI. There may or may not be an erosion of the dorsal aspect of the neck of

the talus in the presence of a subperiosteal osteoid osteoma (Fig. 16–53).

Two lesions often mistaken for bone tumors are the intraosseous ganglion cyst, which is common in the medial malleolus, and posttraumatic subchondral cysts in the dome of the talus (Fig. 16–54); these lesions may grow to be quite large. MRI may document the diagnosis of a subchondral cyst by demonstrating its communication to the articular surface.

Soft Tissue Tumors (Box 16–19)

Benign Soft Tissue Tumors

Benign soft tissue tumors of the foot that occur with relative frequency include ganglion cysts, hemangiomas, lipomas, nerve sheath tumors, plantar fibromatosis, soft tissue chondroma (extraarticular synovial osteochondromatosis), and giant cell tumor of the tendon sheath (extraarticular pigmented villonodular synovitis).[32, 33] MRI is useful to confirm the presence and extent of a soft tissue mass, and determine the precise anatomic location, which aids in surgery; in some cases, the appearance is specific for a particular lesion. The MRI features of all but one of the above listed entities are the same in the foot and ankle as elsewhere in the body and are not discussed in detail here. Plantar fibromatosis is somewhat unique to the foot and is discussed.

Plantar Fibromatosis. Plantar fibromatosis is a be-

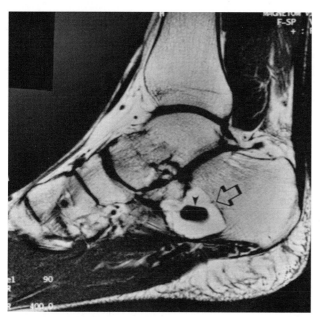

Figure 16–52. INTRAOSSEOUS LIPOMA.
T1 sagittal image, hindfoot. There is a round, high-signal fat mass in the neck of the calcaneus *(open arrow)* that is well circumscribed. In the center of this fatty mass is a focus of low signal *(arrowhead)* that was high signal on STIR and calcified on radiographs. Some people believe that fat fills in around the periphery of preexisting simple bone cysts in the calcaneus to form intraosseous lipomas. This patient also has a radiographically occult fracture in the neck of the talus.

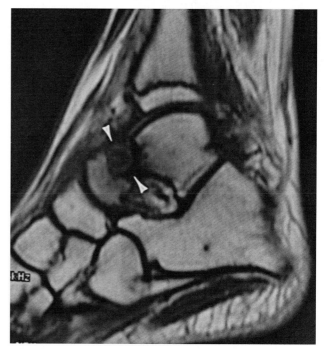

Figure 16–53. OSTEOID OSTEOMA.
T1 sagittal image, ankle. There is a mass eroding the neck of the talus *(arrowheads)* that has a target appearance typical of osteoid osteoma. This is a typical location for subperiosteal osteoid osteoma of the talus.

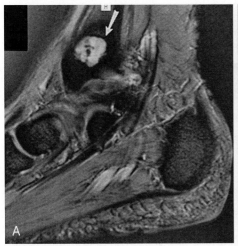
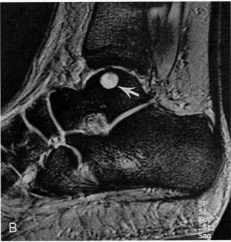

Figure 16–54. BONE TUMOR MIMICKERS.
A, T2* sagittal image, ankle. The lobulated, high-signal lesion in the medial malleolus *(arrow)* was an intraosseous ganglion cyst at biopsy. This is a typical location for this lesion. *B,* T2* sagittal image, ankle. There is a large, round, high-signal lesion in the dome of the talus *(arrow).* These may mimic tumors when large, but this is a subchondral cyst related to previous osteochondral injury. An abnormal low-signal focus in the cartilage overlying the cyst can be seen, which helps to make the diagnosis.

nign proliferation of fibrous tissue along the plantar aspect of the foot, arising in the plantar fascia. It presents as a nodule on the sole of the foot, usually medial in location, and is painless. It develops as either a single or multiple small nodular thickenings of the plantar fascia that appear as low to intermediate signal intensity on *both* T1 and T2W sequences (Fig. 16–55). These lesions often, though not invariably, enhance with intravenous gadolinium. The upper margin may be infiltrative and can grow into the deeper compartments of the foot, whereas the lower margin usually is relatively well defined and outlined by the subcutaneous fat.[34] As long as the MRI signal characteristics and anatomic location are typical of plantar fibromatosis, the lesions often are not surgically removed, unless they are large.

Malignant Soft Tissue Tumors

Synovial Sarcoma. The most common malignant soft tissue tumor of the foot is the synovial sarcoma. It is an extraarticular soft tissue mass which, on conventional radiographs, may show scattered calcifications in approximately 50% of afflicted individuals. It usually affects young adults. It may be infil-

trative and destroy adjacent bone, but also can appear well defined and relatively benign by imaging criteria, sometimes creating a pressure erosion on adjacent bone. Necrosis and hemorrhage may be present and cause a heterogeneous appearance after gadolinium administration. There is essentially nothing specific about the appearance of this lesion, and one must be certain to include this in the differential diagnosis of a nondescript foot mass in a young patient (Fig. 16–56).[32]

Other Sarcomas. Liposarcoma and malignant fibrous histiocytoma are rare below the knee, but if they do occur in the foot/ankle region, they tend to be present at the ankle.

Soft Tissue Tumor Mimickers

Some masses in the foot and ankle are not the result of neoplasm, and MRI can easily differentiate neoplasm from these other entities. Accessory muscles and tears of the anterior tibial tendon are two entities that often present with a mass suspicious for neoplasm based on clinical examination.

Accessory Muscles. Anomalous or accessory muscles in the foot or ankle are relatively common in the population. The accessory soleus and peroneus quartus muscles are the most common accessory muscles encountered in this region. The MRI appearance is diagnostic because the signal and appearance are identical to other muscle on all pulse sequences.[35–37]

The accessory soleus muscle is an anatomic normal variant of the calf musculature that presents as a mass on the medial aspect of the ankle, may be the source of pain secondary to ischemia that occurs during exercise as a form of a localized compartment syndrome, or may compress the posterior tibial nerve in the tarsal tunnel, resulting in tarsal tunnel syndrome. On MRI, it is located medial to the Achilles tendon and has a tendon of its own that inserts either into the Achilles tendon or to the calcaneus (Fig. 16–57).

The peroneus quartus accessory muscle also lies in the posterior ankle, just anterior and lateral to

---

BOX 16–19: COMMON SOFT TISSUE TUMORS, FOOT AND ANKLE

Benign
Ganglion cyst, hemangioma, lipoma, nerve sheath tumors, giant cell tumor of tendon sheath, soft tissue chondroma, plantar fibromatosis
Malignant
Synovial sarcoma
Soft Tissue Tumor Mimickers
Accessory muscles
Accessory soleus
Peroneus quartus
Pressure lesions

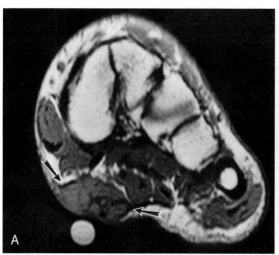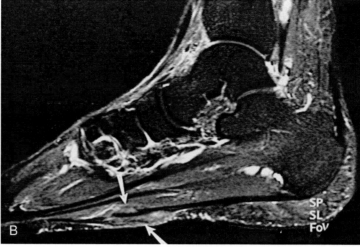

Figure 16–55. PLANTAR FIBROMATOSIS.
A, T1 short-axis axial image, midfoot. There is an intermediate-signal mass *(arrows)* surrounding the plantar fascia. *B,* STIR sagittal image, foot. The mass *(arrows)* is heterogeneous, but generally remains low signal. The plantar fascia courses through the center of the mass.

the Achilles tendon (see Fig. 16–16). Similar to the accessory soleus muscle, the peroneus quartus may present as a mass or be an incidental finding on MRI. Peroneus quartus accessory muscles occur in 13% to 25% of people. They often are asymptomatic, but have been considered responsible for lateral ankle pain and ankle joint instability. It may predispose to subluxation of the peroneal tendons because of its mass effect within the confined space created by the peroneal retinaculum, and subsequent stretching and laxity of the retinaculum. The peroneus quartus runs posteromedial to the peroneus longus and brevis tendons and usually attaches to the retrotrochlear eminence on the calcaneus, which is located posterior to the peroneal tubercle.

The accessory flexor digitorum longus muscle may cause a compressive neuropathy of the posterior tibial nerve in the tarsal tunnel. The tendon from another accessory muscle, the peroneocalcaneus internus, runs parallel to a portion of the flexor

hallucis longus tendon and may simulate a longitudinal split of that tendon.

Pressure Lesions (Box 16–20). Increased stresses on certain musculoskeletal structures can cause changes in those structures that may be confused with pathology, but are really of minimal or no significance. Marrow edema that occurs as a response to increased stresses on bones is such an example and may be difficult to differentiate from infection, early osteonecrosis, or other abnormalities by MRI alone.[38]

Another entity related to chronic stresses is a pressure lesion that may occur in subcutaneous fat at points of increased pressure and chronic repeated friction. Pressure lesions may develop cystic centers and are then called adventitious bursae. These lesions may or may not be symptomatic. Adventitious bursae are bursae that do not initially exist in the body, but form as a response to pressures on the soft tissues. Pressure lesions may mimic a soft tissue tumor, especially before developing cystic changes.

Pressure lesions in the foot occur at pressure points, predictably on the plantar surface of the first or fifth metatarsal heads, which lie lower than the other metatarsal heads, medial to the first metatarsal head in patients with hallux valgus, plantar to the medial aspect of the calcaneal tuberosity, and posterior to the distal Achilles tendon (tendo-Achilles bursa) from ill-fitting shoes. Pressure lesions/adventitious bursae also may occur after surgery to the foot that results in stresses being transferred to a new site, and these are often called "transfer lesions" by orthopedists. Feet that are deformed have pressure lesions occurring in atypical locations, where pressure is greatest.

The lesion is a rounded abnormality in the subcutaneous fat that is low to intermediate signal intensity on T1W MR images and becomes vague in appearance with areas of intermediate and high signal intensity on T2W images (Fig. 16–58). Because these

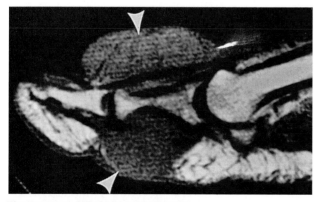

Figure 16–56. SYNOVIAL SARCOMA.
T1 sagittal image, great toe. There is a large, intermediate-signal mass *(arrowheads)* surrounding the great toe. This is a nonspecific MR appearance, but was a synovial sarcoma at surgery.

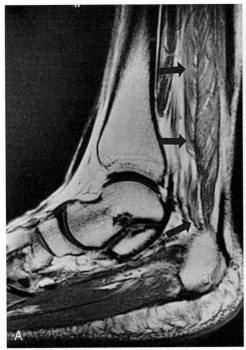 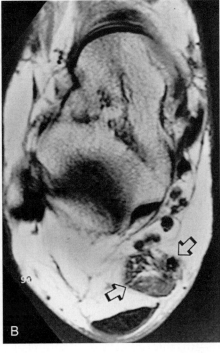

Figure 16–57. ACCESSORY MUSCLE: Soleus.
A, T1 sagittal image, ankle. An accessory soleus muscle is seen on the medial side of the ankle between the Achilles tendon and the osseous structures *(arrows).* It attaches to the top of the posterior calcaneus. *B,* T1 axial image, ankle. The accessory soleus *(open arrows)* is evident medially adjacent to the posterior tibial nerve, artery, and vein.

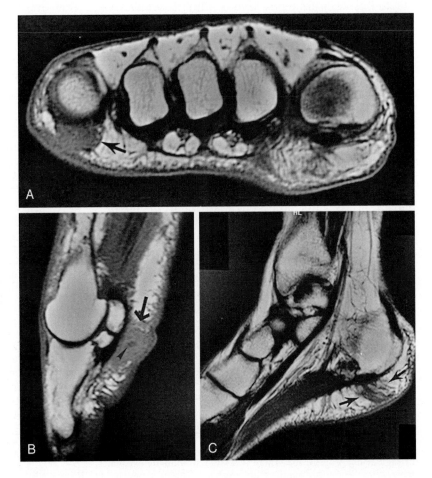

Figure 16–58. PRESSURE LESIONS.
A, T1 short-axis axial image, forefoot. There is a mass *(arrow)* beneath the fifth metatarsal head. *B,* T1 sagittal image, forefoot (different patient than in *A*). An intermediate-signal mass *(arrow)* is present directly beneath the first metatarsal head and sesamoids. There is a low-signal center *(arrowhead),* indicating a cystic center; this is an adventitious bursa. *C,* T1 sagittal image, hindfoot (different patient than in *A* and *B*). There is a pressure lesion with focal intermediate signal interspersed with fat beneath the medial calcaneal tuberosity.

pressure lesions appear as a soft tissue mass, they may be mistaken for significant pathology. The key to diagnosis is that the lesions occur in typical locations, the MRI characteristics are not entirely typical of a true mass lesion, and fat often is intermixed. If these are biopsied, fibrous and fatty tissue is found histologically.

The Diabetic Foot (Boxes 16–21 and 16–22)

Problems in the feet of diabetics are common and often devastating. They have a multifactorial etiology, including small vessel ischemia, neuropathic arthropathy, fractures, and infections. Clinicians treating these patients usually are primarily interested in differentiating osteomyelitis from soft tissue infection, because the patients usually have developed a soft tissue ulcer over a pressure area in the foot. Differentiation is difficult clinically, but is important and affects the therapy the patient will receive, including the length of antibiotic treatment, as well as the decision for surgical debridement. The role of imaging is not only to detect osteomyelitis or soft tissue abscesses, but also to assess the extent of these changes and therefore be useful in the planning of any surgical procedure or biopsy.

Studies have shown MRI to be more cost effective than the standard three-phase radionuclide bone scan and indium-labeled white blood cell scans for diabetic feet infections.[39] MRI is a faster examination to perform, and it shows other lesions of importance to clinical management, such as sinus tracts, cellulitis, abscesses, and tendon abnormalities.

MRI shows changes in the bone marrow from osteomyelitis, consisting of low signal intensity on

T1 sequences, replacing the normal high signal fatty marrow, and high signal intensity on T2 or STIR images (Fig. 16–59).[40–44] Unfortunately, MRI is limited in much the same way as bone scans by the inability to differentiate true osteomyelitis from marrow edema secondary to adjacent soft tissue inflammatory changes ("sympathetic" or reactive

---

BOX 16–21: MARROW SIGNAL ABNORMALITIES IN DIABETIC FEET

- ↑ T1 (fat), ↓ STIR (fat)
  —*Normal*
- ↑ T1 (fat), ↑ STIR
  —*Reactive marrow edema* from adjacent soft tissue inflammation
- ↓ T1, ↓ STIR
  —*Neuropathic,* chronic
- ↓ T1, ↑ STIR
  —*Osteomyelitis* by far most likely diagnosis if there is an overlying ulcer and located at a pressure point
  —*Reactive marrow edema* from adjacent inflammation cannot be excluded
  —*Neuropathic* acute changes most likely if a joint is involved, no overlying ulcer, or does not occur at pressure points

---

BOX 16–22: DIABETIC FEET

Osteomyelitis
- Marrow signal
  —low on T1, high on STIR
- Soft tissue ulcer adjacent to abnormal bone (>90%)
- Occurs at pressure points
  —1st and 5th metatarsal heads, calcaneal tuberosity, distal toes, malleoli
- Nonspecific other possible findings: cortical destruction, periosteal reaction, joint effusion, high signal in soft tissues on STIR from cellulitis/abscesses

Neuropathic Changes
- Marrow signal, low on T1 and either low or high signal (chronic or acute changes, respectively) on STIR
- Abnormalities are joint based; tarsometatarsal joints usually involved
- Bones have deformed shape (fragmentation, resorption)
- Muscles atrophied (high signal on T1 and STIR)
- Nonspecific other possible findings: periosteal reaction, cortical destruction, joint effusion

---

BOX 16–20: PRESSURE LESIONS IN FOOT

Clinical
- Usually asymptomatic, occasionally painful
- Probably related to adventitious bursa formation
- Common locations
  —Plantar to 1st, 5th metatarsal heads
  —Plantar to plantar fascia at calcaneal tuberosity
  —Posterior to distal Achilles (tendo-Achilles bursa)
  —Medial to metatarsal head in hallux valgus
- Histology: fibrous and fatty tissue

MRI
- Low signal all sequences, usually
- Fat may be intermixed in mass
- Often not a true mass appearance on T2
- May have cystic center (↑ signal, T2)

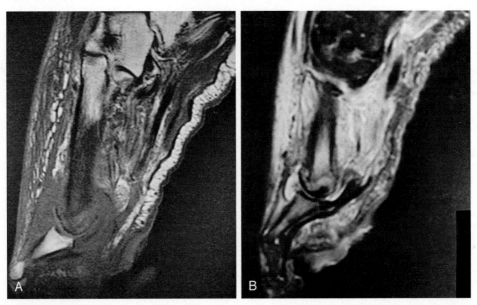

Figure 16–59. OSTEOMYELITIS.
A, T1 sagittal image, first ray. There is an ulcer on the plantar aspect of the first metatarsophalangeal joint and abnormal low signal in the distal two thirds of the shaft of the first metatarsal. The proximal phalanx of the toe is normal fat signal. There is cellulitis involving the dorsal skin and subcutaneous fat. The muscles in the plantar aspect of the foot have fatty infiltration from ischemic or neuropathic changes (denervation). *B,* STIR sagittal image, first ray. The first metatarsal is high signal, compatible with osteomyelitis. The proximal phalanx of the great toe that was normal on T1 is high signal on STIR, indicating reactive marrow edema rather than osteomyelitis. The dorsal cellulitis and the plantar denervated muscle are diffusely high signal.

edema) or from occult fractures with marrow edema, which are common in the neuropathic diabetic foot. Periosteal reaction and cortical destruction may occur with both osteomyelitis and neuropathic changes. If there is normal fatty marrow signal on all pulse sequences, one can be certain there is no osteomyelitis. If marrow signal is abnormal on *both* T1 and STIR images, it may be the result of osteomyelitis, reactive marrow edema from an adjacent soft tissue infection, or acute neuropathic changes. If there is an adjacent soft tissue ulcer or sinus tract and the abnormalities of bone occur at a pressure

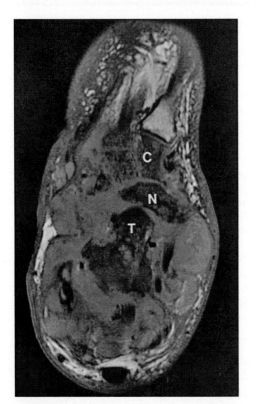

Figure 16–60. NEUROPATHIC CHANGES: Chronic.
T1 long-axis coronal image, foot. The hindfoot and midfoot of this diabetic have disorganization and fragmentation of bones with surrounding soft tissue swelling. The talus (T), navicular (N), and cuneiforms (C) are very low signal and remained low signal on T2W images. The location of abnormalities in the midfoot, no overlying ulcers at pressure points, joints being affected, and low signal on all pulse sequences are typical of chronic neuropathic changes.

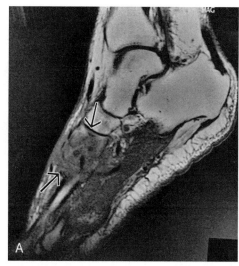
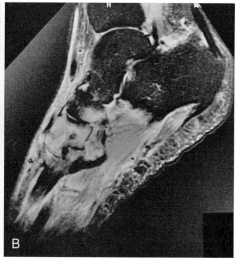

Figure 16–61. NEUROPATHIC CHANGES: Acute.
A, T1 sagittal image, foot. Intermediate signal and bone fragmentation are present in the midfoot of this diabetic patient *(arrows).* *B,* STIR sagittal image, foot. The osseous abnormalities are all high signal. Osteomyelitis could have the same MR features, but this is much more likely to be neuropathic in origin because there is no overlying ulcer or pressure point. Also, the location in the midfoot with multiple joints involved is typical of neuropathic changes.

point, the findings are almost certainly from osteomyelitis even without the presence of cortical destruction. If the T1W images are normal, but T2W or STIR images show high signal in marrow, it is almost certainly from reactive marrow edema and not osteomyelitis (Fig. 16–59).

Location of bone abnormalities in the diabetic foot are very useful for distinguishing neuropathic changes from osteomyelitis. Osteomyelitis occurs at predictable pressure points where soft tissue ulcers develop (plantar to the first and fifth metatarsal heads, calcaneal tuberosity, malleoli, and plantar aspect of distal toes). Patients with foot deformities or previous surgery may have pressure points in different locations than those just listed, so it is important to think about the biomechanics of the specific foot being evaluated in order not to make errors. Neuropathic changes generally are unrelated to soft tissue ulcers, always involve joints, and are most common at the tarsometatarsal joints.

Distinguishing neuropathic changes from osteomyelitis may be difficult with all imaging techniques, including MRI. Classically, MRI shows neuropathic changes as low signal intensity on T1W and T2W (STIR) sequences in bone marrow on both

sides of a grossly disrupted joint space (Fig. 16–60). However, aggressive and active neuropathic changes with bone fragmentation and joint destruction results in high signal intensity marrow edema and soft tissue swelling on T2W images, similar to osteomyelitis.[41] The location of the abnormal bone, the presence or absence of an overlying ulcer, joint involvement, identification of fracture lines, and so forth are the best means of differentiating osteomyelitis from neuropathic changes (Fig. 16–61). Of course, infection superimposed on a neuropathic foot is impossible to distinguish, in general, and serves to keep us humble.

The presence of joint fluid does not make the diagnosis of a septic joint by MRI, because reactive or sympathetic joint effusions are common; however, MRI aids in directing which bones or joints should be biopsied or aspirated.

MRI is valuable in demonstrating the extent of soft tissue abnormality and abscesses, and accuracy may improve with contrast administration. Cellulitis is seen as diffuse contrast enhancement, whereas abscesses show peripheral enhancement with a nonenhancing central portion that can be difficult or impossible to determine without gadolinium.

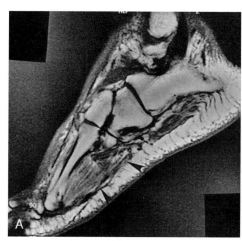
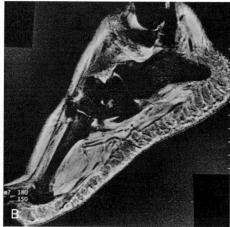

Figure 16–62. DIABETIC MUSCLE CHANGES.
A, T1 sagittal image, foot. There is fatty infiltration of the plantar muscles *(arrowheads)* from denervation or ischemia. *B,* STIR sagittal image, foot. The denervated muscle is high signal on this sequence, not to be confused with infection. There is also dorsal cellulitis that is diffusely high signal.

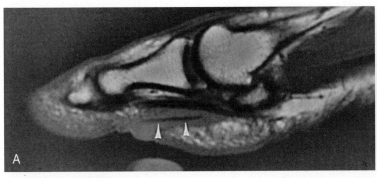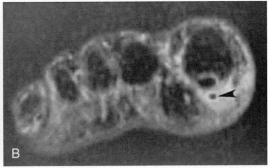

Figure 16–63. FOREIGN BODIES.
A, T1 sagittal image, great toe. A linear, low-signal structure *(arrowheads)* deep to the flexor hallucis tendon was a piece of wood at surgery. It is surrounded by intermediate signal from pus and granulation tissue. *B,* STIR short-axis axial image, forefoot. The wood foreign body *(arrowhead)* remains low signal and is surrounded by high-signal inflammatory tissue.

Other soft tissue abnormalities commonly seen in diabetics' feet include fatty replacement and edema of the muscles (high signal muscle on T1 and high signal on T2W or STIR images), as the result of neuropathic and possibly ischemic changes (Fig. 16–62). High signal on the T2W or STIR images should not be misinterpreted as pyomyositis; fatty infiltration of the atrophied muscles on T1 sequences should allow the proper diagnosis of denervation from neuropathic changes to be made. The Achilles and posterior tibial tendons frequently are partially or completely torn in diabetics, probably from ischemia from microvascular disease.

Foreign Bodies

Foreign bodies are common in the foot, because people inadvertently step on penetrating objects when barefooted. Most foreign bodies are not radioopaque and cannot be seen on radiographs. Small foreign bodies often migrate from the site of entry through the skin to a distant site.

Most foreign bodies are linear and low signal intensity on both T1W and T2W sequences (Fig. 16–63). Soft tissue edema or abscess often is seen surrounding the foreign body, reflecting the inflammatory response to it, and is high signal intensity on T2W sequences. The response to the foreign body is usually much more impressive than the foreign body, which may be easily overlooked.

References

1. Weinstable R, Stiskal M, Neuhold A, et al. Classifying calcaneal tendon injury according to MR findings. *J Bone Joint Surg [Br]* 1991; 73:683–685.
2. Chandnani VP, Bradley YC. Achilles tendon and miscellaneous tendon lesions. *Magn Reson Imaging Clin North Am* 1994; 2:89–95.
3. Dussault RG, Kaplan PA, Roederer G. MR imaging of Achilles tendon in patients with familial hyperlipidemia: comparison with plain films, physical examination and patients with traumatic tendon lesions. *AJR* 1995; 164:403–407.
4. Pavlov H, Heneghan MA, Hersh A, et al. Haglund's deformity: diagnosis and differential diagnosis of posterior heel pain. *Radiology* 1982; 144:83–87.
5. Schweitzer ME, Caccese R, Karasick D, et al. Posterior tibial tendon tears: utility of secondary signs for MR imaging diagnosis. *Radiology* 1993; 188:655–659.
6. Karasick D, Schweitzer ME. Tear of the posterior tibial tendon causing asymmetric flatfoot: radiologic findings. *AJR* 1993; 161:1237–1240.
7. Cheung Y, Rosenberg ZS, Magee T, Chinitz L. Normal anatomy and pathologic conditions of ankle tendons: current imaging techniques. *Radiographics* 1992; 12:429–444.
8. Karasick D, Schweitzer M. The os trigonum syndrome: imaging features. *AJR* 1996; 166:125–129.
9. Rosenberg ZS, Feldman F, Singson RD, et al. Peroneal tendon injury associated with calcaneal fractures: CT findings. *AJR* 1987; 149:125–129.
10. Khoury NJ, El-Khoury GY, Saltzman CL, Kathol MH. Peroneus longus and brevis tendon tears: MR imaging evaluation. *Radiology* 1996; 200:833–841.
11. Tjin A, Ton ER, Schweitzer ME, Karasick D. MR imaging of peroneal tendon disorders. *AJR* 1997; 168:135–140.
12. Schweitzer ME, Eid ME, Deely D, et al. Using MR imaging to differentiate peroneal splits from other peroneal disorders. *AJR* 1997; 168:129–133.
13. Rosenberg ZS, Beltran J, Cheung YY. MR features of longitudinal tears of the peroneus brevis tendon. *AJR* 1997; 168:141–147.
14. Dooley BJ, Kudelkapp P, Menelaus MB. Subcutaneous rupture of the tendon of tibialis anterior. *J Bone Joint Surg [Br]* 1980; 62:471–472.
15. Khoury NJ, El-Khoury GY, Saltman C, et al. Rupture of the anterior tibial tendon: diagnosis by MR imaging. *AJR* 1996; 167:351–354.
16. Erickson SJ, Smith JW, Ruiz ME, et al. MR imaging of the lateral collateral ligament of the ankle. *AJR* 1991; 1546:131–136.
17. Schneck CD, Mesgarzadeh M, Bonakdarpour A, Ross GJ. MR imaging of the most commonly injured ankle ligaments. I: Normal anatomy. *Radiology* 1992; 184:499–506.
18. Schneck CD, Mesgarzadeh M, Bonakdarpour A. MR imaging of the most commonly injured ankle ligaments. II: Ligament injuries. *Radiology* 1992; 184:507–512.
19. Klein MA. MR imaging of the ankle: normal and abnormal findings in the medial collateral ligament. *AJR* 1994; 162:377–383.
20. Rubin DA, Tishkoff NW, Britton CA, et al. Anterolateral soft-tissue impingement in the ankle: diagnosis using MR imaging. *AJR* 1997; 169:829–835.
21. Taillard W, Meyer J-M, Garcia J, Blanc Y. The sinus tarsi syndrome. *Int Orthop* 1981; 5:117–130.
22. Beltran J, Munchow AM, Khabiri H, et al. Ligaments of the lateral aspect of the ankle and sinus tarsi: an MR imaging study. *Radiology* 1990; 177:455–458.
23. Lucas P, Kaplan P, Dussault R, Hurwitz S. MRI of the foot and ankle. *Curr Probl Diagn Radiol* 1997; 26:209–268.

24. Berkowitz JF, Kier R, Rudicel S. Plantar fasciitis: MR imaging. *Radiology* 1991; 179:665–667.
25. Erickson SJ, Quinn SF, Kneeland JB, et al. MR imaging of the tarsal tunnel and related spaces: normal and abnormal findings with anatomic correlation. *AJR* 1990; 155:323–328.
26. Zanetti M, Ledermann T, Zollinger H, Hodler J. Efficacy of MR imaging in patients suspected of having Morton's neuroma. *AJR* 1997; 168:529–532.
27. Zanetti M, Strehle JK, Zollinger H, Hodler J. Morton neuroma and fluid in the intermetatarsal bursae on MR images of 70 asymptomatic volunteers. *Radiology* 1997; 203:516–520.
28. Terk MR, Kwong PK, Suthar M, et al. Morton neuroma: evaluation with MR imaging performed with contrast enhancement and fat suppression. *Radiology* 1992; 189:239–241.
29. Miller TT, Staron RB, Feldman F, et al. The symptomatic accessory tarsal navicular bone: assessment with MR imaging. *Radiology* 1995; 195:849–853.
30. Karasick D, Schweitzer ME. Disorders of the hallux sesamoid complex: MR features. *Skeletal Radiol* 1998; 27:411–418.
31. Haller J, Sartoris DJ, Resnick D, et al. Spontaneous osteonecrosis of the tarsal navicular in adults: imaging findings. *AJR* 1988; 151:355–358.
32. Wetzel LH, Levine E. Soft-tissue tumors of the foot: value of MR imaging for specific diagnosis. *AJR* 1990; 155:1025–1030.
33. Llauger J, Palmer J, Monill JM, et al. MR imaging of benign soft-tissue masses of the foot and ankle. *Radiographics* 1998; 18:1481–1498.
34. Morrison WB, Schweitzer ME, Wapner KL, Lackman RD. Plantar fibromatosis: a benign aggressive neoplasm with a characteristic appearance on MR images. *Radiology* 1994; 193:841–845.
35. Mellado JM, Rosenberg ZS, Beltran J, Colon E. The peroneocalcaneus internus muscle: MR imaging features. *AJR* 1997; 169:585–588.
36. Cheung YY, Rosenberg ZS, Ramsinghani R, et al. Peroneus quartus muscle: MR imaging features. *Radiology* 1997; 202:745–750.
37. Mellado J, Rosenberg ZS, Beltran J. Low incorporation of soleus tendon: a potential diagnostic pitfall on MR imaging. *Skeletal Radiol* 1998; 27:222–224.
38. Mizel MS, Yodlowski ML. Disorders of the lesser metatarsophalangeal joints. *JAAOS* 1995; 3:166–173.
39. Morrison WB, Schweitzer ME, Wapner KL, et al. Osteomyelitis in feet of diabetics: clinical accuracy, surgical utility and cost effectiveness of MR imaging. *Radiology* 1995; 196:557–564.
40. Yuh WT, Carson JD, Baraniewski H, et al. Osteomyelitis of the foot in diabetic patients: evaluation with plain film, TcMDP bone scintigraphy and MR imaging. *AJR* 1989; 152:795–800.
41. Beltran J, Campanini DS, Knight C. The diabetic foot: magnetic resonance imaging evaluation. *Skeletal Radiol* 1990; 19:37–41.
42. Moore TE, Yuh WTC, Kathol MH, et al. Abnormalities of the foot in patients with diabetes mellitus: findings on MR imaging. *AJR* 1991; 157:813–816.
43. Beltran J, Chandnani V, McGhee RA, et al. Gadopentetate dimeglumine enhanced MR imaging of the musculoskeletal system. *AJR* 1991; 156:457–461.
44. Craig JG, Amin MB, Wu K, et al. Osteomyelitis of the diabetic foot: MR imaging-pathologic correlation. *Radiology* 1997; 203:849–855.

FOOT AND ANKLE PROTOCOLS

This is one set of suggested protocols; there are many variations that would work equally well.

ANKLE/HINDFOOT/MIDFOOT: ROUTINE (PAIN)						
Sequence #	1	2	3	4	5	6
Sequence Type	T1	STIR	T1	T2*	T1	T2*
Orientation	Sagittal	Sagittal	Long axis axial	Long axis axial	Short axis axial	Short axis axial
Field of View (cm)	14	14	14	14	14	14
Slice Thickness (mm)	4	4	4	4	4	4
Contrast	No	No	No	No	No	No

ANKLE/HINDFOOT/MIDFOOT: INFECTION/MASS						
Sequence #	1	2	3	4	5	6
Sequence Type	T1	STIR	T1	STIR	T1 fat saturation	T1 fat saturation
Orientation	Sagittal	Sagittal	Long axis axial	Short axis axial	Long axis axial	Sagittal
Field of View (cm)	14	14	14	14	14	14
Slice Thickness (mm)	4	4	4	4	4	4
Contrast	No	No	No	No	Yes	Yes

	ENTIRE FOOT: INFECTION/MASS					
Sequence #	1	2	3	4	5	6
Sequence Type	T1	T1	STIR	STIR	T1 fat saturation	T1 fat saturation
Orientation	Long axis axial	Sagittal	Sagittal	Short axis axial	Sagittal	Long axis axial
Field of View (cm)	14	14	14	14	14	14
Slice Thickness (mm)	4	4	4	4	4	4
Contrast	No	No	No	No	Yes	Yes

	FOREFOOT/TOES: ROUTINE (PAIN)					
Sequence #	1	2	3	4	5	6
Sequence Type	T1	STIR	T1	STIR	T1	T2*
Orientation	Sagittal	Sagittal	Long axis axial	Short axis axial	Short axis axial	Short axis axial
Field of View (cm)	12	12	12	12	12	12
Slice Thickness (mm)	4	4	4	4	4	4
Contrast	No	No	No	No	No	No

	FOREFOOT/TOES: INFECTION/MASS					
Sequence #	1	2	3	4	5	6
Sequence Type	T1	T1	STIR	T1 fat saturation	T1 fat saturation	
Orientation	Sagittal	Long axis axial	Short axis axial	Sagittal	Long axis axial	
Field of View (cm)	12	12	12	12	12	
Slice Thickness (mm)	4	4	4	4	4	
Contrast	No	No	No	Yes	Yes	

	FOREFOOT/TOES: MORTON'S NEUROMA					
Sequence #	1	2	3	4	5	6
Sequence Type	T1	Turbo T2	STIR	T1 fat saturation		
Orientation	Short axis axial	Short axis axial	Long axis axial	Short axis axial		
Field of View (cm)	12	12	12	12		
Slice Thickness (mm)	4	4	4	4		
Contrast				Yes		

Setup for Ankle/Hindfoot/Midfoot

Scout		Final Image
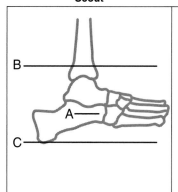	• Sagittal scout • Obtain axial images parallel to axis of calcaneus (line A) • Cover from line B to line C (bottom of calcaneus) • Obtain axial plane as first plane (most valuable) • Base of metatarsals should be included on final images	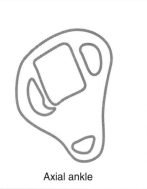 Axial ankle

Scout		Final Image
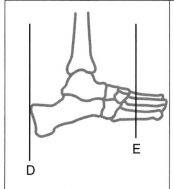	• Sagittal scout • Obtain coronal images perpendicular to axials • Cover from line D to line E to include base of metatarsals	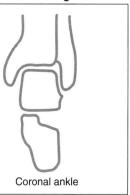 Coronal ankle

Scout		Final Image
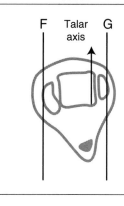	• Axial scout • Obtain sagittal images parallel to talar axis • Cover from line F to line G including malleoli • Obtain sagittals as last plane (least valuable)	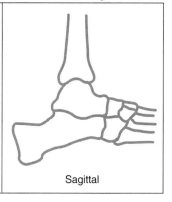 Sagittal

Setup for Entire Foot

Scout		Final Image
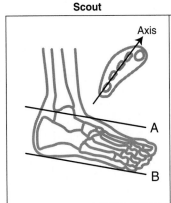	• Short axis axial scout • Obtain long axis coronal images parallel to long axis of foot • Cover from top of talus (line A) to sole of foot (line B) on sagittal scout	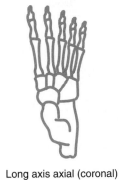 Long axis axial (coronal)

Scout		Final Image
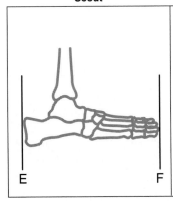	• Long axis coronal scout • Obtain sagittal images parallel to long axis of foot • Cover from line C to D	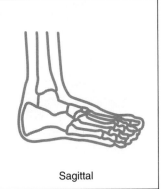 Sagittal

Scout		Final Image
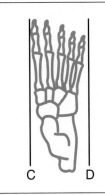	• Sagittal scout • Obtain short axis axial images perpendicular to axis of metatarsals • Cover entire foot from lines E to F	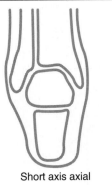 Short axis axial

Setup for Forefoot/Toes

Scout   **Final Image**

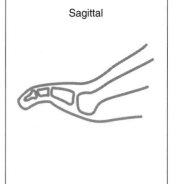

- Short axis axial scout of metatarsals
- Obtain sagittal images perpendicular to line roughly connecting metatarsals 2 through 5 (line A)
- Cover entire width of foot (lines B toC)*

Sagittal

*Include toes and proximal metatarsals in final sagittal and long axis coronal images

Scout   **Final Image**

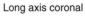
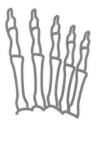

- Short axis axial scout
- Obtain long axis coronal images parallel to line roughly connecting metetarsals 2 through 5 (line A)
- Cover entire foot from lines D to E*

Long axis coronal

*Include toes and proximal metatarsals in final sagittal and long axis coronal images

Scout   **Final Image**

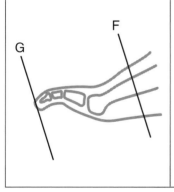
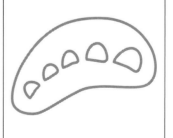

- Sagittal scout
- Obtain short axis axial images perpendicular to axis of metatarsal 2 or 3
- Cover from proximal metatarsal line F through toes (line G)
- Final image should fill the frame

Short axis axial

INDEX

Note: Page numbers in *italics* indicate figures; those followed by t indicate tables; those followed by b indicate boxed material.

A

ABC (aneurysmal bone cyst), 134–135, *136*
  of spine, 312–313
Abductor pollicis longus tendon, 258, *258*
  entrapment and tenosynovitis of, *259*, 259–260, 259b
ABER position, 197
Abscess(es), Brodie's, 107
  cortical, *104*
  epidural, 302–303, *303*, 316, 317b
  in osteomyelitis, *102*, 102–103, *104*, 106, 107, *108*
  medullary, *104*
  muscle, 78, 78b
  soft tissue, *104*
Acetabular labrum, 350–352, *352–354*, 352b
Acetabulum, 334, *335*
Achilles tendon, 395–397, 395b
  Haglund's deformity of, 397, *398*
  normal, 56, *394*, 395, *395*
  paratendinitis of, *60*
  tears of, 396, *396, 397*
  xanthomas of, *63*, 396–397, *397*
ACL. See *Anterior cruciate ligament (ACL).*
Acquired immunodeficiency syndrome (AIDS), infections with, 113
Acromioclavicular joint, anatomy of, 179, *180*
  degenerative changes of, 183, *184*
  stress-related osteolysis in, *163*
Acromiohumeral interval, *180*
Acromion, anatomy of, 179, *180*
  position of, *180*, 183
  shape of, *180–182*, 181–182
  slope of, *182*, 182–183, *183*
Acromioplasty, 209–212
Adductor muscles, metastases to, *84*
  myositis ossificans of, *75*
Adenopathy, epitrochlear, 242
Adhesive capsulitis, 212–213, *213*
AIDS (acquired immunodeficiency syndrome), infections with, 113
ALPSA lesion (anterior labroligamentous periosteal sleeve avulsion), 201b, 203, *206, 207*
Amputation neuroma, 93, *94, 95*
Amyloid, 119–121, 145
  of hip, *120, 147*, 358, *358*
Amyloidosis, 34, *34*
Anconeus epitrochlearis muscle, 233
  accessory (anomalous), *86*
Anemia, aplastic, 41, *42*
  sickle cell, reconversion from, *31, 32*
Aneurysmal bone cyst (ABC), 134–135, *136*

Aneurysmal bone cyst (ABC) *(Continued)*
  of spine, 312–313
Angiomatosis, bacillary, 113
Ankle. See *Foot and ankle.*
Ankylosing spondylitis, 303–305, *305*
Annular ligament, 228, *229*
Annulus fibrosus, anatomy of, 280, *282*
  radial tears of, 281–282, 281b, *283*
Anterior cruciate ligament (ACL), cyst of, 377, *377*
  normal, 376, *376*
  tears of, 376–378, *377–379*
    osseous contusions with, 153, 153b, *154*, 386–387, *387*
    with meniscal tear, 366–367
Anterior interosseous syndrome, *238*, 240, 240b
Anterior labroligamentous periosteal sleeve avulsion (ALPSA lesion), 201b, 203, *206, 207*
Anterior tibial tendon, *394*, 403, *404*, 404b
Aplastic anemia, 41, *42*
Apophyses, 152
Arachnoid cysts, epidural, 316–317, 317b, *318, 319*
  intradural, 322–323
Arachnoid diverticula, 317, 317b, *319*
Arachnoiditis, 303, *303, 304*
Arteriovenous malformations, 142, *144*
Arthritis, 117–124
  approach to imaging of, 117
  coils for, 117
  contrast enhancement of, 117
  due to calcium pyrophosphate dihydrate deposition, 118, *119*
  due to loose bodies, 122, *123*
  hemosiderotic, 119, *120*
  image orientation for, 117
  in amyloid, 119–121, *120*
  in gout, 117–118, *119*
  in hemophilia, 118–119, *120*
  in pigmented villonodular synovitis, 121–122, *122*
  in synovial chondromatosis, 121, *121, 122*
  of elbow, 241
  of hip and pelvis, 353–355, *355*
  of wrist and hand, 273
  positioning for, 117
  pulse sequences for, 117
  regions of interest for, 117
  rheumatoid, 117, *118*
    hypertrophied synovium in, *11*
    of elbow, 241, *241*
    of hip and pelvis, 353
  septic, *110*, 110–111, *111*
Arthrofibrosis, in Hoffa's pad, 378, *379*
Arthrography, magnetic resonance, 13–14
  of elbow, 244

Arthrography *(Continued)*
  of hip and pelvis, 359
  of shoulder, 176, 222
Articular cartilage. See *Cartilage.*
Articular meniscus, 169–170, *170, 171*
Artifact(s), blurring, 6, *8*
  magic-angle, 16, *17*, 57
    in knee, 374, *375*
    in shoulder, *177*, 178–179
  motion, 1, *2*
  susceptibility, *8, 9, 10*, 21
Astrocytomas, 325
Atrophy, marrow, serous, 51–52, *52*
  muscle, fatty, 81, *81*, 81b, *82*
    from nerve abnormalities, 215–217, *217*, 218b
Avascular necrosis (AVN), 46
  of hip and pelvis, 334–337, 335b, *336–339*, 337b, 359
  of humeral head, 218–219, *219*
  of temporomandibular joint, 173
  of wrist, 268–269, *269*, 269b, *270*
Avulsion, 153–157, *156*, 156b, *157*
  chronic, 161–163, *162, 163*
  in immature skeleton, 163–164
  of acetabular labrum, *353*
  of anterior labroligamentous periosteal sleeve, 201b, 203, *206, 207*
  of glenohumeral ligament, 200–201, 201b, *202*
  of hamstring, *347*
  of superior glenoid labrum, *207*, 207–209, *208*, 209b, *210, 211*
Axilla, soft tissue tumors of, benign, 138t
  malignant, 140t
Axillary nerve, compressive neuropathy of, 98
Axons, 89

B

Baastrup disease, 291b, 292–293, *294*
Bacillary angiomatosis, 113
Bacterial myositis, 78, *78*, 78b, 108–109
Baker's cyst, 384
Bankart lesions, 201b, 203, *205–207*
  reverse, 201b, 203, *205*
Bennett lesions, 200, 201b, *202*, 203b
Beta 2-microglobulin deposition, *120*, 121
BHAGL (bony humeral avulsion of glenohumeral ligament) lesions, 200, 201b
Biceps anchor tears, 209, *211*
Biceps femoris tendon, 381
  hematoma around, *72*
Biceps muscle, 232, *233*
Biceps tendon, dislocation of, *62*, 189, 189b, *190*

439

Biceps tendon (Continued)
impingement on, 184
longitudinal split of, 61
normal anatomy of, 56, 56, 177–178, 178, 179, 232, 233
tears of, 61, 189, 189, 189b, 233, 234
Bicipital aponeurosis, 232, 240
Bicipitoradialis bursa, 232, 242, 243
Blurring artifact, 6, 8
Body coils. See Coils.
Bone(s), anatomy of, 151–152
cortical (compact), 151
fibrous lesions of, 133–134, 135
normal appearance of, 14, 14
of elbow, 226–228, 226b, 227–229
of foot and ankle, 417–425
accessory, 417–420, 420b, 421–423
fractures of, 420–422, 422b, 423, 424
osteonecrosis of, 422, 422b, 424
tarsal coalition of, 417, 419–421
tumors of, 422–425, 425, 425b, 426
of hip and pelvis, 334–345
fractures of, 339–343, 339b, 340–344, 344b
herniation pits of, 343–344, 345
normal, 334, 335
tumors of, 344–345, 344b, 345, 346
vascular abnormalities of, 334–339, 335b, 336–340, 337b, 339b
of knee, 386–387, 387
of shoulder, abnormalities of, 217–219, 218, 219, 219b
in instability, 201–203, 201b, 203, 204
of wrist and hand, 265–270
abnormalities of, 266–270, 267–271, 267b, 269b
normal anatomy of, 265–266, 265b, 266
tumors of, 270–271, 271
pitfalls in MRI of, 15
primary lymphoma of, 134
pulse sequences for, 8, 14–15, 14b
sclerotic, 133
trabecular (cancellous), 23b, 24, 151–152
trauma to. See Osseous trauma.
tumors of. See Bone tumors.
Bone bruises. See Bone contusions.
Bone contusions, 152–153, 153, 153b, 154
of knee, 386–387, 387
of shoulder, 218
of wrist, 267, 269
Bone cyst, aneurysmal, 134–135, 136
of spine, 312–313
Bone infarct, medullary, 133, 134, 136
Bone islands, 26, 27, 135
Bone marrow. See Marrow.
Bone tumors, benign and malignant, 40
differential diagnosis of, 132–136, 132–137, 133b–135b
of foot and ankle, 422–425, 425, 425b, 426
of hip and pelvis, 344–345, 344b, 345, 346
of shoulder, 219, 219, 219b
of spine, 312–315, 314–316, 314b, 330
of wrist and hand, 270–271, 271
principles of imaging of, 122, 126
Bony humeral avulsion of glenohumeral ligament (BHAGL) lesions, 200, 201b
Bowing ratio, 263, 263
Bowstringing, 260, 261
Bowtie sign, 367, 368, 372–373, 372b
Brachial plexus, compressive neuropathy of, 98

Brachial plexus (Continued)
neuritis of, 99, 99, 217, 217, 218b
Brachialis muscle, injuries to, 232–233, 233
lymphoma of, 83
myositis ossificans of, 75
normal anatomy of, 232, 233
strain of, 69, 232–233, 233
Brachialis tendon, injuries to, 232–233, 233
normal anatomy of, 56, 56, 232, 233
Brachioradialis muscle, interstitial hemorrhage of, 72
Brodie's abscess, 107
Bruises, bone, 152–153, 153, 153b, 154
of knee, 386–387, 387
of shoulder, 218
of wrist, 267, 269
Bucket handle tear, of glenoid labrum, 207, 207, 209, 210, 211
of meniscus, 367, 368, 369
Buford complex, 197–198, 199, 200, 201b
"Bull's-eye appearance," 28
Bursa(e), bicipitoradialis, 232, 242, 243
greater trochanteric, 349, 349b, 351
iliopsoas, 349, 349b, 350, 351
interosseous, 242
medial collateral ligament, 385, 386
of elbow, 242–243, 243
of hip and pelvis, 349, 349b, 350, 351
of knee, 384–386, 385, 386
pes anserinus, 384–385, 385, 386
popliteal, 384
prepatellar, 384, 385
retrocalcaneal, 397, 398
semimembranosus-tibial collateral ligament, 385, 386
subacromial/subdeltoid, 179–181, 180
bursitis of, 184–185
tendo-Achilles (retro-Achilles), 397, 398
tibial collateral ligament, 385, 386
Bursitis, bicipitoradialis, 242, 243
greater trochanteric, 349, 351
iliopsoas, 349, 350
interosseous, 242
medial collateral ligament, 385, 386
olecranon, 234, 235, 242–243
pes anserinus, 384–385, 385, 386
prepatellar, 384, 385
retrocalcaneal, 397, 398
semimembranosus-tibial collateral ligament, 385, 386
septic, 108
subacromial/subdeltoid, 184–185
subcoracoid, 214, 215
tendo-Achilles (retro-Achilles), 397, 398
Buttocks, soft tissue tumors of, benign, 139t
malignant, 141t

C

Calcaneofibular ligament, 405b, 407, 407, 408
Calcaneus, fracture of, 155
intraosseous lipoma of, 133
tumors of, 424–425, 425, 425b
Calcific myonecrosis, 76, 76
Calcific tendinitis, 62, 64
of shoulder, 214, 214
Calcification, 133
Calcified disks, 289–290, 290
Calcium hydroxyapatite, in tendons, 62, 64

Calcium hydroxyapatite (Continued)
of shoulder, 214, 214
Calcium pyrophosphate dihydrate (CPPD) deposition, 118, 119
Capital femoral epiphysis, slipped, 342–343, 344, 344b
Capitellum, osteochondrosis of, 226
pseudodefect of, 227, 228
Capsule, of shoulder, adhesive capsulitis of, 212–213, 213
in instability, 200, 201b, 202
normal anatomy of, 194
Capsulitis, adhesive, 212–213, 213
Carpal coalition, 269, 271
Carpal instability, 266, 267b
Carpal ligaments, 248–251, 248–252, 248b
extrinsic, 251–252, 252
intrinsic, 248–251, 248–252, 248b
Carpal tunnel, 260, 262
Carpal tunnel syndrome, 91, 262–264, 262b, 263–265
Cartilage, 122–124
abnormalities of, 123, 123–124, 124
approach to imaging of, 117, 122–123
focal defects of, 15, 15
full-thickness defects of, 123, 124
normal appearance of, 15
of hip and pelvis, 352–353, 354
pitfalls in MRI of, 15
pulse sequences for, 14b, 15, 15, 16, 122–123, 124
surface irregularity of, 123
tumors of, 135–136, 135b, 136, 137
Cat-scratch disease, 242
Cavernous hemangiomas, 142, 143
CDH (congenital dislocation of the hip), 355–357, 356, 356b
Cellulitis, 78, 79, 79, 108, 108b, 109
in diabetes, 114, 114
vs. necrotizing fasciitis, 110, 110
Central canal stenosis, 294–296, 295, 296
Central cord syndrome, 311, 312
Chemical fat saturation, 9–12, 11, 12
Chemotherapy, effect on muscle of, 85–87
marrow depletion due to, 41–43, 42, 43, 43b
tumor after, 129
Children, osteomyelitis in, 102, 103, 104, 105
Chondroblastoma, 132
of hip, 344, 346
Chondrocalcinosis, 118, 119
Chondroma, osteo-, 91, 136, 137
Chondromatosis, synovial, 121, 121, 122
of elbow, 241, 242
of hip, 357, 357–358
Chondrosarcoma, 128, 136
myxoid, 148
of hip and pelvis, 344
Chordomas, 315, 316
Clavicle, osteolysis of, 217–218, 218
Climber's elbow, 232–233, 233
Cloaca, in osteomyelitis, 102, 102, 102b, 106, 107, 108
Coils, 3, 4, 20
for arthritis and cartilage imaging, 117
for elbow imaging, 225
for foot and ankle imaging, 393
for hip and pelvis imaging, 333
for infection imaging, 101
for knee imaging, 363
for marrow imaging, 23
for muscle imaging, 65
for osseous trauma imaging, 151
for peripheral nerve imaging, 89

Coils (Continued)
for shoulder imaging, 175
for spine imaging, 279
for temporomandibular joint imaging, 169
for tendon imaging, 55
for tumor imaging, 130–131
for wrist and hand imaging, 247
Compartment syndromes, 76, 76b
acute, 76, 76, 76b
chronic, 76, 76, 76b
exertional, 76, 76b, 77
traumatic, 76, 76, 76b
Compression fracture, vertebral, 39–40, 40b, 41, 159, 160
Compressive myelopathy, disk-related, 288, 288
Compressive neuropathy, in carpal tunnel syndrome, 262–264, 262b, 263–265
of axillary nerve, 98
of lateral femoral cutaneous nerve, 99
of median nerve, 98
at elbow, 239–240, 240b
at wrist, 262–264, 262b, 263–265
of posterior tibial nerve, 91, 99
of radial nerve, 98, 240–241, 240b
of sciatic nerve, 99
of spinoglenoid notch, 214, 216
of suprascapular nerve, 98, 214–215, 214b, 216
of ulnar nerve, 98, 98–99
at elbow, 238–239, 238b, 239
at wrist, 264, 265
Computed tomography (CT), vs. MRI, 3–4
Congenital dislocation of hip (CDH), 355–357, 356, 356b
Contrast enhancement, 4, 12–13, 20
chemical fat saturation and, 11
indications for, 12–13, 12b, 13
of elbow, 225–226
of fibrocartilage, 15, 16
of foot and ankle, 394
of hips and pelvis, 333–334
of infection, 101
of marrow, 23
of muscle abscess, 78, 78b
of myeloma, 37
of peripheral nerves, 89
of shoulder, 175–176
of spine, 13, 280
of synovium, 18, 19
of tumors, 131, 132
of wrist and hand, 248
Contusions, bone, 152–153, 153, 153b, 154
of knee, 386–387, 387
of shoulder, 218
of wrist, 267, 269
muscle, 71b
Conversion, from red to yellow marrow, 24–25, 24b, 25, 25b
Coracoacromial arch, normal anatomy of, 179, 179–181, 180
posttraumatic deformity of, 183
Coracoacromial ligament, anatomy of, 179, 179, 180
thickening of, 183, 184
Coracohumeral ligament, 176
Cortical abscess, 104
CPPD (calcium pyrophosphate dihydrate) deposition, 118, 119
Critical zone, 178
Cross talk, 2, 20
CT (computed tomography), vs. MRI, 3–4
Cubital tunnel, 238, 239
Cubital tunnel syndrome, 238–239, 238b, 239

Cyclops lesion, 378, 379
Cyst(s), 146, 147
aneurysmal bone, 134–135, 136
of spine, 312–313
anterior cruciate ligament, 377, 377
arachnoid, epidural, 316–317, 317b, 318, 319
intradural, 322–323
Baker's, 384
contrast enhancement of, 12–13, 13
degenerative osseous, 184
dermoid, 322
epidermoid, 322
epidural, 316–318, 317b, 318–320
ganglion, 97, 98, 98, 147
intraosseous, of foot and ankle, 425, 426
of wrist and hand, 270–271, 271
suprascapular nerve entrapment from, 214, 216
tarsal tunnel syndrome from, 414, 416
intradural, 320b, 322–323
meniscal, 369–371, 371
paralabral, acetabular, 350, 354
glenoid, 209, 210
perineural (Tarlov), 317, 317b, 320
spinal cord, 323–324, 323b, 324, 324b, 325
subchondral, of hip and pelvis, 344
of talus, 425, 426
synovial, of shoulder, 213, 213
of spine, 292, 294, 316, 317b
of wrist and hand, 273, 274
pisotriquetral, 273, 274
Cystic-appearing masses, 146–148, 146b, 147–149

D

DDH (developmental dysplasia of hip), 355–357, 356, 356b
De Quervain syndrome, 259, 259–260, 259b
Degeneration, of acromioclavicular joint, 183, 184
of hips, 355, 355
of intervertebral disks, 280–293, 281b
compressive myelopathy due to, 288, 288
epidural hematoma due to, 288, 289
marrow with, 28
osseous changes due to, 291–293, 291b, 292–294
protocols for imaging of, 328–329
recurrent, 300–301, 301
vertebral bodies in, 289, 290
of knee, 365, 367
of rotator cuff, 185, 185, 185b
of spine, 291–293, 291b, 292–294
of tendons, 57–58, 58
quadriceps, 58
supraspinatus, 185, 185, 185b
Delayed-onset muscle soreness (DOMS), 66, 67
Deltoid ligament, 404–405, 405
Deltoid muscle, atrophy of, 215–217
Deltoid tendon, normal anatomy of, 177, 177
Demyelination, of spinal cord, 323, 323b, 324b
Denervation, of muscle, 80–81, 81, 81b, 82
Dermatomyositis, 80
Dermoid cysts, 322

Desmoid, of hip, 349–350, 352b
Developmental dysplasia of hip (DDH), 355–357, 356, 356b
Diabetes, foot disease in, 113–115, 113b, 114, 115b, 429–432, 429b, 430, 431
muscle infarction in, 85, 85b, 86
Diastematomyelia, 327, 327
DISI (dorsal intercalated segmental instability), 250–251, 251, 266
Disk(s), intervertebral, annular tears of, 281–282, 281b, 283
bulging, 283, 284, 284b, 285
calcified, 289–290, 290
contour abnormalities of, 282–288
location of, 285–287, 287, 287b
mimickers of, 288, 289, 289b
significance of, 287–288, 288b
types of, 282–285, 284–287, 284b
degeneration of, 280–293, 281b
compressive myelopathy due to, 288, 288
epidural hematoma due to, 288, 289
marrow with, 28
osseous changes due to, 291–293, 291b, 292–294
protocols for imaging of, 328–329
recurrent, 300–301, 301
vertebral bodies in, 289, 290
extrusion of, 283–284, 284, 284b, 286
herniation of, 282, 284b
intraosseous, 306, 307, 308
normal, 280–281, 282
nuclear abnormalities of, 281, 282
postoperative changes in, 299, 300
protrusion of, 283, 284, 284b, 285
sequestered, 284, 284–285, 284b, 287
trauma to, 309, 310
vacuum, 288–289, 290
temporomandibular, 169–170, 170, 171
Disko-osteophytic material, 291
Dislocation, of hip, congenital, 355–357, 356, 356b
of tendon, 62, 62, 62b
biceps, 189, 189b, 190
peroneus, 401–403, 404
patellar, 382–383, 383
osseous contusions with, 153, 154
Disruption. See Tears.
Distal radioulnar joint (DRUJ), 255, 255, 258
Diverticula, arachnoid, 317, 317b, 319
DOMS (delayed-onset muscle soreness), 66, 67
Dorsal intercalated segmental instability (DISI), 250–251, 251, 266
Double posterior cruciate ligament (PCL) sign, 367, 369
Double-line sign, 48, 48
DRUJ (distal radioulnar joint), 255, 255, 258
Duchenne's muscular dystrophy, 80
Dystrophies, 80

E

Echo, 20
Echo time (TE), 4–8, 5b, 21
Echo train, 20
Echo train length (ETL), 5b, 6, 20
ECU (extensor carpi ulnaris) sheath, 255–256, 256, 257
ECU (extensor carpi ulnaris) tendon, dislocation of, 62

ECU (extensor carpi ulnaris) tendon
(Continued)
tenosynovitis or partial tears of, 260,
260
Edema, marrow, 44, 44, 45
epiphyseal, 164, 164b
in osteomyelitis, 106, 107, 108
transient painful, 337–339, 339b, 340
with osteoid osteoma, 132, 132
muscle, 67
neurogenic, from anterior interosseous
nerve syndrome, 238
soft tissue, in osteomyelitis, 106
Elastofibromas, of shoulder, 219–220, 220
Elbow, 225–243
approach to imaging of, 225–226, 226b
arthrography of, 244
articular disorders of, 241, 241, 242
avulsion injuries of, 156, 156b
bones of, 226–228, 226b, 227–229
bursae of, 242–243, 243
climber's, 232–233, 233
coils for, 225
contrast enhancement of, 225–226
epicondylitis of, lateral, 230, 231, 236–
237, 237, 237b, 238
medial, 235–236, 235b, 236
epitrochlear adenopathy of, 242
fractures of, 227–228, 229
golfer's, 235–236, 235b, 236
image orientation for, 225, 226b
ligaments of, 228–232
radial collateral, 228–230, 229–231,
229b
ulnar collateral, 230–232, 230b, 231,
232
Little Leaguer's, 156, 235–236, 235b,
236
loose bodies in, 227, 228, 241, 241, 242
masses of, 241
muscles and tendons of, 232–237, 232b
anterior compartment, 232–233,
232b, 233, 234
lateral compartment, 236–237, 236–
238, 237b
medial compartment, 235, 235–236,
235b, 236
posterior compartment, 233–234,
234, 235
nerves of, 237–241
approach to imaging of, 237–238,
237b, 238
median, 239–240, 240b
radial, 240–241, 240b
ulnar, 238–239, 238b, 239
osteoarthritis of, 241
osteochondritis dissecans of, 226–227,
226b, 227
Panner's disease of, 226, 226b
pigmented villonodular synovitis of,
241, 242
positioning for imaging of, 225
protocols for imaging of, 244–245
pulse sequences for, 225
regions of interest for, 225
rheumatoid arthritis of, 241, 241
synovial osteochondromatosis of, 241,
242
tennis, 236–237, 237, 237b, 238
medial, 235–236, 235b, 236
with radial collateral ligament tear,
230, 231
Enchondroma(s), 135–136, 136
of hand, 270
of hip, 344, 345
of humerus, 201, 219

Endoneurium, 89, 90
Enneking staging system, 125, 126b
Enostosis, 135
Entrapment, of abductor pollicis longus
and extensor pollicis brevis tendons,
259, 259–260, 259b
of median nerve, 98, 239–240, 240b
of posterior tibial nerve, 91, 99
of radial nerve, 98, 240–241, 240b
of suprascapular nerve, 98, 214–215,
214b, 216
of ulnar nerve, 98, 98–99
at elbow, 238–239, 238b, 239
at wrist, 264, 265
Ependymomas, 320, 320b, 325, 326
Epicondylitis, lateral, 236–237, 237,
237b, 238
with radial collateral ligament tear,
230, 231
medial, 235–236, 235b, 236
Epidermoid cysts, 322
Epidural abscess, 302–303, 303, 316,
317b
Epidural cysts, 316–318, 317b, 318–320
Epidural fibrosis, 298, 300, 300–301, 301
Epidural hematoma, 316, 317b
from disk degeneration, 288, 289
from spinal surgery, 300, 301
from trauma, 309, 311
spontaneous, 288, 289, 316
Epidural lipomatosis, 316, 317b, 318
Epidural scarring, 298, 300, 300–301, 301
Epidural space, abnormalities of,
316–318, 317b, 318–320
postoperative changes of, 298, 299b,
300
Epineurium, 89, 90
Epiphyseal marrow edema, 164, 164b
Epiphyses, 152
Epiphysiolysis, 163, 163
Epitrochlear adenopathy, 242
Erlenmeyer flask deformities, 49
ETL (echo train length), 5b, 6, 20
Exertional compartment syndrome, 76,
76b, 77
Extensor carpi ulnaris (ECU) sheath,
255–256, 256, 257
Extensor carpi ulnaris (ECU) tendon,
dislocation of, 62
tenosynovitis or partial tears of, 260,
260
Extensor digitorum manus brevis, 273,
273
Extensor tendons, of ankle, 394
of elbow, 236–237, 237, 237b, 238
of wrist and hand, 258–260, 258–261,
259b
Extrinsic ligaments, of wrist, 251–252,
252

F

Facet joints, degenerative changes of,
291–292, 291b, 293, 294
Fascial herniation, of muscle, 76–77, 77
Fascicles, 90, 90, 91, 91
Fascicular pattern, 90, 90
Fasciitis, necrotizing, 78–79, 78b, 79,
109–110, 110, 110b
plantar, 410–413, 411b, 413, 414
Fast spin echo (FSE) imaging, 6, 20
conventional vs., 6, 7
of bone, 14, 15
parameters for, 5b
pitfalls of, 6, 7, 8

Fast spin echo (FSE) imaging (Continued)
strengths and weakness of, 5b
susceptibility effects in, 10
Fat, in red marrow, 28, 28–29, 29b
Fat saturation, 9–12, 20
for cartilage imaging, 15
for knee imaging, 364, 364–365
for synovial imaging, 18, 19
frequency-selective, 9–12, 11, 12
with STIR, 12
Fat suppression. See Fat saturation.
Fatigue fractures, 159–161, 160, 160b,
161
of femoral neck, 161, 341
of foot and ankle, 422, 424
of hip and pelvis, 339, 339b, 340, 341
vs. tumors, 164, 165
Fatty atrophy, of muscle, 81, 81, 81b, 82
Femoral head, normal anatomy of, 334,
335
osteonecrosis of, 334–337, 335b, 336–
339, 337b
Femoral neck, herniation pits of, 338,
343–344, 345
insufficiency fracture of, 342
stress fracture of, 161, 341
Femur, avulsion injuries of, 155–156,
156b
Erlenmeyer flask deformities of, 49
Fibrocartilage, normal appearance of, 15
pitfalls in MRI of, 15
pulse sequences for, 14b, 15, 16
Fibrolipoma, filum terminale, 320–322,
322
Fibrolipomatous hamartoma, 95–97, 97
of median nerve, 264–265, 266
of sciatic nerve, 349, 349
Fibroma, xantho- (nonossifying), 134
Fibromatosis, 147
plantar, 425–426, 427
Fibrous cortical defect, 134
Fibrous dysplasia, 134, 135
Fibrous histiocytoma, malignant, of hip
and pelvis, 350, 352b
Fibrous lesions, of bone, 133–134, 135
of soft tissue, 145, 147
Fibula, tumors of, 424, 425b
Fibular head, avulsion fracture of, 156
Fibulocollateral ligament, 381, 382
Field of view, 1–2, 20
Filum terminale fibrolipoma, 320–322,
322
Finger(s), glomus tumors of, 272, 273
mallet, 261
tendon abnormalities of, 260, 261
Fistula, in osteomyelitis, 102, 102b
Flexor carpi ulnaris muscle, denervation
of, 81
Flexor digitorum longus tendon, 394, 398
Flexor digitorum profundus muscle,
denervation of, 81
Flexor hallucis longus muscle, strain of,
69
Flexor hallucis longus tendon, normal
anatomy of, 394, 399
tears of, 60, 399, 400
tenosynovitis of, 58, 58, 59, 399–400,
400, 400b, 401
Flexor retinaculum, in carpal tunnel
syndrome, 263, 263–265, 264
normal anatomy of, 260, 262
Flexor tendons, of wrist, bowstringing of,
260, 261
tenosynovitis of, 260
Flip angle, 5b, 8
Fluid signal intensity, 4, 7
Fluid/fluid levels, 134–135, 136

Foot and ankle, 393–437
    accessory muscles of, *403*, 426–427, *428*
    accessory ossicles of, 417–420, 420b, *421–423*
    approach to imaging of, 393–394
    avulsion injuries of, 156, 156b
    bone abnormalities of, 417–425
    coils for, 393
    contrast enhancement of, 394
    diabetic, 113–115, 113b, *114*, 115b, 429–432, 429b, *430*, *431*
    foreign bodies in, 432, *432*
    fractures of, 420–422, 422b, *423, 424*
    image orientation for, 393, 394b
    impingement syndrome of, anterolateral, 407–408, 408b, *410, 411*
        posterior, *400, 406*, 417–419, 420b, *421*
    infection of, 433, 434
    inflammatory conditions of, 407–413
    ligaments of, 403–407
        lateral, 405–407, 405b, *406–408*
        medial, 404–405, *405*
    mass of, 433, 434
    Morton's neuroma of, 415–417, 417b, *418, 419*, 434
    nerve abnormalities of, 413–417
    neuropathic changes in, 429b, *430*, 431, *431*
    os trigonum syndrome of, *400, 406*, 417–419, 420b, *421*
    osteochondritis dissecans of, 420–422, 422b, *423*
    osteomyelitis of, 429–430, 429b, *430*
    osteonecrosis of, 422, 422b, *424*
    pain in, 423, 434
    plantar fasciitis of, 410–413, 411b, *413, 414*
    positioning for imaging of, 393
    pressure lesions of, 427–429, *428*, 429b
    protocols for imaging of, 433–437
    pulse sequences for, 393–394
    regions of interest for, 393–394
    sinus tarsi syndrome of, 408–410, 410b, *411–413*
    sprains of, 407
    tarsal coalition of, 417, *419–421*
    tarsal tunnel syndrome of, 413–415, *415–417*, 415b
    tendon(s) of, *394*, 394–403
        Achilles, *394*, 395–397, *395–398*, 395b
        anterior, 403, *404*, 404b
        anterior tibial, *394*, 403, *404*, 404b
        extensor digitorum longus, *394*
        extensor hallucis longus, *394*
        flexor digitorum longus, *394*, 398
        flexor hallucis longus, *394*, 399–400, *400*, 400b, *401*
        lateral, 400–403, 401b, *402–404*
        medial, 397–400, 398b, *399, 400*, 400b
        peroneal, *394*, 400–403, 401b, *402–404*
        plantaris, *394*, 395, *396*
        posterior, 395–397, *395–398*, 395b
        posterior tibial, *394*, 398, 398b, *399*
    tumors of, osseous, 422–425, *425*, 425b, *426*
        soft tissue, 138t, 140t, 425–429, 426b, *427, 428*
Foramen, sublabral, 197, 198–199, *199*
Foraminal stenosis, 296–297, *297–299*
Foreign bodies, in foot, 432, *432*
    infections due to, 111, *112*

Fovea centralis, 334, 337, *338*
Fracture(s), avulsion, 153–157, *156*, 156b, *157*, 163–164
    Bankart, 201b, 203, *205–207*
        reverse, 201b, 203, *205*
    Hill-Sachs, 201–203, 201b, *204*
    insufficiency, 157–159, *158–160*, 159b
        of hip and pelvis, 339–342, 339b, *342, 343*
    microtrabecular, 152–153, *153*, 153b, *154*
    of elbow, 227–228, *229*
    of foot and ankle, 420–422, 422b, *423, 424*
    of hip and pelvis, 339–343, 339b
        fatigue (stress), 339, 339b, *340, 341*
        insufficiency, 339–342, 339b, *342, 343*
        intertrochanteric, *155*
        protocol for imaging of, 359
        Salter, 339b, 342–343, *344*, 344b
    of olecranon, 228
    of scaphoid, 267, *268*
    of shoulder, 218, *218*
    of spine, 307, *308*
        anterior inferior iliac, *156*
        in spondylolysis, 305–306, 305b, *306, 307*
        vertebral compression, 159, *160*
            osteoporotic vs. pathologic, 39–40, 40b, *41*
    of wrist, 267, *268*
    osteochondral, 164–165, 165b, *166*
        of elbow, 226–227, 226b, *227*
        of foot and ankle, 420–422, 422b, *423*
    pathologic, with Paget's disease, *134*
    radial head, *229*
    radiographically occult, 153, *155*
        of elbow, 227–228, *229*
        of shoulder, 218, *218*
        of wrist, 267, *268*
    Salter, of hip and pelvis, 339b, 342–343, *344*, 344b
    stress (fatigue), 132, 157–161, *158–161*, 158b–161b
        of femoral neck, *161*, 341
        of foot and ankle, 422, *424*
        of hip and pelvis, 339, 339b, *340, 341*
        of tibia, *160*
        vs. tumor, 164, *165*
    supraacetabular, 158, *159*
        insufficiency, 342, *343*
    vertebral compression, 159, *160*
        osteoporotic vs. pathologic, 39–40, 40b, *41*
Freiberg's infraction, 422, *424*
Frequency-selective fat saturation, 9–12, *11, 12*
Frozen shoulder, 212–213, *213*
FSE imaging. See *Fast spin echo (FSE) imaging.*

G

Gadolinium-DTPA (Gd-DTPA) enhancement. See *Contrast enhancement.*
Gamekeeper's thumb, 256–258, *257*, 276
Gammopathies, monoclonal, aggressive, 32, *34–36*, 34–37, 36b
    nonmyelomatous, 32–34
Ganglion cyst(s), 97, 98, *98*, 147
    intraosseous, of foot and ankle, 425, *426*

Ganglion cyst(s) *(Continued)*
    of wrist and hand, 270–271, *271*
    suprascapular nerve entrapment from, 214, *216*
    tarsal tunnel syndrome from, 414, *416*
Gap, 2, 20
Gastrocnemius muscle, exertional compartment syndrome of, *77*
    necrotizing fasciitis of, *79*
Gaucher disease, 48, *49*
Gd-DTPA enhancement. See *Contrast enhancement.*
Gelatinous transformation, 51–52, *52*
Geographic serpentine lines, 46–48, *47*
Giant cell tumor, of patellofemoral compartment, *129*
    of pelvis, 344
    of spine, 313
    of tendon sheath, 62, *64*, 143–145
    of wrist and hand, 272, *272*
GLAD lesions (glenolabral articular disruption), 201b, *207*, 209, *212*
Glenohumeral instability, 193–207, 194b
    anatomic, 194
    anatomy relating to, 194–200
    and impingement, 183
    anterior, 194
    bones in, 201–203, 201b, *203, 204*
    capsule in, 200, 201b, *202*
    defined, 193
    due to ALPSA lesions, 201b, 203, *206, 207*
    due to Bankart lesions, 201b, 203, *205–207*
    due to Bennett lesions, 200, 201b, *202*, 203b
    due to BHAGL lesions, 200, 201b
    due to GLAD lesions, 201b, *207*, 209, *212*
    due to HAGL lesions, 200, 201, 201b, *202*
    due to Hill-Sachs lesions, 201–203, 201b, *204*
    due to SLAP lesions, 201b, *207*, 207–209, *208*, 209b, *210, 211*
    factors in, 194
    functional, 194
    glenohumeral ligaments in, 200–201, *202*
    labrum in, 203–207, *206, 207*
    lesions associated with, 200–207, 201b
    multidirectional, 194
    posterior, 194
    superior, 194
    surgery for, 212
    tendons in, 201b
    types of, 194
Glenohumeral labroligamentous complex, 195–197
Glenohumeral ligaments, humeral avulsion of, 200–201, 201b, *202*
    normal anatomy of, 194–197, *195*, 195b, *196*
Glenoid labrum, ALPSA lesions of, 201b, 203, *206, 207*
    Bankart lesions of, 201b, 203, *205–207*
        reverse, 201b, 203, *205*
    bucket handle tear of, 207, *207*, 209, *210, 211*
    Buford complex of, 197–198, *199, 200*, 201b
    cysts of, 209, *210*
    detached, 207, *207*, 208, *208*
    GLAD lesions of, 201b, *207*, 209, *212*
    in instability, 201b, 203–207, *206, 207*
    noninstability lesions of, *207*, 207–209, 207b, *208*, 209b, *210–212*

Glenoid labrum *(Continued)*
normal anatomy of, 197–200, *197–200,*
197b
partial thickness tear of, 207, *207,* 208–
209, *210*
pulse sequences for, 14b, 15, *16*
SLAP lesions of, 207–209
classification of, 207, *207,* 209b
defined, 201b, 207
normal, 207, *207,* 208
sublabral foramen vs., 197b
with biceps anchor tear, 209, *211*
with bucket handle tear, 207, *207,*
209, *210, 211*
with detached labrum, 207, *207,* 208,
208
with partial thickness tear, 207, *207,*
208–209, *210*
Glenolabral articular disruption (GLAD
lesion), 201b, *207,* 209, *212*
Glomus tumors, of fingers, 272, *273*
Gluteus medius tendon, 347, *348, 351*
Golfer's elbow, 235–236, 235b, *236*
Gout, 117–118, *119*
affecting tendons, 62, *63*
olecranon bursitis in, 242
pseudo-, 118, *119*
tophi in, *63,* 117–118, *119,* 145
Gracilis muscle, pyomyositis of, *78*
Gradient echo (GRE, T2*) imaging, 8–9,
20
of articular cartilage, 15
of bone, *8,* 14–15
of fibrocartilage, *16*
of synovium, 18, *19*
of tendons, *17*
parameters for, 5b
STIR vs., *8*
strengths and weaknesses of, 5b
susceptibility effects in, 9, *10*
Gradient-recalled acquisition–steady state
(GRASS sequence), for cartilage, 124,
124
Grading, of tumors, 125, 126b
Granulocyte colony-stimulating factor, 43
Granulocyte-macrophage colony-
stimulating factor, 43
GRE imaging. See *Gradient echo (GRE,
T2*) imaging.*
Greater trochanteric bursa, 349, 349b, *351*
Groin, soft tissue tumors of, benign, 139t
malignant, 141t
Growthplate, 152
avulsion fractures of, 163–164
physeal bridges of, 163, *164*
traumatic injury of, 163, *163*
Guyon's canal, 264, *265*

H

HAGL (humeral avulsion of
glenohumeral ligament) lesion, 200,
201, 201b, *202*
Haglund's deformity, 397, *398*
Hallux sesamoids, 419–420, *423*
Halo signs, 37, 37b, *39*
Hamartoma, fibrolipomatous, 95–97, *97*
of median nerve, 264–265, *266*
of sciatic nerve, 349, *349*
Hamstring muscles, 346–347, *347*
strain of, *68, 70*
Hamstring tendon, 346–347, *347*
hematoma around, *73*
Hand. See *Wrist and hand.*
Head, soft tissue tumors of, benign, 139t

Head *(Continued)*
malignant, 141t
Hemangioblastomas, 325
Hemangioma(s), cavernous, 142, *143*
intramuscular, 82, *82*
intraosseous, 133, *133*
of spine, 312, 313–314, *314*
marrow with, *28*
soft tissue, 142, *143*
spinal, 312, 313–314, *314*
tarsal tunnel syndrome from, *417*
Hematoma(s), 71–74, 71b, *72–74,*
142–143, *144*
around biceps femoris tendon, *72*
around hamstring tendon, *73*
epidural, 316, 317b
from disk degeneration, 288, *289*
from spinal surgery, 300, *301*
from trauma, 309, *311*
spontaneous, 288, *289,* 316
of muscle, 71–74, 71b, *72–74*
Hematomyelia, 310–311, *312,* 313b, 323,
323b
Hematopoiesis, increased demand for, 31
Hematopoietic growth factors, 43, *43*
Hemophilia, 118–119, *120*
Hemorrhage, in spinal cord, 310–311,
312, 313b, 323, 323b
muscle, into tumor, 73, *74*
intraparenchymal or interstitial, 70–
71, *72*
Hemorrhagic tumor, 142, *145*
Hemosiderin deposition, 51, *51,* 51b
in hemophilia, 119, *120*
in pigmented villonodular synovitis,
121–122, *122*
Hemosiderotic arthritis, 119, *120*
Herniated nucleus pulposus (HNP), 282
Herniation, disk, 282, 284b
intraosseous, 306, *307, 308*
muscle, 76–77, *77*
Herniation pits, *338,* 343–344, *345*
High-intensity zones, 281b, 282, *283*
Hill-Sachs lesions, 201–203, 201b, *204*
Hip(s) and pelvis, 333–358
approach to imaging of, 333–334, 334b
arthritis of, 353–355, *355*
articular cartilage of, 352–353, *354*
avascular necrosis of, 334–337, 335b,
336–339, 337b, 359
avulsion injuries of, 155, *156,* 156b
bursae of, 349, 349b, *350, 351*
coils for, 333
contrast enhancement of, 333–334
degenerative joint disease of, 355, *355*
developmental dysplasia of, 355–357,
356, 356b
fracture(s) of, 339–343, 339b
fatigue (stress), 339, 339b, *340, 341*
insufficiency, 339–342, 339b, *342,*
343
intertrochanteric, *155*
protocol for imaging of, 359
Salter, 339b, 342–343, *344,* 344b
herniation pits of, *338,* 343–344, *345*
idiopathic transient osteoporosis of,
44–45, *45,* 164, 337–339, 339b, *340*
image orientation for, 333, 334b
labrum of, 350–352, *352–354,* 352b
Legg-Calvé-Perthes disease of, 337,
337b, *338, 339*
ligamentum teres of, 350
muscle and tendon abnormalities of,
345–348, 346b, *347, 348*
nerves of, 348–349, *349*
normal anatomy of, 334, *335*

Hip(s) and pelvis *(Continued)*
osseous structures of, 334–345
fractures of, 339–343, 339b, *340–344,*
344b
herniation pits of, *338,* 343–344, *345*
normal, 334, *335*
tumors of, 344–345, 344b, *345, 346*
vascular abnormalities of, 334–339,
335b, *336–340,* 337b, 339b
osteonecrosis of, 334–337, 335b, *336–*
339, 337b, 359
positioning for imaging of, 333
pulse sequences for, 333
regions of interest for, 333
slipped capital femoral epiphysis of,
342–343, *344,* 344b
tumors of, intraarticular, *357,* 357–358,
357b, *358*
osseous, 344–345, 344b, *345, 346*
soft tissue, 139t, 141t, 349–350, 352b
Histiocytoma, malignant fibrous, of hip
and pelvis, 350, 352b
HIV (human immunodeficiency virus),
infections with, 113
HNP (herniated nucleus pulposus), 282
Hodgkin's lymphoma, 39
Hoffa's pad, arthrofibrosis in, 378, *379*
Human immunodeficiency virus (HIV),
infections with, 113
Humeral avulsion of glenohumeral
ligament (HAGL) lesion, 200, 201,
201b, *202*
Humeral head, avascular necrosis of,
218–219, *219*
Humerus, avulsion injuries of, 156, 156b
chronic, *162*
enchondroma of, *201, 219*
Hydrosyringomyelia, 323, 323b
Hydroxyapatite crystals, in tendons, 62,
64
Hyperemia, marrow, 44–45, *44–46,* 44b

I

Idiopathic inflammatory polymyopathies,
79–80, *80*
Idiopathic transient osteoporosis of hip
(ITOH), 44–45, *45,* 164, 337–339,
339b, *340*
Iliofemoral ligament, 345
Iliopsoas bursa, 349, 349b, *350, 351*
Iliopsoas tendon, 352, *352*
Iliotibial band (ITB) friction syndrome,
381–382, *383*
Image noise, 1, *2,* 20
Image orientation, for arthritis and
cartilage, 117
for elbow, 225, 226b
for foot and ankle, 393, 394b
for hips and pelvis, 333, 334b
for infection, 101
for marrow, 23
for muscle, 65
for osseous trauma, 151
for peripheral nerves, 89
for shoulder, 175, 176b
for spine, 279, 280b
for temporomandibular joint, 169
for tendons, 55
for tumors, 131
for wrist and hand, 247, 248b
Imaging matrix, 1, *3,* 20
Impaction injuries, 152–153, *153–155,*
153b
Impingement, ankle, anterolateral,
407–408, 408b, *410, 411*

Impingement *(Continued)*
  posterior, *400, 406,* 417–419, 420b, *421*
  shoulder, 181–185
    causes of, 181–183, *181–184,* 181b
    defined, 181
    effects of, 181b, 183–184, 184b
    instability and, 183
    posterosuperior, 190–191, 190b, *191*
    subcoracoid, 191, *192*
    surgery for, 209–212
    symptoms of, 181b
Infants, developmental dysplasia of hip in, 355–357, *356,* 356b
  osteomyelitis in, 102, 104
Infarction, bone marrow, 32b, 46–48, 46b, *47, 48*
  medullary bone, 133, *134,* 136
  muscle, 85, 85b, *86*
  spinal cord, 323b, 324–325, 324b, *325*
Infection(s), 101–115
  approach to imaging of, 101, 101b
  cellulitis as, 78, 79, *79,* 108, 108b, *109*
  in diabetes, 114, *114*
  coils for, 101
  contrast enhancement for, 13, 101
  due to foreign bodies, 111, *112*
  image orientation for, 101
  myositis due to, 78, *78,* 78b, 108–109
  necrotizing fasciitis as, 78–79, 78b, *79,* 109–110, *110,* 110b
  of foot and ankle, 415, *416*
    diabetic, 113–115, 113b, *114,* 115b, 429–430, 429b, *430*
  of muscle, *78,* 78–79, 78b, *79*
  of spine, 301–303, 301b, *302, 303,* 330
  of wrist and hand, 273–274, *274,* 276
  osteomyelitis as, 101–108
    abscess/phlegmon in, *102,* 102–103, *104,* 106, 107, *108*
    acute, 105–107, *107*
    adult pattern of, 104–105
    childhood pattern of, 104, *105*
    chronic, 107–108, *108*
    chronic recurrent multifocal, 113
    cloaca in, 102, *102,* 102b, 106, 107, *108*
    contiguous spread of, 103b, 105, *105*
    direct implantation of, 103b, 105, *106*
    fistula in, 102, 102b
    hematogenous seeding of, 103–105, 103b, *105*
    in AIDS, 113
    in diabetes, *114,* 114–115, 115b, 429–430, 429b, *430*
    infantile pattern of, 104
    involucrum in, 102, *102,* 102b, *103*
    joint effusion in, 107, *108*
    marrow edema in, 106, *107, 108*
    MRI findings in, 106b
    routes of contamination for, 103–105, 103b, *105, 106*
    sequestrum in, 101–102, *102,* 102b, 107, *108*
    sinus tract in, 102, 102b, *103,* 107, *108*
    subacute, 107, *108*
    subperiosteal fluid collection in, 107
    ulcers in, 106
  positioning for imaging of, 101
  pulse sequences for, 101
  regions of interest for, 101
  septic arthritis as, *110,* 110–111, *111*
  septic tenosynovitis/septic bursitis as, 108, *109*

Infection(s) *(Continued)*
  soft tissue, 108–110, 108b, *109, 110,* 110b
  with acquired immunodeficiency syndrome, 113
Inflammatory conditions, of foot and ankle, 407–413
  of spine, 301–305, 301b, *302–305*
Inflammatory myopathies, 77–80, *78–80,* 78b
Inflammatory neuritis, 99, *99*
Infraction, Freiberg's, 422, *424*
Infrapatellar plica, 383–384
Infraspinatus muscle, atrophy of, *217*
Infraspinatus tendon, in posterosuperior impingement, 190–191, 190b, *191*
  normal anatomy of, 176–177, *177,* 178, *179*
  tears of, 190, *190*
Injury(ies). See also *Trauma.*
  avulsion, 153–157, *156,* 156b, *157*
    chronic, 161–163, *162, 163*
    in immature skeleton, 163–164
    of acetabular labrum, 353
    of anterior labroligamentous periosteal sleeve, 201b, 203, *206, 207*
    of glenohumeral ligament, 200–201, 201b, *202*
    of hamstring, *347*
    of superior glenoid labrum, *207,* 207–209, *208,* 209b, *210, 211*
  chronic repetitive (stress), 132, 157–161, *158–161,* 158b–161b
  impaction, 152–153, *153–155,* 153b
Instability, carpal, 266, 267b
  distal radioulnar joint, 255, *255*
  dorsal intercalated segmental, 250–251, *251,* 266
  glenohumeral. See *Glenohumeral instability.*
  scapholunate, 250–251, *251*
Insufficiency fractures, 157–159, *158–160,* 159b
  of hip and pelvis, 339–342, 339b, *342, 343*
Interdigital neuroma, 98, 145, 415–417, 417b, *418, 419,* 434
Intermediate TR, short TE sequence, 4–6, 5b
Interosseous bursa, 242
Interspinous ligaments, 308, *309*
Intervertebral disk(s), annular tears of, 281–282, 281b, *283*
  bulging, 283, *284,* 284b, *285*
  calcified, 289–290, *290*
  contour abnormalities of, 282–288
    location of, 285–287, *287,* 287b
    mimickers of, 288, *289,* 289b
    significance of, 287–288, 288b
    types of, 282–285, *284–287,* 284b
  degeneration of, 280–293, 281b
    compressive myelopathy due to, 288, *288*
    epidural hematoma due to, 288, *289*
    marrow with, *28*
    osseous changes due to, 291–293, 291b, *292–294*
    protocols for imaging of, 328–329
    recurrent, 300–301, *301*
    vertebral bodies in, 289, *290*
  extrusion of, 283–284, *284,* 284b, *286*
  herniation of, 282, 284b
    intraosseous, 306, *307, 308*
  normal, 280–281, *282*
  nuclear abnormalities of, 281, *282*
  postoperative changes in, 299, *300*

Intervertebral disk(s) *(Continued)*
  protrusion of, 283, *284,* 284b, *285*
  sequestered, *284,* 284–285, 284b, *287*
  trauma to, 309, *310*
  vacuum, 288–289, *290*
Intradural space, 319–323, 320b, *321, 322,* 330
Intrathecal nerve roots, after spinal surgery, 298–299, *300*
Intrinsic ligaments, of wrist, 248–251, *248–252,* 248b
Inversion recovery imaging. See *STIR imaging.*
Inversion time (TI), 5b, 6
Involucrum, in osteomyelitis, 102, *102,* 102b, *103*
Irritation, neuroma from chronic, 93, *94*
Ischemia, marrow, 46–48, 46b, *47, 48*
  muscle, 85, 85b, *86*
ITB (iliotibial band) friction syndrome, 381–382, *383*
ITOH (idiopathic transient osteoporosis of hip), 44–45, *45, 164,* 337–339, 339b, *340*

J

Joint effusion(s), due to foreign bodies, 111, *112*
  in osteomyelitis, 107, *108*
  in septic arthritis, 110–111
  of elbow, 241
  of hip, 355, *355*
Joint involvement, with tumors, 127, *129*
Jumper's knee, 384, *385*

K

Kienböck's disease, 268–269, 269b, *270*
Kiloh-Nevin syndrome, *238,* 240, 240b
Knee(s), 363–391
  approach to imaging of, 363–365, *364*
  avulsion injuries of, 156, 156b, *157*
  bones of, 386–387, *387*
  bursae of, 384–386, *385, 386*
  coils for, 363
  contrast enhancement of, 365
  contusions of, 386–387, *387*
  fat suppression for imaging of, *364,* 364–365
  jumper's, 384, *385*
  ligament(s) of, 376–382
    anterior cruciate, 376–378, *376–379*
    lateral collateral, 380–382, *382, 383*
    medial collateral, 378–380, *380–382*
    meniscofemoral, *373,* 373–374, *374*
    posterior cruciate, 378, *379, 380*
    transverse, *373,* 373
  meniscus(i) of, 365–376
    anterior and posterior horns of, 365, *366*
      speckled, *373,* 373
    chondrocalcinosis of, *119*
    cysts of, 369–371, *371*
    discoid, 371–373, *372,* 372b
    flipped, anterior, 367, *369*
      medial, 369, *370*
    myxoid (intrasubstance) degeneration of, 365, *367*
    normal, 365, *366*
    pitfalls in imaging of, 373–37*?,* *376,* 376b
    pulse sequences for, 1*?,* 364, *364*
    tear(s) of, 366–369

Knee(s) *(Continued)*
    approach to imaging of, 14b, 15, 363, *364*
    bucket-handle, 367, *368, 369*
    medial flap, 369, *370*
    oblique or horizontal, 367, *367*
    radial (free-edge, parrot beak), 367–369, *370*
    vertical longitudinal, 367, *368*
    with ACL tear, 366–367
    osteochondritis dissecans of, 165, *166*
    patella of, 382–383, *383*
    patellar tendon of, 384, *385*
    positioning for imaging of, 363
    protocols for imaging of, 389–391
    pulse sequences for, 14b, 15, 363–365, *364*
    soft tissues of, *387*, 387–388, *388*
    synovial plicae of, 383–384, *384*

L

Labrum, acetabular, 350–352, *352–354, 352b*
    glenoid, ALPSA lesions of, 201b, 203, *206, 207*
        Bankart lesions of, 201b, 203, *205–207*
            reverse, 201b, 203, *205*
        bucket handle tear of, 207, *207*, 209, *210, 211*
        Buford complex of, 197–198, *199, 200,* 201b
        cysts of, 209, *210*
        detached, 207, *207,* 208, *208*
        GLAD lesions of, 201b, *207*, 209, *212*
        in instability, 201b, 203–207, *206, 207*
        noninstability lesions of, *207*, 207–209, 207b, *208*, 209b, *210–212*
        normal anatomy of, 197–200, *197–200,* 197b
        partial thickness tear of, 207, *207,* 208–209, *210*
        pulse sequences for, 14b, 15, *16*
        SLAP lesions of, 207–209
            classification of, 207, *207,* 209b
            defined, 201b, 207
            normal, 207, *207,* 208
            sublabral foramen vs., 197b
            with biceps anchor tear, 209, *211*
            with bucket handle tear, 207, *207,* 209, *210, 211*
            with detached labrum, 207, *207,* 208, *208*
            with partial thickness tear, 207, *207,* 208–209, *210*
Lacertus fibrosus, 232, 240
Lateral collateral ligament (LCL), of ankle, 405–407, 405b, *406–409*
    of knee, 380–382, *382, 383*
Lateral epicondylitis, 236–237, *237,* 237b, *238*
    with radial collateral ligament tear, 230, *231*
Lateral femoral cutaneous nerve, compressive neuropathy of, 99
Lateral recess stenosis, 296, *297*
Lateral ulnar collateral ligament (LUCL), insufficiency of, 230
    normal anatomy of, 228–229, *229*
LCL (lateral collateral ligament), of ankle, 405–407, 405b, *406–409*
    of knee, 380–382, *382, 383*
Legg-Calvé-Perthes disease, 337, 337b, *338, 339,* 352

Leiomyosarcoma, *131*
Leukemias, 30, 32, *33*
Ligament(s), annular, 228, *229*
    anterior cruciate, cyst of, 377, *377*
        normal, 376, *376*
        tears of, 376–378, *377–379*
            osseous contusions with, 153, 153b, *154,* 386–387, *387*
            with meniscal tear, 366–367
    calcaneofibular, 405b, 407, *407, 408*
    carpal, 248–251, *248–252,* 248b
        extrinsic, 251–252, *252*
        intrinsic, 248–251, *248–252,* 248b
    coracoacromial, anatomy of, 179, *179, 180*
        thickening of, 183, *184*
    coracohumeral, 176
    deltoid, 404–405, *405*
    fibulocollateral, 381, *382*
    glenohumeral, humeral avulsion of, 200–201, 201b, *202*
        normal anatomy of, 194–197, *195,* 195b, *196*
    iliofemoral, 345
    interspinous, 308, *309*
    lateral collateral, of ankle, 405–407, 405b, *406–409*
        of knee, 380–382, *382, 383*
    lunotriquetral, *248,* 248–250, 248b, 251, *252*
    medial collateral, bursa of, 385, *386*
        of ankle, 404–405, *405*
        of knee, 378–380, *380–382*
    meniscofemoral, *373,* 373–374, *374*
    normal appearance of, 15–16
    nuchal, 308, *309*
    of ankle, 403–407
        lateral, 405–407, 405b, *406–408*
        medial, 404–405, *405*
    of elbow, 228–232
        radial collateral, 228–230, *229–231,* 229b
        ulnar collateral, 230–232, 230b, *231, 232*
    of Humphrey, 373–374
    of knee, 376–382
    of Wrisberg, 373–374, *374*
    of wrist and hand, extrinsic, 251–252, *252*
        intrinsic, 248–251, *248–252,* 248b
        lunotriquetral, *248,* 248–250, 248b, 251, *252*
        radioulnar, 255, *255*
        scapholunate, 248–251, *248–251,* 248b
        ulnar collateral, *253,* 256
    pitfalls in MRI of, 16, *17*
    posterior cruciate, 378, *379, 380*
        double, 367, *369*
    posterior longitudinal, ossification of, 318
    pulse sequences for, 14b, 16
    radial collateral, 228–230, *229–231,* 229b
    radiolunotriquetral, 251, *252*
    radioscaphocapitate, 251, *252*
    radioulnar, 255, *255*
    scapholunate, 248–251, *248–251,* 248b
        ganglion cysts of, *271*
    spinous, normal, 308, *309*
        ossification of posterior longitudinal, 318
        trauma to, 307–309, 309b, *310*
    sprains of, medial collateral, 379, *380, 381*
        radial collateral, 230

Ligament(s) *(Continued)*
    spring, 404
    supraspinous, normal, 308, *309*
        torn, *310*
    talofibular, 405b, 407, *407–409*
    talonavicular, 404
    tear(s) of, anterior cruciate, 376–378, *377–379*
        osseous contusions with, 153, 153b, *154,* 386–387, *387*
        with meniscal tear, 366–367
        deltoid, 405, *405*
        fibulocollateral, 381, *382*
        lunotriquetral, 251, *252*
        medial collateral, 379, *381*
        posterior cruciate, 378, *380*
        radial collateral, 229–230, *230, 231*
        radioulnar, 255, *255*
        scapholunate, *250,* 250–251, *251*
        talofibular, 407, *409*
        tibiofibular, 407, *407*
        ulnar collateral, of elbow, 231–232, *232*
            of thumb, 256–258, *257,* 276–277
        tibial collateral, bursa of, 385, *386*
        tibiocalcaneal, 404–405, *405*
        tibiofibular, 405–407, 405b, *406, 407*
        tibiotalar, 404–405, *405*
        transverse, 373, *373*
        ulnar collateral, of elbow, 230–232, 230b, *231, 232*
            of thumb, 256–258, *257*
            of wrist, *253,* 256
Ligamentum flavum, normal, 309
    torn, *310*
Ligamentum teres, 350
Lipoma(s), *11*
    intradural, 320–322, *322, 326*
    intramuscular, 82, *83*
    intraosseous, 132–133, *133*
        of calcaneus, 424, *425*
    of hip, 349, 352b
    soft tissue, 137, *142*
Lipomatosis, epidural, 316, 317b, *318*
Lipomyelomeningoceles, 320
Liposarcoma, of hip and pelvis, 350, 352b
    soft tissue, 137, *142, 143*
Lister's tubercle, 258, *258*
Little Leaguer's elbow, 156, 235–236, 235b, *236*
Long head of the biceps. See *Biceps tendon.*
Long TR, long TE sequence, 4, 5b, 6b, *7*
Loose bodies, 122, *123*
    in elbow, 227, *228,* 241, *241, 242*
    in rheumatoid arthritis, 117, *118*
    in synovial chondromatosis, 121, *121*
Lower extremity, fatigue fractures of, 160b
    soft tissue tumors of, benign, 138t
        malignant, 140t
LUCL (lateral ulnar collateral ligament), insufficiency of, 230
    normal anatomy of, 228–229, *229*
Lunate, osteonecrosis of, 268–269, 269b, *270*
    type II, 269–270, *271*
Lunotriquetral ligament, *248,* 248–250, 248b, 251, *252*
Lymph nodes, with tumor, 129
Lymphoma, intramuscular, 82, *83*
    of bone, *39,* 40, 134

M

Macroglobulinemia, Waldenström's, 34, *34*

Magic-angle phenomenon, 16, *17*, 57
  in knee, 374, *375*
  in shoulder, *177*, 178–179, 185
Magnetic resonance arthrography, 13–14
  of elbow, 244
  of hip and pelvis, 359
  of shoulder, 176
Magnetic resonance imaging (MRI),
    applications of, 18–19
  fat saturation in, 9–12, *11*, *12*
  gadolinium in, *4*, *11*, 12–13, 12b, *13*
  lack of motion in, 1, *2*
  of articular cartilage, 15, *15*
  of bone, *14*, 14–15
  of fibrocartilage, 15, *16*
  of muscle, 16, *18*
  of synovium, 16–18, *19*
  of tendons and ligaments, 15–16, *17*
  pulse sequences in, 4–9, 5b
    fast (turbo) spin echo, 5b, 6, *7*, *8*, *10*
    gradient echo (T2*), 5b, 8–9, *8–10*
    inversion recovery (STIR), 5b, 6–8, *7*, *8*, *12*
    proton (spin) density, 4–6, 5b
    spin echo, 4–6, 5b, *6*, 6b, *7*
    T1, 4, 5b, *6*, 6b, *7*
    T2, 4, 5b, 6b, *7*
  signal and resolution in, 1–3, *2–4*, 2b
  three-dimensional, 8, *9*
  tissue contrast in, 3–13
  vs. computed tomography, 3–4
Malignant fibrous histiocytoma (MFH), of
    hip and pelvis, 350, 352b
Malignant melanoma, 82, *84*, 143, *145*, 145–146
Malleolar fossa, 407, *407*, *408*
Mallet finger, *261*
Mandibular condyle, 169, *170*
Marrow, after spinal surgery, 298
  approach to imaging of, 23
  coils for, 23
  contrast enhancement of, 23
  conversion of, 24–25, 24b, *25*, 25b
  depletion of, 41–44, 41b
  edema of, 44, *44*, *45*
    epiphyseal, 164, 164b
    in osteomyelitis, 106, *107*, *108*
    transient painful, 337–339, 339b, *340*
    with osteoid osteoma, 132, *132*
  focal areas of fat in, *28*, 28–29, 29b
  hemosiderin deposition in, 51, *51*, 51b
  heterogeneity of, 25–26, 25b, *28*, 28–29, *29*, 29b
  hyperemia of, 44–45, *44–46*, 44b
  image orientation for, 23
  in aplastic anemia, 41, *42*
  in diabetes, 113b, *114*, 114–115
  in Gaucher disease, 48, *49*
  in leukemias, 30, 32, *33*
  in lymphoma, *39*, 40
  in monoclonal gammopathies, aggressive, 32, *34–36*, 34–37, 36b
    nonmyelomatous, 32–34
  in multiple myeloma, 30
  in osteopetrosis, 48–51, *50*
  in osteoporosis, aggressive (disuse), *28*
    regional migratory, 45, *46*
    transient, of hip, 44–45, *45*
  in Paget's disease, 48, *50*
  in vertebral bodies, 291, 291b, *292*
  in vertebral compression fracture, 39–40, 40b, *41*, *42*
  infarction of, 32b, 46–48, 46b, *47*, *48*
  ischemia of, 46–48, 46b, *47*, *48*
  metastases to, 37–39, *38–40*
  normal, anatomy and function of, 23–26, 23b

Marrow *(Continued)*
  MRI of, 14, *14*, 25b, 26–29, *26–29*, 29b
  of pelvis and hips, 334
  pitfalls in MRI of, 15
  positioning for imaging of, 23
  primary tumors of, 40
  proliferative disorders of, 29–37, 30b
    benign, 29–34, *30–33*, 31b, 32b
    malignant, *34–36*, 34–37, 36b
  pulse sequences for, 8, 14–15, 14b, 23
  reconversion of, 25, 30–32, *31*, 31b, *32*, 32b
  red (cellular, active, myeloid, hemato-
      poietic), anatomy and function of, 23b, 24, 24b
    conversion to yellow of, 24–25, 24b, *25*, 25b
    focal areas of, *27*, 28, 29, *29*
    MRI of normal, *26*, *27*, 27–28
    reconversion of yellow to, 25, 30–32, *31*, 31b, *32*, 32b
    variations in normal, 25–26, 25b, *26*
  regeneration of, 43, 43b
  regions of interest for, 23
  replacement disorders of, 37–40, 37b
  serous atrophy (gelatinous transforma-
      tion) of, 51–52, *52*
  vascular abnormalities of, 44–48, 44b
  with chemotherapy, 41–43, *42*, *43*, 43b
  with radiation therapy, 43–44, *44*
  yellow (fatty, inactive), anatomy and
      function of, 23b, 24, 24b
    conversion from red, 24–25, 24b, *25*, 25b
    normal, MRI of, 26, *26*, *27*
    reconversion from red to, 25, 30–32, *31*, 31b, *32*, 32b
Mass(es). See also *Tumor(s)*.
  cystic-appearing, 146–148, 146b, *147–149*
  of elbow, 241
  of foot and ankle, 415, *416*
  of wrist and hand, 276
Mastocytosis, *30*
Matrix, imaging, 1, *3*, 20
Medial collateral ligament (MCL), bursa
    of, 385, *386*
  of ankle, 404–405, *405*
  of knee, 378–380, *380–382*
Medial epicondylitis, 235–236, 235b, *236*
Medial patellar plica, 383–384, *384*
Medial tendon, *235*, 235–236, 235b, *236*
Medial tennis elbow, 235–236, 235b, *236*
Median nerve, compressive neuropathy
    of, 98, 239–240, 240b
  fibrolipomatous hamartoma of, *97*, 264–265, *266*
  normal anatomy of, 239, 260–262, *262*
    of elbow, 239–240, 240b
    of wrist and hand, 260–262, *262*
      in carpal tunnel syndrome, 260–265, *262–265*, 262b
  pseudoneuroma of, 262–263
Medullary abscess, *104*
Medullary bone infarct, 133, *134*, 136
Melanoma, malignant, 82, *84*, 143, *145*, 145–146
Meningioma, 319, 320b, *321*
Meningocele(s), lateral thoracic, 317–318
  postoperative, 298, *299*
  pseudo-, 309, 318
  sacral, 316–317, 317b, *319*
Meniscocapsular separation, 379–380, *381*, *382*
Meniscofemoral ligament, 373, 373–374, *374*

Meniscus(i), 365–376
  anterior and posterior horns of, 365, *366*
    speckled, 373, *373*
  articular, 169–170, *170*, *171*
  chondrocalcinosis of, *119*
  cysts of, 369–371, *371*
  discoid, 371–373, *372*, 372b
  flipped, anterior, 367, *369*
    medial, 369, *370*
  myxoid (intrasubstance) degeneration
      of, 365, *367*
  normal, 365, *366*
  pitfalls in imaging of, 373–376, *373–376*, 376b
  pulse sequences for, 14b, 15, 363–364, *364*
  tear(s) of, 366–369, 367b
    approach to imaging of, 14b, 15, 363, *364*
    bucket handle, 367, *368*, *369*
    medial flap, 369, *370*
    oblique or horizontal, 367, *367*
    radial (free-edge, parrot beak), 367–369, *370*
    vertical longitudinal, 367, *368*
    with ACL tear, 366–367
Meniscus homologue, 255, *256*
Mesotendon, 56, *58*
Metastases, in tumor staging, 125, 126, 126b, *127*
  skeletal, 37–39, *38–40*
  to muscle, 82, *84*
  to spine, 314–315, 320b, 323, 325, 330
  to subarachnoid space, 323
MFH (malignant fibrous histiocytoma), of
    hip and pelvis, 350, 352b
Microfibrils, 55
β2-Microglobulin deposition, *120*, 121
Microtrabecular fractures, 152–153, *153*, 153b, *154*
"Mini-brain" pattern, 34, *35*
Monoclonal gammopathies, aggressive, 32, *34–36*, 34–37, 36b
  nonmyelomatous, 32–34
Morton's neuroma, 98, 145, 415–417, 417b, *418*, *419*, 434
Motion artifact, 1, *2*
MRI. See *Magnetic resonance imaging (MRI)*.
Multiple myeloma, 30, 34–37, *35*, *36*, 36b, 314
Multiple sclerosis, 323
Muscle(s), 65–87
  abnormalities of, 65–87
  abscess of, 78, 78b
  accessory (anomalous), 85, *86*
    of foot and ankle, *403*, 426–427, *428*
    of wrist and hand, 272–273, *273*
  adductor, metastases to, *84*
    myositis ossificans of, *75*
  anconeus epitrochlearis, 233
    accessory (anomalous), *86*
  approach to imaging of, 65
  biceps, normal anatomy of, 232, *233*
  brachialis, injuries to, 232–233, *233*
    lymphoma of, *83*
    myositis ossificans of, *75*
    normal anatomy of, 232, *233*
    strain of, *69*
  brachioradialis, interstitial hemorrhage
      of, *72*
  chemotherapy effect on, 85–87
  coils for, 65
  compartment syndromes of, 76, *76*, 76b, *77*

Muscle(s) (Continued)
  contrast enhancement of, 65
  contusions of, 71b
  delayed-onset soreness of, 66, 67
  deltoid, atrophy of, 215–217
  denervation of, 80–81, 81, 81b, 82
  dystrophies of, 80
  edema of, 67
  extensor digitorum manus brevis, 273, 273
  fascial herniation of, 76–77, 77
  fatty atrophy of, 81, 81, 81b, 82
  flexor carpi ulnaris, denervation of, 81
  flexor digitorum profundus, denervation of, 81
  flexor hallucis longus, strain of, 69
  gastrocnemius, exertional compartment syndrome of, 77
    necrotizing fasciitis of, 79
  gracilis, pyomyositis of, 78
  hamstring, 346–347, 347
    strain of, 68, 70
  hematoma of, 71–74, 71b, 72–74
  hemorrhage of, into tumor, 73, 74
    intraparenchymal or interstitial, 70–71, 72
  image orientation for, 65
  infarction of, 85, 85b, 86
  infraspinatus, atrophy of, 217
  ischemia to, 85, 85b, 86
  MRI appearance of, 16, 65, 65
  myopathies of, 80
    inflammatory, 77–80, 78–80, 78b
  myositis ossificans of, 71b, 73–75, 75
  necrotizing fasciitis of, 78–79, 78b, 79
  normal, 65, 65
  obturator, strain of, 69, 348
  of elbow, 232–237, 232b
    anterior compartment, 232–233, 232b, 233, 234
    lateral compartment, 236–237, 236–238, 237b
    medial compartment, 235, 235–236, 235b, 236
    posterior compartment, 233–234, 234, 235
  of foot and ankle, accessory, 426–427, 428
    in diabetes, 431, 432
  of hip and pelvis, 345–348, 346b, 347, 348
  paraspinous, strain of, 311, 313
  pectoralis, injuries of, 220, 220
  peroneus longus, herniation of, 77
  peroneus quartus, accessory, 403, 426–427
  piriformis, 347–348
  popliteal, strain of, 68
  positioning for imaging of, 65
  primary diseases of, 80
  pulse sequences for, 14b, 16, 18, 65
  pyomyositis of, 78, 78, 78b
  radiation effect on, 85–87, 86
  rectus femoris, hematoma of, 73
    strain of, 67, 67
  regions of interest for, 65
  rhabdomyolysis of, 84–85
  sartorius, metastases to, 84
  soleus, accessory, 426, 428
    denervation of, 91
  strains of, 66–70, 67–70
    brachialis, 69, 232–233, 233
    obturator, 69, 348
    of hip and pelvis, 346–347, 346b, 347

Muscle(s) (Continued)
  paraspinous, 311, 313
  popliteal, 68
  rectus femoris, 67, 67
  supinator, lipoma of, 83
    syndrome of, 240–241
  supraspinatus, overdevelopment of, 183
  surgery effect on, 85–87
  tears of, 66–70, 67–70
    chronic, 73, 74
    grading of, 67–68, 68–70
    healing of, 68–70
    pectoralis, 220, 220
  teres minor, atrophy of, 215–217, 217
  tibialis anterior, denervation of, 82
  trauma to, 66–77
    compartment syndromes due to, 76, 76, 76b, 77
    delayed-onset soreness due to, 66, 67
    direct, 70–75, 71b, 72–75
    fascial herniation due to, 76–77, 77
    hematoma due to, 71–74, 71b, 72–74
    hemorrhage due to, 70–71, 72
    indirect, 66–70, 66b, 67–70
    miscellaneous, 75–77, 76, 76b, 77
    myositis ossificans due to, 73–75, 75
    spinal, 311, 313
  triceps, 233
  tumors of, 81–84, 82–85, 82b
    hemorrhage into, 73, 74
  vastus intermedius, edema of, 67
Muscular dystrophies, 80
Myelin sheaths, 89
Myeloma, multiple, 30, 34–37, 35, 36, 36b, 314
Myelomalacia, 323, 324, 324, 325
Myelopathy, compressive, disk-related, 288, 288
  progressive posttraumatic myelomalacic, 323, 324
Myonecrosis, calcific, 76, 76
Myopathies, 80
  inflammatory, 77–80, 78–80, 78b
Myositis, bacterial, 78, 78, 78b, 108–109
Myositis ossificans, 71b, 73–75, 75
Myotendinous junction, 67
Myxoid chondrosarcoma, 148
Myxomas, 84, 85
  intramuscular, 146, 148

N

Navicular, accessory, 419, 422
Neck, soft tissue tumors of, benign, 139t
  malignant, 141t
Necrosis, avascular, of hip and pelvis, 334–337, 335b, 336–339, 337b, 359
  of humeral head, 218–219, 219
  of temporomandibular joint, 173
  of wrist, 268–269, 269, 269b, 270
  in nerve sheath tumors, 95, 96
Necrotizing fasciitis, 78–79, 78b, 79, 109–110, 110, 110b
Neonates, developmental dysplasia of hip in, 355–357, 356, 356b
  osteomyelitis in, 102, 104
Neoplasms. See Tumor(s).
Nerve(s), abnormalities of, muscle atrophy from, 215–217, 217, 218b
  axillary, compressive neuropathy of, 98
  encasement in tumors of, 99, 99
  lateral femoral cutaneous, compressive neuropathy of, 99
  median, compressive neuropathy of, 98, 239–240, 240b

Nerve(s) (Continued)
  fibrolipomatous hamartoma of, 97, 264–265, 266
  normal anatomy of, 239, 260–262, 262
    of elbow, 239–240, 240b
    of wrist and hand, 260–262, 262
      in carpal tunnel syndrome, 260–265, 262–265, 262b
  pseudoneuroma of, 262–263
  of elbow, 237–241
    approach to imaging of, 237–238, 237b, 238
    median, 239–240, 240b
    radial, 240–241, 240b
    ulnar, 238–239, 238b, 239
  of foot and ankle, 413–417
  of hip and pelvis, 348–349, 349
  of shoulder, 214–217, 214b, 216, 217, 217b, 218b
  of spine, trauma to, 311–312, 313
  of wrist and hand, 260–265
    median, 260–265, 262–265, 262b
    ulnar, 264, 265
  peripheral. See Peripheral nerve(s).
  peroneal, ganglion cyst of, 98
  posterior tibial, compressive neuropathy of, 91, 99
    neuroma of, 94
  pseudotumors of, 98, 98
  radial, compressive neuropathy of, 98, 240–241, 240b
    normal anatomy of, 240
  radiation effect on, 99
  sciatic, 348–349, 349
    compressive neuropathy of, 99
    neuritis of, 93
    neuroma of, 95
    normal, 90, 90
  spinoglenoid notch, compression of, 214, 216
  suprascapular, entrapment of, 98, 214–215, 214b, 216
  trauma to, 92, 92, 93
  tumors of, 92–98, 94–98, 95b
  ulnar, compressive neuropathy of, 98, 98
    at elbow, 238–239, 238b, 239
    at wrist, 264, 265
    neuritis of, 92, 93, 238
    neuroma of, 94
    normal anatomy of, 91, 238, 239, 264, 265
    surgical transposition of, 93
Nerve entrapment, of median nerve, 98, 239–240, 240b
  of posterior tibial nerve, 91, 99
  of radial nerve, 98, 240–241, 240b
  of suprascapular nerve, 98, 214–215, 214b, 216
  of ulnar nerve, 98, 98–99
    at elbow, 238–239, 238b, 239
    at wrist, 264, 265
Nerve root(s), avulsion of, 311–312, 313
  intrathecal, after spinal surgery, 298–299, 300
Nerve sheath(s), 89–90, 90
Nerve sheath tumors, 93–95, 95b, 96, 97, 148, 149
  of spine, 319, 320b, 321
  tarsal tunnel syndrome from, 414, 416
Nerve syndromes, anterior interosseous, 238
  posterior interosseous, 240–241
Neural foramen stenosis, 296–297, 297–299

Neurapraxia, 92
Neurilemoma, 93–95, 95b, *96, 97,* 148
Neuritis, brachial, 99, *99,* 217, *217,* 218b
  from chronic subluxation, 92, *93*
  inflammatory, 99, *99*
  posttraumatic, 92, *92*
  ulnar, *92, 93,* 238
Neuroarthropathy, in diabetes, 115, 115b
Neurofibromas, 93–95, 95b, *96,* 148
  intramuscular, 84
Neurogenic edema, from anterior
  interosseous nerve syndrome, *238*
Neuroma(s), 92–93, *94, 95*
  Morton's (interdigital), 98, 145, 415–
    417, 417b, *418, 419,* 434
  pseudo-, of median nerve, 262–263
Neuropathy(ies), compressive, in carpal
    tunnel syndrome, 262–264, 262b,
    263–265
  of axillary nerve, 98
  of lateral femoral cutaneous nerve,
    99
  of median nerve, 98
    at elbow, 239–240, 240b
    at wrist, 262–264, 262b, *263–265*
  of posterior tibial nerve, *91,* 99
  of radial nerve, 98, 240–241, 240b
  of sciatic nerve, 99
  of spinoglenoid notch, 214, *216*
  of suprascapular nerve, 98, 214–215,
    214b, *216*
  of ulnar nerve, 98, *98*
    at elbow, 238–239, 238b, *239*
    at wrist, 264, *265*
  in diabetic foot, 429b, *430,* 431, *431*
  of elbow, 237–241
    approach to imaging of, 237–238,
      237b, *238*
    median, 239–240, 240b
    radial, 240–241, 240b
    ulnar, 238–239, 238b, *239*
  unexplained, 99
Neurovascular bundle, tumor encasement
    of, *99*
Neurovascular involvement, with tumors,
    127, *129*
Newborns, developmental dysplasia of
    hip in, 355–357, *356,* 356b
  osteomyelitis in, 102, 104
Noise, image, 1, *2,* 20
Normal texture sign, 130
Nuchal ligament, 308, *309*
Nucleus pulposus, abnormalities of, 281,
    282
  anatomy of, 280, *282*
  herniated, 282

O

Obesity, marrow conversion with, 31–32
Obturator muscle, strain of, *69,* 348
OCD (osteochondritis dissecans),
    164–165, 165b, *166*
  of elbow, 226–227, 226b, *227*
  of foot and ankle, 420–422, 422b, *423*
Olecranon, bursitis of, 234, *235,* 242–243
  fractures of, 228
OPLL (ossification of posterior
    longitudinal ligament), 318
Os acromiale, 183, *183*
Os styloideum, 266, *267*
Os trigonum syndrome, *400, 406,*
    417–419, 420b, *421*
Osseous degeneration, of spine, 291–293,
    291b, *292–294*

Osseous structures. See *Bone(s).*
Osseous trauma, 151–165
  acute, 152–157
  anatomic basis for, 151–152
  approach to imaging of, 151
  coils for, 151
  contusion due to, 152–153, *153,* 153b,
    154
  differential diagnosis of, 164, 164b, *165*
  due to avulsion injuries, 153–157, *156,*
    156b, *157*
    chronic, 161–163, *162, 163*
    of immature skeleton, 163–164
  due to impaction injuries, 152–153,
    153–155, 153b
  due to stress injuries, 132, 157–161,
    158–161, 158b–161b
  fractures due to. See also *Fracture(s).*
    avulsion, 153–157, *156,* 156b, *157,*
      163–164
    fatigue, 159–161, *160,* 160b, *161*
    insufficiency, 157–159, *158–160,*
      159b
    microtrabecular, 152–153, *153,* 153b,
      154
    radiographically occult, 153, *155*
    stress, 132, 157–161, *158–161,* 158b–
      161b
  image orientation for, 151
  imaging options for, 152
  in osteochondritis dissecans, 164–165,
    165b, *166*
  osteolysis after, 161–163, *163*
    of clavicle, 217–218, *218*
  overview of, 152
  positioning for imaging of, 151
  pulse sequences for, 151
  repetitive, 157–164
    to immature skeleton, *163,* 163–164,
      164
  to spine, 307, *308*
Osseous tumors, benign and malignant,
    40
  differential diagnosis of, 132–136, *132–*
    137, 133b–135b
  of foot and ankle, 422–425, *425,* 425b,
    426
  of hip and pelvis, 344–345, 344b, *345,*
    346
  of shoulder, 219, *219,* 219b
  of spine, 312–315, *314–316,* 314b, 330
  of wrist and hand, 270–271, *271*
  principles of imaging of, *122,* 126
Ossicles, accessory, of foot and ankle,
    417–420, 420b, *421–423*
Ossification of the posterior longitudinal
    ligament (OPLL), 318
Osteitis, 105
  in diabetes, 114
Osteoarthritis. See *Arthritis.*
Osteochondritis dissecans (OCD),
    164–165, 165b, *166*
  of elbow, 226–227, 226b, *227*
  of foot and ankle, 420–422, 422b, *423*
Osteochondroma, *91,* 136, *137*
Osteochondromatosis, synovial, of elbow,
    241, *242*
  of hip, *357,* 357–358
Osteochondrosis, of capitellum, 226
Osteoid osteoma, 132, *132*
  of spine, 312, 313, *314*
  of talus, 425, *425*
Osteoid/chondroid tumor matrix, 133
Osteolysis, posttraumatic, 161–163, *163*
  of clavicle, 217–218, *218*
Osteoma, osteoid, 132, *132*

Osteoma *(Continued)*
  of spine, 312, 313, *314*
  of talus, 425, *425*
Osteomyelitis, 101–108
  abscess/phlegmon in, *102,* 102–103,
    104, 106, 107, *108*
  acute, 105–107, *107*
  adult pattern of, 104–105
  childhood pattern of, 102, *103,* 104,
    105
  chronic, 107–108, *108*
  chronic recurrent multifocal, 113
  cloaca in, 102, *102,* 102b, 106, 107, *108*
  contiguous spread of, 103b, 105, *105*
  direct implantation of, 103b, 105, *106*
  fistula in, 102, 102b
  hematogenous seeding of, 103–105,
    103b, *105*
  in AIDS, 113
  in diabetic foot, *114,* 114–115, 115b,
    429–430, 429b, *430*
  infantile pattern of, 102, 104
  involucrum in, 102, *102,* 102b, *103*
  joint effusion in, 107, *108*
  marrow edema in, 106, *107, 108*
  MRI findings in, 106b
  routes of contamination for, 103–105,
    103b, *105, 106*
  sequestrum in, 101–102, *102,* 102b,
    107, *108*
  sinus tract in, 102, 102b, *103,* 107, *108*
  subacute, 107, *108*
  subperiosteal fluid collection in, 107
  ulcers in, 106
Osteonecrosis, 32b, 46–48, 46b, *47, 48*
  Kienböck's, 268–269, 269b, *270*
  of foot and ankle, 422, 422b, *424*
  of hip and pelvis, 334–337, 335b, *336–*
    339, 337b, 359
  of humeral head, 218–219, *219*
  of temporomandibular joint, 173
  of wrist, 268–269, *269,* 269b, *270*
Osteopetrosis, 48–51, *50*
Osteophytes, 291
Osteoporosis, aggressive (disuse), *28*
  idiopathic transient, of hip, 44–45, *45,*
    164, 337–339, 339b, *340*
  insufficiency fractures due to, of hip
    and pelvis, 339–342, 339b, *342,*
    343
  regional migratory, 45, *46*
  vertebral compression fractures due to,
    39–40, 40b, *41*

P

Paget's disease, 48, *50,* 133, *134*
Pain, in foot and ankle, 415, *416*
Panner's disease, of elbow, 226, 226b
Pannus, 117
Paragangliomas, 319–320, 320b, *322*
Paralabral cysts, acetabular, 350, *354*
  glenoid, 209, *210*
Parameniscal cyst, 369–371, *371*
Paraspinous muscles, strain of, 311, *313*
Paratendinitis, 59, *60*
Pars interarticularis, osseous defect in,
    305–306, 305b, *306, 307*
Parsonage-Turner syndrome, 99, *99,* 217,
    217, 218b
Patella, dislocation of, 382–383, *383*
  osseous contusions with, 153, *154*
Patellar tendon, 384, *385*
Patellofemoral compartment, giant cell
    tumor of, *129*

PCL (posterior cruciate ligament), 378, *379, 380*
 double, 367, *369*
Pectoralis muscle, injuries of, 220, *220*
Pelvic insufficiency fractures, *158, 159*
Pelvis. See *Hip(s) and pelvis.*
Perineural cysts, 317, 317b, *320*
Perineurium, 89, *90*
Peripheral nerve(s), 89–99
 abnormalities of, 90–99, *91,* 92b
 advantages of MRI of, 89
 coils for, 89
 compressive neuropathy and entrapment syndromes of, *98,* 98–99
 contrast enhancement of, 89
 fascicles of, 90, *90, 91, 91*
 fibrolipomatous hamartoma of, 95–97, *97*
 image orientation for, 89
 inflammatory neuritis of, 99, *99*
 neurofibroma and neurilemoma of, 93–95, 95b, *96, 97*
 neuromas of, 92–93, *94, 95*
 normal anatomy and MRI appearance of, 89–90, *91*
 positioning for imaging of, 89
 pseudotumors of, 98, *98*
 pulse sequences for, 89
 radiation effect on, 99
 subluxation of, 92, *93*
 surgical transposition of, 92, *93*
 trauma to, 92, *92, 93*
 tumor encasement of, 99, *99*
 tumors of, 92–98, 148, *149*
 unexplained neuropathy of, 99
Peroneal nerve, ganglion cyst of, *98*
Peroneal tendons, *394,* 400–403, 401b, *402–404*
Peroneus brevis splits, 401, 401b, *403*
Peroneus longus muscle, herniation of, *77*
Peroneus quartus muscle, accessory, *403,* 426–427
Pes anserinus bursa, 384–385, *385, 386*
Phased array coil, 3
Phlegmon, in osteomyelitis, 103
Physeal bridges, posttraumatic, 163, *164,* 267–268
Physeal injuries, 163, *163*
 of wrist, 267–268
Physeal scar, 26, *27*
Physis, 152
 avulsion fractures of, 163–164
Pigmented villonodular synovitis (PVNS), 121–122, *122,* 143, *146*
 of elbow, 241, *242*
 of hip, 357
 vs. hemosiderotic arthritis, 119
Piriformis syndrome, 347–348
Pisotriquetral synovial cyst, 273, *274*
Pivot-shift phenomenon, 386
Plantar fasciitis, 410–413, 411b, *413, 414*
Plantar fibromatosis, 425–426, *427*
Plantaris tendon, normal, *394,* 395, *396*
 tears of, 387–388, *388*
Plasma cell dyscrasias, 32, *34–36,* 34–37, 36b
Plicae, medial patellar, 383–384, *384*
Polymyalgia rheumatica, *80*
Polymyopathies, idiopathic inflammatory, 79–80, *80*
Popliteal artery, pulsation from, 374, *374*
Popliteal bursa, 384
Popliteus muscle, strain of, *68*
Popliteus tendon, pseudotear of, 374–376, *376*

Popliteus tendon *(Continued)*
 tears of, 381, *382*
Positioning, 1
 for arthritis and cartilage, 117
 for elbow, 225
 for foot and ankle, 393
 for hip and pelvis, 333
 for infection, 101
 for knee, 363
 for marrow, 23
 for muscle, 65
 for osseous trauma, 151
 for peripheral nerves, 89
 for shoulder, 175
 for spine, 279
 for temporomandibular joint, 169
 for tendons, 55
 for tumors, 130–131
 for wrist and hand, 247
Posterior cruciate ligament (PCL), 378, *379, 380*
 double, 367, *369*
Posterior interosseous nerve syndrome, 240–241
Posterior longitudinal ligament, ossification of, 318
Posterior spinous processes, degenerative changes of, 291b, 292–293, *294*
Posterior tibial nerve, compressive neuropathy of, *91,* 99
 neuroma of, *94*
Posterior tibial plateau, avulsion fracture of, *156*
Posterior tibial tendon, *394*
 tears of, *60, 398,* 398b, *399*
Posterosuperior impingement, 190–191, 190b, *191*
Posttraumatic osteolysis, of clavicle, 217–218, *218*
Prepatellar bursa, 384, *385*
Pressure lesions, of foot and ankle, 427–429, *428,* 429b
Prestyloid recess, 255, *256*
Progressive posttraumatic myelomalacic myelopathy, 323, *324*
Pronator syndrome, 239–240, 240b
Proton density imaging, 4–6, 5b, 21
Pseudogout, 118, *119*
Pseudomeningocele, 309, 318
Pseudoneuroma, of median nerve, 262–263
Pseudotumors, of nerves, 98, *98*
Pubic symphysis, stress reaction of, *340*
Pulse sequence(s), 4–9, 5b, 21
 defined, 4
 "designer," 29
 fast (turbo) spin echo, 5b, 6, *7, 8, 10*
 for arthritis, 117
 for cartilage, 14b, 15, *15, 16,* 117, 122–123, 124
 for elbow, 225
 for foot and ankle, 393–394
 for hips and pelvis, 333
 for infection, 101
 for knee, 14b, 15, 363–365, *364*
 for marrow, 23
 for muscle, 65
 for osseous trauma, 151
 for peripheral nerves, 89
 for shoulder, 175
 for spine, 279–280
 for temporomandibular joint, 169
 for tendons, 55
 for tumors, 131
 for wrist and hand, 247–248
 gradient echo (T2*), 5b, 8–9, *8–10*

Pulse sequence(s) *(Continued)*
 inversion recovery (STIR), 5b, 6–8, *7, 8,* 12
 number of, 4
 parameters for, 5b
 proton (spin) density, 4–6, 5b
 spin echo, 4–6, 5b, *6,* 6b, *7*
 strengths and weakness of, 5b
 T1, 4, 5b, *6,* 6b, *7*
 T2, 4, 5b, 6b, *7*
Pump bumps, 397, *398*
PVNS. See *Pigmented villonodular synovitis (PVNS).*
Pyomyositis, 78, *78,* 78b

Q

Quadriceps tendon, degeneration and partial tear of, *58*
 MRI of normal, 56, *56*
Quadrilateral space syndrome, 215–217, *217,* 217b

R

RA. See *Rheumatoid arthritis (RA).*
Radial collateral ligament (RCL) complex, 228–230, *229–231,* 229b
Radial head, fracture of, *229*
Radial nerve, compressive neuropathy of, 98, 240–241, 240b
 normal anatomy of, 240
Radiation therapy, effect on muscle of, 85–87, *86*
 effect on nerves of, 99
 marrow depletion due to, 43–44, *44*
 tumor after, 129–130, *130*
Radiolunotriquetral ligament, 251, *252*
Radioscaphocapitate ligament, 251, *252*
Radioulnar joint, distal, 255, *255, 258*
Radioulnar ligaments, 255, *255*
Radius, fracture of distal, *155*
RCL (radial collateral ligament) complex, 228–230, *229–231,* 229b
Reconversion, of yellow to red marrow, 25, 30–32, *31,* 31b, *32,* 32b
Rectus femoris muscle, hematoma of, *73*
 strain of, 67, *67*
Regeneration, marrow, 43, 43b
Regions of interest, for arthritis, 117
 for elbow, 225
 for foot and ankle, 393–394
 for hip and pelvis, 333
 for infections, 101
 for marrow, 23
 for muscles, 65
 for shoulder, 175
 for spine, 279–280
 for temporomandibular joint, 169
 for tendons, 55
 for tumors, 131
 for wrist and hand, 247–248
Repetition time (TR), 4–8, 5b, 21
Resolution, 2–3, 2b, *4,* 21
Retinaculum(a), 62
 flexor, in carpal tunnel syndrome, 263, *263–265,* 264
 normal anatomy of, 260, *262*
Retro-Achilles bursa, 397, *398*
Retrocalcaneal bursa, 397, *398*
Retroperitoneum, soft tissue tumors of, benign, 139t
 malignant, 141t
Rhabdomyolysis, 84–85

Rheumatoid arthritis (RA), hypertrophied synovium in, *11*
 of elbow, 241, *241*
 of hip and pelvis, 353
Rice bodies, 117, *118, 264*
Rotator cuff, degeneration of, 185, *185,* 185b
 normal anatomy of, 176–177, *177*
 tears of, full-thickness, 185b, 186–189, *187–189*
  massive, 191–193, *192,* 213, *213*
  partial thickness, *185,* 185–186, 185b, *186*
  surgery for, 209–2214
Rotator interval, *179,* 193, *193,* 193b
Ruptures. See *Tears.*

S

Sacral insufficiency fracture, 342, *342, 343*
Sacral meningoceles, 316–317, 317b, *319*
Sacroiliac joints, infection of, 353–355, *355*
 normal, 353, *354*
Sacroiliitis, 353–355, *355*
Salter fractures, of hip and pelvis, 339b, 342–343, *344,* 344b
SAPHO syndrome, 113
Sarcoma, after chemotherapy, 129
 after radiation therapy, *130*
 after surgery, *130*
 chondro-, *128,* 136
  myxoid, *148*
  of hip and pelvis, 344
 grading of, 125, 126b
 leiomyo-, *131*
 lipo-, of hip and pelvis, 350, 352b
  soft tissue, 137, *142, 143*
 local extent of, 126
 of foot and ankle, 426, *427*
 of spine, 315
 soft tissue, 82–84
 staging of, 125, 126b
 synovial, *129*
  of foot and ankle, 426, *427*
  of hip and pelvis, 350, 352b
Sartorius muscle, metastases to, *84*
Scaphoid, fracture of, 267, *268*
 osteonecrosis of, 268, *269,* 269b
Scapholunate advanced collapse (SLAC) wrist, 251, *251,* 267b
Scapholunate ligament, 248–251, *248–251,* 248b
 ganglion cysts of, *271*
SCFE (slipped capital femoral epiphysis), 342–343, *344,* 344b
Scheuermann's disease, 306, *307*
Schmorl's nodes, 306, *308*
Schwann cells, 89
Schwannomas, 93–95, 95b, *96, 97,* 148
 tarsal tunnel syndrome from, 414, *416*
Sciatic nerve, 348–349, *349*
 compressive neuropathy of, 99
 neuritis of, *93*
 neuroma of, *95*
 normal, 90, *90*
Sclerotic bone, 133
Semimembranosus-tibial collateral ligament bursa, 385, *386*
Septic arthritis, *110,* 110–111, *111*
Septic bursitis, 108
Septic tenosynovitis, 108, *109*
Sequestrum, in osteomyelitis, 101–102, *102,* 102b, 107, *108*

Seroma, after sarcoma excision, *130*
Serous atrophy, 51–52, *52*
Serpentine lines, geographic, 46–48, *47*
Sesamoids, hallux, 419–420, *423*
Sharpey's fibers, 280
Shin splints, 161, *162*
Short tau inversion recovery imaging. See *STIR imaging.*
Short TR, short TE sequence, 4, 5b, *6,* 6b, *7*
Shoulder, 175–220
 acromion of, anatomy of, 179, *180*
  position of, *180,* 183
  shape of, *180–182,* 181–182
  slope of, *182,* 182–183, *183*
 acronyms and eponyms of, 201b
 adhesive capsulitis of, 212–213, *213*
 ALPSA lesions of, 201b, 203, *206, 207*
 approach to imaging of, 175–176
 Bankart lesions of, 201b, 203, *205–207*
  reverse, 201b, 203, *205*
 Bennett lesions of, 200, 201b, *202,* 203b
 BHAGL lesions of, 200, 201b
 bones of, abnormalities of, 217–219, *218, 219,* 219b
  in instability, 201–203, 201b, *203, 204*
 Buford complex of, 197–198, *199, 200,* 201b
 bursitis of, 214, *215*
 calcific tendinitis of, 214, *214*
 capsule of, adhesive capsulitis of, 212–213, *213*
  in instability, 200, 201b, *202*
  normal anatomy of, 194
 coils for, 175
 contrast enhancement of, 175–176
 contusions of, 218
 coracoacromial arch of, normal anatomy of, *179,* 179–181, *180*
  posttraumatic deformity of, 183
 cysts of, paralabral, 209, *210*
  synovial, 213, *213*
 fractures of, 218, *218*
 frozen, 212–213, *213*
 GLAD lesions of, 201b, *207,* 209, *212*
 glenohumeral ligaments of, humeral avulsion of, 200–201, 201b, *202*
  normal anatomy of, 194–197, *195,* 195b, *196*
 HAGL lesions of, 200, 201, 201b, *202*
 Hill-Sachs lesions of, 201–203, 201b, *204*
 image orientation for, 175, 176b
 impingement of, 181–185
  causes of, 181–183, *181–184,* 181b
  defined, 181
  effects of, 181b, 183–184, 184b
  instability and, 183
  posterosuperior, 190–191, 190b, *191*
  subcoracoid, 191, *192*
  surgery for, 209–212
  symptoms of, 181b
 instability of, 193–207, 194b
  anatomic, 194
  anatomy relating to, 194–200
  and impingement, 183
  anterior, 194
  bones in, 201–203, 201b, *203, 204*
  capsule in, 200, 201b, *202*
  defined, 193
  due to ALPSA lesions, 201b, 203, *206, 207*
  due to Bankart lesions, 201b, 203, *205–207*

Shoulder *(Continued)*
  due to Bennett lesions, 200, 201b, *202,* 203b
  due to BHAGL lesions, 200, 201b
  due to GLAD lesions, 201b, *207,* 209, *212*
  due to HAGL lesions, 200, 201, 201b, *202*
  due to Hill-Sachs lesions, 201–203, 201b, *204*
  due to SLAP lesions, 201b, *207,* 207–209, *208,* 209b, *210, 211*
  factors in, 194
  functional, 194
  glenohumeral ligaments in, 200–201, *202*
  labrum in, 203–207, *206, 207*
  lesions associated with, 200–207, 201b
  multidirectional, 194
  posterior, 194
  superior, 194
  surgery for, 212
  tendons in, 201b
  types of, 194
 labrum of, ALPSA lesions of, 201b, 203, *206, 207*
  Bankart lesions of, 201b, 203, *205–207*
   reverse, 201b, 203, *205*
  bucket handle tear of, *207, 207,* 209, *210, 211*
  Buford complex of, 197–198, *199, 200,* 201b
  cysts of, 209, *210*
  detached, *207, 207, 208, 208*
  GLAD lesions of, 201b, *207,* 209, *212*
  in instability, 201b, 203–207, *206, 207*
  noninstability lesions of, *207,* 207–209, 207b, *208,* 209b, *210–212*
  normal anatomy of, 197–200, *197–200,* 197b
  partial thickness tear of, *207, 207,* 208–209, *210*
  pulse sequences for, 14b, 15, *16*
  SLAP lesions of, 207–209
   classification of, *207, 207,* 209b
   defined, 201b, 207
   normal, 207, *207,* 208
   sublabral foramen vs., 197b
   with biceps anchor tear, 209, *211*
   with bucket handle tear, *207, 207,* 209, *210, 211*
   with detached labrum, *207, 207, 208, 208*
   with partial thickness tear, *207, 207,* 208–209, *210*
 MR arthrography of, 176, 222
 nerve abnormalities of, 214–217, 214b, *216, 217,* 217b, 218b
  Parsonage-Turner syndrome of, 217, *217,* 218b
 pectoralis muscle injuries of, 220, *220*
 positioning for imaging of, 175
 postoperative, 209–212
 protocols for imaging of, 222–223
 pulse sequences for, 175
 quadrilateral space syndrome of, 215–217, *217,* 217b
 regions of interest for, 175
 rotator cuff of, degeneration of, 185, *185,* 185b
  normal anatomy of, 176–177, *177*
  tears of, full-thickness, 185b, 186–189, *187–189*

Shoulder (Continued)
  massive, 191–193, 192, 213, 213
  partial thickness, 185, 185–186,
    185b, 186
  surgery for, 209–214
  rotator interval of, 179, 193, 193, 193b
  SLAP lesions of, 207–209
    classification of, 207, 207, 209b
    defined, 201b, 207
    normal, 207, 207, 208
    sublabral foramen vs., 197b
    with biceps anchor tear, 209, 211
    with bucket handle tear, 207, 207,
      209, 210, 211
    with detached labrum, 207, 207, 208,
      208
    with partial thickness tear, 207, 207,
      208–209, 210
  suprascapular nerve entrapment of,
    214–215, 214b, 216
  tendons of, calcific tendinitis of, 214,
    214
    impingement on, 183–184
    normal anatomy of, 176–179, 177–
      179
    tears, degeneration, and dislocation
      of, 185–193
      infraspinatus, 190, 190–191, 190b,
        191
      long head of biceps, 189, 189,
        189b, 190
      massive rotator cuff, 191–193, 192,
        213, 213
      subscapularis, 172, 191, 191b
      supraspinatus, 185–189, 185b
  tumors of, osseous, 219, 219, 219b
    soft tissue, 138t, 140t, 219–220, 220
Sickle cell anemia, reconversion from,
  31, 32
Signal, 1–2, 2, 2b, 3
Signal acquisitions, 2
Signal averages, 2, 21
Signal drop-off, 3, 4
Signal intensity, 3–4
  fluid, 4, 7
  tissue, 4, 6b
Signal-to-noise ratio (SNR), 2, 20
Sinus tarsi syndrome, 408–410, 410b,
  411–413
Sinus tract, in osteomyelitis, 102, 102b,
  103, 107, 108
Skeletal metastases, 37–39, 38–40
Skier's thumb, 256–258, 257, 276
SLAC (scapholunate advanced collapse)
  wrist, 251, 251, 267b
SLAP lesions, 207–209
  classification of, 207, 207, 209b
  defined, 201b, 207
  normal, 207, 207, 208
  sublabral foramen vs., 197b
  with biceps anchor tear, 209, 211
  with bucket handle tear, 207, 207, 209,
    210, 211
  with detached labrum, 207, 207, 208,
    208
  with partial thickness tear, 207, 207,
    208–209, 210
Slice thickness, 1–2, 21
Slipped capital femoral epiphysis (SCFE),
  342–343, 344, 344b
SNR (signal-to-noise ratio), 2, 20
Soft tissue, abscess of, 104
  edema of, in osteomyelitis, 106
  foreign bodies in, 111, 112
  infection of, 108–110, 108b, 109, 110,
    110b

Soft tissue (Continued)
  injury to, 152, 152
  of knee, 387, 387–388, 388
  tumor(s) of, 137–148
    amyloid, 145, 147
    benign, 138t–139t
    cystic-appearing, 146–148, 146b,
      147–149
    differential diagnosis of, 137–148
    distribution by anatomical site and
      age of, 138t–141t
    fibrous, 145, 147
    giant cell, 143–145
    gouty tophi as, 145
    hemorrhagic, 142, 145
    in pigmented villonodular synovitis,
      143, 146
    intramuscular myxoma as, 146, 148
    lipomatous, 137, 142, 143
    malignant, 140t–141t
    melanoma as, 143, 145, 145–146
    of foot and ankle, 138t, 140t, 425–
      429, 426b, 427, 428
    of hip and pelvis, 139t, 141t, 349–
      350, 352b
    of shoulder, 138t, 140t, 219–220,
      219b, 220
    of wrist and hand, 138t, 140t, 271–
      273, 271–273
    principles of imaging of, 126, 137
    vascular, 137–142, 143, 144
    with high signal on T1W images,
      137–143, 137b, 142–145
    with low signal on T2W images,
      143–146, 146, 146t, 147
Soleus muscle, accessory, 426, 428
  denervation of, 91
Spin density imaging, 4–6, 5b
Spin echo imaging, 21
  fast (turbo). See Fast spin echo (FSE)
    imaging.
  parameters for, 5b
  strengths and weaknesses of, 5b
  tissue signal intensity with, 4, 6b
  types of, 4–6, 6, 7
Spinal canal, 315–327
  epidural space of, 316–318, 317b, 318–
    320
  intradural space of, 319–323, 320b,
    321, 322, 330
  stenosis of, 294–296, 295, 296
Spinal cord, compression of, 330
  cysts of, 323–324, 323b, 324, 324b, 325
  demyelination of, 323, 323b, 324b
  edema of, 311, 312
  hemorrhage in, 310–311, 312, 313b,
    323, 323b
  infarction of, 323b, 324–325, 324b, 325
  lesions of, 323–325, 323b, 324–326,
    324b
  tethered, 325–327, 326, 327, 327b
  trauma to, 310–311, 312, 313b
  tumors of, 323b, 324b, 325, 326
Spinal stenosis, 293–297, 294b, 295–299
Spinal surgery, changes after, 298–299,
  299, 299b, 300
  failed, 299–300, 301
Spine, 279–332
  ankylosing spondylitis of, 303–305,
    305
  anterior inferior iliac, avulsion fracture
    of, 156
  approach to imaging of, 279–280, 280b
  arachnoiditis of, 303, 303, 304
  cervical, compressive myelopathy of,
    288

Spine (Continued)
  degenerative changes of, 287, 287b,
    328
  disko-osteophytic material in, 291
  stenosis of, 295, 298
  coils for, 279
  contrast enhancement of, 13, 280
  disk degeneration of, 280–293, 281b
    annular tears in, 281–282, 281b, 283
    calcified disks due to, 289–290, 290
    compressive myelopathy due to, 288,
      288
    contour abnormalities in, 282–288
      location of, 285–287, 287, 287b
      mimickers of, 288, 289, 289b
      significance of, 287–288, 288b
      types of, 282–285, 284–287, 284b
    epidural hematoma due to, 288, 289
    marrow with, 28
    normal disk vs., 280–281, 282
    nuclear abnormalities in, 281, 282
    osseous changes due to, 291–293,
      291b, 292–294
    protocols for imaging of, 328–329
    recurrent, 300–301, 301
    vacuum disks due to, 288–289, 290
    vertebral bodies in, 289, 290
  epidural abscess of, 302–303, 303
  fracture of, 307, 308
    anterior inferior iliac, 156
    in spondylolysis, 305–306, 305b,
      306, 307
  image orientation for, 279, 280b
  infection of, 301–303, 301b, 302, 303,
    330
  inflammatory changes of, 301–305,
    301b, 302–305
  intraosseous disk herniations of, 306,
    307, 308
  kissing, 291b, 292–293, 294
  ligaments of, normal, 308, 309
    ossification of posterior longitudinal,
      318
    trauma to, 307–309, 309b, 310
  lumbar, degenerative changes of, 282,
    283, 285–287, 285–287, 287b, 292–
    294, 329
    normal, 282
    stenosis of, 296–299
  meningocele of, postoperative, 298, 299
  metastases to, 314–315, 320b, 323, 325,
    330
  osseous degeneration of, 291–293,
    291b, 292–294
  pars interarticularis of, osseous defect
    in, 305–306, 305b, 306, 307
  positioning for imaging of, 279
  postoperative changes of, 298–301,
    299–301, 299b, 329
  protocols for imaging of, 328–332
  pulse sequences for, 279–280
  regions of interest for, 279–280
  spinal canal of, 315–327
    epidural space of, 316–318, 317b,
      318–320
    intradural space of, 319–323, 320b,
      321, 322, 330
    stenosis of, 294–296, 295, 296
  spondylodiskitis of, 301–302, 301b,
    302
  spondylolysis and spondylolisthesis of,
    305–306, 305b, 306, 307
  stenosis of, 293–297, 294b, 295–299
  thoracic, degenerative changes of, 329
  trauma of, 306–312, 309b
    epidural fluid collections due to,
      309, 311

Spine (Continued)
  osseous, 307, 308
    protocols for imaging of, 329
    to cord, 310–311, 312, 313b
    to disks, 309, 310
    to ligaments, 307–309, 309, 310
    to muscles, 311, 313
    to nerves, 311–312, 313
    vascular abnormalities due to, 309–310, 311
  tumors of, cord, 323b, 324b, 325, 326
    intradural, 319–322, 320b, 321, 322
    nerve sheath, 319, 320b, 321
    osseous, 312–315, 314–316, 314b, 330
Spinoglenoid notch nerve compression, 214, 216
Spinous processes, posterior, degenerative changes of, 291b, 292–293, 294
Split fat sign, 95, 96, 97
"Spoiler" pulse, 9
Spondylitis, ankylosing, 303–305, 305
Spondylodiskitis, 301–302, 301b, 302
Spondylolisthesis, 305
Spondylolysis, 305–306, 305b, 306, 307
Sprain, ankle, 407
  of medial collateral ligament, 379, 380, 381
  of radial collateral ligament, 230
Spring ligament, 404
Staging, of tumors, 125–129, 126b, 127b, 128, 129
Stener lesion, 257, 257–258
STIR imaging, 6–8, 20
  fast spin echo vs., 7
  fat saturation with, 12
  gradient echo vs., 8
  of articular cartilage, 15, 15
  of bone, 8, 14
  of muscle, 16, 18
  parameters for, 5b
  strengths and weaknesses of, 5b
Strains, 66–70, 67–70
  brachialis, 69, 232–233, 233
  obturator, 69, 348
  of hip and pelvis, 346–347, 346b, 347
  paraspinous, 311, 313
  popliteal, 68
  rectus femoris, 67, 67
Stress fractures, 132, 157–161, 158–161, 158b–161b
  of femoral neck, 161, 341
  of foot and ankle, 422, 424
  of hip and pelvis, 339, 339b, 340, 341
  of tibia, 160
  vs. tumors, 164, 165
String sign, 95, 96, 97
Subacromial/subdeltoid bursa, 179–181, 180
Subacromial/subdeltoid bursitis, 184–185
Subarachnoid space, metastases to, 323
Subchondral cysts, of hip and pelvis, 344
  of talus, 425, 426
Subcoracoid bursitis, 214, 215
Subcoracoid impingement, 191, 192
Sublabral foramen, 197, 198–199, 199
Subluxation, neuritis from, 92, 93
  of tendon, 62, 62b
Subperiosteal fluid collection, in osteomyelitis, 107
Subscapularis recess, 214, 215
Subscapularis tendon, dislocation of, 62
  normal anatomy of, 176, 177, 178, 178, 179
  tears of, 191, 191b, 192
Superior labrum tear propagating anterior and posterior to biceps anchor. See SLAP lesions.

Supinator muscle, lipoma of, 83
Supinator syndrome, 240–241
Supraacetabular fractures, 158, 159
  insufficiency, 342, 343
Suprapatellar plica, 383–384
Suprascapular nerve entrapment, 98, 214–215, 214b, 216
Supraspinatus muscle, overdevelopment of, 183
Supraspinatus tendon, calcium hydroxyapatite in, 64
  impingement on, 183–184
  magic angle phenomenon of, 177, 178–179
  normal anatomy of, 176–177, 177, 178–179, 179, 179b
  tears, degeneration, and dislocation of, 185–189, 185–189, 185b
Supraspinous ligament, normal, 308, 309
  torn, 310
Surface coils. See Coils.
Surgery, muscle after, 85–87
  shoulder after, 209–212
  spinal changes after, 298–301, 299–301, 299b, 329
  tumor after, 129–130, 130
Susceptibility effects, 8, 9, 10, 21
Synovial chondromatosis, 121, 121, 122
  of elbow, 241, 242
  of hip, 357, 357–358
Synovial cysts, of shoulder, 213, 213
  of spine, 292, 294, 316, 317b
  of wrist and hand, 273, 274
  pisotriquetral, 273, 274
Synovial herniation pits, 338, 343–344, 345
Synovial osteochondromatosis, of elbow, 241, 242
  of hip, 357, 357–358
Synovial plicae, of knee, 383–384, 384
Synovial sarcoma, 129
  of foot and ankle, 426, 427
  of hip and pelvis, 350, 352b
Synovitis, due to foreign bodies, 111, 112
  in septic arthritis, 110–111
  pigmented villonodular, 121–122, 122, 143, 146
    of elbow, 241, 242
    of hip, 357
    vs. hemosiderotic arthritis, 119
Synovium, hypertrophied. See Rheumatoid arthritis (RA).
  normal appearance of, 16
  pitfalls in MRI of, 18
  pulse sequences for, 14b, 18, 19
Syrinx, 323–324, 323b, 324

T

Talofibular ligaments, 405b, 407, 407–409
Talonavicular ligament, 404
Talus, osteochondral injury of, 420–422, 422b, 423
  subchondral cyst of, 425, 426
  tumors of, 425, 425, 425b
Target sign, in nerve sheath tumors, 95, 96
Tarlov cysts, 317, 317b, 320
Tarsal coalition, 417, 419–421
Tarsal sinus, 408–410, 410b, 411–413
Tarsal tunnel syndrome, 413–415, 415–417, 415b
TE (echo time), 4–8, 5b, 21
Tears, biceps anchor, 209, 211
  bucket handle, of glenoid labrum, 207, 207, 209, 210, 211

Tears (Continued)
  of meniscus, 367, 369, 3665
  ligament, anterior cruciate, 376–378, 377–379
    osseous contusions with, 153, 153b, 154, 386–387, 387
    with meniscal tear, 366–367
  deltoid, 405, 405
  fibulocollateral, 381, 382
  lunotriquetral, 251, 252
  medial collateral, 379, 381
  posterior cruciate, 378, 380
  radial collateral, 229–230, 230, 231
  radioulnar, 255, 255
  scapholunate, 250, 250–251, 251
  talofibular, 407, 409
  tibiofibular, 407, 407
  ulnar collateral, of elbow, 231–232, 232
    of thumb, 256–258, 257, 276–277
  meniscal, 366–369, 367b
    approach to imaging of, 14b, 15, 363, 364
    bucket handle, 367, 368, 369
    medial flap, 369, 370
    oblique or horizontal, 367, 367
    radial (free-edge, parrot beak), 367–369, 370
    vertical longitudinal, 367, 368
    with ACL tear, 366–367
  muscle, 66–70, 67–70
    chronic, 74
    grading of, 67–68, 68–70
    healing of, 68–70
    pectoralis, 220, 220
  of acetabular labrum, 350–352, 352–354
  of glenoid labrum, bucket handle, 207, 207, 209, 210, 211
    in ALPSA lesions, 201b, 203, 206, 207
    in Bankart lesions, 201b, 203, 205–207
      reverse, 201b, 203, 205
    in GLAD lesions, 201b, 207, 209, 212
    in SLAP lesions, 197, 201b, 207, 207–209, 208, 209b, 210, 211
    partial thickness, 207, 207, 208–209, 210
  plantar fascia, 411b, 413, 414
  rotator cuff, full-thickness, 185b, 186–189, 187–189
    massive, 191–193, 192, 213, 213
    partial thickness, 185, 185–186, 185b, 186
  rotator cuff interval, 193, 193, 193b
  tendon, 59–62
    Achilles, 396, 396, 397
    anterior tibial, 403, 404, 404b
    biceps, 61, 189, 189, 189b, 233, 234
    complete, 57, 59–62, 61
    extensor, 236–237, 237, 237b, 238
    extensor carpi ulnaris, 256, 257
    factors predisposing to, 59b
    flexor hallucis longus, 60, 399, 400
    gluteus medius, 347, 348, 351
    hamstring, 346–347, 347
    infraspinatus, 190, 190
    medial, 235–236, 235b, 236
    partial, 57, 59, 60, 61
    peroneus, 401, 401b, 402, 403
    plantaris, 387–388, 388
    popliteus, 381, 382
    posterior tibial, 60, 398, 398b, 399
    subscapularis, 191, 191b, 192
    supraspinatus, 185–189, 185–189, 185b

Tears (Continued)
    triceps, 233–234, *234, 235*
    triangular fibrocartilage, 253–255, *254*
Temporal bone, 169, *170*
Temporomandibular joint (TMJ), 169–173
    abnormal, 170–173, 171b, *172*
    approach to imaging of, 169
    avascular necrosis of, 173
    degenerative changes of, *172*, 173
    internal derangements of, 171–173, *172*
    normal, 169–170, *170, 171,* 171b
    protocols for imaging of, 173b
Tendinitis, 57
    calcific, 62, *64*
        of shoulder, 214, *214*
    para-, 59, *60*
Tendo-Achilles bursa, 397, *398*
Tendon(s), 55–62
    abductor pollicis longus, 258, *258*
        entrapment and tenosynovitis of, *259,* 259–260, 259b
    abnormalities of, *57,* 57–62, 57b
    Achilles, 395–397, 395b
        Haglund's deformity of, 397, *398*
        normal, 56, *394, 395, 395*
        paratendinitis of, *60*
        tears of, 396, *396, 397*
        xanthomas of, *63,* 396–397, *397*
    approach to imaging of, 55
    biceps, dislocation of, *62,* 189, 189b, *190*
        impingement on, 184
        longitudinal split of, *61*
        normal anatomy of, 56, *56,* 177–178, *178, 179,* 232, *233*
        tears of, *61,* 189, *189,* 189b, 233, *234*
    biceps femoris, 381
        hematoma around, *72*
    brachialis, injuries to, 232–233, *233*
        normal anatomy of, 56, *56,* 232, *233*
    calcium hydroxyapatite in, 62, *64*
    coils for, 55
    contrast enhancement of, 55
    degeneration of, 57–58, *58*
        supraspinatus, 185, *185,* 185b
    deltoid, normal anatomy of, 177, *177*
    dislocation of, 62, *62,* 62b
        biceps, 189, 189b, *190*
        peroneus, 401–403, *404*
    extensor, of ankle, *394*
        of elbow, 236–237, *237,* 237b, *238*
        of wrist and hand, 258–260, *258–261,* 259b
    extensor carpi ulnaris, 255–256, *256, 257*
        tenosynovitis or partial tears of, 260, *260*
    flexor, of wrist and hand, bowstringing of, 260, *261*
        tenosynovitis of, 260
    flexor digitorum longus, 398
    flexor hallucis longus, normal anatomy of, *394,* 399
        tears of, *60,* 399, *400*
        tenosynovitis of, 58, *58, 59,* 399–400, *400,* 400b, *401*
    gluteus medius, 347, *348,* 351
    gout affecting, 62, *63*
    hamstring, 346–347, *347*
        hematoma around, *73*
    high signal within, *56,* 56–57, 56b
    iliopsoas, 352, *352*
    image orientation for, 55
    infraspinatus, in posterosuperior impingement, 190–191, 190b, *191*
        normal anatomy of, 176–177, *177, 178, 179*

Tendon(s) (Continued)
    tears of, 190, *190*
    longitudinal split, 59, *61*
    medial, *235,* 235–236, 235b, *236*
    meso-, 56, *58*
    normal, anatomy of, 55–56, *56*
        MRI of, 15–16, *56,* 56–57, 56b, *57*
    of elbow, 232–237
        anterior compartment, 232–233, 232b, *233, 234*
        lateral compartment, 236–237, *236–238,* 237b
        medial compartment, *235,* 235–236, 235b, *236*
        posterior compartment, 233–234, *234, 235*
    of foot and ankle, *394,* 394–403
        anterior, 403, *404,* 404b
        lateral, 400–403, 401b, *402–404*
        medial, 397–400, 398b, *399, 400,* 400b
        posterior, 395–397, *395–398,* 395b
    of hip and pelvis, 345–348, *347, 348*
    of shoulder, calcific tendinitis of, 214, *214*
        impingement on, 183–184
        normal anatomy of, 176–179, *177–179*
        tears, degeneration, and dislocation of, 185–193
    of wrist and hand, 258–260, *258–261,* 259b
    paratendinitis of, 59, *60*
    patellar, 384, *385*
    peroneal, *394,* 400–403, 401b, *402–404*
    pitfalls in MRI of, 16
    plantaris, normal, *394,* 395, *396*
        tears of, 387–388, *388*
    popliteus, pseudotear of, 374–376, *376*
        tears of, 381, *382*
    positioning for imaging of, 55
    posterior tibial, *394*
        tears of, *60, 398,* 398b, *399*
    pulse sequences for, 14b, 16, *17,* 55
    quadriceps, degeneration and partial tear of, *58*
        MRI of normal, 56, *56*
    regions of interest for, 55
    rotator cuff, degeneration of, 185, *185,* 185b
        normal anatomy of, 176–177, *177–179*
        tears of, full-thickness, 185b, 186–189, *187–189*
            massive, 191–193, *192,* 213, *213*
            partial thickness, *185,* 185–186, 185b, *186*
        surgery for, 209–214
    subluxation of, 62, 62b
    subscapularis, dislocation of, *62*
        normal anatomy of, 176, 177, 178, *178, 179*
        tears of, 191, 191b, *192*
    supraspinatus, calcium hydroxyapatite in, *64*
        impingement on, 183–184
        magic angle phenomenon of, *177,* 178–179
        normal anatomy of, 176–177, *177, 178–179, 179,* 179b
        tears, degeneration, and dislocation of, 185–189, *185–189,* 185b
    tears of, 59–62
        Achilles, 396, *396, 397*
        anterior tibial, 403, *404,* 404b
        biceps, *61,* 189, *189,* 189b, 233, *234*

Tendon(s) (Continued)
    complete, *57,* 59–62, *61*
    extensor, 236–237, *237,* 237b, *238*
    extensor carpi ulnaris, 256, *257,* 260, *260*
    factors predisposing to, 59b
    flexor hallucis longus, *60,* 399, *400*
    gluteus medius, 347, *348*
    hamstring, 346–347, *347*
    infraspinatus, 190, *190*
    massive rotator cuff, 191–193, *192,* 213, *213*
    medial, 235–236, 235b, *236*
    partial, *57,* 59, *60, 61*
    peroneus, 401, 401b, *402, 403*
    plantaris, 387–388, *388*
    popliteus, 381, *382*
    posterior tibial, *60,* 398, 398b, *399*
    subscapularis, *172,* 191, 191b
    supraspinatus, 185–189, *185–189,* 185b
    triceps, 233–234, *234*
    tendinitis of. See *Tendinitis.*
    tenosynovitis of. See *Tenosynovitis.*
    teres minor, normal anatomy of, 176, 178, *179*
    tibial, anterior, *394,* 403, *404,* 404b
        posterior, *394,* 398, 398b, *399*
    triceps, 55, *56,* 233–234, *234, 235*
    tumors of, 62, *64*
    xanthomas of, 62, *63*
Tendon sheath, anatomy of, 55–56
    giant cell tumor of, 62, *64,* 143–145
        of wrist and hand, 272, *272*
    normal, MRI of, 57
    tenosynovitis of, 59
Tennis elbow, 236–237, *237,* 237b, *238*
    medial, 235–236, 235b, *236*
    with radial collateral ligament tear, 230, *231*
Tenosynovitis, *57,* 58–59, *58–60,* 58b
    De Quervain, *259,* 259–260, 259b
    of abductor pollicis longus, *259,* 259–260, 259b
    of extensor carpi ulnaris, 260, *260*
    of flexor digitorum, 260
    of flexor hallucis longus, 58, *58, 59,* 399–400, *400,* 400b, *401*
    septic, 108, *109*
    stenosing, 58, 58b, 59, *59*
        of flexor hallucis longus, 399, *400*
Teres minor muscle, atrophy of, 215–217, *217*
Teres minor tendon, normal anatomy of, 176, 178, *179*
Tethered cord, 325–327, *326, 327,* 327b
TFCC (triangular fibrocartilage complex), 252–256, *253–257,* 253b
Thigh splints, 161, *162*
Three-dimensional (3D) volume imaging, 8, *9*
    of articular cartilage, 15
Thumb, gamekeeper's (skier's), 256–258, *257,* 276
    ulnar collateral ligament of, 256–258, *257*
TI (inversion time), 5b, 6
Tibia, stress fracture of, *160*
    tumors of, 424, 425b
Tibial collateral ligament bursa, 385, *386*
Tibialis anterior muscle, denervation of, *82*
Tibialis anterior tendon, *394,* 403, *404,* 404b
Tibialis posterior tendon, *394,* 398, 398b, *399*

Tibiocalcaneal ligament, 404–405, *405*
Tibiofibular ligaments, 405–407, 405b, *406, 407*
Tibiotalar ligament, 404–405, *405*
Tissue contrast, 3–13
  fat saturation in, 9–12, *11, 12*
  gadolinium in, *4, 11,* 12–13, 12b, *13*
  pulse sequences in, 4–9, 5b
    fast (turbo) spin echo, 5b, 6, *7, 8, 10*
    gradient echo (T2*), 5b, 8–9, *8–10*
    inversion recovery (STIR), 5b, 6–8, *7, 8,* 12
    proton (spin) density, 4–6, 5b
    spin echo, 4–6, 5b, *6,* 6b, *7*
    T1, 4, 5b, *6,* 6b, *7*
    T2, 4, 5b, 6b, *7*
Tissue signal intensity, 4, 6b
TMJ. See *Temporomandibular joint (TMJ).*
T1 halo sign, 37, 37b, *39*
T1-weighted imaging, 4, *6, 7,* 21
  of bone, 14
  of fibrocartilage, 14, *16*
  of muscle, 16, *18*
  of synovium, 18, *19*
  of tendons, *17*
  parameters for, 5b
  strengths and weaknesses of, 5b
  tissue signal intensity with, 6b
Tophi, gouty, *63,* 117–118, *119,* 145
TR (repetition time), 4–8, 5b, 21
Transfer lesions, 427–429, *428,* 429b
Transverse ligament, 373, *373*
Trauma. See also *Injury(ies).*
  compartment syndrome due to, 76, *76,* 76b
  marrow edema due to, *44*
  muscle, 66–77
    compartment syndromes due to, 76, *76,* 76b, *77*
    delayed-onset soreness due to, 66, *67*
    direct, 70–75, 71b, *72–75*
    fascial herniation due to, 76–77, *77*
    hematoma due to, 71–74, 71b, *72–74*
    hemorrhage due to, 70–71, *72*
    indirect, 66–70, 66b, *67–70*
    miscellaneous, 75–77, *76,* 76b, *77*
    myositis ossificans due to, 73–75, *75*
    spinal, 311, *313*
    strains due to, 66–70, *67–70*
  osseous, 151–165
    acute, 152–157
    anatomic basis for, 151–152
    approach to imaging of, 151
    coils for, 151
    contusion due to, 152–153, *153,* 153b, *154*
    differential diagnosis of, 164, 164b, *165*
    due to avulsion injuries, 153–157, *156,* 156b, *157*
      chronic, 161–163, *162, 163*
      of immature skeleton, 163–164
    due to impaction injuries, 152–153, *153–155,* 153b
    due to stress injuries, 132, 157–161, *158–161,* 158b–161b
    fractures due to, avulsion, 153–157, *156,* 156b, *157,* 163–164
      fatigue, 159–161, *160,* 160b, *161*
      insufficiency, 157–159, *158–160,* 159b
      microtrabecular, 152–153, *153,* 153b, *154*
      radiographically occult, 153, *155*
      stress, 132, 157–161, *158–161,* 158b–161b
Trauma *(Continued)*
    image orientation for, 151
    imaging options for, 152
    in osteochondritis dissecans, 164–165, 165b, *166*
    osteolysis after, 161–163, *163*
    osteolysis of clavicle due to, 217–218, *218*
    overview of, 152
    positioning for imaging of, 151
    pulse sequences for, 151
    repetitive, 157–164
    to immature skeleton, *163,* 163–164, *164*
  soft tissue, 152, *152*
  spinal, 306–312, 309b
    epidural fluid collections due to, 309, *311*
    osseous, 307, *308*
    protocols for imaging of, 329
    to cord, 310–311, *312,* 313b
    to disks, 309, *310*
    to ligaments, 307–309, *309, 310*
    to muscles, 311, *313*
    to nerves, 311–312, *313*
    vascular abnormalities due to, 309–310, *311*
  to ligaments, spinal, 307–309, *309, 310*
  to nerves, 92, *92, 93*
    spinal, 311–312, *313*
  to wrist, 276
Triangular fibrocartilage complex (TFCC), 252–256, *253–257,* 253b
Triceps muscle, 233
Triceps tendon, 56, *56,* 233–234, *234, 235*
Trochanters, 334
Tropocollagen, 55
Trough sign, 201b
Trunk, soft tissue tumors of, benign, 139t
  malignant, 141t
T-sign, *232*
T2 halo sign, 37, 37b, *39*
T2-weighted imaging, 4, *7,* 21
  of bone, 14, *15*
  parameters for, 5b
  strengths and weaknesses of, 5b
  tissue signal intensity with, 6b
T2*-weighted imaging, 8–9, 20
  of articular cartilage, 15
  of bone, 14–15
  of fibrocartilage, *16*
  of synovium, 18, *19*
  of tendons, *17*
  parameters for, 5b
  STIR vs., *8*
  strengths and weaknesses of, 5b
  susceptibility effects in, 9, *10*
Tumor(s), 125–148
  after chemotherapy, 129
  after radiation, 129–130, *130*
  after surgery, 129–130, *130*
  approach to image interpretation for, 131–132
  approach to imaging of, 130–131
  bone (osseous), benign and malignant, 40
    differential diagnosis of, 132–136, *132–137,* 133b–135b
    of foot and ankle, 422–425, *425,* 425b, *426*
    of hip and pelvis, 344–345, 344b, *345, 346*
    of shoulder, 219, *219,* 219b
    of spine, 312–315, *314–316,* 314b, 330
    of wrist and hand, 270–271, *271*
Tumor(s) *(Continued)*
    principles of imaging of, *122,* 126
  cartilaginous, 135–136, 135b, *136, 137*
  coils for, 130–131
  contrast enhancement for, 131
  cystic-appearing malignant, 146–148, *148*
  encasement of nerves in, 99, *99*
  extent of, extraosseous, 127, *128*
    intraosseous, 126–127, *128*
    local, 126–127, *128*
  giant cell, of patellofemoral compartment, *129*
    of pelvis, 344
    of spine, 313
    of tendon sheath, 62, *64,* 143–145
    of wrist and hand, 272, *272*
  glomus, of fingers, 272, *273*
  grading of, 125, 126b
  image orientation for, 131
  intramuscular, 81–84, *82–85,* 82b
    hemorrhage into, 73, *74*
  joint involvement with, 127, *129*
  lymph nodes with, 129
  marrow edema due to, *45*
  metastases of, in tumor staging, 125, 126, 126b, *127*
    skeletal, 37–39, *38–40*
    to muscle, 82, *84*
    to spine, 314–315, 320b, 323, 325, 330
    to subarachnoid space, 323
  nerve, 92–98, *94–98,* 95b
  nerve sheath, 93–95, 95b, *96, 97,* 148, *149*
    of spine, 319, 320b, *321*
    tarsal tunnel syndrome from, 414, *416*
  neurovascular involvement with, 127, *129*
  of foot and ankle, osseous, 422–425, *425,* 425b, *426*
    soft tissue, 138t, 140t, 425–429, 426b, *427, 428*
  of hip and pelvis, intraarticular, *357,* 357–358, 357b, *358*
    osseous, 344–345, 344b, *345, 346*
    soft tissue, 139t, 141t, 349–350, 352b
  of shoulder, osseous, 219, *219,* 219b
    soft tissue, 138t, 140t, 219–220, *220*
  of spine, cord, 323b, 324b, 325, *326*
    intradural, 319–322, 320b, *321, 322*
    nerve sheath, 319, 320b, *321*
    osseous, 312–315, *314–316,* 314b, 330
  of tendon, 62, *64*
  of tendon sheath, giant cell, 143–145
  of wrist and hand, osseous, 270–271, *271*
    soft tissue, 138t, 140t, 271–273, *271–273*
  positioning for imaging of, 130–131
  principles of imaging of, 126–130, *127–131,* 127b
  pseudo-, of nerves, 98, *98*
  pulse sequences for, 131
  recurrent, 130, *131*
  regions of interest for, 131
  soft tissue, 137–148
    amyloid, 145, *147*
    benign, 138t–139t
    cystic-appearing, 146–148, 146b, *147–149*
    differential diagnosis of, 137–148
    distribution by anatomical site and age of, 138t–141t

Tumor(s) *(Continued)*
  fibrous, 145, *147*
  giant cell, 143–145
  gouty tophi as, 145
  hemorrhagic, 142, *145*
  in pigmented villonodular synovitis, 143, *146*
  intramuscular myxoma as, 146, *148*
  lipomatous, 137, *142, 143*
  malignant, 140t–141t
  melanoma as, 143, *145*, 145–146
  of foot and ankle, 138t, 140t, 425–429, 426b, *427, 428*
  of hip and pelvis, 139t, 141t, 349–350, 352b
  of shoulder, 138t, 140t, 219–220, 219b, *220*
  of wrist and hand, 138t, 140t, 271–273, *271–273*
  principles of imaging of, 126, 137
  vascular, 137–142, *143, 144*
  with high signal on T1W images, 137–143, 137b, *142–145*
  with low signal on T2W images, 143–146, *146*, 146t, *147*
  staging of, 125–129, 126b, 127b, *128, 129*
  stress fracture mimicking, 164, *165*
Tumor matrix, osteoid/chondroid, 133
Turbo spin echo imaging. See *Fast spin echo (FSE) imaging.*

U

Ulcers, in diabetes, 114, *114*
  in osteomyelitis, 106
Ulnar collateral ligament (UCL), of elbow, 230–232, 230b, *231, 232*
  of thumb, 256–258, *257*
  of wrist, *253, 256*
Ulnar nerve, compressive neuropathy of, 98, *98*
  at elbow, 238–239, 238b, *239*
  at wrist, 264, *265*
  neuritis of, *92, 93,* 238
  neuroma of, *94*
  normal anatomy of, *91,* 238, *239,* 264, *265*
  surgical transposition of, *93*
Ulnar tunnel syndrome, 264, *265*

Ulnar variance, 265, 265b, *266*
Ulnolunate impaction, 266–267, *268*
Upper extremity, soft tissue tumors of, benign, 138t
  malignant, 140t

V

Vascular abnormalities, of marrow, 44–48, 44b
  of osseous structures of hip and pelvis, 334–339, 335b, *336–340,* 337b, 339b
  with spinal trauma, 309–310, *311*
Vascular malformations, 137–142, *143, 144*
Vastus intermedius muscle, edema of, *67*
Vertebral bodies, degenerative changes of, 291, 291b, *292*
  vacuum, 289, *290*
Vertebral compression fracture, 39–40, 40b, *41,* 159, *160*
Volume coils, 3
Voxels, 1–2, *3,* 21

W

Waldenström's macroglobulinemia, 34, *34*
Weighting, 3, 21
  proton (spin) density, 4–6, 5b
  T1, 4, 5b, *6,* 6b, *7*
  T2, 4, 5b, 6b, *7*
  T2*, 8–9, 20
Wrist and hand, 247–274
  anomalous muscles of, 272–273, *273*
  approach to imaging of, 247–248, 248b
  arthritis of, 273
  bone contusions of, 267, *269*
  carpal coalition of, 269, *271*
  carpal instability of, 266, 267b
  carpal tunnel of, 260, *262*
  carpal tunnel syndrome of, 262–264, 262b, *263–265*
  enchondromas of, 270
  extensor carpi ulnaris sheath of, 255–256, *256, 257*
  fibrolipomatous hamartoma of, 264–265, *266*
  fractures of, 267, *268*

Wrist and hand *(Continued)*
  ganglion cysts of, 270–272, *271, 272*
  Guyon's canal of, 264, *265*
  infection of, 273–274, *274,* 276
  ligament(s) of, extrinsic, 251–252, *252*
    intrinsic, 248–251, *248–252,* 248b
    lunotriquetral, *248,* 248–250, 248b, 251, *252*
    radioulnar, 255, *255*
    scapholunate, 248–251, *248–251,* 248b
    ulnar collateral, *253,* 256
  masses of, 276
  meniscus homologue of, 255, *256*
  nerve(s) of, 260–265
    fibrolipomatous hamartoma of, 264–265, *266*
    median, 260–265, *262–265,* 262b
    ulnar, 264, *265*
  os styloideum of, 266, *267*
  osseous structures of, 265–270
    abnormalities of, 266–270, *267–271,* 267b, 269b
    normal anatomy of, 265–266, 265b, *266*
    tumors of, 270–271, *271*
  osteonecrosis of, 268–269, *269,* 269b, *270*
  physeal injuries of, 267–268
  protocols for imaging of, 276–277
  scapholunate advanced collapse (SLAC), 251, *251,* 267b
  synovial cysts of, 273, *274*
  tendons of, 258–260, *258–261,* 259b
  trauma screening for, 276
  triangular fibrocartilage complex of, 252–256, *253–257,* 253b
  tumors of, osseous, 270–271, *271*
    soft tissue, 138t, 140t, 271–273, *271–273*
  type II lunate of, 269–270, *271*
  ulnar variance of, 265, 265b, *266*
  ulnolunate impaction of, 266–267, *268*

X

Xanthofibroma, 134
Xanthoma, of Achilles tendon, 62, *63,* 396–397, *397*

ISBN 0-7216-9027-0